Never Again

Marilyn Emerson

Never Again

Published by 21st Century Press
Springfield, MO 65807

21st Century Press is a Christian publisher dedicated to publishing books that have a high standard of family values. We believe the vision for our company is to provide families and individuals with user-friendly materials that will help them in their daily lives and experiences. It is our prayer that this book will help you discover Biblical truth for your own life and help you meet the needs of others. May God richly bless you.

21st Century Press
2131 W. Republic Rd, MB 211
Springfield MO 65807
email: lee@21stcenturypress.com

ISBN TP: 978-1-951774-55-4
ISBN Ebook: 978-1-951774-56-1

Printed in the United States of America

21stCENTURY
PRESS
READING YOU LOUD AND CLEAR

Contents

Contents

FOREWORD

Why was the COVID-19 pandemic so much more significant than the fact of people getting sick and dying around the world at the same time? How did it happen and why? What were the reasons it was deliberately perpetrated globally? How did all the circumstances surrounding the pandemic prepare our world for a complete totalitarian takeover, with eventually only one despot and one agenda allowed for the entire globe? These questions, along with many others, will be discussed at length and answered with a Christian World View in this treatise.

At first, the author was simply a follower of Christ with a gift of discernment to correlate current world events with the truths of Scripture. From the beginning of the early global changes we saw about three years ago, it became clear almost immediately that there were a lot of questions being asked, but no real answers were forthcoming from leadership. The more questions, the more the stonewalling. It seemed this was due either to government leaders not knowing the answers or to leaders not being willing to share the answers. Granted, it took some time to figure out what was happening and why, but there usually wasn't even a consensus among leaders on the answers.

There were deliberate efforts to induce fear and panic over the dire prospects we faced. The fear-mongering was coming from people in the medical arena that most of us had never heard much about, but wouldn't our doctors tell us the truth about the real dangers and prognosis of this previously unknown virus? Who would have a better idea of the facts than a medical doctor and scientist heading the National Institute of Allergies and Infectious Diseases (NIAID)? This man had been involved in medicine and scientific research for decades. When he surfaced in the Trump Administration as the authority on COVID-19, without so much as an invitation, he was somehow placed on the COVID -19 task force, and from that point took it upon himself to be the "official spokesman" on all things COVID. Nothing much was known about him by the United States' John Q. Public, certainly, few of us knew his real track record throughout those decades in the NIAID, which was far less than stellar.

Continued questions were being asked. As the disease clearly began spreading almost as rapidly as was predicted, many theories were proffered as to the origin of the virus. Today, even though Communist China continues to deny that it originated from the Wuhan Institute of Virology (WIV), whether accidentally or intentionally, there is still no proof, but there is clearly a large passel of circumstantial evidence. The fact is, the CCP (Communist Chinese Party), three years later, still denies an objective and open investigation, suggesting there was much to hide, but they've been allowed to hide it.

There are questions in every realm of the pandemic we must investigate from many angles because the answers are so entwined and indivisible with one another they resemble a head full of dreadlocks! However, the most overarching question we must address at length is, "What is the driving force behind all of the problem questions? It is imperative to understand this answer, since all other pieces of the puzzle have been directly related to it. The answer lies with the now well-known "Globalist Elites". For many years, there has been a public denial of the existence and power of this group, such that Wikipedia and other social media sources say the idea is part of the New World Order "conspiracy theory." Be assured by the best-known "elites," they are neither theory nor part of a secret plot. At an earlier time, they were not operating overtly, but those days are gone. Globalist elites are meeting annually, and their numbers have grown exponentially. They are not hiding their agenda or their intentions and are very verbal about both. For anyone to deny their existence is much like the ostrich with its head buried in the sand. So, first of all, this book will show clear identification of this group, its power and wealth, and its agenda in detail, as well as how the pandemic was both a harbinger and a means to their ends. Indeed, it will show how well this agenda fits into the prophesied future events detailed in Scripture.

Following the unveiling of the "elites" agenda, we will be able to see the many far-reaching effects of the global pandemic and understand how each piece of it furthered the realization of their agenda. Pieces of the puzzle include all of the measures thrust upon most of the world to divide and isolate people, and the reasons for perpetrating global immunization, social distancing, mandatory masking, and even mandates themselves. Well-renowned and respected doctors and scientists who disagreed with these measures and other directives were threatened, persecuted, and faced the risk of losing licenses and livelihoods for telling the truth. Outstanding and venerable Journals of Medicine and Science suddenly denied well-known truths and backed the narrative of the elites officially. The illegitimate and manipulative means of initiating experimental vaccines were all led and forced by Big Pharma, with the cooperation of almost every health-related agency in the United States and internationally. The plan was to have 100% global compliance for a mandated drug with the intent of global control over personal freedom. There is far more in this realm regarding loss of freedom of personal choices.

We must also discuss many specifics of this puzzle that will blow the lid off the idea that this pandemic was merely an unfortunate global happening that accidentally and tragically occurred and changed the course of history for the betterment of mankind. It was no such thing. Instead, it was in the making several decades ago with a progressive plan in place. Legislation that would protect Big Pharma was placed early on to enable drugs and vaccines to enter the market on "Emergency Use Authorization" so they didn't have to pass through the rigorous testing and safety concerns before they could be authorized by the FDA for use. At the same time, the pharmaceutical companies could not be held accountable legally for adverse effects.

The specifics of protecting the already enormous wealth and power of the globalist elites include the full compliance of all health agencies, governments, scientific establishments, hospitals, universities, Big Pharma, Big Tech, and Big Business to ensure that there were no influences able to refute their agenda or ask too many questions. Many individuals have written post-COVID articles and books detailing the efforts they made to tell and defend the truth, only to be censored on social media and often removed from it completely. That truth proves the severity of efforts to keep the public in the dark, suppression of anything potentially hazardous to the narrative (suppression of our freedoms of speech, of religion, of public assembly, the press, and personal security).

Many laws were violated to mandate dos and don'ts to be obeyed or risk fines and imprisonment. Our laws have, by virtue of our Constitution, been made by our legislative bodies, not presidents, governors, mayors, or departments of health. That is NOT their job. It most assuredly is not the job of an overzealous, irresponsible government employee. Standard operating procedures were entirely ignored and no one spoke up to defend them. Such was the degree of authoritarian behavior that was allowed, partly because it was done so overtly and authoritatively! These pandemic overlords nearly got by with murder, oh wait— they did quite literally get by with murder. This was done by barring effective medicines to enable the use of the experimental, impractical, expensive, and toxic treatments that killed many. They mandated immunizations for certain essential groups, such as medical personnel and the military. Many in those groups and many others whose employers mandated them died from those COVID immunizations as surely as if they'd been targeted with a weapon. Many more have chronic health issues, that may be permanent, which they never had before.

This is, after all, just an introduction to this book. It is the intent and hope of the author for you, the reader, to understand some hard truths about the nature of the origin and reality of the COVID-19 pandemic. By understanding that, it will be easy to see how this story dovetails with the predictions of Scripture for the end times. It will enable all of us to better prepare for the coming of our Lord for His Church because that day is ever nearer. Globalist elites believe their ideas are uniquely their own, but our God knew what they would be doing to prepare the world for His judgment and the coming of the one world government with its evil ruler Millenia ago. This world is now rushing ahead to that soon day.

INTRODUCTION

For almost 3 years, we watched a world gone mad; a world that few of us knew how to relate to or understand had been thrust upon us. All the rules we knew for navigating in our world had been thrown out and replaced with mandates that left us all scratching our heads in frustrated confusion. Suddenly, we were told to listen only to certain "expert" individuals and agencies that were supposed to have all the answers to our questions about a frightening new disease, about which few actually agreed. Answers to our questions changed regularly, and it was difficult to determine who we should believe or look to for the answers, or indeed, were there any responsible answers? In fact, a good number of people wondered if there were answers at a time when common sense and the ability to reason had abandoned the globe.

Those of God's people who have trusted His Son, Jesus Christ, as their Lord and Savior need not despair at all the confusion, chaos, and deception. The apostle Paul wrote to Timothy, his son in the faith, to share what the Lord had shown him regarding "the last days" spoken of in many places in Scripture. Paul assured Timothy he would see sinful, chaotic, and confusing things he called "perilous times." Then Paul gave a lengthy list of the things Timothy should look for in his first century of "last days" and understand they would get progressively worse just before the Lord returned. Note what Paul wrote:

> "You should know this, Timothy, that in the last days there will be very difficult (perilous) times. People will love only themselves and their money. They will be boastful and proud, scoffing at God, disobedient to parents, and ungrateful. They will consider nothing sacred. They will be unloving and unforgiving; they will slander others and have no self-control. They will be cruel and hate what is good. They will betray their friends, be reckless, be puffed

> up with pride, and love pleasure rather than God. They will act religious, but they will reject the power that could make them godly. Stay away from people like that…Ever learning, but never able to come to the knowledge of truth."
>
> —2 Timothy 3:1-5, 7 (NLT)

We could explore and expand eloquently on all of the above areas mentioned, and create an entire blueprint of what ungodly people will say and do in these last days. Since we've all seen the depravity of unregenerate humanity at length, that much description isn't necessary at this time. However, as we begin to discuss these things in our first chapter, please remember that God told us it would be easy to identify people who perpetrate the evils above in the last days. We have no need to be shocked at the degree and intensity of the evil we see, but we do need to watch out for them, know what is happening, and avoid being deceived by them, as so many were during the events of these last three years. When in doubt, we must run to our Savior for the answers we seek and trust Him to guide us through the morass of our times.

> Know this also, as Scripture warns, "Stay alert! Watch out for your great enemy, the devil. He prowls around like a roaring lion, looking for someone to devour."
>
> —I Peter 5:8 (NLT)

We are all well aware that as children of God, there is nothing our enemy would rather do than deceive us, whether, it be with temptation, causing us to doubt what God has told us, or make us fear what our future holds. Whatever he can use to deceive us or defeat us, he will use. Never doubt Satan has been ever busier in the affairs of this world, still hoping to be the ultimate victor, using all the world has to offer with a majority of evil men and women with evil goals and motives. Indeed, after our Lord has raptured His church, and removed the presence of His Holy Spirit from this earth, Satan will establish his seven-year reign on earth and empower a man, Antichrist, to carry on the present evils with new vengeance and exponential forms of evil, even as our Lord prophesied Millennia ago. This time of Satanic control will make the last three years look like a picnic in the park!

In the Old Testament scriptures, many were the times the Kings set Watchmen to guard the walls of the cities to be sure they were not invaded without knowing it, and were prepared to defend the kingdom from any and all attacks. Many of God's prophets spoke about these watchmen.

> "I have posted Watchmen on your walls, (Jerusalem); they will never be silent day or night. You who call on the Lord, give yourselves no rest."
>
> —Isaiah 62:6 NLT

This author has felt compelled by the Lord to write about all that has happened in our world and proclaim His Word to all who would hear it. First, the truth of the situation needed to be proclaimed so that people would NOT believe the lies of the enemy, and would not be in abject fear or panic over these circumstances. Second, we must understand that our God is NOT shocked or taken by surprise. All of these circumstances are just a part of His preparation for the end days coming nearer. Hence, the title of this book, *Watchman, What of the Night?* We must all become watchmen and proclaim the things we see and hear in truth and in light of these coming days.

THEREFORE, Jesus said, **"WATCH! THAT NO MAN DECEIVE YOU!" Matthew 24:4 NLT**

Part I

The Power and Wealth of the Small Majority

Chapter 1

Understanding Globalist Elites

Since the beginning of time, every civilization has had a very small minority within its society having the power and wealth to control the majority of that society. Some sociologists and political scientists still believe this idea is mere theory, without substance in reality. However, all the great empires were led predominantly by despots with a handful of powerful officers, ruling over all the masses primarily with harsh tactics. The ideas of freedom and a democratic government with elected leaders is a reasonably recent development in history. This concept has generally worked far better for a majority of people. However, in recent decades a few citizens with positions in corporations, or on corporate boards have acquired enormous percentages of global wealth and power. Having majority influence over policy-planning networks through the generous financial support of foundations or leadership positions with think tanks or policy-discussion groups, members of the "elite" exert significant power over corporate and governmental decisions. Current "elites" wield this power and influence in business and politics internationally.

Today, power, wealth, and control are concentrated globally in a small group of individuals and groups, primarily independent of national and local governments. This is the same group of high-level individuals who did the lion's share of planning and executing the COVID-19 pandemic while manipulating massive international changes in global governance, and forcing the people of the world to accept them as the new normal. Power-driven elites tend to be united in their goals and agendas, while the non-elites are diverse and powerless. Elite's interests are generally unified due to common backgrounds and positions and the defining characteristics of power, wealth, and control.

Elites oppose "pluralism," which holds that people of different beliefs, backgrounds, and lifestyles can coexist in the same society and participate equally in the political process. It's a tradition that gives multiple major social groups and interests representation within more powerful ruling sets or governments.[1] Pluralism contributes to more palatable political and economic outcomes for all the collective needs of society. Elites are people who hold leading positions in key organizations in society and strive to be politically influential to enable personal agendas. They have preeminent roles in setting agendas, producing knowledge, constructing institutions, making and implementing strategic decisions, and assessing policy outcomes. In other words, individuals and diversities are anathema to elites. Consequently NO regime today, national or global, can thrive if it lacks substantial endorsement from elite circles.

The World Economic Forum (WEF), founded and led by Klaus Schwab, has been the primary force of the Globalist Elites. However, at the age of 88 years with 55 years as Executive Chairman, Schwab announced his immediate step-down April 21, 2025. Eighty-year-old Peter Brabeck-Letmathe has been appointed as acting CEO and the WEF's objectives, plans, and future will continue, but it will also strive to remain relevant to changing global issues. Meanwhile the WEF has met almost annually in Europe since 1910. Each January, several thousand leading business executives, politicians, journalists, and other elites flock to a tiny alpine village in Davos, Switzerland, for the WEF's exclusive, invitation-only annual meeting. TV, radio, and print reporters fawn over the so-called 'good and the great.' People such as Jamie Dimon, CEO of JP Morgan Chase, and Microsoft founder Bill Gates, were both present January 15-19, 2024 and both were seen on television. On the surface, ideas and discourse might seem like a normal business meeting, but if you could scratch the surface, you would see something quite different. The WEF was started as a policy think tank in London, England, and was anything but random. However, in 1971, with the help of the European Commission (EC), Klaus Schwab, then a business professor at the University of Geneva, founded the European Management Forum and invited 450 business executives to a conference in Davos. The idea was to get European leaders to learn about how American business works. There was institutional backing, which attracted business leaders and later, politicians. One of the most shocking things about Schwab is the enormity of what he has achieved.

There are some global concerns, however, about the WEF's future health since Schwab's recent resignation. Current leadership states it has no serious concern. The WEF has a highly qualified acting CEO for the interim as the board seeks a permanent replacement. Most believed Schwab was like a monarch who would continue his role until his death. Schwab also employed family members in high-ranking posts within the not-for-profit organization. Insiders refused to speak on the record because they feared reprisals such as being banned from WEF events, or even being fired for talking. Other insiders, both current and former employees, anonymously compare Schwab to Russia's dictator. According to a *Guardian* newspaper report, "Klaus picked his leaders using the same criteria Putin uses to pick deputies for the state duma: loyalty, guile, sex appeal," the paper quoted one of the sources as saying.

By 1987, WEF was the official name, and since then, has been an international driving force. It's stated mission is "improving the state of the world by engaging business, political, academic, and other leaders of society to shape global, regional, and industry agendas." The Forum states that the world is best managed by a self-selected coalition of multinational corporations, governments and civil society organizations.

(CSOs), which it expresses through initiatives like the "Great Reset" and the "Global Redesign." The foundation is mostly funded by its 1,000-member multinational companies. Schwab grew WEF's

$6,000 startup capital in 1971 into a $390 million/year business. Today, WEF's annual meeting serves more billionaires and CEOs than any other event on earth. Schwab tightly controlled the whole succession discussion until very recently, when allegations and accusations of sexual misconduct, a culture of harassment and discrimination within the WEF, and questions about financial practices all surfaced. Reuters reported WEF hired external lawyers to investigate these claims. They "did not find it (WEF) had committed any legal violations, nor did they substantiate allegations of misconduct against Schwab." Interestingly, the immediate resignation came within the same month of their report! There had been no plans of such a decision.

The WEF and its annual meeting in Davos have received criticism over the years, including allegations of the organization's corporate capture of global and democratic institutions, institutional whitewashing initiatives, the public cost of security, the organization's tax-exempt status, unclear decision processes and membership criteria, a lack of financial transparency, and the environmental footprint of its annual meetings. Most notable, on several occasions, the WEF has championed a number of highly controversial issues, including the war on terrorism, boycotting Israel, North Korea's nuclear testing, Brexit, President Xi Jinping of the People's Republic of China (PRC) in his defense of the global economic scheme, criticism of the U.S., Populist's movements, global warming/climate change mitigation, etc. This is a short list.

There is so much more to this organization of elites but we must press on to the connection between COVID-19 and the Global Elites.

Globalist Elites and the COVID-19 Pandemic

In New York City on October 18, 2019, long before the world at large had any idea of the possibility of a pandemic existing, a high-level, live-simulation exercise was conducted to 'prepare public and private leaders for a pandemic response. The Johns Hopkins Center for Health Security, in partnership with the World Economic Forum and the Bill and Melinda Gates Foundation, hosted "Event

201." The exercise brought together business, government, security, and public health leaders to address a "hypothetical global pandemic scenario." It also featured a live virtual experience from 8:50 AM to 12:30 PM EDT to "engage stakeholders worldwide and members of the public in a meaningful conversation of difficult high-level policy choices that could arise in the midst of a severe pandemic."[1]

The reason for this exercise was the supposed growing numbers of epidemics in recent years, with about 200 events annually someplace, including Ebola, Zika, MERS, and SARS. Also, "collective vulnerability to the social and economic impacts of infectious disease crises appears to be increasing. Experts suggest there is a growing likelihood of one of these events becoming a global threat—or an 'event 201' pandemic—that would pose disruptions to health and society and cause average annual economic losses of 0.7% global Gross Domestic Product (GDP), similar in scale to climate change."[2]

Arnaud Bernaert, Head of Shaping the Future of Health Care, World Economic Forum, claimed we were in a new era of increased epidemic risk. That meant necessary public/private cooperation would be more challenged even though it was most essential to decrease the risk and impact. Consequently, it was the ideal time to ramp up the cooperation between national governments, key international institutions, and critical industries, and increase our global abilities for preparedness and response. In other words, since elites had already planned the disaster they were prepared to deliver, it was also the best possible time to induce global cooperation. This would enable elites to carry out all of the lucrative plans for dealing with the mess they were going to make!

There are International Health Regulations (IHR) that applied to no fewer than196 nations around the globe, legally committed to preventing and responding to all acute public health risks. These formerly established regulations would minimize public health risks and allow no 'unnecessary interference' with international traffic and trade. "We live in an increasingly interconnected world, and we must help all United Nations' member states align with the IHRs and be prepared to prevent, detect, and respond to acute outbreaks," said Chris Elias, President of Global Development at the Gates Foundation. "If we fail to do so, the world will be unprepared for the next pandemic."[3]

Clearly, IHRs were developed by the United Nations. 194 of the 196 nations are also members of the World Health Organization. Developed in 2005, these regulations provide a legal framework that defines countries' rights and obligations in handling public health events and emergencies having the potential to cross borders. The obligations for countries include the mandatory reporting of public health events and include criteria for determining whether or not a particular event constitutes a "public health emergency of international concern." All countries must designate a National IHR Focal Point for communications with WHO, to establish and maintain core capacities for surveillance and response, including designated points of entry. Additional provisions outline the areas of international travel and transport such as the health documents required for international travel. All of these international regulations were clearly planned and meant to remove the opportunities for national sovereignty to determine such areas.

"In this new era of extreme pandemic threat, public/private cooperation is essential for an effective response," said Tom Inglesby, Director of the Johns Hopkins Center for Health Security. "While governments and public health systems are already strained due to the increase in dangerous outbreaks, experts agree that a severe, fast-spreading, human-to-human pandemic incident could happen at any time. We believe this well-crafted, thorough, and realistic, tabletop exercise will provide leaders with a deeper understanding of the impact of epidemics on their communities and inspire them to take important steps to advance prevention and response."[4]

Now that we can visualize the upshot of this "pandemic visualization exercise," we can see an enormously large amount of preliminary expectation prior to the actual pandemic. Note the following observations from this brilliant piece of subterfuge:

- Each of the speakers quoted and the participants in this exercise were designated Global Elites, including the WEF itself which was sponsoring and operating the charade, and all were WEF members. The Gates Foundation also partners consistently with the WEF.
- It was held in New York City to draw the US into the enormity of the possibility/ (probability) of pandemic, and to increase press coverage.
- It was stated that the world has seen a huge number of epidemics in recent years; (what constitutes a 'huge' number?) First, there have always been epidemics, many in history were far more lethal and enduring than recent ones. Second, we're talking pandemic which was already planned and they knew when and from where it was coming very soon!
- The entire article speaks about "experts," all of which were part of the whole WEF/WHO system. They could only speak expertly because they knew what was coming!
- They also push the non-reality of climate change, another big agenda item, while correlating the effect of a pandemic on that supposed change.
- We were in a new era of epidemic risk, because they were planning the pandemic for a plethora of their own reasons.
- The constant speak of ramping public/private cooperation was necessary to make their plans of pandemic ensue successfully. 'Preparedness' and 'response' are key words used for psychological manipulation—preparing people to accept the coming demands.
- Preparing for potential disruptions to health and society, economic changes, and new rules in the interest of public safety, are all psychological preparation.

- International Health Regulations, formulated by the UN in 2005, are legally binding and imply that every nation must comply with them. They have been followed for years and are not likely ever to change, unless they become even more restrictive. They are completely incidental to the making of all the newly-planned rules for public health safety for the pandemic.
- So-called "experts" agree that a "severe, fast-spreading human-to-human pandemic" could happen at any time! Of course they agree, it's already been established.
- At least 16 participants in this exercise were from a broad range of backgrounds and industries. That doesn't make them "experts." It makes them globalist co-conspirators of the same ilk! [(4)]

COVID-19 and the Whistle-blowers

There are so many roads to travel in identifying all of the details we need to see regarding the pandemic. Many doctors, nurses, scientists, journalists, and others began to understand what was happening very early in the pandemic. Many discoveries were made, including unprecedented vice, lies, deception and fraud that surfaced with reference to COVID-19. These professionals began looking at the visible aspects, the signs and symptoms of the coronavirus, and began treating infected patients to the best of their knowledge and abilities. Soon, counter measures for treating the illness were being pushed instead of the ones being used effectively by medical staff and saving peoples' lives as they have always done. These courageous health professionals offered their patients safe, effective, inexpensive, and life-saving treatments for COVID. Dr. Peter McCullough was one of those physicians who did his homework, because he was also a renowned researcher in his own right. "According to Dr. McCullough, 'Powerful multi-drug regimens reduced hospitalizations by 87% and deaths by 75%.'"[5] He and many of his colleagues dared to speak out against the ill-advised protocols public health groups had recommended. Their measures had caused more misery and death than the pandemic itself.

Another physician, Dr. Peter Breggin, MD and his wife Ginger Ross Breggin who were also researchers were hearing the stories about the obviously irrational, contradictory, and harmful public health policies implemented for the treatment of COVID-19. They began inquiring and investigating the sources. Eventually, what they learned grew so deep and wide in scope it became an entire book, entitled, *COVID19—The Global Predators; We Are Their Prey!* Much of the information in this chapter will be summarized from their observations and diligent research. Another three, highly-respected physicians wrote their observations and experience in the introduction of their book including:

- Peter McCullough, MD, MPH who spent much time, effort, and money refuting the touted and ineffective public health measures. He wrote medical journal articles proving the effectiveness of protocols used well over 6 months with excellent results, only to have them censored. Subsequently, he lost his University Research position and nearly lost his license because the establishment couldn't allow the truth to be published or even known.
- Elizabeth Lee Vleit, MD, acting physician, and President/ CEO of the Truth for Health Foundation. Dr. McCullough and Dr. Vleit wrote a patient guide and a patient treatment guide, available to the public online to disseminate the truth about COVID. Dr. McCullough acted as Senior Medical Advisor for this foundation, which is now stronger and more widely known than ever.
- Vladimir "Zev" Zelenko, MD, who is a strong vocal defender of human rights, and spoke against the globalists' agenda of the mass murder of thousands with these destructive protocols. He authored the Zelenko Protocol for the early treatment of COVID-19, saving thousands of lives at home and around the world.

One of the most basic public health principles is, "The more society can function normally during a pandemic—the better the people will manage to survive." This age-old axiom was turned on its head in 2020 by the pandemic perpetrators, "The more society can be frightened, isolated, controlled, and suppressed—the safer it will be from the virus." This upside-down principle became abundantly clear as the driving force in the pandemic.

From the earliest beginning, the origin of SARS-CoV-2 was blatantly and continuously denied, when it was crystal clear to anyone with a brain—the source was China. That's where it first surfaced, and quickly began to spread, first throughout Wuhan, and then through the whole country, long before it presented anywhere else. One thing was certain. It was the obvious product of long and frequent collaboration of both U.S. and Chinese gain-of-function research. Each were creating deadly SARS-CoV viruses in American and Chinese labs. The origin of SARS-CoV-2 was easily traced and documented in multiple scientific publications.

Most of those studies were funded, at least in large part, by the National Institutes of Health (NIH) and Anthony Fauci's National Institute of Allergy and Infectious Diseases (NIAID). Many of the Chinese/American gain-of-function projects were funded collaborations paid for by the NIH and the NIAID. Other same-source funding supported individual American and Chinese Communist Party (CCP) researchers creating dangerous viruses. When Anthony Fauci was questioned about this information before a US Senate committee hearing, he lied under oath saying that neither NIH nor NIAID funded gain-of-function research conducted in either China or the United States. As of the end of 2021 (two years into the pandemic), "NIAID and NIH continued to fund these deadly gain-of-function experiments in American labs,"[6] Other United States agencies have also contributed funding to gain-of-function research, including, quite ominously, the shadowy Defense Advanced Research Projects Agency (DARPA) which is a part of the Department of Defense (DOD).

Before continuing to expose more of what was happening in our own nation we must pause for a brief understanding of the term "gain-of-function" as it's necessary to understanding the depth of the scientific depravity that has been happening at least as far back as the Obama administration, who, to his credit, tried to outlaw it. Gain-of-function 'medical' research genetically altars a pathogen in a way that might or might not enhance the biological functions of their gene constructions. This may affect how virulent the pathogen is, the speed of its transmission, the types of hosts most easily infected, etc. This type of experimentation is expected to ***increase*** the transmissibility and/or the virulence of the pathogens. It is also intended to reveal targets to better predict emerging infectious diseases and in turn get the jump on developing vaccines and other therapeutics.

On the surface, depending on who is arguing the concept, this may sound like a good idea. But here is an example. Influenza B can ONLY infect humans and harbor seals. Introducing a mutation of Influenza B to rabbits in a controlled lab situation would be considered a gain-of-function experiment because the virus didn't have that function previously. In theory, such experiments could help reveal which parts of the viruses' genome (all the genetic information of an organism) will correspond to the species it can infect, enabling the creation of antiviral medicines which could block that function.

Here's the rub! Many forms of gain-of-function research, especially work involving certain selected COVID-19 agent pathogens, carry built-in biosafety and biosecurity risks. There are some groups designated to lessen the risks while allowing its potential benefits, however, there are still far too many bioethical questions and concerns present. Critics call gain-of-function experimentation "engineered doomsdays." Gain-of-function is an enormously misleading euphemism for taking viruses out of nature, making them more infectious or virulent, commonly turning formerly harmless viruses into deadly human pathogens capable of killing millions, all for the benefit of producing more worthless money-making vaccines with which to line more globalist pockets, just like they did with the COVID19 vaccines. The real terminology should be gain-of-lethal-function!!

Going back to these discoveries and all that had been treasonously perpetrated on Americans and the nations, the Breggins' felt it was imperative in mid-April of 2020, to send this information to President Donald Trump. They published a blog video about Anthony Fauci and the NIAID's funding of the US/ CCP collaboration in the making of these deadly viruses. When the information reached the President two days later, he canceled all funding for collaborative viral research. However, even with that prompt action, there is clear reason to believe Fauci again found ways around that prohibition. That has historically been his continued modus operandi. Not long after, the Breggins discovered most of the relevant and identifiable institutions in the West, including the NIH, the NIAID, the FDA, the CDC, WHO, most major social media, many scientific and medical establishments, tech companies, universities, governments, and multiple globalist billionaires were suppressing and continued to suppress the early and highly effective treatments for COVID-19.

This begs the question: Why did the globalist elites continue to violently suppress early home treatments, causing morbidity and mortality of millions of people? The answers quickly became clear. Money, money, and more money. One of the most important reasons for a global pandemic was to produce money-making vaccines and force the global masses to take them. They knew exactly how to make this happen quickly. Pharmaceutical companies were already preparing vaccines for COVID-19 long before it surfaced .Both Pfizer and Moderna were already under contract and in production. Others would follow shortly. Normally, it would take years to do clinical trials, and get a new drug or vaccine through the FDA authorization process.

Prior planning and knowledge of exactly how the COVID-19 vaccines could be rolled out early in the pandemic was common knowledge for the globalist vaxbackers. An Emergency Use

Authorization (EUA) legislation was passed after the events of 9/11, in 2004, but many events had led to its passing long before 2004. Major health issues contributed to this including:

- The use of Thalidomide for morning sickness in pregnancy led to tens of thousands of severe birth defects and a public health disaster.
- The 1976 Influenza A or swine flu—then President Ford instigated the first-ever national vaccination program. After millions had taken that vaccine, a pandemic never happened, but the vaccine caused thousands of cases of Guillain-Barré syndrome, often causing paralysis and death.
- The AIDS crisis was an early precursor of EUA authority in the 1980s. "Public health experts" suggested the use of DDI,(didanosine) an experimental drug having no FDA approval. Dr. Anthony Fauci proposed using it while further study continued. This idea looked good to President George H.W. Bush, whose support caused the FDA to try it due to the need. It caused severe side effects.
- Then came 9/11 and the War on Terror, followed by the numerous anthrax mail attacks. The Project Bioshield Act of 2004 designated billions of dollars "for purchasing vaccines in preparation for a bioterror attack, and for stockpiling emergency countermeasures. To be able to act rapidly in an emergency, Congress allowed FDA to authorize formally unapproved products for emergency use against a threat to public health and safety (subject to a declaration of emergency by HHS). The record indicates that Congress was focused on the threat of bioterror specifically, not on preparing for a naturally-occurring pandemic."[7]

Interestingly, the FDA's new authority wasn't used much for the next 16 years. However, with an amendment to the original legislation, it was used preemptively to prepare for some countermeasures in case they were needed in MERS, Zika, Ebola, and other epidemics—none of which ever happened in the U.S. In February of 2020, the planned-for pandemic surfaced as a national health emergency warranting the emergency use of *in vitro* ("in glass") test tubes as opposed to *in vivo* ("in body") diagnostics and the now necessary vaccinations. Later in March, other pandemic declarations made it necessary to approve other countermeasures. "Since then, the FDA has issued nearly 400 EUAs for personal protective equipment, medical equipment, in vitro diagnostic products, drug products, and most notably, vaccines...An EUA had never been granted for a brand-new vaccine before; this, combined with the stakes of administering a vaccine to people who are otherwise healthy, led the FDA to commit itself to heightened standards of review."[8]

Why was this EUA so pivotal to the globalist elites? The EUA also empowers the government to finance drug company costs for the development of vaccines and rush them onto the market at breakneck speed without standard FDA approval as safe and effective. The catch was that under the EUA. the US could not finance and rush through the experimental and potentially lethal vaccines unless there were NO safe and effective treatments already in place.

Consequently, Bill Gates, Anthony Fauci, and the drug companies, with their greedy investors, had to continue doing everything in their power to *DISCREDIT* any existing treatment options that were both safe and effective. At ANY time they failed to suppress all effective treatments, their mountainous ambitions for more money, power, and control from the unwarranted experimental mass jabs would simply collapse. The use of hydroxychloroquine and ivermectin drugs being used in home treatment for COVID-19 were proven successful at reducing hospitalizations and deaths by large percentages. However, the globalist elites suppressed and then banned this information wherever it surfaced by forcing unneeded, unproven, and dangerous vaccines on the entire world. As unconscionable as it sounds, most of the wealthiest and most powerful people and organizations in the world would rather allow people to die without treatment that works, than lose their much planned-for and anticipated pandemic opportunities. Even if it requires coercing every person on the planet to be experimentally vaccinated, they will make it happen, while the government must pay all their expenses and protect them from appropriate law suits for all the damage done. Absolutely NO accountability exists.

Confronting the Criminals

On June 28, 2021, Dr. Peter McCullough, MD, sent the Breggins this important analysis:

> "We are more than six months into the largest mass vaccine program in US history. There have been NO press briefings to the public on overall vaccine safety by the CDC, FDA, NIH, or the White House Task Force. The silence has been deafening despite 411,391 adverse event reports to the CDC with 54,606 urgent care visits, 23,257 hospitalizations, and 6,985 deaths to date. No analysis of these adverse event reports has been given to our terrified citizens who are being forced to gamble their health and their lives on unsafe, experimental vaccines or lose the right to exercise their Constitutional rights to travel, go to work, go to school, or to public or private events.
>
> If there was complete reporting of *every* vaccine-related safety event, the already huge numbers of injured and dead from the vaccine would be at least ten-fold or greater. At this rate, since the launch of the mass-vaccination program, there will be more casualties and damage to the health of Americans attributable to the vaccines than to the COVID-19 respiratory illness during the same period."[9]
>
> As of early 2024, that prediction was as bad in totality as Dr. McCullough's predictions. In fact, considering the number of continuing and ongoing issues of post COVID

and Long COVID yet to surface in the unforeseeable future, the damage done exponentially exceeds his predictions. In many cases, the illnesses and deaths can't all be proven to be initiated by the vaccines, but in most cases, the circumstantial evidence of onset times, are 99% certain. A family member who lost a loved one under these obvious circumstances, will never believe anything else! Yet, the CDC, WHO, and so-called health experts vehemently deny these facts. As of January, 2026, these groups have finally begun to accede to the extensively clear presence of proven facts. Permanent multi-faceted damages, disabilities, and deaths continue. Many cannot be proven without autopsies, but all recorded evidences from health records, and testimonials of family members have continued.

Knowing all this, the deplorable and depraved actions of the globalist elites who planned and executed the pandemic beginning years ago, had and still have NO compunction for what they did and are still trying to do, even though the EUA status is over. Reformulated vaccines have since been marketed and even though the pandemic itself is long over, with its current status being no more dangerous than any other infectious virus, the push to sell vaccine is still alive and well. We know the globalist elites and all cooperative parties deliberately carried out a well-planned, long-term strategy to vaccinate the world for massive increases in their wealth, power, and control. "COVID-19 was about forcing humanity to submit to experimental, dangerous, and expensive vaccines, then using it as a basis of justification for increasing totalitarian power."[10]

The Breggins "uncovered how a loose but well-coordinated array of billionaires, tech companies, public health schools and authorities, major worldwide corporations, and their allies had been planning for all this as early as 2016. They made a financial killing on what they defined and repeatedly predicted as the inevitable and soon-to-arrive pandemic. At least four years ahead of the pandemic, globalists began making massive marketing expenditures to prepare the world for accepting dangerously rushed vaccine programs in the future. The propaganda splurge was stunning. Even before 2017 was over, they were already predicting and prepping the world specifically for a SARS-CoV pandemic through which to impose their vaccines on humanity at the first possible opportunity. As early as January 2017, the 'Global Predators (the term used by the Breggins), planned for the financial windfall to come specifically from making and marketing untried, highly dangerous mRNA and DNA vaccines. They already had programs called 'platforms' in the early stages of development with Moderna and Pfizer that would in 2020 be named and unveiled as 'Operation Warp Speed.'"[11]

This name was used regularly by the globalists when they began to collect corporate, philanthropic, and government financing, all of which was the foundation of Klaus Schwab's 'Great Reset', announced in 2020 as the new global financial future to come. The entire program was done without any input from or involvement with any actual government body, court of law, or citizen's groups putting ANY approval or restrictions on their stunning and high-handed plans.

It is important to note from the start of COVID-19 in 2020, collaborating globalists included America's top Tech corporations, including Microsoft (Bill Gates), Apple (Tim Cook), Alphabet (Google and U-Tube), Facebook (Meta/Mark Zuckerberg, and Twitter (Jack Dorsey and a company full of idealists). Almost every single American billionaire, in CEO and power positions, remains deeply ensconced today in the predatory morass of globalists. These include Jeff Bezos, Bill Gates, Warren Buffet, the Waltons, Steve Balmer, Larry Page, and Michael Bloomberg. Note also that each one is also deeply invested in the People's Republic of

China and its CCP. Elon Musk, current CEO of Twitter is the topmost billionaire, but he tends always to ride the prevailing wave of the moment. Anthony Fauci and Bill Gates are nearly joined at the hip in word and deed.

Tedros Adhanom Ghebreyesus, a former Ethiopian, public-health official is the director-general of the World Health Organization (WHO) since 2017 and is also an extremely liberal globalist player. Fauci and Tedros are two of the most powerful voices for the wealthiest globalists; both are close to Gates and even closer to the Communist Chinese, the largest globalist influence of all. Tedros regularly and consistently predicts another pandemic worse than COVID-19 and easily more deadly. Who would know better? Because the WHO is just another offshoot of the UN, it is supposed to be nothing more than an advisory board having no power to demand the recommendations they make be enforced. Because globalists want to use it to mandate directives, there is now a global movement of the people of the world to expose this usurped role of the WHO *clearly*, to protect us all from the WHO's huge power grab.

In addition to the corruption of the globalist elites and their recent crimes, we must be clear about other areas affected influencing the health and well-being of us all. America's top two schools of public health, Harvard and Johns Hopkins, wholly supported the wealthy global army of billionaire voices and are proceeding into the future with all of the globalist plans. These schools have traditionally printed the most highly respected medical and scientific journals including: The Lancet, the New England Journal of Medicine (NEJM), and the Journal of the American Medical Association (JAMA). However, all of these have cooperated fully with the globalist agenda, exonerating the Chinese Communists, preventing early treatments, and forcing experimental drugs onto humanity. They heavily encouraged crushing freedom-loving Western peoples with antiquated and ineffective public health measures. They squelched any normalcy of individual lives, society and our economy. Finally, each rejected the formerly effective and highly respected physicians they formerly touted as the best and further blocked them from publishing anything contrary to the globalist narratives.

Additionally, "all the old and supposedly 'progressive' radio and TV media unflinchingly supported the globalist elites, while protecting Communist China. They include ABC, NBC, CBS, National Public Radio, CNN, and MSNBC. They all continue today to various degrees to reject the known source of the SARS-CoV-2 virus as being from the Wuhan Institute of Virology in Communist China. They dub this truth as 'racist' and 'conspiratorial.' The old establishment print media, including the Washington Post (WP), the Wall Street Journal (WSJ), the New York Times (NYT), and USA Today act in harmony with their radio and T.V. buddies."[12] It must still be true that money talks and a lot of money speaks so loudly, we can barely hear the truth. Note also: the lion's share of large, especially ivy-league, American universities are closely tied to the wealthy globalists and very often to the CCP. The problem is so egregious that many of these well-known institutions are under federal investigation for their Chinese ties.

Naturally, many key politicians are also in bed with the Chinese, not the least of which was the entire family of former President Biden. The entire 'progressive' Socialist political establishment in power during his administration become completely entwined with the highest circles of worldwide industry, finance, and the Chinese government. There is no misunderstanding of the stated goals of the CCP. It regularly declares its plans to merge the entire world into a Chinese Empire of Communism with its own supreme ruler, much like it had in its earlier glory days.

Anyone in the West who continues to deny this stated

goal, lives in delusion. Ignoring the statement and determined power behind it, with cooperation and mutual ties, we all could find ourselves in the ultimate state of full servitude and in a certain death trap if that trend either continues or returns in the near future.

"Even Pope Francis became a Communist collaborator, both in action and by open declaration. Prior to his recent resignation, he had pushed the Catholic Church as far to the left as he possibly could…Every global predator we could name is financially wedded to, and filled with admiration for, not the United States or other Western democracies, but to Communist China and its totalitarianism. This ultimate realization from our (Breggins) research was totally dismaying."[13]

COVID-19 policies aimed at and caused the massive destruction and even shutdown of Western economies. The full intention of globalist elites has been to intimidate and harm all democratic republics, including the US, the UK, Germany, and Australia. Their stated goal is to vastly increase top-down governments, moving at the least to authoritarianism, and at the best to full-on totalitarianism all over the globe. Big Tech, Big Pharma, and Big Business continue their assertions that a one-world government is a conspiracy theory not to be taken seriously, while simultaneously touting the New World Order as its goal! It is one of the main goals of the World Economic Forum as touted by Klaus Schwab and the globalist elites, along with the Global Reset to help make it happen. There is definitely a Master Plan, to be further detailed in a later chapter.

Meanwhile, we have shown the nature of the criminals driving the pandemic and some of the things associated with the pandemic goals of the globalist elites.

CHAPTER 2

Who Are the Leading Criminals?

> There will be terrible times in the last days. People will be lovers of themselves, lovers of money, boastful, proud, abusive, disobedient to their parents, ungrateful, unholy, without love, unforgiving, slanderous, without self-control, brutal, not lovers of the good. Treacherous, rash, conceited, lovers of pleasure rather than lovers of God. Having a form of godliness but denying its power. Have nothing to do with such people. Always learning but never able to come to a knowledge of the truth...while evil people and impostors will go from bad to worse, deceiving and being deceived.
>
> (2 Timothy 3:1-5; 7; 13)

Klaus Schwab

In the last chapter, we saw Klaus Schwab as the mastermind behind the World Economic Forum, but who was he really? A brief history of the man's earlier years may help us understand him better. Schwab was born in Ravensburg, Germany in 1938 but his parents were both of Swiss lineage. Schwab himself said, "The legacy of the wartime situation had a huge impact on me. I became very interested in reconciliation and dialogue. We had to create a new Europe based on these two things."[1] Schwab has two doctoral degrees, one in mechanical engineering; the other in economics and social sciences. The young man spent a year at Harvard University and then became the youngest professor at the University of Geneva.

While in Geneva, Schwab worked in the just-emerging field that applied academic analysis to the world of business. He developed his "stakeholder theory;" this underlying principle was the foundation for all his future work at the World Economic Forum he founded forty years later. He believed companies not only serve shareholders but all the stakeholders of their organization. That means all the social groups connected directly or indirectly to the enterprise, dependent on its success and prosperity, includes not just shareholders and creditors but also employees, customers, suppliers, the state, and the society in which the enterprise is active.

In relation to the WEF, Schwab saw it as 'the glue' between different stakeholders in society. "The World Economic Forum is not a decision-making body. It is a platform for initiatives, programs and taskforces. It gives each of our participants the possibility to shape their own opinion based on the latest strategic insights. I believe fundamentally in the inter-relationship between economic development and social progress. I feel that governments today alone cannot address global challenges, nor can business alone, nor can non-governmental organizations (NGOs). At the World Economic Forum we had to create platforms for the three main pillars of society; that is government, business, and civil society, to interact and confront the issues which we have on the global agenda."[2]

If you did not understand what Klaus Schwab said, don't worry. These high-level speeches always contain a plethora of words, representing some pie-in-the-sky ideas that no one really understands. They simply pretend to 'get it' and this format is largely what Schwab was known for. Extremely intelligent people tend to treat thoughts like complete philosophies, and call them theories because there is no means of proof! The probable reason for the success of the Forum is its motto, simply "committed to improving the state of the world." In 1971, Klaus brought together 400 wealthy men and women, each influential in their individual fields, for a conference. This group was already prestigious, so it helped to fulfill the WEF mission by blending business, political, academic and other leaders of society by shaping global, regional, and industry agendas.

Klaus Schwab had an inexhaustible list of professorships and honorary doctorates from no fewer than 18 foreign universities and wrote several books. There are 16 national distinctions, and 14 selected awards. His wife and two grown children also worked in the Forum. However, current information does not include them since Klaus stepped down. The full extent of the nature of the dangerous ideas coming from the mind of this man can be inspected from his books, which include: *The Fourth Industrial Revolution.* Warning: This is not recommended reading unless needed to induce sleep! Political scientist Klaus-Gerd Giesen argued that the dominant ideology of this book is transhumanism. It can be defined as a philosophical and intellectual movement which advocates for the enhancement of the human condition by developing and making widely available sophisticated technologies that can greatly enhance longevity, cognition, and well-being. According to Schwab, the Fourth Industrial Revolution will be driven largely by the convergence of digital, biological, and physical innovations. Technologies, such as artificial intelligence (AI), genome editing, augmented reality, robotics, and 3-D printing, are rapidly changing the way humans create, exchange, and distribute value. Indeed, it's a rare day when evidence of the advancement of these very entities is not seen or heard.

"Our ability to edit the building blocks of life (DNA) has recently been massively expanded by low-cost gene sequencing and techniques such as CRISPR; artificial intelligence is augmenting processes and skill in every industry.

"Neurotechnology is making unprecedented strides in how we can use and influence the brain as the last frontier of human biology; automation is disrupting century-old transport and manufacturing paradigms; and technologies such as blockchain, are used in executing cryptocurrency transactions. Smart materials are redefining and blurring the boundary between the digital and physical worlds."[3]

All of the above areas of technological advancement are perceived by globalist elites as positives in almost every way, but underneath all of them lie some monstrous possible effects for the whole human race. There are a few potential benefits, but the probable harms far outweigh the benefits. Klaus acknowledged this revolution could produce far greater inequalities, especially in a huge disruption of labor markets. As greater automation replaces labor, it will change production across the entire economy. There is no doubt that the disparity of manned jobs to tech jobs will be far greater than in any of the previous three industrial revolutions. Having a net increase in safe and rewarding jobs hardly makes up for all the loss to those people who will never be "techy!" The inability to fairly distribute the supposed benefits will result in even greater global challenges. With a global governance under an entire reset, there is little likelihood of human equality anywhere. With individual freedoms gone, and the ability to make one's own decisions also gone, welcome to global socialism.

In 2020, Klaus Schwab rolled out his "Great Reset" plans. In the beginning, the ideas were so preposterous, the idea was dubbed a "conspiracy theory" started by "right wing" and "religious kooks!" Very quickly we all understood it was not a conspiracy theory, nor was it perpetrated by anyone in the conservative camp. President Biden officially proclaimed it the national policy of the United States. He and his climate change "czar," John Kerry, immediately began to set our nation on a catastrophic course, that would look like a runaway train before the collisions even started.

Since Schwab hatched the idea, we need to look somewhat at length about what this plan entails, and exactly how close it resembles the days of the prophesied and imminent Tribulation under the Antichrist. On 12/21/2011, just before Christmas and during the Obama Administration, the UN General Assembly and its Security Council unanimously adopted a pledge entitled, "Transforming Our World: The 2020 Agenda for Sustainable Development." It was primarily drafted to address climate change concerns, but it turned out to be nothing more than a gigantic wish list for the dream of a better world! When you see the terms of the pledge, you can easily recognize the brain and ideology of Klaus

Schwab behind it. There were five main ideas listed as follows:

- "All countries and all ***stakeholders***, acting in collaborative partnership will implement this plan."
- "The ***stakeholders*** are the assorted globalist elites who are not representing the interests of governments or, in most cases, corporations, but themselves. This pledge has 59 numbered points to its vision, with an additional 17 goals including numerous subgoals, adding up to 169 targets. It is nothing but a complete babble of political nonsense being used to blind the world at large to their massive ambitions!"
- Within this document there is no mention of "liberty." There are three mentions of "freedom," but they are not in the context of our universal, God-given, or even natural freedoms. Instead, they are "in accordance with national and international legislation and agreements."
- "There are 23 mentions of "rights" as a justification for various goals such as gender equality."
- "It has NO concept whatsoever of 'individual freedom' or 'political liberty' as we in the United States know it. These concepts have absolutely no place in globalist thinking. Globalist elites all desire totalitarianism. Globalists want to impose their brand of 'justice' on the world; it's nothing but a ruse they use to exploit all of humanity."[4]

This was a foundational document, meant to put into circulation the world-wide ideas Klaus Schwab fleshed out in his book, *The Great Reset.* Interestingly, the term did not originate with Schwab. It was coined in a little-known book by Richard Florida published in 2010, but was quickly adopted by Klaus Schwab. He showcased COVID-19 in his own book, and it is easy to see how much the pandemic inspired him, gave him renewed hope for his whole agenda and further energized all the globalist elites who had planned heavily on it to do just that. In addition, the book inspired politically motivated people everywhere and established Schwab as the "greatest intellectual" in the whole of globalism, as well as the "intellectual backbone" of American policy under President Joseph Biden.

Schwab then declared that globalism is NOT compatible with patriotic democracies. This is where the real rubber met the road for him; it meant by default—there is no place within the 'great reset' for patriotic democracies. He buried another statement within his book: "the three notions of economic globalization; political democracy and nation states are mutually irreconcilable"—which of course is true. The citizens of a patriotic, democratic republic would NEVER willingly and knowingly submit to governance by globalist elites. This readily explains why globalists HATE America as the most powerful democratic republic and the beacon of liberty. America remains the greatest roadblock to globalist ambitions, no matter who else espouses them. Naturally, the American threat was especially felt by globalists when President Donald J. Trump was elected twice. He embodies the spirit of freedom and liberty, in a strong democratic republic. An American majority was drawn the first time and is currently more profoundly drawn to a cheerleader, fellow citizens, their country's history, its tradition of greatness and their liberty above anything globalism could offer. When President Trump was elected the first time despite the carefully planned fraud of the Clinton camp, there was hope for better days and positive advances were made before the onset of the pandemic. This author believes that our God allowed the whole fraudulent Biden administration to give Americans further understanding of just how horrid a liberal freehand could be with no hope for better in sight. All the unlawful efforts of liberals to prevent President Trump from further leadership failed stunningly. It also enabled him to review all that had been done and give him the opportunity to wisely prepare for continued leadership the second time. It was even abundantly clear how much our Father God led and protected him at every turn from the enormous efforts made to keep him from re-entering a new administration.

The exact opposite was true under the Biden Administration. Globalist elites and left-wing liberalism/socialism managed to cheat President Trump out of his second term in office with every known trick in the books, because they could not further their agenda with him in charge. Biden and his well-known handlers shifted almost every political policy Americans held to further the globalism agenda. He was literally placed into office, with the corrupted efforts of American liberal socialists with the support of the globalist elites to push their global reset, open our borders, encourage blatantly illegal immigration, set sanctuary cities, perpetrate rampant crime, destroy our economy, and revive the asinine, climate change policies which have no foundation in truth. He winked at, aided, and abetted Communist China in playing their dangerous games as the largest globalist influence of all. Globalism and the great reset made huge strides in a very short time. Fortunately, with this destruction, bedrock, grass-roots Americans got their eyes opened to the agenda and what it was going to mean if it continued.

Thankfully, for the first time in too long, patriots finally realized failure to act, would likely change our country as we know it to one we wouldn't even recognize, and one that would be nearly impossible to fix.

Finally, we will see in a future chapter much more about the Great Reset, and its influence in end times events, but let's sum up the globalist leadership of Klaus Schwab and the ongoing WEF agenda. Remember, Communist China and the CCP is regarded as the biggest Globalist Elite of all. Schwab was a devotee of Xi Jinping, the CCP's President of the People's Republic of China, having a personal net worth of 1.3 billion dollars. Klaus made this fact publicly clear, especially in 2021 when Xi was shown exaggerated esteem as a speaker at the World Economic Forum's Davos meeting. Klaus actually "invoked COVID-19 as a blessing to his cause." He added, "The COVID19 pandemic has demonstrated that no institution or individual alone can address the economic, environmental, social, and technological challenges of our complex, interdependent world."[6] But, confusingly, Schwab never named anyone to actually take charge of it all. He did, however, go out of his way to curry favor with Xi Jinping and frequently apologized for the CCP, which was clearly one of his most preferred stakeholders!

Dr. Peter Breggins declared, "In essence, COVID-19 gave Schwab the opportunity to honor in public the MOST powerful and violent dictator in the world…The fawning over him so overtly and unashamedly was a sickening sight to behold."[7]

Anthony Fauci

How do people or even governments ever make a determination when faced with a myriad of criminals, who is the worst of the worst? In the case of globalist elites it is not as hard to pick one. While Schwab was dealt with first because he was part of the whole foundation of diabolical ideas which could ultimately hurt millions of people. He was still part of a very large, ongoing process and the depth of that damage is yet to be determined. However, it isn't difficult to say Anthony Fauci very literally murdered millions through his pride, self-absorption, deceit, and greed throughout the pandemic years, but also through several other previous laboratory shenanigans with flu and HIV/Aids epidemics where he was also the primary cause of hundreds of thousands of deaths due to his high-handed, and really bad health decisions. Let's look first at some of his notorious history and then again at his performance throughout the COVID-19 pandemic.

At the beginning of the pandemic, few average Americans being introduced to Anthony Fauci, had a clue who he was or knew anything about him unless they traveled in scientific circles. Taken at face value, he was not imposing, but a smallish, slender, bespeckled older man. Gray hair, an almost unassuming look and a slight smile were meant to appear innocent, yet wise. For what it's worth, personally, the look he had felt false; for someone who was supposed to be THE authority on the pandemic, at least initially, he did not exude the confidence he should have shown. Watch the eyes! He presented himself as a rather meek personage, one we were supposed to believe would make hard but compassionate healthcare decisions. However, when other authorities began challenging him with hard questions the façade fell off! He had been the director of one of the 27 Institutes in the National Institutes of Health (NIH), namely the National Institute of Allergy and Infectious Diseases (NIAID), for forty years. This fact supposedly made him an "expert;" the expert many politicians were looking to for guidance on COVID-19. Initially, Fauci appeared to exemplify the professional scientist and public servant. However, within days he very deliberately usurped total authority over the entire pandemic scene as if God Himself had personally ordained him.

As Dr. Breggin commented, "'Science' and 'Authority' are not compatible. The area of public health is chaotic and constantly changing with unknown or untold human, unpredictable factors. The idea of ONE person being 'The Authority' is not defensible or justifiable. We should all perceive that any person crashing into the spotlight like Fauci did, as a scientific authority, is trying to manipulate people with unproven arguments. From a professional health perspective most of his arguments were only partially true at best and almost certainly not in our best interests. Many of us became concerned, especially those of us in the medical profession, when Fauci so frequently contradicted his own words and was clearly and consistently promoting the agendas of Big Pharma. In the beginning, few of us imagined that tracking his ideas would lead straight to Bill Gates and then to all the other globalist elites. The Breggins NEVER imagined finding Fauci DIRECTLY funding gain-of-function projects and making deadly viruses with American researchers at America's Universities (with mostly American taxpayer money). Worse, they found these research scientists openly and proudly collaborating with the mightiest global predator of all, the CCP. These treasonous acts ultimately fueled the CCP's chilling biological weapons strategy called,

'UNRESTRICTED

WARFARE!' " [8]

"Another severely damaging crime was committed by Fauci on October 31, 2020, just 72 hours before presidential election day. Anthony Fauci was a career Senior Executive Service (SES)-level, government employee who under the federal Hatch Act was NOT permitted to use this title when involved in political activities. In pure defiance of that law, at a hyper-critical point in American history, before a highly-contested election, Fauci interfered with the election by issuing dire warnings about COVID-19 and President Trump's handling of it. The Washington Post, in obvious cahoots with Fauci and the globalist elites, offered threatening headlines. The Washington Post went on to repeat and explain the ominous headlines. Fauci, a leading member of the government's response team said the US needed to make an 'abrupt change' in public health practice and behaviors (meaning a change in US leadership) which was both profoundly political and illegal." [9]

The illegal damage was done—and Fauci's statements dittoed and reinforced those made by candidate Joe Biden who in a debate stated that under another Trump administration we were all facing "a dark winter." This same anti-Trump warning was of course published by the liberal mainstream media far and wide. Clearly this was an issue of far greater scope than some Democrats unseating the Republican incumbent! This was international globalism illegally doing everything in their power to remove an enemy so they could continue their agendas without pushback.

About this same time, Ginger Breggin unearthed a startling discovery in her research. A 2015 scientific publication disclosed something so bizarre she could hardly believe it was real. The paper was published by Vinset D. Menechery and colleagues at the University of North Carolina and was entitled, "A SARS-like Cluster of Circulating Bat Coronaviruses Shows Potential for Human Emergence." This was both shocking and incriminating because it showed, prior to the emergence of COVID-19, OUR US scientists were already collaborating with and funding two of China's top gain-of-function scientists who were making SARS-CoV pathogens.

A second follow-up paper verified Chinese and American scientists continued working closely together to create what was obviously a precursor to SARS-CoV-2. Incidentally, it was also considered a potential "biological weapon!"

You can now clearly understand from this discovery, Americans were working with Chinese to insert the deadly spike protein, we've all now learned about, into an otherwise harmless coronavirus to enable it to penetrate human cells and cause a SARS-CoV pandemic! This research was largely funded by Anthony Fauci's NIAID as well as several other Institutes within the NIH Institutes, with predominantly misappropriated money. This gain-of-function research was done with the full cooperation of the CCP regime scientists and American scientists, from various university laboratories. Other funding came from various American institutions including Harvard University and the FDA's National Center for Toxicological Research, and more.

There is proof these agencies were all collaborating with Chinese researchers at the Wuhan Institute of Virology. Their gain-of-function research provided the scientific basis for China's 'biological warfare' program! Is that not breathtaking? Supposedly smart scientists working for years with our #1 enemy to help them develop weapons to use against us is criminal treason and a capital crime! Worse, not one of them has yet been charged, much less convicted. Anthony Fauci provided the lion's share of the funding for these crimes from American taxpayer dollars! His persistent support of all collaboration with the Chinese was done knowingly and he intentionally funded the CCP, its military, its biological warfare program, and its ability to engineer the SARS-CoV2, causing COVID-19. This was pure, unadulterated TREASON.

When the Breggins published this information on their website in April of 2020 and made a U-Tube video about the whole disaster, it had 40,000 views over-night. One year later, U-Tube, of the Big Tech scene, used that video as an excuse to take down the Breggins' channel. After the take-down, they sent the video to every scientific, media, and political contact they had available to them, including close contacts in President Trump's circle. The President promptly canceled the funding for collaboration with China, but it did NOT stop Fauci. Later in June, when Fauci was asked by a Congressional Committee member why the funding was canceled, Fauci said he didn't know why!!! As usual, the main stream media did not support the President's decision. But this episode points clearly to the fact that Fauci is a cold-blooded, bold-faced liar also, who could and would skirt any question about his actions, anytime.

Naturally, this information triggers a plethora of questions. "Why were the Breggins the ***first*** whistleblowers? Why was there no national display of utter outrage over these heinous crimes and only scant support for our President? Certainly, the Breggins had no difficulty understanding the enormity of the implications for America and for the world. The depth of the evil and the horrifying threat to our nation was overwhelming. Had anything close to this happened a couple decades before and been discovered, there is no doubt of thorough investigations and charges would have been brought promptly. However, under the thinly veiled authority behind the pandemic, essentially nothing was done. Even today, nearing 2026, we have yet to hear publicly of ANY charges filed, any indictments, and certainly no trials or demands for retribution have been made since then. It's a new day, and a very dangerous era we entered. Rumors have surfaced after the pandemic ended that the US Military has held many military tribunals on the charges of treason and more. However, if they happened, it is not public knowledge. The rumors are assumed true because the criminal parties and many of the Deep State perpetrators have more or less disappeared into the woodwork and necessary appearances seem to look like their dopplegangers.

The agenda for all this expensive and deadly pandemic really boils down to the development of new vaccines! Remember, development of the vaccines for COVID-19 was already 10 years old when the pandemic started! A $10 million dollar award from NIH was given to a program to be led by Ralph Baric at the University of North Carolina School of *Global* Public Health. The whole justification for this ominous project was, among other things, to develop VACCINES! The Breggins said, "As eerily unreal as it seemed to us, our research for this book moved us inexorably toward the solid conclusion that COVID-19 was ALWAYS about making fortunes from rushed-through vaccines while weakening America and strengthening globalism."[10]The Fauci-funded research of Ralph Baric actually goes all the way back to 2008 when infectious clones of infectious human coronaviruses were made. Once again it was supported with NIH grants and funds from "Vaccines for Global Health" to the University of North Carolina School of Public Health. Who could ever imagine how many deadly SARS-CoV viruses have been engineered since 2008 and now lurk in laboratories around the world!

"In February of 2020, a Chinese researcher published a study confirming the novel coronavirus was man-made in a Chinese laboratory; shortly, that paper disappeared from all the usual search engines."[11] Predictably, China has used our technology, but in this event, they didn't have to steal it; Anthony Fauci gave it to them along with US taxpayer money to further develop it. The travesty of this is absolutely breath-taking. Ever since Mao Tse-Tung, there has been ongoing development of Chinese bioweapon warfare which is 100% tied inexplicably to the CCP military, part of China's Military-Civil Fusion. That means that Fauci, his NIAID and NIH, while colluding with China, consistently provided that violent dictatorship with a significant upgrade in its military threat toward the US and the world. The well-known and stated intent of the People's Liberation Army is to be a "world-class military," second to none by 2049. This is exponentially worse than if a spy went over to China and whispered military secrets in Xi's ears!! America's national security has definitely been breached.

The question arises from those who simply can't understand why; "Was Fauci just simply naïve, innocent or uninformed of all this?" ***NOT A CHANCE!*** Fauci had already done roughly the same thing in the lab with the highly pathogenic H5N1 influenza virus. Regarding this viral research, Fauci said, "the potential benefits and risks of these experiments MUST be discussed and understood by '*MULTIPLE STAKEHOLDERS'* (an array of global elites) including the '*GENERAL PUBLIC'* (representative 'experts'). You cannot find in this statement one single hint of a democratic republic in which the people, through voting and other lawful means, control the major direction taken by society."[12] In other words, Anthony Fauci has been a notoriously premeditating, avaricious and egregious criminal for decades. Even though a vast number of people knew of his criminal history, he was NEVER arrested, and always protected by the globalist elites as long as he did what they expected of him.

There is absolutely NO question of whether Fauci knew. He has always been fully aware of what he was doing! The identical behaviors of thwarting the law, cheating colleagues out of recognition for things he wanted credit for, pathologic lying to cover what he intended and then did it anyway, as well as a myriad of other immoral and unethical endeavors over the course of his career. There is no regard for patriotism toward one's own country, and though Fauci has never been as wealthy as the globalist elites, he embodies all their traits of pride, greed, and craving of greater honor, power, and control exactly as they have. It can't be a matter of poor judgment either, because he has proven too shrewd, too deceitful, and too worldly for that. Fauci is almost larger-than-life within a large group of individuals and entities who accept his behaviors as normal because they do the same things while pursuing their various global enterprises to accumulate greater wealth, position, and power. Most of the globalist elites share his willingness to ignore or to sacrifice the interests of their own nations in the pursuit of more wealth, more personal power, and ego strutting. President Joe Biden was a deep admirer of Fauci, leaving him with plenty of wiggle room in his administration. "The NIH is an enormous "stakeholder" and Fauci more than directed his portion of it. In fact, the NIH owns hundreds of patents and has enormous power and financial interests in Big Pharma, including a patent on Moderna's COVID-19 vaccine."[13] "A public citizen asked, 'Does Anthony Fauci own half of the patent for Moderna's COVID vaccine? An NIH scientist who developed key vaccine technology confirmed it and added, 'the patent gives us leverage'."[14] Under the Emergency Use Authorization (EUA) regarding drugs and vaccines, Fauci and colleagues made "investments" into pharmaceutical companies with our US taxpayer's money, but these so-called "investments" are really like "gifts" from us to them since that money is "awarded." This is how the whole system works: Moderna's vaccine was highly touted 'in advance' by Bill Gates; so Moderna received a grant of almost a half-billion dollars ($438 million) from a US government agency. The Biomedical Advanced Research and Development Authority (BARDA) 'awarded' it to Moderna to accelerate the development of its vaccine. Other agencies also contributed their own large sums to support their own vested interests. In any other arena these various maneuvers would be considered "money laundering!" Many white-shirt criminals have done jail time for a lot less!

At the same time Pfizer's vaccine, also promoted by Bill Gates in 2017, was and still is Moderna's prime competitor, however, since globalist elites help fund all of Big Pharma, all the individual companies tend to happily share in the generosity rather than competing with each other. The Gates Foundation was also heavily vested in mRNA vaccines up to $1.75 billion dollars as of December 2020. More on Gates later, but we see Pfizer's and Moderna's vaccines were the first and second COVID vaccines authorized by the FDA through the Emergency Use Authorization (EUA). The Communist Chinese Party (CCP) is also heavily vested in Pfizer's vaccines. The US, Germany, and the CCP all partnered with Pfizer and worked together on the mRNA vaccine. Once again, US Globalist corporations were bilking America while fueling the CCP with money and dangerous biomedical "know-how." In addition, the United States government is also heavily vested in Pfizer through the Department of Health and Human Services (HHS), and the Department of Defense. A $1.95 billion-dollar agreement was made by our DOD to produce 100 million doses of COVID-19 vaccine (that isn't a true vaccine—more on that later), also approved under the EUA. It is especially important to note—the US was already buying Pfizer's vaccine rabidly for a full FOUR MONTHS BEFORE the FDA approved it!

Anthony Fauci made $417,608 annually as a government employee with extremely generous benefits and retirement before COVID. There is supposed to be a ceiling on how much additional money can be made from patents and other remunerations for government employees. We will probably never know the extent of Fauci's twisted motives and greed, nor the full extent of the evil he very literally personifies. He has also exponentially increased the power and wealth of his "baby," the NIAID, together with other parts of the NIH, because he fully wrapped himself in an unearned cloud of 'glory.' We know of his history with other lucrative biological and financial motives, so it is highly likely he has considerable hidden ideological motives not yet unearthed. We know he has grandiose plans in conjunction with Klaus Schwab for an authoritarian or totalitarian global government which will make all humankind "safe from viruses" by limiting the activities of people in nature, no matter how high the cost to our entire civilization.

We can only ask ourselves just how deep is Fauci's betrayal of America. Bottom line—Fauci is not nearly the most powerful of the globalist elites. Instead he acts as their mouthpiece, speaking on their behalf.

More on Anthony Fauci—His History Before Covid Began

Long before most people knew anything about Fauci, he was involved in a maelstrom of highly-questionable, public health problems he supposedly led from the science/laboratory perspective. He made a number of very bad health-based decisions. He was literally responsible for the deaths of thousands of citizens who were treated erroneously and flippantly for their illnesses and died. Clearly Fauci was already notorious, but not nearly enough people were aware of it in time to cut short similar bad choices made with COVID-19. During the 1980s HIV / Aids crisis Fauci was directly responsible for betraying HIV patients around the world. There were strong implications of treason and criminal conspiracy to commit mass murder already on the books from that tragedy.

Fauci has been as good as immune from the effects of even the harshest criticisms largely because he's been so well protected by globalist elites in bureaucracy and media. However, in the retro analysis, his notorious background and the resulting controversies completely exhibit the same attitude and behaviors we saw in his handling of COVID-19; they simply hadn't changed at all. Back in the 1980s, Fauci took the world stage as the AIDs Czar. Soon, rabid accusations of his sacrificing the lives of AIDs patients to the interests of Big Pharma were heard. There was outrage over his handling of HIV. In 1988, an AIDs activist addressed an open letter to Fauci accusing him of murder. The letter was entirely true. There were riots and demonstrations in front of the NIAID offices where no fewer than 1000 people marched on Fauci.

"Under Fauci's leadership, the FDA approved an extremely lethal experimental drug called Azidothymidine (AZT), also known as Retrovir. It had just been introduced to delay the development of AIDs in HIV patients. Conditions were fraught with chaos and controversy. AZT was one of the most toxic, expensive, and controversial drugs in the history of medicine."[15]The similarity of the AZT story to Fauci's known manipulation of the COVID-19 treatment protocols already effectively being used, in favor of REMDESIVIR, is spooky enough to send chills down all our spines. Fauci fiercely forced the use of this experimental, ultra- expensive, toxic, and ineffective drug for COVID treatment. It was never adequately tested in trials. He BANNED the good, effective, inexpensive, tried and true drugs offering less hospitalization and less deaths so the money could freely flow from the horrible and deadly use of Remdesivir instead. This drug had to be given by IV and was the only drug of choice ALLOWED. Thousands of COVID patients were hospitalized with treatable symptoms, given Remdesivir, and died. But once again, under the EUA status of pandemic, it was the Mother Lode for Big Pharma. The same astronomical cost for its use, was exactly like that of AZT's expense in the 80s.

Costs for AIDS patients in the 80s made it the MOST EXPENSIVE drug ever marketed and given to AIDS patients who were already disease-poor and lacking insurance. Simple use of proven Sulfa drugs worked better than AZT! The most common illness infecting HIV patients with deficient immune systems and pneumocystis pneumonia (PCP), was caused by a FUNGUS! It wasn't generally a problem in people with healthy immune systems, but Bactrim (Sulfa) had been used for 20 years+ and clinical trials had confirmed its use for PCP was safe and effective. Quack Dr. Fauci opposed the use of Bactrim, pushing his AZT. He refused to allow its use for two years while clinical trials were being completed to use Bactrim. In that two years, 17,000 patients died needlessly!

Not since that tragedy have American physicians been so stymied by government interference, until COVID-19. But, this time the government and Fauci went even further overboard. They thoroughly kiboshed the use of the good, cheap, and effective drugs doctors like Peter McCullough, MD and a host of others had been using with their patients for many months at home reducing the numbers of hospitalizations and deaths exponentially. No good and proven meds like ivermectin and hydroxychloroquine (HCQ) were allowed; and only the one very bad drug was allowed. It was a heinous travesty beyond belief. Can anyone even imagine the frustration and anger of physicians, whose hands were completely tied from treating COVID-19 effectively as they had already done previously? Worse still, if any medical personnel had the audacity to write about it, or try to expose it, they were treated as the criminals, at risk of losing their licenses, their livelihoods, and banned from any of the professional medical journals that exposed the travesty.

Even the HIV/AIDS malpractice charge didn't stop Fauci! When the deadly Ebola epidemic hit Africa, Fauci FOUGHT all US efforts to quarantine any heavily exposed persons, (especially health care workers returning to the States). He exerted enormous efforts to stop Governors of States from protecting their citizens against the spread of Ebola. Similarly, Fauci tried to stop President Trump from banning travel from China to America early in the onset of COVID-19. In both cases, Fauci's agenda was clear. In the case of the Ebola quarantine, he wanted everyone to feel the need for vaccines so they could resume their normal lives. In the case of the early COVID, knowing full well it had originated in China, the agenda was to let it spread far and wide so everyone would run for the vaccines once they became available. In either case it was never about saving lives. Anthony Fauci has a long history of friendship with Big Pharma and the globalists' network. He constantly spoke from both sides of his mouth, and his words were couched in hyperbole. He spoke of his public health collaborations as if they were the final word on truth when in fact his relationships were with some of the greediest corporations on the planet. Every word and action was manipulation designed to protect and exponentially increase all their profits.

Fauci always claimed he "helped" the FDA bypass the lengthy approval processes for new drugs and vaccines, then reassured his vast audiences there was no reduction in safety. That is absolutely impossible and nothing but a bold-faced lie. Clinical studies can last for years if there are reasons to repeat parts of them or make changes in the product to get a better version, etc. When all those precautions established to ensure safety and efficacy are dropped, all responsibility for problems, horrid side effects, including disability and death are also dropped. All safety, efficacy, and accountability simply evaporates. Fauci also said, "Infectious diseases will continue to pose a significant threat to public health and 'ECONOMIES OF COUNTRIES WORLDWIDE.'" Obviously, Fauci planned ahead and knew his 'surprise' would disrupt the economies of the entire globe. How did he know? Plans were already formulated for the massive lock downs.

For now, this is just the tip of the iceberg concerning the criminality of Anthony Fauci. It is enough for the reader to get a glimpse of the depths of his evil and treacherous depravity, as well as how he worked and maybe continues to work under cover within the globalist leadership to help accomplish all their goals. The depths to which this paragon of evil has gone is second only to the powerful globalist elites actually running the whole agenda. We will see more of the specific crimes he committed in a later chapter. It suffices to say this devil evidences not a shred of a conscience in everything he does; there is no moral or ethical compass by which he lives. Even if he were to die tomorrow, the trail of blood he is responsible for shedding rivals the worst despots of all history.

Bill Gates and the Bill and Melinda Gates Foundation

The Bill and Melinda Gates Foundation is a nonprofit organizational trust, claiming to fight poverty, disease, and inequity around the world by its own motto and according to Google which is part of Big Tech globalism protecting its own. Its owners were Bill Gates, Melinda French Gates, and Warren Buffet. The foundation gives grants to people and organizations, most often by invitation and depending on whether the money goes toward the goals of the foundation. Under this structure, the foundation has given away more than $59 billion dollars to "cure disease, save lives, and help the world's neediest people." My goodness, they sound like some of the most charitable people on the planet, but most of these grants are given to entities like drug companies to make more drugs and vaccines in particular. In turn, these grants make Bill Gates billions more than was ever granted. Globalists connected with Big Pharma all make billions, and as of the end of COVID-19, trillions of dollars were and continue to be made from the vaccine business. Warren Buffett gave another $50.7 billion to the foundation. Naturally, most people know Gates best as the co-founder of the software giant, Microsoft, but he spent most of his time with foundation concerns. In 2020, he considered his major focal points climate change, global health and development, and education. On June 23, 2021, Buffett resigned as trustee for the foundation. At age 95, he is still the chairman and CEO of Berkshire Hathaway (holding company), since 1970, and is the 8th richest person in the world. He plans to retire as CEO at the end of 2025, retaining his chairman position. Buffet lives on only 1% of his wealth and gives 99% to charitable causes. Granted, almost anyone could live on 1% of billions! While he easily falls into the globalist category, he doesn't operate his businesses as most of them do. He lives very modestly for all his wealth in the same house he first owned in Omaha, NE. However, while he is a very generous philanthropist, his many causes, such as depopulation, don't generally reflect Biblical values!

It would appear that Bill Gates is both an entrepreneur and philanthropist extraordinaire and has only the highest of charitable goals, but that is light years from the truth. "Gates provided his perspective on a range of issues in a substantial interview published in the March 27, 2014, issue of *Rolling Stone* magazine. In the interview, Gates provided his perspective on climate change, his charitable activities, various tech companies and people involved in them, and the state of America. In response to a question about his greatest fear when he looks 50 years into the future." Gates stated, "There'll be some really bad things that'll happen in the next 50 or 100 years, but hopefully none of them on the scale of, say, a million people you didn't expect to die from a pandemic, or nuclear, or bioterrorism…'" [16]

"During the COVID-19 pandemic, Gates was widely looked at by media outlets as an expert on the issue, despite not being a public official or having any prior medical training. His foundation did, however, establish the COVID-19 Therapeutics Accelerator in 2020 to hasten the development and evaluation of new and repurposed drugs and biologics to treat patients for COVID-19. As of February 2021, Gates expressed that he and Anthony Fauci frequently talked and collaborated on matters including vaccines and other medical innovations to fight the pandemic."[17]At least as far back as 2016, Bill Gates has heavily promoted vaccines for the world to save lives, especially in poorer and more underdeveloped countries. The same year he declared, "We must make this the decade of vaccines!" The bottom line—he believes the entire world should be given a vaccine for every known pathogen possible because only then, will we have the health to master all the other pressing world problems. He has touted this agenda for at least 20+ years. Because of the exponential increase in life-threatening side effects and deaths from the COVID-19 "vaccines," which again are not vaccines in the true sense of the word, have caused a very large number of people to avoid them altogether, and even to literally become anti-vaxxers! This constant push to take dangerous vaccines has changed a lot of minds and made many people think twice about receiving them ever again. In spite of that, Bill Gates, at the Davos conference in January, 2024, was still pushing vaccines as hard as ever. Along with the majority of globalist elites, Gates once again stated an oft repeated goal to "urgently reduce the world population." This was/is a blatant oxymoron. Promoting vaccines to keep people from getting ill and dying, when his real goal was/is to decrease the surplus population! In the Bible that is called "speaking with a forked tongue!"

These injectables of the pandemic era were never FDA approved for safety and effectiveness because they were too toxic, with adverse effects clearly known ahead of 'Operation Warp Speed.' Proof of injury and death from the vaccines abounds via documentation and the Vaccine Adverse Effects Reports System. More importantly, the Pfizer Documents from the COVID-19 vaccine trials clearly exhibit the whole truth. The 'vaccines' given throughout the pandemic months were toxic in so many ways, there was no way to list them effectively in Vax Fact Sheets, or consider any possible informed consent. Literature written since the end of the pandemic review the vaccines made since the EUA, for previous lack of effective clinical trials. These supposed reviews claim the toxicity is no longer present, however all of these claims came primarily from main-stream and social media, all of which are still being controlled by Big Tech companies, and supported by globalist elites. Consequently, even today (end of 2025), the push continues. However, with the appointment of Robert Kennedy, Jr to the office of HHS Secretary in the current Trump Administration, progress is being made to thwart the constant vaccine agenda, as well as many other health-related travesties which have been perpetrated on Americans. It is still difficult to see truth on the web from a plethora of health agencies, which begs us to be conscientious consumers.

Throughout the pandemic days, Bill Gates had a vested interest in suppressing criticism and spent millions to that end. In short, vaccines and their manufacture substantially contributed to his global foundation and to his personal goals for the world. He remains a vaccine tycoon; one who has no qualms about gaining global support for his very lucrative business. For those who would simply chalk up his vast endeavors to philanthropy, please note his own comments:

- We fund research to create intellectual property so that anything invented with our money and going to richer countries brings a huge return on our money—not a philanthropic philosophy!
- Then we have more money to do more research for the benefit of poor countries at a lower cost. This sounds noble, but it still pads the multi-million-dollar investments by volumes. It's more like a Robin Hood philosophy because it makes all illegalities sound noble.
- It is not philanthropy when the person in question is already one of the richest and most powerful people in the world. When ONE person is already worth billions of dollars becomes THE "Moving Force" within a single industry and specialized sector of health such as making vaccines and continuously cements that position, getting ever wealthier in the process, his power is almost impossible to challenge. That doesn't help people!! Instead it presents the worst and most enormous public health risks to the entire global community.
- This problem alone is just a small piece of the overall power Bill Gates exudes in just the vaccine monopoly. With globalist elites, it's a runaway train, with no power to challenge or halt it.

•

President Trump could see what was happening with all the money and power thrown into this vast vaccine agenda. With the World Health Organization (WHO) also throwing its weight behind Big Pharma they ensured everyone would be subjected to these vaccines whether they liked it or not. So our President stopped further US financial support to the WHO, knowing Communist China was its next greatest supporter. So Bill Gates became WHO's largest donor. WHO promptly deleted some and redefined other scientific concepts to promote Bill Gates, the CCP and Big Pharma. The United Nations established WHO for disseminating health information, not to manipulate health policy and directives. Redefinition of tried-and-true health rules made us all dizzy-here are clear examples:

1. Coronaviruses lived on surfaces until they didn't!
2. Masks didn't work until they did and then they didn't after all!
3. There is asymptomatic transmission of COVID-19, except there isn't!
4. Lock downs work to control the virus, except they didn't!
5. All these people are sick without symptoms until oops—PCR tests are now wildly inaccurate; they were never intended to be diagnostic tools!
6. Everyone is in danger of the virus, except those who don't get sick!
7. It spreads in schools, except it rarely did!

Just one big, very fishy, inconsistent mess continued perpetually, but the narratives were never allowed questions or subject to criticism!

After all this, WHO simply deleted the well-established fact of

"Natural Immunity" from its entire website—a change wiping out over 100 years of medical advances in immunology and epidemiology! One Reddit subscriber said it this way, "When the existing textbooks students use in college contradict the latest official pronouncements from 'healthcare' authorities, during a crisis in which the ruling class is clearly attempting to seize permanent power; we've got a problem." But why? Bill Gates and his vaccine monopoly had no intention of waiting around for people to develop their own natural or so-called "herd or community immunity," We all needed to feel so helpless and hopeless without the possibility of attaining herd immunity, we would all rush right out and gladly procure our vaccines. So the true definition of natural immunity, proven over time and experience, was no longer acceptable. According to WHO, this immunity could only be achieved through immunization! We are NOT joking!! Science became nothing more than a marketing tool in the hands of Bill Gates and the globalist elites, and another step closer to their ideal goal of totalitarian rule.

There is exponentially more about Bill Gates and his marriage to Big Pharma as well as his other criminal behaviors. Though he speaks in the forums and to the general public about all his wonderful plans and goals to better the plight of humanity, what he really means by betterment isn't even close to an improvement—but a disaster for those he supposedly helped. They follow the exact same lines as the other globalist elites, and he is very serious about attaining them, though he sounds so deceptively reasonable and caring. He had and still has a silver tongue, but it is every bit as noxious as those of the others' tongues. We have only to look at the history of Bill Gates in business from High School forward and through all the Microsoft years to watch the sickening progression of the tycoon. It is common knowledge that many of Gate's business practices were far from honest and far more than just competitive. He continued in them "until 1998, when the US Department of Justice, along with twenty individual states, sued Microsoft for breach of anti-trust laws. Gates had never been particularly well-loved, but that case turned him into one of the most despised people on the planet...When he was called to make a deposition, he seemed surly, and unresponsive, refused to give straight answers, and at one point even tried to quibble over the definition of the word 'we.' The trial had become a disaster, and the government was talking about splitting Microsoft into two separate companies. Everything was finally falling apart. Shortly afterward, Bill Gates announced that he would be donating one hundred million dollars to fund vaccines for children."[18] Thus, computers took a back seat for Bill Gates, and "philanthropy" became his new power focus!

Big Pharma's Criminality is Second to None

Since Big Pharma is one of the biggest globalist elites on the planet, for which the most uninformed American would quickly agree, this chapter must be included when the subject is the criminals! A British gentleman named Peter Gotzsche wrote a brilliant expose entitled, *Deadly Medicines and Organized Crime—How Big Pharma Has Corrupted Healthcare.* It was written in 2013 and today, a decade later, all that he has said is exponentially truer. His treatise said, "Activities by major pharmaceutical companies include corruption, fraud, bribery, and omission of data to market their products. While all drugs have side effects, not all have benefits. The influx of money by Pharma undercuts regulation, education, and scientific integrity."[19] Prescription drugs are the third leading cause of death after heart disease and cancer. Gotzsche exposed the pharmaceutical industries and their 'charade' of fraudulent behaviors, both in research and in marketing where the morally depraved disregard for human lives is the norm. He convincingly drew close comparisons with the tobacco conglomerates, revealing the extraordinary truth behind efforts to confuse and distract the public and their politicians. "The main reason we take so many drugs is not that drug companies don't sell drugs; they sell lies about drugs. This is what makes drugs so different from anything else in life...virtually everything we know about drugs is what the companies have chosen to tell us and our doctors…the reason patients trust their medicines is that they extrapolate the trust they have in their doctors into the medicines they prescribe."[20] Most patients don't realize that although their doctors may know a lot about them and their diseases, including human physiology and psychology, they often have very little knowledge about the drugs they prescribe except what has been carefully concocted, dressed up for marketing, and cleverly presented to them by representatives of the drug industry.

Peter Gotzsche is an outspoken and knowledgeable critic who wrote his book to "influence policy towards much more transparency…he indicated he had to publish a book because it was much too difficult to publish his criticism in medical journals."[21] The political clout Big Pharma enjoys is second to none, because the pharmaceutical industry is one of the most powerful forces in America. In a Congress of 100 Senators and 435 members of the House for a total of 535 Congressional men and women, Big Pharma has more than 1,800 well-paid lobbyists on Capitol Hill as of June, 2023. Pfizer, the same company that produced one of the two most touted COVID-19 vaccines and was in constant collaboration with its donors, such as Bill Gates, Anthony Fauci, India, and the CCP ranks as the #1 most powerful pharmaceutical company in the world. India is the biggest vaccine exporter in the world; exporting 65-70% of the WHO's vaccine requirements. In 2022 alone, Pfizer's company revenue broke the $100 billion-dollar barrier, a first in the industry, largely as a result of the robust sales of COVID-19 products. Pfizer also has the biggest CEO-to-Employee pay ratios at almost 500:1.

A 2019 Gallup poll found the pharmaceutical industry "the most poorly-regarded industry in Americans' eyes." The critique of Big Pharma included their seemingly neverending price increases, massive lobbying influence, their role in the heinous opioid crisis, and their obnoxious advertising strategies; proving distrust of the pharmaceutical industry is far reaching and well-deserved. "New reports indicate big drug companies are now fighting to weaken the parts of the 'Build Back Better Act' which were intended to deliver relief to families and give Medicare the power to negotiate for lower prescription drug prices. As Big Pharma continues its fight against Medicare negotiation, here are four big reasons why America's families reject drug companies' claims and are demanding action:

- **HIGH PRICES—**'Drug Companies Hiked the Prices of Nearly 1,000 drugs in January (2021).' More than 900 brand name drugs experienced the highest price increases in over a decade. 'Americans Don't Trust Pharmaceutical Companies on Pricing.' 75% of Americans don't trust them to price their products fairly and believe it's due to Big Pharma's greed. They also report the huge company profits are the major factor contributing to soaring costs.

- **POWER AND INFLUENCE—**'The Pharmaceutical Industry Spent Over $250 Million Trying to Kill Medicare Negotiations.' That money was spent on lobbying, devoting three lobbyists to each member of congress (1,605 lobbyists to cheat seniors out of lowered drug costs). 72% of Americans say Big Pharma has too much influence over the federal government.

- **INNOVATION LIES—**'Drug Companies' Stock Buybacks and Dividends Exceed Research and Development Spending.' Over a four-year period (2016-2020), 14 companies spent $56 billion dollars more on buybacks and dividends than they spent on R&D in the same period. The majority of Americans (roughly 70%) are not convinced the industry's argument that drug price negotiation will harm its ability to fund R&D.

- **SKY-HIGH PROFITS—**'Drug Companies Enjoy the Highest Profits of Any Major Industry.' Big Pharma companies have profit margins nearly three times the average for the S&P 500. In 18 years (2000-2018), 35 large drug companies raked in a combined revenue of $11.5 TRILLION with a gross profit of $8.6 TRILLION. Drug companies could lose $1Trillion and still be the most profitable industry."[22]

Once again, we can understand more about the corruption of Big Pharma with all of the above information, and we haven't even touched the crimes of the COVID-19 era and forward. We've already seen the connections made by all the previously discussed globalist elites, but those connections have existed for years and go deeper every year. Given what we know already about Anthony Fauci and his 36+ years of dealing with infectious diseases, we need to understand how impossible it would be in all those years to fulfill his role without deep indebtedness and major pandering to Big Pharma. Dr. Peter Breggins worked as a consultant for the National Institute of Mental Health for just 2 years and said, "It was completely clear to me from the very beginning that governmental health officials are manipulated like puppets by Big Pharma, their lobbyists, and politicians in order for their influence and pocketbooks to grow. Anthony Fauci was certainly no exception and he knows how to play their game expertly."[23] Should this chapter continue, there is enough documented information of the corruption of Big Pharma in general, but the details even of what has been done in the realm of vaccines alone could fill volumes. It suffices for the moment to simply establish Big Pharma as one of the main criminal entities we must consider in conjunction with all the other globalist elites. Dr. Peter Breggins continually calls them 'Predators' throughout his book by the same name, *Global Predators*. This title could simply not be more apt as we go forward. We have not by any means exhausted the depths of the criminals involved, but we can't finish the chapter without looking at the biggest predator and criminal of all. China, better known as the Peoples' Republic of China would be daunting by its sheer population, size, and history, but the ruling entity is the Chinese Communist Party (CCP), headed by one of the most egregious dictators in the world—Xi Jinping.

The Chinese Communist Party

People have been doing biotechnology and other related

sciences meticulously, day after day, for decades. It would seem impossible to tell such outrageous lies about a novel coronavirus being developed from infected bats. Even more outrageous, their infected bodies in a local marketplace subsequently infected humans and started a global pandemic! An asinine story like that should have rendered the entire scientific community a sorry bunch of morons! However, for significant time, the world bought it, if not for the sake of an explanation, for keeping diplomacy intact with the CCP liars. However, even the normal, John Q. Public heard this story and knew the improbability of such a thing even being considered as truth! However, that was just one of the stories about the origin of the SARS-CoV-2 pathogen perpetrated by the CCP which we're all supposed to swallow because it came from China. For real biotechs, the story was absolutely preposterous, yet CCP and other globalist elites in cahoots with China, as much as swore on Marx's grave it happened just that way for some time!

Even ending 2025, the origin of the pandemic is still hotly debated whenever it resurfaces, because in so doing, the issue is said to never be settled for sure, no matter how much evidence exists to disprove it. Granted, the CCP has never fully cooperated with any official investigators who might have shown proof, but that would never happen either. Disclosure is NOT a Chinese word! However, because of all the known circumstantial evidence pointing specifically to a lab leak from the Wuhan Institute of Virology (WIV), everyone but the CCP and the other elites know it's so. The only real question is whether the leak was accidental or intentional. Based on all other evidence, that really isn't a question either!

The Select Subcommittee on the Coronavirus Pandemic held a hearing on "Investigating the Origins of COVID-19" in Washington March, 2023, to gather facts on the origin. Several witnesses testified to how the science, the facts, and the evidence certainly added up to a lab leak in Wuhan. The group agreed, knowing the origin of COVID-19 was "fundamental" to predicting and preventing future pandemics. However, knowing the history, nature, characteristics, and agenda of the CCP, there will never be a possibility of prediction and prevention with the CCP! Leadership wants to protect our health and national security in preparing the United States for the future. But realistically, no one can ascertain a clear view of the future. Despite all the treaties, summits, leadership meetings or promises, it's nearly impossible to plan around an atheistic, brutal, immoral, unethical, and totalitarian despot like Xi Jinping. A loose cannon would be more predictable! Worse, most of the world is deathly afraid of the CCP and what it is capable of doing. No one wants to come out forcefully against the probability the SARS-CoV-2 was intentionally leaked. However, even if it wasn't intentional, given the nature and danger of these viruses, there should have been safety measures and constant surveillance on these labs to prevent ANY accidents from happening. We know that was not true, and we know that other "accidents" in other Chinese labs had happened previously. We know they were involved in gain-of-function research to find ways to make the viruses more infectious and deadly than were their original form. We can prove Drs. Fauci and Collins of the NIAID and the NIH respectively, used unverified data to dismiss the lab leak theory in favor of natural transmission, which was highly improbable and grossly incorrect. Jamie Metzl testified, "China's government (aka, the CCP) destroyed samples, hid records, imprisoned Chinese journalists, prevented Chinese scientists from saying or writing anything on pandemic origins without prior governmental approval, actively spread misinformation, and prevented an evidence-based investigation."[24]

We know Big Tech and the mainstream media constantly downplayed—and even denied—the scientific evidence of COVID-19 emerging from the WIV. Nicholas Wade testified to, "the campaign to discredit the lab leak theory. Scientists stayed in line with the natural origin camp led by Drs. Fauci and Collins because of their dependence on government grants and because the media completely failed to challenge the 'approved' narrative."[25] All the witnesses agreed, however, that the possibility of COVID-19 originating from a lab is NOT a conspiracy theory.

The most telling testimony about CCP involvement in the whole charade was from Dr. Robert Redfield, former director of the US Centers for Disease Control and Prevention (CDC). He was asked by Rep. Debbie Lesko (R-CO) if we could have any certainty that the virus did not come from the Wuhan lab and that US funding was not used for the coronavirus research. Dr Redfield replied, "Absolutely, we cannot do that…but in September 2019 (now declassified), three things happened in that lab. One, they deleted the sequences. That is highly irregular—researchers don't usually like to do that. Second, they 'commanded' the command and control of the lab from civilian authority to military control. Highly unusual. And the third thing they did, which I think is really telling, is they let a contractor re-do the ventilation system in that lab. There is strong evidence there was a significant event in that laboratory in September 2019."[26]

Going back to the CCP, we see some of the multiple proven facts of its total involvement in the pandemic from before it ever started. Since at least December of 2019 if not much sooner, CCP officials lied about the human-to-human transmission of the SARS-CoV-2. They told the world the pathogen was NOT easily transmitted and NOT very contagious when they were already certain it was both. Beijing sent the lies through the WHO (another major globalist elite) and to health authorities of other nations, deliberately leading them to pay scant attention to the real story, thus causing only minimal precautions or planning. On top of the previous deception, CCP leaders were in the process of locking down Wuhan and other large cities, indicating they believed lockdowns would be effective to slow or stop transmission in China. At the exact same time, they were pressuring other countries to accept passengers from China on international flights without any restrictions or quarantines, when they clearly knew it would likely be spread to the ends of the earth. That means that without ANY doubt, the millions of deaths outside of China were intentional and even pre-planned— MURDER in the First Degree!

Many people will simply not believe that the CCP could be so vicious and calculating, but there just isn't any doubt. The CCP uses the "Soviet" empirical framework called "Comprehensive National Power" to rank the strength of all countries. The CCP has clearly stated it wants the #1 rating or rank. That can be done in one or both of two ways: Increasing CCP power or decreasing powers of all other nations. Therefore, once COVID-19 had infected China, its leadership used the disease to weaken everyone else. It has become abundantly clear that the CCP is prepared to either devastate or eliminate any country that stands in the way of its goal. Researchers in China publicly discuss bioweapons in its journals. The CCP has a National Defense University with an authoritative journal called the *Science of Military Strategy*. In the 2017 edition, a new kind of biological warfare was mentioned—'specific, ethnic, genetic attacks.' "China's national strategy of 'military-civil fusion' makes biology a huge priority, and the Peoples' Liberation Army could be at the forefront of expanding and exploiting this knowledge."[27]

Their intent is proven by Beijing's constant efforts to collect genetic profiles of any foreigner possible, while withholding any transfer of Chinese profiles outside of China. Clearly, the CCP 'military-civil fusion' strategy is not only far-reaching but holds some dark and secret military intentions. One wonders if such an attack of specialized pathogens is possible. The answer is "YES!" Technicians are capable of building a DNAbased weapon that can target a 'single person', so there is no doubt that weapons to target a specific ethnic group are also possible. Given this development, the next pathogen released from China could leave Chinese people immune while sickening and killing other specific groups of people. It could be called the CCP's 'civilization killer'!

The PLA's keen interest in global genetics can be noted in strategic literature and research materials dating from 2010 to the present. Those 'specific, ethnic, genetic attacks' were mentioned in a 2017 textbook—almost 7 years ago, long before COVID19. Chinese military scholars and scientists are exploring new directions in military innovation. "China has been leading the world in the number of trials of the CRISPR gene-editing technology in humans. A Chinese scientist, He Jiankui, has supposedly been able to gene-edit some embryos that became the world's first genetically modified humans. This news provoked serious concerns and backlash around the world and in China. However, there are reasons to be skeptical that China will overcome its history and track record of activities that are at best ethically questionable, or at worst cruel and unusual, in healthcare and medical sciences. Also, the intersection of biotechnology and AI has promise along with huge potential danger. In 2016, the potential strategic value of genetic information led the CCP to launch the National Gene Bank, which intends to become the world's largest repository of such data. The effort is administered by BGI, in Beijing, and now has a global presence in California and Australia...US policymakers are concerned, if not troubled by the company's easy access to genetic information of Americans. It raises questions about its linkage to human rights abuses, including the 'FORCED' collection of genetic information from Uighurs (a minority people group in Xinjiang,China, who are Muslim). There are also links between BGI's research and military research activities."[28]

It is increasingly important to keep a careful watch on the Chinese military's interests in biotechnology as an emerging area of their warfare, guided by strategists who talk about potential genetic weapons and the possibilities of a 'bloodless victory.' The tools of CRISPR technology to edit genes are still novel but advancing rapidly. In the process, the CCP's total lack of transparency and uncertainty of ethical considerations in China's research initiatives raise the risks of significant potential technological surprises.

The American death toll from COVID-19 officially crossed over the one million mark long before the pandemic was over, unless you question its accuracy—a topic for later discussion. President Biden was NOT curious or concerned about this travesty and basically dropped the matter as no longer relevant, as if to say there is no need for focusing further on the casualties. What is done is done and we move on. Therefore, Xi Jinping was quite certain he would suffer no penalty, or even a reprimand for murdering this vast number of Americans, not to mention all those of the remaining countries. Therefore why would he have any qualms or compunction about spreading another disease, particularly if it furthered his very ambitious and driving goal of world dominance? It appears there is no available deterrence or fear of consequences for him. The word 'accountability' is not in his vocabulary either!

Interestingly, since America continued to view the obvious evidence of the CCP surveilling our nation with satellites and balloons, analysts state the initial moments of a war with China will be fought in "low-earth orbit" as both sides move to either shoot down or disable the craft of the other. Indeed, it already happened. A full-scale exchange of attacks could be preceded by another virus, gene-edited to attack only foreigners, identified from the gene bank! COVID-19 definitely proved the effectiveness of biological warfare. We all can certainly remember the crippling effects this warfare had globally on the nations in ways too numerous to discuss here. Though over all, the world moved on to recovery, many of those effects are still affecting the lives of people today all over the world.

The Bottom Line—China is potentially ready for anything! The CCP has no compunction about what they can do or not do to realize their goals. Their own people are completely expendable. The remaining globalist elites, in an effort to stay on their perception of the winning side, will do all in their power to cooperate and yes, help China meet its goals. They have no idea they too are just as expendable as the Chinese people in the end. Some would ask, "What about the U.N.'s Biological Weapons Convention (BWC)?" "It prohibits the development, production, acquisition, transfer, stockpiling, and use of biological and toxic weapons." This document was the first multilateral disarmament treaty banning an entire category of 'weapons of mass destruction' (WMD). It reached almost universal membership, including China. Its enforcement began March 26, 1975. The Convention, like many rules made by the United Nations, DID NOT include national inspections, so this treaty has no power to stop the CCP from doing any of these things. Even with China's initial agreement, and more specifically its total lack of compliance with any global rule, there is no inspection or any other authority that could force their compliance.

Yet another global problem is the continuing international 'assumption' that COVID=19 was merely a natural occurrence and that the CCP really had no proven initiation of the pandemic. After all, its people were massively affected as well. But, like the proverbial ostrich with its head perpetually in the sand, the international community continues to play the dangerous game of would-be cooperation with China to prevent another pandemic. Its long past time for the global community to admit that the CCP both manufactured and deliberately spread COVID-19. Governments should be taking the necessary steps to deter the CCP and building their defenses against the next product of China's biological weapons labs. REMEMBER—COVID-19 emerged ready, not only to sicken, but to kill! This is no longer a matter of science-fiction, but a biotechnological reality. Before closing this chapter on the globalist criminals, we must realize it's obvious there are thousands of elites we hear less about. Even though they walk in other areas of governance, business, public health, technology, etc., some do it more quietly and even more graciously, but make no mistake. The underlying characteristics, agendas, and thought processes mesh well, simply because their main goals are still money, power, control, and acknowledgment of their status. On those things they can most certainly agree to work together. They don't know it, of course, but they are just fulfilling Almighty God's prophesied agenda for His time of judgment on this earth. He already planned such a time of a one-world system which they regularly tout, and an ultimate master-mind who will put his man in the driver seat. It won't be called a New World Order or the Great Reset, but they are coming imminently in God's time. Unless these power mongers have recently read God's Word, they have NO idea what this time will really look like, but assuredly, it will NOT resemble what they imagine. Scripture is loaded with clear evidence of God's plans for evil men and women. Let us have a quick look at the ultimate end of each one.

"Do not fret because of those who are evil or be envious of those who do wrong; for like the grass they will soon wither, like green plants they will soon die away...The wicked plot against the righteous and gnash their teeth at them; but the Lord laughs at the wicked, for He knows their day is coming...I have seen a wicked and ruthless man flourishing like a luxuriant native tree, but he soon passed away and was no more; though I looked for him, he could not be found" Psalm 37:1-2; 12-13; 35-36.

"Woe to those who call evil good and good evil, who put darkness for light and light for darkness, who put bitter for sweet and sweet for bitter...I will punish the world for its evil, the wicked for their sins. I will put an end to the arrogance of the haughty and will humble the pride of the ruthless" Isaiah 5:20; 13:11.

CHAPTER 3

COVID-19 And the Globalists

John Kerry and Joseph Biden

Interesting that these two names should pop up right after the CCP! This exceedingly corrupted pair of political criminals have been hanging around for decades exploiting anyone or anything they could exploit to get whatever they wanted. Naturally, what they wanted was more power and more money. They both operated within their own family corruptions, using political position to climb their political and corporate ladders. Both have a long history of not only cooperating with but fraternizing with the CCP. Both have been and still are Benedict Arnolds. They clearly have no love of our nation, nor do they espouse our nation's values or its Constitutional structure.

Obviously, they are NOT alone in these sentiments or actions, but their examples near the top of the large list of American criminals still operating.

John Kerry is a member of the Forbes family and grew up as a child of military personnel in Massachusetts and Washington D.C. He's an attorney, a politician, a Democrat, an activist and until January, 2024 was President Biden's Climate Czar, or the 'Special Presidential Envoy for Climate.' He left the Biden Administration after just three years. That might sound impressive, but in reality quite deceiving and rather useless in terms of real work. A supposed major concern was the reduction of fossil-fuel energy internationally. However, before taking the 'czar' position, he made millions from his stock in various energy-industry companies. He also owned millions of dollars in oil and gasoline stocks, while acting in his various political roles. He represented Massachusetts in the US

Senate for 28 years, was Secretary of State in the Obama administration, and was the Democratic nominee for president of the US in the 2004 election, losing to George W. Bush. This seems like a stellar life of accomplishment! Here's the real rub![1]

After graduating from Yale, Kerry served in the US Naval Reserve and was in South Viet Nam just four months, sustaining three wounds in combat with Viet Cong. He received three Purple Heart medals, a Silver Star, and Bronze Star medals for valorous conduct in separate engagements. However, when Kerry returned to the U.S., he promptly became an 'outspoken opponent of the Viet Nam War and activist' while attending law school. Later in a political battle, it was revealed he was of Jewish ancestry and the priesthood. Paternal great grandparents converted to Catholicism and he was unaware of it. Maternal grandparents were Winthrop/ Forbes, Bostonians with a long line of politicians and businessmen. The extended family acquired most of its wealth trading opium, tea, and various other commodities with China. The other major source of wealth was building railroads and waterways.

Kerry has two daughters by his first wife whom he divorced in 1988 and that marriage was annulled in 1997. She later died of cancer and he remarried a widow with three sons. He was the wealthiest Senator serving at the time due in large part to his wife's fortune. In 2011, his personal assets ranged from $230-$320 billion. His history and records were painted by the mainstream media as stellar, sounding like the man actually walked on water! However, let the real records show, comrades testify, and men and women who were there tell their story. Kerry was really wounded very minimally for those three Purple Hearts with nary a limp. No duty time was lost for any 'injury'. His descriptions of his courageous efforts defy the truth. Many who also served maintain that Kerry's own description of his exploits proved major breeches of standing procedures and were often against orders. Others in the Delta who served appropriately well said they knew of no one else who had served only four months and racked up five prestigious medals!

Kerry himself stated his main motivation for going to 'Nam' was actually REVENGE for the loss of a close friend who served there. The late Admiral Elmo R. Zumwalt Jr. who had been the Chief Naval Officer in Viet Nam at the same time, had a very different take on Kerry's recollections, "Young Kerry created great problems for me and the other top brass, by killing so many non-combatant civilians and going after other non-military targets. We had virtually to straitjacket him to keep him under control."[2] He was putting himself in for medals every time he bumped his head... then he used those three Purple Hearts to request the trip home eight months before his tour of duty ended. He then got a desk job working under an Admiral until he applied for early discharge to run for office. Telling his many stories, polishing his undeserved medals, and playing the role of 'war hero' was just the political ticket he needed. "He looks like the All-American, but in reality, he is truly anti-American and is a communist sympathizer. In 1971, he conducted a massive interference in foreign policy on Viet Nam by meeting with North Vietnamese delegations in Paris to discuss how to stop the war. That alone is grossly illegal and traitorous."[3]

As a young Naval Lieutenant returning from Vietnam, he was already a trouble-making 'progressive', eager to bash America and favor Communist regimes. He testified as a returning veteran (of a whole four months) before a Congressional Committee and made all Americans feel ashamed and guilty for being Americans. He described 'hear-say only' atrocities supposedly committed that he had NOT personally seen, though he personally performed many of them. Even then he hated America so much he used every bit of deceit he could find to disillusion millions of other Americans, while building his own political future. His whole family has been involved with the Biden family in profit-making schemes with the CCP for decades. Their children were partners in CCP deals. With 'progressive' leaders like him, America could fall to the CCP.

More recently, Kerry proclaimed his "Zero War," high-profile declaration of war against climate change (a standard among all globalist elites) and treated it exactly like a war. He was one of many using the COVID-19 debacle to justify radically transforming America and the world, and fully supported the Great Reset as U.S. policy. At every opportunity he spouted the identically same jargon of all the other globalist elites. He avidly supported the partnerships between profit-making corporations and governments. Because of the globalists' staunch commitment to whatever corruption is required, there are no warnings raised about the real dangers inherent in blurring the system of checks and balances within government that do not allow exploitation of its citizens. Slave labor was fine in the CCP because it put Americans out of work. He/they did business with any of the brutal despots who violently abuse their own people.

To date, only severe sanctions, generally imposed by conservative Americans have kept these 'predators' from massively abusing the weak, poor, or enslaved. The Great Reset continually touts its care of the disenfranchised but it is not now nor will it ever be a humanitarian movement. That concept like many others touted, is nothing but pie-in-the-sky rhetoric designed to sound beneficial while meaning absolutely nothing, or the exact opposite. The most interesting and somewhat gratifying thing about elites, as previously pointed out, is they are so focused on their own money and power, they haven't noticed they have no plan for resolving their own inevitable conflicts either with each other or ultimately with the CCP! During God's appointed time of Tribulation, there will be just one ruler supreme, the Antichrist. If the CCP holds, it will NOT be them, neither will it be any of these globalists running this era. Scripturally, this leader will rise up from the masses with so much charisma that almost all people will listen to him and laud him. What a rude awakening that will be!

On November 24, 2020, President Joe Biden presented John Kerry as the new "climate envoy," a cabinet-level post that allowed him membership on Biden's National Security Council and along with it some big clout at the top of the State Department with its new Secretary of State. In his formal acceptance speech Kerry invoked "God." It was a total farce and deliberate blasphemy. He explained that science would work in God's service, but it was clear that any God-fearing person MUST see science as God's instrument. What he really meant was any God-fearing person must see him, John Kerry, as God's emissary of science! to America and the world. Kerry addressed the WEF the very same day. Its president asked Kerry if the WEF was expecting too much of President Biden. Kerry answered, "No, it's not too much. The Great Reset will happen with even greater speed and intensity than most people imagine." Then Kerry added "In effect, citizens of the US have already accepted the Great Reset by electing Biden, because of the inability of democratic governments to deliver."[4] In the first place, America didn't elect Joe Biden as President, globalists backed the fraud of liberal socialists and the Deep State to steal the election. It might look like President Biden accomplished this but he wasn't personally capable. The globalist predators including the Deep State are driving the progressive runaway train as fast and furiously as they can. However, they didn't plan on Patriot Americans being sick of the whole vicious lie. Finally, after stepping down from his manufactured position under Biden, he altruistically declared he would remain committed globally to his climate change beliefs and work tirelessly to spread the word. Interestingly, at now age 83, there is little proof he continued in any capacity. Even before the 2024 re-election of President Trump, for all intent and purposes, Kerry dropped mostly out of sight.

Joseph Biden

The other half of this demonic duo is Joseph Robinette Biden, Jr. This man's early life and ancestry gives hints of who he is and the behaviors that developed his current character and demeanor. Joe was firstborn of four siblings in a Catholic family. There was earlier political leaning from his maternal great grandfather who had been a Pennsylvania state senator. It was also a family of avid sportsmen. Biden's father led an affluent lifestyle as a young adult, sailing yachts, riding to the hounds, flying airplanes and driving fast cars. Early in Joe's life his father co-owned a good business with plenty of money and perks to fly frequently from Boston to Scranton, PA, home of the Finnegans, his maternal grandparents. After WWII, his father's business failed and the family moved back to Scranton where Joe attended a series of Catholic schools.

Several times in his youth, Joe considered becoming a priest! Except for his apparent piety, it would have been destined to failure! By high school age, the family settled in Delaware, his home today. Joe played football and baseball well; excelling in sports gave Joe a way of gaining social acceptance despite a severe stuttering problem from early age. Biden was never an outstanding student, even near the bottom of his class in law school, but was considered a natural leader among classmates.

In 1964, Biden met and dated Neilia Hunter from an affluent New York family; they married two years later. Law School was at Syracuse University to be near Neilia. "He told her he aimed to become a senator by the age of 30 and then president."[5] However, by his own description, he found law school to be "the biggest bore in the world" and he said he pulled many all-nighters just to get by. He relied on the notes of other students for classes that he skipped as well as help from his fiancé in studying. During his first year in law school, "Biden submitted a fifteen-page paper for a legal methods course that was found to have contained 'academic plagiarism' of five pages of a recently published article in the Fordham Law Review. A report from the law school faculty said that Biden should be failed in the course as a result. In response, Biden said the copying was inadvertent due to his not knowing the proper rules of citation."[6] Biden was permitted to retake the course after receiving an "F," which was later dropped from his record.

There were a few instances on his record of segregation reform. He was involved in at least one demonstration against the last segregated theater in Wilmington, DE. During the summer of 1962, while in college, Biden worked as the only white lifeguard at a swimming pool in a black Wilmington neighborhood. He later credited that job with increasing his awareness of racial issues.

Concerning military draft, Biden received five "2-S" student deferments, the last one coming in 1968 at the peak of the Viet Nam War. As he was about to graduate from law school, he received a draft notice but was medically deferred to "1-F" status due to having asthma—as a teenager. That was questioned by many, since he was heavily involved with sports with no apparent difficulty, and young men facing draft were commonly looking for ways to avoid it, especially during that era. At least he did not take part in anti-war demonstrations as Kerry so vigorously did! He was busy with law school, marriage and family. Joe and Neilia had three children: Joseph R. (Beau) Biden III in 1969, Robert Hunter in 1970, and Naomi Christina in 1971.

Early law practice saw him change from Republican, to an Independent as a public defender, to Democrat politically, however he was not enamored with corporate law, and criminal law didn't pay enough. In 1969, he ran locally as a Democrat for New Castle County Council and won it handily, but was already talking about running for US Senate in a couple years. Sure enough, in 1972, he ran for the US Democratic Senator from Delaware against an elderly Republican incumbent, and against all odds; he won with a small margin. This was probably due to his beautiful young family, a popular and energetic campaign, and a charismatic ability to connect with voters. Just a few weeks after the election, Biden's wife and one-year old daughter Naomi were killed in an automobile accident. Neilia was hit by a tractor-trailer truck and within a few days the driver was cleared of any wrongdoing. Beau and Hunter were taken to the hospital in fair condition—Beau had a broken leg and some wounds, and Hunter a minor skull fracture and head wounds. Biden actually considered resigning his senate seat to care for his sons, but was persuaded not to quit by Senate Majority Leader, Mike Mansfield.

"In later years, Biden said on several occasions the truck driver had been driving drunk prior to his wife's collision, and several media outlets reported it as fact. The driver died in 1999, but his daughter sought to have his name cleared again and to get an apology from Biden."[7] Subsequently, the original accident investigator had become a Delaware Superior Court Judge and again cleared the driver of the truck of any wrongdoing. Biden actually did call the man's daughter to apologize personally and she accepted it. With national attention, Biden was sworn into office one month later in his boys' presence as well as extended family members. "He was just 30 years old, the minimum age to become a senator, however the accident left him beyond angry and in a crisis of faith, saying he had not known he was capable of such rage. To be at home with his sons, he made a ninety-minute each way, daily commute by Amtrak to Washington, throughout his Senate career. Initially, Joe had trouble focusing on his work and appeared to just go through the motions of being a senator in his memoirs. He noted staffers were taking bets on how long he would last. A single father for five years, he left standing orders he should be interrupted in the Senate at any time, if his sons called."[8]

During those first years in the Senate, Biden focused on consumer protection, environmental issues and called for far greater governmental accountability. He supported legislation dedicated to campaign finance reform. How times changed his idealism and good sense. Interestingly, those were not typical Democratic issues. Two years later, he started dating, with no intention of remarriage. But in 1975, Joe met Jill Jacobs, a teacher from Pennsylvania, on a blind date. Biden credited her with renewing his interests in life and politics. She was supposedly hesitant to marry, entering a life in the spotlight, and raising his two sons. However, they were married two years later by a Catholic priest in the UN Chapel in NYC and honeymooned in Hungary behind the Iron Curtain. They had one daughter, Ashley Blazer, born in 1981, and they maintained the appearance of regular attendance at Mass (Data verified per Wikipedia).

Many political analysts have been unimpressed with Biden's senate and vice-presidential track records. He spent 16 years as Chairman of the Senate Judiciary Committee where he was recognized for writing and directing the *Violence Against Women Act.* He was committed to criminal justice reform, foreign policy, and civil rights. He also chaired the Senate Foreign Relations Committee giving him involvement in shaping US foreign policy, especially in matters related to arms control, nuclear proliferation, and international relations. That may have been a bad fit for him! As the Vice President in 2008, he represented the US on a plethora of diplomatic missions, and advocated for important policy initiatives. However, as the backup for a strong, and extremely liberal president, he had opportunity to witness and learn a lot about bad policies being inflicted on the citizens of the US. Through these years in particular, Biden had opportunity, continually afforded him, to rub shoulders with a great number of powerful and despotic leaders with whom he was more than merely acquainted. When President Obama had exhausted his two terms in office, he had no intention of truly bowing out of the scene, and Joe Biden was designated to continue Obama's radical agenda, most of which the American public had not accepted. The leaning of our foreign policy toward one world governance was not what most Americans desired. MAGA was the desired focus.

After Biden's tenure as the VP, he, in association with his brother and son, Hunter, began wheeling and dealing in the international market. He liked the connections he'd made as Senator and VP with the wealthy globalist elites and their agenda; if they did business with elites, they too could make a lot of money. Biden had traded favors with the CCP in various arenas already. The highly-shady reputation of son, Hunter, and his businesses were/are connected to Joe's and vice versa. Proof of this information is documented from Hunter's notorious laptop details. They've spent years as international hustlers and became a grave globalist threat, specifically because of Joe's documented subservience to the CCP. He liked money, and never cared much for hard work to get it—bribery worked better. One report by the House Oversight and Accountability Committee made it abundantly clear on the extent of its concern.

When Biden became president, with continually mounting evidence of the Bidens' Influence Peddling, the Committee "accelerated its investigation of the Biden family's domestic and international business practices to determine whether the Biden family was targeted by foreign actors. President Biden was already compromised and our national security threatened. Records obtained through the Committee's subpoenas to date revealed that the Bidens and their associates have received over $20 million in payments from foreign entities."[9]

The details of this timeline are summarized in terms of the countries involved and the amounts of money that made their way into Biden accounts from 2009 to August, 2023. It's a somewhat lengthy record, but extremely necessary to verify this author's research and verify the lengthy illegal involvement of the President.

- January 2009—Obama Admin began
- November 1, 2013—Hunter Biden, business assoc., and CCP investors agreed to create Bohai Harvest Equity Investment Fund Mgmt. Co., LTD., controlled by the Bank of China, to focus on mergers and acquisitions, and investments in and reforms of state-owned enterprises.
- December 4, 2013—VP Biden traveled with Hunter Biden on AF2 to China and met CEO of BHR, Jonathan Li. Shortly after, BHR's business license was approved and Hunter Biden became a board member.
- February 5, 2014—Hunter Biden met Kazakhstani oligarch Kenes Rakishev at the Hay Adams Hotel in Washington D.C. In email correspondences with Devon Archer surrounding the meeting, he requested Secretary of State John Kerry visit Kazakhstan. Archer replied, "If we have some business started as planned, I will ensure its planned soonest." Rakishev was a Kazakhstan oligarch and millionaire and was a director at Kazakhstan's state-owned oil company KazMunayGas and also maintained close ties to Karim Massimov, who became prime minister on April 2, 2014.

- February 14, 2014—Russian oligarch Yelena Baturina—the wealthiest woman in Russia, then married to the former mayor of Moscow—wired the Rosemont Seneca Thornton bank account $3.5 million. Its beneficiary was Rosemont Seneca Partners, chaired by Hunter Biden.
- March 11, 2014—Russia—Rosemont Seneca Thornton transferred $2,752,711 to a Rosemont Seneca Bohai bank account. On the same day $750,000 of the original wire from Baturina was sent to Devon Archer from Rosemont Seneca Thornton. Rosemont Seneca Bohai was an entity used by both Hunter Biden and Devon Archer. In his testimony to the Committee, Archer confirmed that he and Hunter Biden were 50-50 owners in Rosemont Seneca Bohai. Rosemont Seneca Bohai was opened in Delaware on February 13, 2014—the day before the $3.5 million was wired from Yelena Baturina. The bank records can be found in the third bank records memo.
- April 1, 2014—Russia and Kazakhstan—In the Spring of 2014, after Yelena Baturina sent the $3.5 million wire to Rosemont Seneca Thornton and around the same time that Kenes Rakishev wired money to Rosemont Seneca Bohai for Hunter Biden's sports car, Vice President Biden attended dinner with Yelena Baturina, Kenes Rakishev, Karim Massimov, Hunter Biden, Devon Archer, and others at Café Milano in Washington, D.C., Joe stayed for dinner. Devon Archer provided this information during his transcribed interview.
- April 15, 2014—Ukraine—Burisma, a Ukrainian energy company, appointed a Biden business associate to their board of directors.
- April 22, 2014—Kazakhstan—Kenes Rakishev's Singapore company wired $142,300 through his Latvian company to a Rosemont entity. The details can be found in the third bank records memorandum.

- April 22,2014—Ukraine—Vice President Biden traveled to Ukraine and gave an anti-corruption speech. (that's rich!)
- April 23, 2014—Kazakhstan—The Rosemont entity wired $142,300 to a car dealership in New Jersey for a new sports car for Hunter Biden. The details can be found in the third bank records memorandum.
- May 12, 2014—Ukraine—Burisma announced Hunter Biden joined its board of directors.
- May 21, 2014—Romania—Vice President Biden visited Romania and delivered a speech to the Romanian Prime Minister, judges, prosecutors, and leaders of the Romanian Parliament.
- September 12, 2014—China-BHR—BHR invested $1.7 million in CCP-linked petroleum and chemical company.
- December 9, 2014—China-BHR—Hunter Biden and business associate invested $484,920 into BHR.
- December 22, 2014—Kazakhstan—Kenes Rakishev's Kazakhstani oil company and Burisma joined with a CCP-linked company and announced a transnational financial agreement.
- April 16, 2015—Ukraine and Kazakhstan—On April 16, 2015, Vice President Joe Biden attended a dinner with Karim Massimov, Vadym Pozharsky, Hunter Biden, Devon Archer, and others at Café Milana in Washington D.C. Devon Archer provided this information during his transcribed interview.
- September 15, 2015—China-BHR—BHR joined with a CCP-linked entity to acquire US-based Henniges Automotive in a deal reportedly worth $600 million.
- September 28, 2015—Romania—Vice President Biden invited Romanian President Klaus Iohannis to the White House. A readout of the meeting states, the "Vice President welcomed

President Iohannis' focus on anti-corruption efforts and rule of law as a means to strengthen national security and promise greater investment and economic growth." President Iohannis said the Vice President "voiced satisfaction over Romania's progress with the fight against corruption."

- November 2, 2015—Ukraine—Vadym Pozharskyi suggested high-level US officials come to Ukraine and talk with Prosecutor General Viktor Shokin and President Petro Poroshenko about Mykola Zlochevsky's investigations. Prosecutor General Shokin investigated Burisma and Burisma's owner, Zlochevsky for fraud. Prosecutor General Shokin was the Ukrainian government official Vice President Biden demanded Poroshenko fire.
- November 5, 2015—Romania—Romanian businessman, Gabriel Popoviciu, began making deposits into Robinson Walker, LLC's bank account. Robinson Walker, LLC was an entity owned by a Biden associate, Rob Walker. Popoviciu's company sent Robinson Walker the first wire for $179,836.86. From November 2015 to May 2017, Popoviciu's company paid Robinson Walker, LLC over $3 million. Biden family accounts received approximately $1.038 million from the Robinson Walker, LLC account after Popoviciu's deposits. Sixteen of the seventeen payments from Popoviciu's company to Robinson Walker, LLC were made while Joe Biden was Vice President. Details can be found in the Second Bank Records Memorandum.
- November 6, 2015—Ukraine—Amos Hochstein, a high-level US government official working in the Obama-Biden Administration, met with Hunter Biden and discussed Burisma.
- November 9,2015—Romania—Rob Walker's account wired Hunter Biden $59,900. Details found in the Second Bank Records Memorandum.

- November 11, 2015—Ukraine—Amos Hochstein met with Vice President Biden in the West Wing.
- November 12, 2015—Ukraine—Amos Hochstein called Hunter Biden.
- November 13, 2015—Romania—Hunter Biden met with the US Ambassador to Romania.
- November 13, 2015—Ukraine—VP Biden touched down in Ukraine last night. Initial notes from the road: "Last night, I landed in Kyiv, Ukraine—a nation in transition. This is the fifth time I've visited this region as Vice President. And over the course of the next couple days, I'll be meeting with Ukrainians who have stood up and actively participated in efforts to fix the country they love—reformers from the government, the Ukrainian legislature, and civil society. I'll have a long working lunch and a bilateral meeting with Prime Minister Yatsenyuk. I'll speak before the Rada—the Ukrainian legislature. And I'll get to meet with Mayor Klychko of Kyiv." The notes in their entirety were meant to be read and be inspiring to the reader; containing beautiful, flowery, supportive statements about the people of Ukraine he and his son used to gain more wealth.
- November 14, 2015—Ukraine—Vadym Pozharskyi emailed Hunter Biden confirmation that the Vice President would be traveling to Ukraine.
- November 14, 2015—Romania—Hunter Biden met with the Ambassador of Romania to the United States.
- November 15, 2015—Romania—Hunter Biden traveled to Romania.
- December 4, 2015—Ukraine—Mykola Zlochevsky and Vadym Pozharsky complained about constant 'government pressures' and urged Hunter Biden to call the Vice President

of the US, Joe Biden. Devon Archer testified that Hunter Biden, Zlochevsky, and Pozharsky 'called D.C.' Devon Archer provided this information during his transcribed interview.

- December 7, 2015—China-CEFC—Hunter Biden and CEFC Chairman Ye Jianming began communicating regarding a possible US partnership.
- December 7 ,2015—Romania—Robinson Walker, LLC wired Hunter Biden $59,725. Details found in the Second Bank Records Memorandum.
- December 7, 2015—Ukraine—Vice President arrived in Ukraine, where he demanded Prosecutor General Shokin be fired if Ukraine wants $1 billion in international Monetary Fund (IMF) loans
- December 9, 2015—Ukraine—Vice President Biden departed Ukraine and got a commitment from President Poroshenko that Prosecutor General Shokin would be fired.
- December 17, 2015—Ukraine—Vice President Biden hosted a holiday party at the Vice-Presidential residence, which Amos Hochstein and Hunter Biden both attended.
- December 23, 2015—Romania—Robinson Walker, LLC wired Hunter Biden $60,091.24. Details found in the Second Bank Records Memorandum.
- January 20, 2016—Ukraine—Vice President Biden met with President Poroshenko in Switzerland at the WEF where Biden reinforced the linkage between the loan guarantee and the necessary reforms.
- February 4, 2016—Ukraine—Mykola Zlochevsky gave Hunter Biden unspecified, extravagant birthday gifts.
- February 11,2016—Ukraine—Vice President Biden and President Poroshenko conducted a call.

- February 12, 2016—Romania—Robinson Walker, LLC wired Hunter Biden's Owasco P.C. $61,126.24. Details found in the Second Bank Records Memorandum.
- February 16, 2016—Ukraine—President Poroshenko asked Prosecutor General Shokin to resign.
- February 18, 2016—Ukraine—Vice President Biden called President Poroshenko to thank him for calling on Prosecutor General Shokin to resign.
- February 19, 2016—Ukraine—President Poroshenko said he received Prosecutor General Shokin's letter of resignation.
- March 24, 2016—Romania—Robinson Walker, LLC wired Owasco P.C. $61,816.05. Details found in the Second Bank Records Memorandum.
- March 29, 2016—Romania—Hunter Biden met again with US Ambassador to Romania.
- March 29, 2016—Ukraine—Ukrainian Parliament approved President Poroshenko's firing of Prosecutor General Shokin.
- May 23, 2016—Romania—Robinson Walker, LLC wired Owasco P.C. $123,830.80. Details found in the Second Bank Records Memorandum.
- May 23, 2016—Romania—Robinson Walker, LLC wired Owasco P.C. $53,419.74. Details found in the Second Bank Records Memorandum.
- July 11 2016—Romania—Robinson Walker, LLC wired Owasco P.C. $116,860.93. Details found in the Second Bank Records Memorandum.
- August 31, 2016—Romania—Robinson Walker, LLC wired Hunter Biden $20,000. Details found in the Second Bank Records Memorandum.

- September 22, 2016—Robinson Walker, LLC wired Owasco P.C. $32,092.81. Details found in the Second Bank Records Memorandum.
- September 29, 2016—Robinson Walker, LLC wired Hunter Biden $20,000. Details found in the Second Bank Records Memorandum.
- October 11, 2016—Robinson Walker, LLC wired Owasco P.C. $41,638.12. Details found in the Second Bank Records Memorandum.
- November 1, 2016—China-BHR—BHR agreed to purchase Lundin Mining Corp's minority stake in African cobalt/copper mine, Tenke Fungurume Mining S.A. for $1.14 billion.
- November 15, 2016—Romania—Robinson Walker, LLC wired Hunter Biden $122,179. Details found in the Second Bank Records Memorandum.
- January 1, 2017—China-BHR—BHR invested $460 million in a Chinese facial recognition company.
- January 20, 2017—Important Date—Obama-Biden Administration ended.
- February 2, 2017—Romania—Robinson Walker, LLC wired unspecified Biden account $20,000. Details found in the Second Bank Records Memorandum.
- February 10, 2017—Romania—Robinson Walker, LLC wired unspecified Biden account $420,000. Details found in the Second Bank Records Memorandum.
- February 13, 2017—Romania—Robinson Walker, LLC wired Hallie Biden $10,000. Details found in the Second Bank Records Memorandum.
- February 16, 2017—China-CEFC—Chairman Ye Jianming gave Hunter Biden a diamond worth $80,000 after having dinner together in Miami, FL.

- February 16, 2017—Romania—Robinson Walker, LLC wired unspecified Biden account $20,000. Details found in the Second Bank Records Memorandum.
- February 27, 2017—Romania—Robinson Walker, LLC wired Hunter Biden $14,000. Details found in the Second Bank Records Memorandum.
- March 1, 2017—China-CEFC—Chairman Ye Jianming's company wired $3 million to Robinson Walker, LLC an entity owned by a Biden Associate, Rob Walker. Details found in the Second Bank Records Memorandum.
- March 6, 2017—China-CEFC—Robinson Walker wired unspecified Biden account $5,000. Details found in the First Bank Records Memorandum.
- March 13, 2017—China-CEFC—Robinson Walker wired unspecified Biden account $25,000. Details found in the First Bank Records Memorandum.
- March 20, 2017—China-CEFC—Robinson Walker wired Hallie Biden $25,000. Details found in the First Bank Records Memorandum.
- March 27, 2017—China-CEFC—Robinson Walker wired Hunter Biden's Owasco P.C.$50,000. Details found in First Bank Records Memorandum.
- March 29, 2017—China-CEFC—Robinson Walker wired an account associated with Hunter Biden—$100,000. Details found in First Bank Records Memorandum.
- March 31,2017—China-CEFC—Robinson Walker wired Owasco P.C. $50,000. Details found in the First Bank Records Memorandum.
- March 31, 2017—China-CEFC—Robinson Walker wired Owasco P.C. $100,000. Details found in the First Bank Records Memorandum.

- April 3, 2017—China-CEFC—Robinson Walker wired James Biden's JBBSR INC $50,000. Details found in the First Bank Records Memorandum.
- April 3, 2017—China-CEFC—Robinson Walker wired JBBSR INC $50,000. Details found in the First Bank Records Memorandum.
- April 14, 2017—China-CEFC—Robinson Walker wired a company associated with Hunter Biden $10,692. Details found in the First Bank Records Memorandum.
- April 18, 2017—China-CEFC—Robinson Walker wired Owasco P.C. $300,000. Details found in the First Bank Records Memorandum.
- April 20, 2017—China-CEFC—Robinson Walker wired JBBSR INC $120,000. Details found in the First Bank Records Memorandum.
- April 21, 2017—China-CEFC—Robinson Walker wired unspecified Biden account $25,000. Details found in the First Bank Records Memorandum.
- April 24, 2017—China-CEFC—Robinson Walker wired JBBSR INC $125,000. Details found in the First Bank Records Memorandum.
- May 13, 2017—China-CEFC—Email between Biden business associates about the ownership of the CEFC deal, mentioned "10 held by H for the big guy?"
- May 17, 2017—China-CEFC—Robinson Walker wired unspecified Biden account $15,000. Details found in the First Bank Records Memorandum.
- May 18, 2017—China-CEFC—Robinson Walker wired JBBSR INC $15,000. Details found in the First Bank Records Memorandum.

- June 2, 2017—Romania—Robinson Walker, LLC wired Owasco P.C. $61,726.87. Ledger proof.
- June 6, 2017—China-CEFC—Hunter Biden sent a message to James Gilliar discussing their CEFC deal. He said, "Why in God's name would I give this marginal bully the keys to my family's only asset?" Copy of message proof.
- July 30, 2017—China-CEFC—In a WhatsApp message to a Chinese company, Hunter Biden stated, "Please have the director call me-not James or Tony or Jim-have him call me tonight. I am sitting here with my father and we would like to understand why the commitment made has not been fulfilled. I am concerned that the Chairman has either changed his mind and broken our deal without telling me or that he is unaware of the promises and assurances made have not been kept. Tell the director that I would like to resolve this now before it gets out of hand. And now means tonight. And Z if I get a call or text from anyone involved in this other than you Zhang or the Chairman, I will make certain that between the man sitting next to me and every person he knows and my ability to forever hold a grudge you will regret not following my direction. All too often people mistake kindness for weakness-and all too often I stand over top of them saying I warned you. From this moment until whenever he reaches me." Hunter Biden went on to say, "Ok my friend-I am sitting here waiting for the call with my father. I sure hope whatever it is you are doing is very, very important."
- August 2, 2017—China CEFC—Arrangement between CEFC and Biden family changed as original Biden associates were removed. Hunter Biden wrote "The chairman changed that deal after we met in MIAMI TO A MUCH MORE LASTING AND LUCRATIVE ARRANGEMENT to create a holding company 50% owned by ME and 50% owned by

him. Consulting fees are one piece of our income stream but the reason this proposal by the chairman was so much more interesting to me and my family is that we will also be partners in the equity and profits of the JV's investments."

- August 2, 2017—China-CEFC—The joint entity, Hudson West III, LLC was formed, with 50% owned by CEFC agent Gongwen Dong and 50% owned by Hunter Biden.
- August 3, 2017—China-CEFC—In a WhatsApp exchange, Hunter Biden told CEFC associate Gongwen "Kevin" Dong, "The Bidens are the best I know at doing exactly what the Chairman wants from this [partnership]." Gongwen Dong was a business associate of Chairman Ye Jianming who executed numerous transactions on the Ye's behalf.
- August 4, 2017—China-CEFC—CEFC wired $100,000 to Hunter Biden's company, Owasco, P.C. Details found in the First Bank Records Memorandum.
- August 8,2017—China-CEFC—CEFC wires $5 million to Hudson West III.
- August 27, 2017—(China-CEFC)—Message from Gongwen Dong (aka Kevin) "I will pick you up at 12 pm at the lobby of your hotel. The luncheon will start at 12:30 pm." Answer from Hunter Biden, "Where is luncheon Kevin? My uncle will be here with his BROTHER who wants to say hello to the Chairman. He is here to visit my daughter." Message return from Kevin, "The chairman invited you to his new home in NYC, 15 CPW." Message returned from Hunter Biden, "So please give me location and time. Jim's BROTHER if he comes just wants to say hello, he will not be stopping for lunch." China-CEFC—entry note: Hunter Biden communicated over WhatsApp to CEFC associate Gongwen Dong.
- September 3, 2017—Important Date—Joe Biden received $40,000 in laundered China money from the account of his

brother, James Biden, and his sister-in-law, Sarah Biden, in the form of a personal check (shown)

- September 21, 2017—China-CEFC—Hunter Biden requested keys made for his office be shared with his Chinese partners: "Joe Biden, Jill Biden, Jim Biden, and Gongwen Dong (Chairman Ye CEFC emissary)"; and adjusted his business signage listing The Biden Foundation and Hudson West (CEFC US) on the sign.
- November 8,2017—China-CEFC—Patrick Ho, a CEFC agent in America, arrested at JFK airport on suspicion of bribery and money laundering on behalf of CEFC China.
- February 13, 2018—Kazakhstan—The US Treasury's Financial Crimes Enforcement Network (FinCEN) issued a notice accusing Rakishev's Latvian company of money laundering.
- March 1, 2018—China-CEFC—Ye Jianming detained by Chinese authorities for "suspected economic crimes." His whereabouts remained unknown.
- March 1, 2018—Important Date—Bank records revealed a $200,000 direct payment from James and Sara Biden to Joe Biden in the form of a personal check. In 2018, James Biden received $600,000 in loans from, Americore—a financially distressed and failing rural hospital operator. According to bankruptcy court documents, James Biden received these loans "based upon representations that his last name, 'Biden,' could 'open doors' and that he could obtain a large investment from the Middle East based on his political connections." On March 1, 2018, Americore wired a $200,000 loan into James and Sara Biden's personal bank account-not their business bank account. On the same day, James Biden wrote a $200,000 check from this same personal bank account to Joe Biden.

- March 23, 2018—China-CEFC—Hudson West III LLC and CEFC began to dissolve.
- December 5, 2018—China-CEFC—Patrick Ho is convicted for violating the Foreign Corrupt Practices Act in a multinational bribery scheme and money laundering offenses.
- March 19, 2019—China-CEFC—Patrick Ho was sentenced to three years after he was found to have bribed officials in Africa in pursuit of oil deals to benefit CEFC China, as well as laundering money through various international accounts to perpetuate these business dealings.
- April 25, 2019—Important Date—Joe Biden announced his presidential campaign.
- July 26, 2019—China-BHR—Hunter Biden received a $10,000 wire from Wang Xin, an employee at BHR. The wire originated in Beijing and Joe Biden's Wilmington; Delaware home was listed as the beneficiary address.
- August 2, 2019—China-BHR—Hunter Biden received a $250,000 wire from Jonathan Li and Tan Ling. The wire originated in Beijing and Joe Biden's Wilmington, Delaware home was listed as the beneficiary address.
- September 21, 2019—Important Date—Joe Biden responded to reporters in Iowa inquiring about his relationship to Hunter Biden's foreign business ventures: "I have never spoken to my son about his overseas business dealings." (Biden immediately made a comment on Fox news accusing Trump of abusing his power to smear him!")
- October 13, 2019—Important Date— "Hunter neither played a role in the formation or licensure of [BHR], nor owned any equity in it while his father was Vice President. He served only as a member of its board of directors, which he joined

based on his interest in seeking ways to bring Chinese capital to international markets. It was an unpaid position… To date, Hunter did not receive any compensation for being on BHR's board of directors. He did not receive any return on his investment; there were no distributions to BHR shareholders since Hunter obtained his equity interest. Moreover, Hunter played no role in directing or making BHR's investments. Hunter intends to resign from the BHR board of directors on or by October 31,2019"—spokesman for Hunter Biden December 8, 2019—Important Date— "I don't know what he was doing," Joe Biden said of his son's work for Burisma, a Ukrainian energy company, in an interview. "I know he was on the board. I found out he was on the board after he was on the board, and that was it."(a pathologic liar!)

- June 13, 2020—Ukraine—Ukrainian law enforcement announced $6M bribery scheme by Mykola Zlochevsky in order to end the probe of the Burisma founder.
- June 30, 2020—Important Date—FBI FD-1023 form was created. An FD-1023 form was generated by the FBI to memorialize information obtained from a confidential human source. This confidential human source told the FBI that an oligarch had told the CHS he bribed then-Vice President Biden for $5 million (and $5 million for his son, Hunter Biden) in exchange for certain actions related to Ukraine.
- October 22, 2020—Important Date—During an October presidential debate, Joe Biden responded to a question about election security: "I have not taken a penny from any foreign source ever in my life."
- October 22, 2020—Important Date—During the same October presidential debate, Joe Biden also said, "My son has not made money, in terms of things about, what are you talking about? China. The only guy who made money in

China is [President Trump]."

- October 23, 2020—China-CEFC—Tony Bobulinski was interviewed by the FBI and details on how the Bidens' dealt with CCP-linked entities began when Joe Biden was Vice President of the United States. The Bidens were paid shortly after Joe Biden left the vice presidency for their work.
- March 16, 2023—Important Date—The Oversight and Accountability Committee released its first bank records memorandum revealing over $1 million in payments from a Chinese company to the Bidens through an associate.
- March 17, 2023—Important Date—When asked about his family dealings and whether Biden family members received money from his son's business associates, Joe Biden responded, "That's not true."
- April 24, 2023—Kazakhstan—Former Kazakhstan Prime Minister Karim Massimov, who attended dinner with then-Vice President Biden in 2015, was sentenced to 18 years in prison for treason, abuse of power, and attempting a coup.
- May 10, 2023—Important Date—The Oversight and Accountability Committee released its second bank records memorandum revealing the Bidens' influence peddling schemes in Romania and China.
- June 22, 2023—Hunter Biden Criminal Investigation—The Committee on Ways and Means released IRS whistleblower testimony about the Department of Justice's politicization and misconduct with respect to allegations against Hunter Biden.
- July 19, 2023—Hunter Biden Criminal Investigation—The House Oversight Committee held a hearing with two IRS whistleblowers who testified about the Department of Justice's misconduct and politicization in] the Biden criminal

investigation. Key takeaways from the hearing can be found as follows: The Biden family set up over 20 shell companies, mostly during Joe Biden's vice presidency. IRS confirmed. Bank records obtained show the Biden family, their business associates, and their companies received over $10 million from foreign nationals and their related companies. The Bidens engaged in many intentionally complicated financial transactions through their associations to hide payments and avoid scrutiny. Both Committee and whistleblowers have confirmed Hunter received millions from China, Ukraine, and Romania. IRS whistleblowers presented evidence of Joe Biden's knowledge and involvement in his family's business schemes. IRS whistleblowers provided evidence of the Justice Department's politicization and misconduct in the Biden criminal investigation. IRS whistleblowers confirm they were not allowed to follow evidence that could have led to Joe Biden. Attorney General Merrick Garland may have perjured himself. IRS whistleblowers faced retaliation from the federal government for providing evidence of politicization, misconduct, and wrongdoing. All three House Committees involved are working to present facts to the American people that the Biden Admin continues to deny even when faced with overwhelming evidence!

- July 20, 2023—Important Date—Senator Chuck Grassley released an unclassified FBI-generated record describing an alleged criminal scheme involving then-Vice President Joe Biden and a Ukrainian business executive. Senator Grassley acquired the record, an FD-1023, via legally protected disclosures by Justice Department whistleblowers.

- July 24, 2023—Important Date—Business Insider reveals Hunter Biden's gallery sold art to major Democratic donor and Biden-appointed commissioner Elizabeth Hirsh Naftali. Naftali was appointed by President Biden to the Commission for the Preservation of America's Heritage Abroad. This is the same Commission President Obama appointed Eric Schwerin, Hunter Biden's longtime business associate, to in 2015. This comes after President Biden "pledged that there would be an 'absolute wall' between his official duties and his family's private business interest."

- July 25, 2023—Important Date—Washington Examiner reveals Alexander Mackler, a close associate of the Biden family and former Biden Staffer, spent years working in the U.S. attorney's office. According to Mackler's Linked-in, part of his tenure was under U.S. Attorney David Weiss. He also had overlap with the months when whistleblowers said the office took up an investigation of Hunter Biden. "Mackler also appeared to have a close personal relationship with Hunter Biden. In emails found on Hunter Biden's laptop, Mackler corresponded frequently with Hunter Biden and his business associates and even referred to Hunter Biden fondly as a 'brother' in October 2018."
- July 26, 2023—Hunter Biden Criminal Investigation—Hunter Biden's Sweetheart Plea Deal: obtained a copy of Hunter Biden's sweetheart plea deal.
- July 26, 2023—Hunter Biden's Criminal Investigation—Hunter Biden's Sweetheart Plea Deal Hearing Transcript: U.S. District Judge Maryellen Noreika refused to rubberstamp Hunter Biden's sweetheart plea deal. At the hearing, the Justice Department admitted that Hunter Biden's sweetheart plea deal was unprecedented. Hunter Biden also admitted that he made money from China, contradicting Joe Biden's claims that his son never made money in China. Hunter Biden also admitted that his former business partner was CCP-linked Ye Jianming. The hearing transcript is available at this same website for the sake of completing this document.

- July 31, 2023—Ukraine—The House Oversight Committee held a transcribed interview with Devon Archer, Hunter Biden's former business associate. During the transcribed interview, Archer testified that Joe Biden was "the brand" that Hunter Biden sold around the world to enrich the Biden family. Archer also admitted that Burisma would have gone out of business if 'the brand' had not been attached to it." Key excerpts and the full transcript can also be found on this website.
- August 9, 2023—Russia, Ukraine, and Kazakhstan—Chairman Comer released a third bank records memorandum detailing how the Bidens and their business associates received millions from oligarchs in Russia, Kazakhstan, and Ukraine during Joe Biden's vice presidency. After Hunter Biden received millions of dollars in payments, then-Vice President Joe Biden dined with his son's foreign associates in Washington D.C. That memo can be found at this website.
- August 14, 2023—Hunter Biden Criminal Investigation—Chairman Comer released the transcript for the former FBI supervisory special agent (SSA), who worked for the FBI for 20 years and retired in June 2022. He corroborated IRS Supervisory Special Agent Gary Shapley's testimony that FBI headquarters tipped off Secret Service headquarters and the Biden transition team about the planned Hunter Biden interview during U.S. Attorney for Delaware David Weiss' investigation. The former FBI SSA and Shapley were told not to approach Hunter Biden but wait for his call. Instead of receiving a call from Hunter Biden, they received a call from his attorney and were never able to interview Hunter Biden during the investigation. The transcript can be found at this website. This completes the Oversight and Accountability Committee's full report on President Joe Biden and his son, Hunter Biden that details the proof of most of the illegal and certainly criminal activities that to this day have never been tried, charged, or prosecuted in a

court of law. Neither have the charges of treason for operating criminally in cooperation with foreign countries and their representatives who clearly showed and reported on many occasions they are NOT friends of our United States.[10]

There are a few additional comments about Joe Biden that complete his identification as a full-on globalist elite, not to mention a traitor to our nation. He doesn't have the extreme wealth of many, but not for want of trying! He also doesn't have the mental capacity to wield, as many of them have, but he had the power as President of the United States, making him sought after to keep the globalist agenda running along the approved track for the New World Order and the Global Reset which made him important to other globalists.

Given all the now known cooperation with the CCP, its very clear why he made many of the decisions regarding China the way he did. For example, when President Trump was dealing with the whole COVID-19 pandemic, Joe Biden called him a "Xenophobe" for labeling the SARS-CoV-2 the "China Virus" and belittled him for shutting down all traffic from China as soon as the pandemic was confirmed. Biden also pushed the whole fraudulent Russia scandal probe of President Trump while keeping China completely out of the scandal. When Biden was the Vice President, there was documented scandal of his dealings, along with Hunter even then; it has NOT gone away or been erased.

Continued proof as above and more has always been available, but the politicization of our nation's Justice Department, the FBI, the CIA, and Secret Service had his increased influence on keeping the criminal facts and the degeneration of his administration closely guarded at all times. The globalist elites NEEDED him right where he was to forward their agenda even if he couldn't think clearly, speak well, remember anything or remain standing! There were plenty of books and articles written about Joe's scandals long before the last election occurred, and he was NOT favored to win the election while sitting at home sheltering in his basement. But "somehow" he wound up in the oval office! Note also there was and continues to be a total "blackout" on the Biden family crimes in all of the main-stream media. As all the above evidence suggests, Joe Biden is completely incapable of telling the truth. There is constant denial by main-stream media (Big Tech globalists run this) of election fraud that enabled Biden's win. Despite this narrative, "a recent poll found that in the 2020 election, 1-in-5 people (20%) who voted by mail committed some type of voter fraud, by their own admission."[11] That was just on mail-in ballots alone.

The Biden family gave the CCP special trade regulatory concessions that even American companies didn't have and couldn't obtain. As of October 2, 2020, there were 217 CCP companies listed on U.S. exchanges with a total market value of $2.2 Trillion dollars! President Trump tried to stop the bleeding and made lobbyists furious. No wonder "slippery," lackluster Joe Biden became the Democrat candidate for president and WON! But, he looked lustrous to the globalist predatory billionaires and corporations. There is so much more that could be said about President Biden, but it should be noted above that business with Asian nations and China continued while he was in office.

Enter, the CCP's spy balloons in American airspace over Alaska. At first military officials assigned little importance to this because it was done before, watched and monitored. NORAD, however, continued to track and assess the balloon's path and activities. Initially, it was not assessed to be a security risk. But "it was never done so brazenly or so far before. The debris from the balloon could endanger lives on the ground. It was a massive orb, carrying a payload the size of three coach buses. It took 7 days from when the balloon first entered U.S. airspace before an F-22 fighter jet fired a heat-seeking missile into the balloon on the opposite end of our country, sending its equipment and machinery tumbling into the Atlantic Ocean. The balloon's week-long journey…left a wake of shattered diplomacy, furious reprisals from Biden's political rivals and a preview of a new era of escalating military strain between the world's two largest economies. It also raised questions about why it wasn't shot down sooner and what information, if any, it scooped up along its path."[12]

Five days into the balloon's journey, intelligence said it needed to come down but they had to wait until it was over water to be safe enough for people on the ground and still recover its payload as intactly as possible. Beijing insisted on Friday that the device was simply a weather balloon drifted off course, but the US government was confident the balloon was being used for surveillance, because it carried equipment not normally associated with standard weather balloons. The US also observed small motors and propellers on the balloons, leading officials to believe Beijing had some control over its path. US officials said the balloons were a part of a fleet of Chinese spy balloons that had been spotted across five continents over the last several years.

Meanwhile, this balloon caused an hours-long grounding of commercial flights around Billings, MT, and people started watching it, as the military worked to respond. Jets flew everywhere. US officials spoke to their Chinese counterparts throughout the week, making it clear the balloon was likely to be shot down. The entire operation was monitored and planned for best outcome. Waiting to carry out the plan allowed the US to 'study and scrutinize the balloon and its equipment' and learn technical things about the balloon and its surveillance capabilities.[13] A number of legislators believed President Biden failed to act soon enough or decisively enough to bring them down and that he downplayed their significance considerably. Of course he did! He was NOT about to compromise his own connections with China to take care of his responsibility to the safety and security of his own country. There is no wonder at all why the globalist elites were determined to see Joe Biden elected as the next president in the midst of the pandemic whether legally or not. They simply could NOT allow President Donald J. Trump to remain in the White House. Joseph Biden would play their desired game as long as the money rolled in. Public health officials kept saying "Watch the Science!" But it wasn't about science at all; instead we only needed to "Watch the Money!"

"When justice is done, it is a joy to the righteous but terror to evildoers," Proverbs 21:15 ESV

"For I the Lord love justice; I HATE robbery and wrong…" Isaiah 61:8a ESV

"But the cowardly, the unbelieving, the vile, the murderers, the sexually immoral, those who practice magic arts, the idolaters and ALL liars—they will be consigned to the fiery lake of burning sulfur. This is the second death." Revelation 21:8 ESV

"Do NOT be deceived, God is NOT mocked; for whatever a person sows, this he will also reap." Galatians 6:7 NASB

CHAPTER 4

Globalists Involved With the COVID-19 Pandemic

LeBron James—Major Sports Influencer

During the pandemic, there was constant liberal media influence, misinformation, and a steady and constant threat to our nation's foundations. Professional sports teams often allowed players and management to disparage our flag and our nation because the CCP would handsomely pay them for it, while these same people NEVER showed such disrespect for the CCP! They did this because these same people gleaned great benefits from CCP's markets and its governmental generosity buys them loyalty. If you have something big to offer, they'll gladly foot the bill. The same was true in spades for those brilliant, US. scientists who sold their very souls to the CCP for the many lucrative benefits they were offered. Never mind loyalty to one's own nation whenever MONEY is involved.

In LeBron James' early professional years, he was a highly-likable basketball star from Akron, Ohio, now 40+ years old. As a champion in high school, his team won three Ohio State championships in four years and he was the national high-school basketball player of the year his senior season. In 2003, James was selected by the Cleveland Cavaliers/NBA and signed an unprecedented $90 million endorsement contract with the Nike shoe company before he ever played a pro game! Awards were gleaned every year as a young pro athlete, including two MVPs. By the end of the 2009-10 season, LeBron was arguably the most sought-after free agent in NBA history, and with his contract expired, he signed with Miami Heat, excelling there.

After returning to Ohio, the Cavaliers did very well, and LeBron continued racking up MVPs and big wins, finally signing with the

Los Angeles Lakers. Then he suffered a personal injury that ended his13 personal playoffs-streak. The next season was disrupted by the pandemic, causing a 4-month suspension and a shortened season but he gave a dominant performance. In addition to all his NBA achievements, James was a member of the US Men's Olympic Basketball team that won the bronze at the 2004 Games, the gold at the 2008 Games, and gold at the 2012 Games. He also published a memoir.

Interestingly, LeBron was born to a 16-year old mother and his father, having an extensive criminal record, was not involved in his life. Life was often a struggle when he grew up and they moved often so his mom could keep steady work. His mother Gloria realized her son would be better off in a more stable family environment and allowed him to move in with the family of Frank Walker, a local youth football coach who introduced LeBron to basketball when he was only nine years old. He began playing team basketball in the fifth grade. James and three of his teammates chose to attend a private Catholic high school with a majority of white students, a move that stirred some local controversy. By 16 years old, LeBron was 6 feet-7 inches and appeared on the cover of Sports Illustrated, becoming the first high school underclassman to do so. At that time, James' playing abilities and a few controversies over receiving gifts caused him some grief and a loss or two, but he signed with the NBA. He used some marijuana, which he said was to help him cope with the stress resulting from the constant media attention he received. This young man also played outstanding football in high school, such that some sports analysts, football critics, high school coaches and former and current players speculated that James could have played in the NFL as well!

He was a good kid who held good American values and had no problem saying so. He supported a suffering home state with his sympathies. James went to the Miami Heat club so he could win championships and fans forgave him as his fame skyrocketed. He went back to Ohio, and later signed with the Los Angeles Lakers. James married his high school sweetheart Savannah in 2023 in San

Diego, CA. They have two sons, Bronny and Bryce and a daughter Zhuri. He invests heavily in his health, to the tune of about $1.5 million per year for personal chefs, athletic trainers, and physical therapies.

For many years, James' public image was stellar, considered to be the "face of the NBA." His opinions often yielded significant influence on people who made important league decisions. He was ranked by *Forbes* as one of the world's most influential athletes and listed by *Time* as one of the 100 most influential people in the world. He was adored by fans in earlier years, but fans are fickle and often express their distaste when they aren't happy. On July 20, 2019, James joined teammates "taking the knee" during the national anthem to humiliate America and its values. Here is the strong evidence that an abundance of wealth, fame, and power it produces, nearly always corrupts, even for those who started out with good values. Throughout his career, James has taken public stances on controversial issues, and has mentioned his feeling of obligation to effect change using his status. The 2019 demonstration of "taking the knee," however, delighted his "potential partners" in the CCP. Additionally, he thrilled the CCP even more when he publicly humiliated Houston Rockets' General Manager Daryl Morey over his support of Hong Kong protestors against the CCP. The hometown boy had joined the ranks of the Globalist Elites, the biggest game on the whole planet. However, in February of 2022, political commentator Bill Maher called James hypocritical because he refused to take a critical stance towards the Chinese government's human rights abuses.[1]

James continues to sign endorsement contracts for a number of "globalist" corporations including all the major Big Tech companies and Nike, and supports most of the WEF ideas and agenda, as well as the major billionaire individuals. As of 2024, at the age of 39, he had, according to *Forbes*, a net worth of $1 billion dollars. "Now his controversial comments further his brand power in the CCP. He gets $32 million from Nike annually. He criticizes free speech in America and tells America to lay off the CCP. After his criticism of

Morey, the NBA threw Morey under the bus and supported James' criticism of him."[2] It's likely, of course, that the CCP provides under-the-table incentives to James, just as they do for every other globalist cooperative; such incentives are not available in America. With his 'at least' three mansions, and his extremely expensive manner of living, James quickly became accustomed to the extra dough! Even the entire NBA is unwilling to risk CCP censure and it clearly believes the leadership in America, except for Conservatives and Trump backers will not punish its defense of the CCP. It's crystal clear the CCP managed to corrupt a willing and wealthy young man, and turned him into an avid supporter of the globalist mindset and lifestyle, making him a critic of the country that gave him all the glorious opportunities he's had for 39 years. Much worse, the NBA backers of the CCP's major assets also act as its supporters. As the big money keeps rolling along with the power and glory it grows, it's highly unlikely that any of this story will change.

Michael Bloomberg—Major Business Influencer

An American businessman, politician, philanthropist, and author, Michael Bloomberg is 83 years old, has a long history of public service, and is also the majority owner (88%), co-founder, and CEO of Bloomberg L.P. He also served as mayor of New York City for three terms and was a Democratic presidential candidate in the 2020 election. In addition to all of that, Michael has strong ties to the CCP; when he spoke out in defense of the CCP too early in the race, it cost him the presidential bid in 2019.

Bloomberg spoke on November 21-23, 2019 at the New Economy Forum in Beijing and under CCP influence figuratively slapped President Trump in the face. At that time he mentioned his funding partners including 3M, Exxon Mobile, FedEx, HSBC, Hyundai, Master Card, and others. "The CCP's violent dictator Xi Jinping stood by grinning widely as Bloomberg stood fawning over the Communists. It was a sickening 'lovefest' of global predators."[3]

"A little more than a year later, on January 14, 2021, the Bloomberg report supported President Trump's second impeachment and expedited conviction of Trump while supporting Xi Jinping, and increasing trade with China, the arch global predator. Xi Jinping must have smiled and shaken his head at the infidelity and stupidity of rich Americans! Although Bloomberg held a November, 2020 conference, done virtually due to COVID, he had it co-hosted by the CCP as he did in 2019. He didn't have to be in Beijing to get the full cooperation of one of the most murderous regimes in the history of the world!"[4]

We have seen two prominent and treacherous examples of American globalists, one from the corrupted field of professional sports, and one from the ultra-socialist, corrupted political arena.

"According to *Bloomberg News*, a CCP participant at the (WEF) forum boasted how his country had continued to cooperate with America despite President Trump's policies to the contrary. Xie Zhenhua, China's former top climate diplomat, said U.S./China climate cooperation continued despite Trump's efforts…Even after the U.S. federal government signaled its intended withdrawal from the Paris climate agreement, China and the U.S. maintained cooperation at local levels, through think tanks, and the private sector. This was not mere braggadocio. Xie Zhenhua confirmed how China's tentacles reach far deeper into our American society than any presidential policy could easily destroy."[5]

To show we are not blowing smoke, we should add that Bill Gates was a co-chair of the forum. Another co-chair was Henry M. Paulson, former U.S. Treasury Secretary under George W. Bush (2006-2009), but at the time, an active member of Biden's transition team. His presence in both Democratic and Republican administrations serves to remind us that the Bush family, Bill Gates, and Bloomberg are all globalists with a lot in common, including a fear and hatred of President Trump and populism in general. Globalists Bill Clinton, 42nd President of the U.S., his wife, Hillary R. Clinton, former U.S. Secretary of State during Obama's years, were all speakers. Janet Yellen, former chair of the U.S. Federal Reserve Board of Governors, announced as Biden's future Secretary of the Treasury, was also present. Global corporate executives were also well represented with the president and CEO of McDonalds Corporation, the executive chairperson of IBM, the CEO of Master Card, the president and CEO of FedEx, a chief executive of Prudential PLC, the CEO of Goldman Sachs, the CEO of Honeywell, and numerous others.

Naturally, pharmaceutical industry executives were present, most notably Moderna CEO Stéphane Bancel. Moderna is a young, wealthy, and powerful company that is one of Bill Gates' and hence Anthony Fauci's favorites. Both gave Moderna's vaccine a very large push.

International political leaders were strongly represented as well, including the Prime Minister of India, Tony Blair, former Prime Minister of the United Kingdom, and His Majesty Abdullah II bin Al Hussein, King of Jordan. Bankers with top positions in the past and the present with the European Bank, Bank of England, Reserve Bank of India, Credit Suisse, and the People's Bank of China were all represented.

Finally, there was another attendee that should definitely surprise most people. There is an agency called The *U.S. Defense Advanced Research Projects Agency*— (DARPA). More surprising still, it has a very shadowy and secret history of human experimentation, including recent efforts in support of Elon Musk's research in mind control through computer and brain interfacing. The Breggins have been very critical of Musk's work for good reasons. One of those reasons involves Regina Dugan, CEO of Wellcome Leap, a nonprofit started by the Wellcome Trust. It is an enormous charity started by Henry Wellcome, the pharmaceutical giant. Wellcome Leap identifies itself as a high-tech government research program doing experimental mind control and compares itself to a DARPA-type project for global health. Wellcome Leap cannot disguise its joy at all the opportunities presented to it by the COVID-19 tragedy. They will 'thrive' on the need for "Apollo-like programs for vaccines, therapeutics, testing, and new health advances for the future.

We have noted all the globalists actively meeting and planning to do everything in their power to fund and control the global future of the world. It is absolutely appalling and also threatening to watch and listen to Americans like the Clintons, Bloomberg, and Gates, along with corporate heads of some of the largest companies in the world. Add the entire cabal of their COVID-19 activists like Peter Daszak, the gross apologist for the CCP and President of Eco-Health Alliance. Tedros, director general of WHO, a lackey that has almost no real medical background, is the icing on the globalist cake. All are celebrating the return to business as usual with China. The CCP remains the greatest military, economic, and political threat to the free world and to all humanity.

Any thinking person can readily see why the enormous globalist system is so wealthy and powerful, and will stop at nothing to control the world, hated President Trump's successes and the great accomplishment of the promises he made. There was so much improvement for Americans, globalists were threatened by it, therefore they launched open attacks on Trump and backed all the 'progressive' powers that were available to get rid of Trump. Bloomberg very vocally and openly chose China's CCP over his own homeland of America. The conferences frequently held in globalist arenas deliberately perpetuated lies about the origin of COVID-19 and defended China, openly and adamantly denying it had come out of Chinese labs. Continued huge climate change resolutions were another huge topic of these conference agendas and everyone involved was on its bandwagon. They have never backed their agendas with real scientifically proven facts, but climate control is another area where globalists see a huge opportunity to control the masses.

Commentator Laura Ingraham of Fox News declared Bloomberg's Virtual forum, held during COVID-19 was aimed at crushing individual liberty and subjugating people to the whims of the wealthy international community of globalists. Her program critique actually showed that predatory globalism is getting increased scrutiny. "At this moment, planning is under way by the wealthiest and most powerful people on Earth about how you should live your life; how nations should be structured and societies reorganized to promote global harmony through a 'world-wide distribution of assets'...so much more clarity on the entire globalist agenda was being clearly given."[6]

American Billionaire Globalists Aren't Rare

The United States as of 2024 has 1,135 billionaires. Of the 16+ top billionaires, 14 of them qualified as globalist predators, though that number may well be higher one year later. That would be true even if the only qualifier was heavy investments in the CCP! Five years ago, according to the following tally reported by Peter Breggins, the top 16 richest Americans were as follows:[7]

1. Jeff Bezos—Owner of Amazon and the Washington Post
2. Bill Gates—Director of the Bill and Melinda Gates Foundation
3. Warren Buffett—Former Co-Trustee of 3 in Gates Foundation and much more
4. Larry Ellison—Owner of Oracle, the ONLY one who openly voices his values and has taken steps to separate himself from the horde. He has deep concerns about the CCP and supported President Trump
5. Mark Zuckerberg—Owner of Facebook (Meta)
6. 1 of 3 - Walton family members, owners of Walmart—investments in CCP are in the billions and growing, including 19+ stores already built in Wuhan
7. 2 of 3 - Walton family members, owners of Walmart—investments in CCP are in the billions and growing, including 19+ stores already built in Wuhan
8. 3 of 3 - Walton family members, owners of Walmart—investments in CCP are in the billions and growing, including 19+ stores already built in Wuhan

9. Steve Balmer—Owner of Microsoft

10. Larry Page—Owner of Alphabet/Google

11. Sergey Brin –Owner of Alphabet/Google

12. Michael Bloomberg—Director of New Economy Forum

13. Charles Koch—Owner of Koch Enterprises—Donates to Republicans and says he's Libertarian, but all other investments promote globalism

14. Julia Koch and family—Owners of Koch Enterprises

15. Mackensie Bezos—Her ex, Jeff Bezos, retains voting rights of her Amazon shares, so she is not held responsible for Amazon globalism, and is not a predator

16. Phil Knight and family—Owners of Nike with heavy investments in the CCP

Elon Musk is at the top of American billionaires, but he is a maverick investor/owner and not considered a globalist. It is also worth reporting former President Donald Trump and his supporters managed very well against such David/Goliath odds! We Americans still have strength and will to keep our country but we MUST not give up!

As of 2026, other top contenders of the 16 mentioned have also been in and out of these positions.

It is especially important to note—nearly all of the above predators have an almost uniform attachment to the CCP which is very concerning to liberty-loving Americans. However, any predators operating in the international arena are automatically drawn in to the CCP connection. It seems they cannot avoid ending up profiting from a partnership with the CCP. It has become abundantly clear a great deal of seductive courting is used by the CCP, encouraging predators to believe their financial and political future lies in the vast Chinese market. Possibly, even their safety may rely on staying on good terms with the CCP monstrosity.

Another thing that must be observed about the power of the globalists and their corporations was their agenda to put Donald Trump and his administration out of business. Trump represented the most gigantic hurdle to getting Americans and hence all other national entities moving forward with their globalist agenda. This drive to undermine his administration started long before COVID-19. However there can be no question of their planning for and instigation of the pandemic to take him down. American politics suffered interference from international and globalist entities operating within the United States using everything they had in their power. Probably the biggest mode of interference was Big Tech, because almost every tech entity was based in the United States and owned by American globalists.

Just to show why there was so much accusation of misinformation on the various mainstream and social media platforms, we need to look at the top eleven U.S. corporations in 2022, their ranking and their net worth. They are all responsible for full-on hostility toward Donald Trump and any of his supporters. It should be understood, that all of the top 100 US corporations continuously jockey for rank and worth. In January, 2025, they were listed as follows:[8]

1. Twitter—worth $50 billion then; thankfully it's now under the conservative control of Elon Musk, and much damage has been corrected—current worth $12.32 billion (about 20% of what Musk paid for it.)

2. Netflix—worth $61 billion—current worth $418.41 billion

3. Adobe—worth $64 billion—current worth $190.42 billion

4. Starbucks—worth $84 billion—current worth $111.95 billion

5. Nike—worth $91 billion—current worth $111.93 billion

6. Intel—worth $169 billion—current worth $240 billion
7. Facebook—worth $405 billion—current worth $527 billion
8. Amazon—worth $425 billion—current worth $1.8 trillion
9. Microsoft—worth $507 billion—current worth $1 trillion
10. Alphabet/Google—worth $574 billion—current worth $1.8 trillion
11. Apple—worth $750 billion—current worth $2.4 trillion

The top five Most Valuable American Companies today are now Apple, Microsoft, Alphabet, Inc., Amazon, and Nvidia. This simply shows the enormous amount of money being made primarily in the Technology sectors. Those company CEOs, as you might imagine, are also the wealthiest globalists in the world; some of them have also reached financial status as trillionaires. No wonder they think they can walk on water and call all the shots!

Dissemination of Misinformation by Globalists

All of these American corporations are owned by billionaire predators as we saw previously. The information our government has about any of us is readily available. Your name, personal information, how you vote, what party you belong to, and a whole lot more are known. Naturally it was not surprising if we posted information, even if we knew it to be true, it would go through a sophisticated monitoring process. There was a standard narrative on each media site of what information was acceptable for posting. If your post didn't match or agree with the narrative, you might be warned the first time, or later, you might have your next post omitted. If you persisted, you could be blacklisted, or you could be banned from that site altogether. If a select group of "fact-checkers" deemed it misinformation, again, based on the accepted narrative, it was not allowed. Never mind that the "fact-checkers" were hired as henchmen of Big Tech itself, so it was not facts that were checked, but conformity with the narrative that was checked. Very probably, this was not the first time for many of us, but it certainly was THE WORST time ever in our country having our freedom of speech deliberately censored because Big Tech (aka globalist corporate heads) didn't like it. You'll remember the President of the United States, who widely used the Twitter platform to communicate with the American people, was banned from it as well.

Market responses to Twitter's violent Trump suppression confirmed that MANY wealthy persons and corporations were and are globalist predators. Together, these eleven corporations were so powerful, they succeeded in deleting Presidential communications which clearly contributed in untold ways to Trump's election loss, forcing him out of office, and disenfranchising over half of American voters. In short, Donald Trump and his supporters had over half of America's biggest and most valuable companies actively fighting against them, not to mention the liberal political machinations of fraud. Yet, despite all the forceful denials, swearing it wasn't so, there is still plenty of evidence Trump legally won his second term! No matter how much swearing and even legal denial of actual court cases, the majority of conservative Americans and a good many others will never be convinced it wasn't so. Subsequently, far more positive proof has been found, and is well-documented.

Another thing that must be clearly understood has everything to do with the globalist narrative. It had been decided BEFORE the Pandemic was globally unleashed, just exactly what it should look like in terms of mandatory public health care mandates. The masking, social distancing, vaccinations, etc. "had all been decided for us, and practiced at the Event 201 pandemic exercise of October 18, 2019, knowing where and when it was actually coming! Naturally, that fact has vociferously been denied by its globalist organizers who said they ran the exercise 'just in case,' because the world had seen a growing number of epidemic events." Globalists maintained the specifics of the exercise should not be taken as predictions for the COVID-19 pandemic, but that is not the same information later proven by Anthony Fauci's documentation! Not surprisingly, that bit of unsolicited documentation has been scrubbed from the internet and simply could not be found anywhere! In spite of that, no one should ever take all the known information about the pandemic, as in adding 2 + 2 and not get 4!

CHAPTER 5

What Is the True Globalist Agenda?

What Schwab, Global Predators, and the CCP Have in Common

At first blush, it seems very odd to most of us that so many powerful business-oriented globalists want to hobnob with the likes of the most evil and destructive dictator in the world. However, we recall the CCP believes its government MUST seize any and every opportunity afforded it to dominate and ultimately CONTROL ALL HUMAN ACTIVITIES! Remember, no other ultimate goal will be enough for them—it must be THE #1 ruling empire of the whole world. According to what followers of the God of the Bible believe, there will be a one-world government, but it will not originate in China and it will not be led by Xi Jinping or any other Chinese dictator. But of course, they don't know that. Therefore, it uses its own corporations to infiltrate the "Western" hemisphere, especially, but also the world. In China, all corporations must answer to the CCP and aid the cause of "unrestricted warfare" against the United States and the world.

Globalist predators envision themselves in a world where they, the business leaders, "partner" with governments all over the world (fusion). The CCP is so large and powerful that it welcomes its leadership and influence. They still don't have a clue that this will eventually take globalists off the map entirely. Fauci has helped the CCP develop its biological warfare. Google has profoundly aided the CCP in developing its massive surveillance of the Chinese people. During COVID-19, globalists learned they could bully governments into making the desired changes they wanted to see under the guise of public health. They wielded enormous influence in getting Joe Biden into the presidency. Since they have so much money, power, and control, they really believe this "partnership" with the CCP will give them more of the same, but they are sadly delusional if they think, even for a moment, the CCP won't destroy them all in the end. There will be no such thing as sharing the wealth, power, and control for China.

The Real Schwab and His Global Reset

As we discussed earlier, Klaus Schwab touts a basic program called "stakeholder capitalism; supposedly it was followed by the Biden administration. It all sounds highly humanitarian in the surface wording of what corporations would look like. It is most like a very "progressive" government in partnership with corporations, but it isn't anything close to a "free market" with healthy competition. In Schwab's dreamland perfection, the Bank of America CEO, Brian Moynihan and his associates are best suited to set world priorities. It is NOT an associative capitalism—it's an associative world government or "New World Order" masquerading as capitalism. The more serious problem is that individual capitalists are the true entrepreneurs that actually generate creativity and wealth. With freedom capitalism gone, all of humanity would slow to a slight crawl!

This is where Schwab was able to push his Global Reset plans. The COVID-19 pandemic provided a unique opportunity to "THINK ABOUT THE KIND OF FUTURE WE WANT." (paraphrased, that would be 'we're thinking about the kind of world globalists want.') *Time* magazine partnered with the WEF to ask leading 'thinkers' to share ideas for how to 'transform' the way we live and work. This is all elementary "pie-in-the-sky" dreaming that's been given serious political theory and even concrete programs, but all of these share disastrous prospects as follows:[1]

- Schwab's own 'stakeholder capitalism' which means many individual interests other than the corporation's own profits MUST be adhered to by that capitalist owner. All other stakeholders such as (e.g.) Black Lives Matter, or climate change advocates have their own 'profit' motives, no matter how awful or destructive those motives might be, even if the profit is nothing more than the ability to express rage or simply glean corporate handouts. The corporations make all the sacrifices, while bowing to the 'progressive' Marxist stakeholders. (Communism revisited)

- Since the ideology of the great reset changes continuously, depending on the latest ideas of the 'great thinkers', it should accomplish the following:
- Redesigning capitalism to utilize 'social values'
- 'Reimagining' capitalism
- Fixing the global economy or Making a 'sustainable' future
- Developing a new, more effective 'green deal'
- Fixing racial inequality,
- Revolutionizing E-commerce,
- Building a better tech industry
- Smashing the 'glass ceiling' for women
- Changing 'how' we work
- Helping all people adapt to changes and threats more quickly

What is not mentioned are what becomes of individual freedoms or political liberty, the true drivers of all human progress. There will be no building of stronger democratic republics. We can find NO mention of ANY form of religion. Patriotism and nationalism are naughty words. American history, culture, traditions, values, and mores are forever ERASED from our thoughts. There is a great deal of this being done in our country already. Our history books very often neglect to tell the truth and if it's told, or discussed, it's not about the greatness of our nation. Instead, 'progressive' writers seek to undermine everything good and focus on past or current problems dealt with incorrectly and are now bigger problems.

The world will be the globalist wolfpack's playground. Everything that America is or has ever been will be gone in globalist dreams. Current American politicians, that is those who call themselves 'progressive' have no idea what real progress should look like, and are already playing the globalist game. President Biden and many like him or worse have already abandoned our America, and work to give it all away in exchange for the globalist narrative. They want business/government fusions to make them wealthier, full of themselves, and more powerful. Read the mainstream media outlets and follow the narrative. Until President Trump was re-elected, 'progressives' got us closer to destruction every day. Thankfully, this administration has halted or rescinded most of the destructive policies Biden and the Deep State made. However, down the road, when/if 'progressive' leadership returns, their dream of a New World Order which they still tout unashamedly whenever someone listens, will resume. Barring our Lord's return, America has at least one more chance to plug the dam and stanch the oncoming floods in this administration. Beyond that, we certainly have no guarantee of the present optimism continuing. Conservative Christians are increasingly under attack, and the Enemy, along with his powerful forces is relentless. However, we "look up, for our redemption draws near." It will come as an astronomical shock to all these globalists who have planned for the New World Order, which they will get, but it will be nothing like they have imagined it would be.

Now, we can clearly document Klaus Schwab's real intentions of "predatory capitalism" with a speech he gave in June of 2020 in the midst of COVID-19 after struggling 50 years to be heard on his global reset. He's talking about top-down governmental control. Those are just fancy words for 'totalitarianism'. "To achieve a better outcome, the world must act jointly and swiftly to revamp all aspects of our societies and economies, from education to social contracts and working conditions. Every country from the United States to China, MUST participate, and every industry, from oil and gas to tech MUST be transformed. In short, we need a "Great Reset" of capitalism."[2] Notice the MUSTS! The United States would never have participated in this Great Reset under such terms with President Trump, but President Biden was placed BECAUSE he was all in. Given his previously documented thirst for wealth, power, and control, he had no problem complying, and given another term in office he may have succeeded. Thankfully, that wasn't God's plan for our nation.

It behooves us all to beware! As we experienced during the Pandemic, there are plenty of people, too numerous to count, who have no compunction about subjecting the entire world to suffering and death, believing, it will eventually fall into line behind the globalist elites. Elites rejoiced every day over Biden's weakening of America with COVID-19 and the Great Reset. Our nation's major newspapers were All mouthpieces for extreme progressivism and global propaganda. "A great and wonderful exception was/is the *Epoch Times*, a conservative news source that prints plain truth every day. It printed an excellent article on this same subject and its reputation has grown in its strength and determination to remain a beacon of patriotism and love of liberty.[3] This article was an excellent overview of the whole sordid mess with its author revealing what was evolving with the Great Reset, including Anthony Fauci's contribution as a 'progressive theorist.' Smith also decried Canadian Prime Minister Trudeau for calling COVID-19 "an opportunity for a reset to reimagine economic systems that actually address global challenges like poverty, inequality, and climate change."[3]

Pope Francis is a Globalist Elite

An impressive number of Roman Catholics and others have voiced their concerns about the Pope because of his globalist politics. A series of articles on *Breitbart* were written by Thomas D. Williams, who has had a long career as a theologian, ethicist, and professor. He said both Biden and the Pope take money from and defer to the CCP regularly. There is abundant proof of this most disturbing fact in one of Williams' articles. In another article, Cardinal Joseph Zen, the former bishop of Hong Kong, declared the "renewed Vatican-China deal" was a "complete defeat for faithful Catholics." Smith also reported, "China's most famous civil rights activist joined the chorus of critics who denounced the recent deal between the Vatican and Chinese Communist Party (CCP) as a 'betrayal' of Chinese Catholics."[4]

The Pope has been seriously criticized for his "extension of a controversial and secret 2018 agreement with the CCP about the renaming of Catholic bishops in China. In this agreement, the Pope gave the CCP the power to choose the Catholic bishops in China in exchange for very large undisclosed sums of money.

Finally, author Smith reported U.S. Senators pressed the Pope to denounce the religious persecution of the Uyghur Muslims the CCP had interred behind barbed wire in China, (the CCP has carried this genocidal campaign on for years because it's an unwanted minority group in China). However, the Pope had already forfeited the freedom of his own Church in China by allowing the CCP to appoint its bishops. There was no end to the Pope's compromises to the CCP. Fortunately, Pope Francis aged out and resigned. The new Pontiff, Pope Leo XIV, is believed to think and feel much as Francis did, however, it's a bit early to say. According to early interviews, Pope Leo appears more religiously conservative and traditional, but leans left politically, not agreeing with many of our President's policies. As to his position on the global stage, only time will tell. The global rhetoric heard about governance has not been openly discussed, but it will depend a great deal on his treatment of the globalist agenda, especially the biggest globalist!

Transhumanism—More of the Global Reset

Another major Schwab brainstorm, of which he is an avid proponent, is transhumanism. He has promoted the concepts of technology and artificial intelligence (AI) as part of his Fourth

Industrial Revolution for several years. More currently he wants to utilize technological interventions that can transform our brains and behaviors to make us, in fact, LESS human. The greater question: is it transhumanism or the 'living dead?' Less human is also less able to have any real spontaneous emotions or loving connections with other humans. In other words, we're looking at ROBOTS! Just as it was in Marxism, it is always cynical, and the 'progressive' coverup for plain old global exploitation of humanity by a self-appointed elite.

Transhumanism is both inhuman and utopian. No matter the technique used, all exhibit the same effects:

- Blunting of the human mind
- Compromising free will
- Dulling or killing any form of spirituality
- Always rendering humans more docile, apathetic, pliable and easy to lead

Transhumanism includes any and all attempts to connect the human brain directly to super computers. There are far too many moral and ethical concerns to all of this; however, there are none believed strong enough to hold up the global reset, if someone chooses to do it. Deep brain stimulation and other forms of psychiatric surgery have tried to influence emotions and human conduct by mutilating the brain. According to Dr. Beggins, who has an in-depth history of work in the field of psychiatry, there is an amazing film called *The Minds of Men* by Aaron and Melissa Dykes. Dr Breggins is featured in this film discussing the history of mind control through technology, and he is actively and legally opposed to any such efforts. He has also been critical of Elon Musk's proposals and experiments connecting the human brain directly to supercomputers.[5]

The Silence of Cities and the Culture of Death

Another equally distressing aspect of Schwab's global reset goes farther yet. During the COVID-19 pandemic, he became even more convinced that the lockdowns vastly improved cities all over the world. He said the lockdowns reduced human activity and actually impacted the planet Earth's crust! The earth could get a much-needed rest! He claimed noise pollution dropped by 50%. Lower background noise meant smaller earthquakes were detected and offered insight to scientists on seismic threats.

The global reset plans include limiting the number of people all over the planet through various means of population control, (a goal that was clear long before the planned epidemic started). Ideally, after depopulation, the remaining population will be docile citizens (probably programmed to be so), ready to serve the globalist elites in whatever capacity they are needed while globalists grow ever more wealthy, more glorious, and more powerful. Granted, most depopulation efforts would NOT be agreeable to productive, happy people, so apparently, they don't expect any such people. The evidence of depopulation efforts became very clear during the COVID-19 Pandemic. Any sanctity of human life was clearly missing for all those who espoused the 'healthcare' options offered. Certainly, effective treatments were banned, and toxic injectables forced on a great many people who would NOT have taken them voluntarily. This will all be discussed at length in later chapters.

The truly tragic essence in all of this— globalists WORSHIP DEATH! Naturally, that would NOT be their own death, but the death of humanity at their own hands. That's one of the reasons the use of transhumanism is no problem for them. This thought process explains a lot more about their EVIL and its Real Source in the End Times. It explains their history of the millions of murders, abortions, euthanasias, the promotion of psychiatric drugs and interventions of the not-so-distant past. Legalized marijuana, and other recreational drugs today work so well, and blind so many, the strategy of that is clear. Humans are only truly equal in death. They can appear perfect in death. The insanity of these plans will always push humanity closer and closer to death, and the more massive the death becomes, the better. Premature death due to new pandemics is not a tragedy to them, but an opportunity to make more money; whether killing more people either with super bugs or the toxic vaccines they make to fight them, since both techniques work equally well toward the goal. Beyond these easy techniques for killing, massive death will happen either by extinction or by transhumanism into the inhumanism of completely compliant robots, if their goals are allowed to continue.

The Global Reset Destroys all Traditional Norms

Globalist elites enlisted Prince Charles (now King Charles) as the Big Broadcaster of introduction to the Great Reset among the media. He faithfully parroted the enormous opportunity COVID-19 had given the world to "reset the global economy and prioritize sustainable development without further harming the planet."[6] (Never mind the harm for the people).Then Charles basically quoted the notorious World Economic Forum script. He declared the pandemic had 'forced' global governments to put their own economies aside to the betterment of global economies and demonstrated big changes were possible. He failed to mention it was one of the major points of instigating the pandemic in the first place. The pandemic did not afford economic or any other kind of opportunity to anyone but the globalists!! This was exactly how all globalists viewed COVID-19; it's touted for its usefulness, and necessary for conditioning people to accept their hideous changes, while happily embracing their own impossible dreams.

Next in the change process there will be no further political distinctions between 'left' and 'right', 'conservative' and 'liberal', etc. Right now, politics play little to no role in globalist thinking. Those labels only matter to the extent of determining which ones more closely promote the agenda of the globalists. Religion is NOT a consideration because it's simply a moot point. Anyone with strong faith, such as Christians or Muslims, is unlikely to buy into the globalist narrative anyway, so they are definitely among the expendable. Except for the Marxism of the CCP, and radical Jihadists of Islam, globalist "predators" are totally ideologically and spiritually without foundational roots. They may masquerade as politicians according to the current audience, but they have no deeply binding ideology aside from becoming more wealthy, recognizable and powerful. Globalist predators were compared aptly to viruses, by Dr. Breggins. "They have no divisions, no citizenship, no political affiliations, no understanding of the harm they do, and no respecter of persons. We are ALL prey to both predators and viruses!"[7]

How Globalists Pervert Capitalism

As the saying goes, "There is a fly in the ointment." Sometimes there is a very big difference of opinion; the more money involved, the more the potential differences. Even though all globalists are supposedly following the same narrative, things still go badly wrong at times! For example: Bill and Melinda Gates may share a common foundation and the foundation appears to be quite functional. However, Bill and Melinda had enough differences of opinion to get divorced, and Warren Buffett (the foundations third trustee) left the foundation. Naturally, the real effects of these serious splits are mostly unknown. While they are still globalist billionaires, it sure didn't buy them personal happiness. Infidelity was a rumored issue as well.

Then, there are the Clintons. There isn't time or paper enough to cover that subject, but we know of a certainty with all their fame and history, there are many flies in that ointment. While they don't fully fit the definition of globalists, there are many similarities. They are poor by globalist standards with an estimated net worth of only $120 million. Even as seniors, they still hold political aspirations of office. As is true of most foundations, it is a 501c3, not for profit organization touting the motto "making a difference in people's lives across the U.S. and around the world." One program of the foundation is the Clinton Global Initiative (CGI) that "brings together established and emerging global leaders (because you can't run with the globalists unless you speak their language) to create and implement solutions for the world's most pressing challenges. CGI works with partners to develop Commitments to Action. These are new, specific, and measurable actions in climate resilience, health equity, and inclusive economic recovery and growth."[7] Doesn't that sound as altruistic as anything can? However, when Hillary ran for president against Donald Trump, she was well beyond certain she would win that election hands down. The reason for that was because CGI worked with Dominion Voting Machines in election fraud (yes, proven) to help her out. Contrary to publicly stated goals, touted in glowing global terms, foundations are about so much more than what is stated.

One of the most notorious criminals of all time, Mr. George Soros, now including his son, Alexander his successor, can take the prizes away from any Mafia family on a record for evil. By the way, he regularly donated BIG money to the Clinton foundation. Soros, by his frequent declarations, hates America passionately and he hates her free enterprise system of business. More than all that, he hates Donald Trump. Soros masquerades as an idealistic "progressive," but he's made it his personal quest to destroy America. He partnered with the Chinese Communist Party and designated China as a ringleader in the New World Order. He looms largely in his avowed predatory habits. Evil and Soros are solid bed partners. He easily gloats about having destroyed the economies of several southeast Asian countries. Soros says, "I am basically there to make money. I cannot and do not look at the social consequences of what I do."[8] Soros made his billions by looking for vulnerable countries and institutions, then destroying them, while making financial bets on their decline. He famously 'broke' the British pound, sold it short, and made $1 billion dollars.

One of his worst-case treacheries was his aiding and abetting the breakdown of law and order in America by funding lawless District Attorneys, urban rioters, Black Lives Matter, Antifa, and more, effectively eliminating law enforcement and releasing criminals without bond. He heavily funded Democrats against President Trump for his second term. The question is "WHY?" Why did the Clintons, and Bill Gates both accept his donations and disclose them? Globalists act as though they are fearless and shameless about anything and everything they do. As villainous and evil as Soros is, (actively vying with the devil himself in media), he is NEVER attacked by the mainstream media, by universities, by Big Tech, or any other globalist entity. His actions are either supported or systematically hidden from public awareness. Here is further revelation on Soros. Right in the middle of the ongoing concerns with potentially massive voter fraud involving U.S. voting systems, Soros named Lord Mark Malloch Brown president of his Open Society Foundation. Here's the kicker—Brown was 'leaving' a job as CEO of Smartmatic, the same manufacturer of the voting machines conservative media accused of rigging the election against Trump! Hmmm! Clearly, this was NO accident! Brown worked for Soros' cause, so Soros rewarded and protected him. Anyone can see just how the globalist predators live and work.

We could certainly look at this mere bit of factual evidence and say "Money is the root of All evil!" But that is not true and not what the Holy Scriptures say either. They say, "The LOVE of money is the root of ALL evil." How true it is! Money itself has no intrinsic value in or of itself. It is simply a much sought after tool men use liberally to buy all the things they crave, such as recognition, control, and power. It is simply a driving LUST for power over the masses. There are some very large egos involved and most want their fair share of fame, the extreme of which is to be worshiped in a 'godlike' fashion; enter the coming Anti-Christ! In America, COVID-19 was used as the justification for increasing uncontrolled government power at every level of authority (extreme anti-Constitutionalism). However money talks if you have it, and talks all the time if you have a lot of money!

BEWARE! Scripture talks about being as wise as serpents (who is the most famous serpent you've ever heard of?), and as harmless as doves. Beware of any fast talking, filthy-rich people who continually spout their ideals but have no intention of working for anything or anyone except themselves. If our treasured concepts of liberty, freedom, and democracy are belittled, or worse are absent, they are enemy agents. They are capable of talking faster and spending far more than any of us to get what they want and will stop at nothing to procure it.

Big Tech and Major Universities are Big Globalists Too

Everyone today talks about technology, even BIG TECH blows its own horn, but do we understand what that really means? Generically, it is widely defined as the MOST prosperous and influential technological companies in the IT industry. Sometimes, they are also called the Big Five, including Alphabet (Google), Apple, Meta, Amazon, and Microsoft. It further refers to digital product and service companies which have a significant market share in their respective category, for example Tencent or Facebook, basically a part of one of the Big Five and are equivalents of them. In China, Baidu, Alibaba, Tencent, and Xiaomi (BATX0) are also equivalents. Big Tech can also include smaller tech companies with high valuations such as Netflix or Nvidia, or non-tech companies with high-tech practices, such as automaker Tesla.

The term "Big Tech" first appeared in media reports circa 2013, as some economists saw signs of these companies becoming dominant with little regulation. It became popular around 2017 following the investigation into Russian interference in the 2016 U.S. elections. As to the role these companies played with access to such huge amounts of user data and their ability to influence their users came, Big Tech came under Congressional review. The Big Five are dominant players in their respective areas of technology. Artificial intelligence, cloud computing, consumer electronics, ecommerce, home automation, online advertising, self-driving cars, social networking, software, and streaming media are popular examples. They are among the most valuable public companies with a maximum market capitalization of from $1 to $3 trillion U.S. dollars. The Big Tech companies are considered among the most prestigious employers in the world. They are now so powerful they are often criticized for creating a new economic order called "surveillance capitalism."[9] They serve billions of users and are able to influence user behavior and control enormous amounts of user data.

Consequently, it's imperative we understand what this means to our nation and to each of us as individual users. As we've shown before, these companies are owned by globalist elites, and are therefore globalist as well. This fact should give us pause, and cause for much thought. If this globalist 'order' is surveillance-oriented at its most basic function, there is NOTHING unknowable and therefore readily usable. We saw the damage this entity did in monitoring and controlling information fully to the advantage of the globalists who ran the whole pandemic narrative to say what they wanted said, and censor whatever didn't fit their programmed narrative. Those of us who knew and understood what was really happening were unable to get that information disseminated. Citizens everywhere suffered for the lack of true information. Truth was never reported or allowed unless by virtue of much smaller, non-corporate media doing their best to keep information lines open. This happened exactly as planned for the duration of the pandemic to accomplish all that globalist elites wanted accomplished. Freedom of speech is one of our rights under our Constitution in America that was almost completely denied us.

The bigger and more unscrupulous the business, the more it can dominate government; not only its normal regulators, but the entire Congress and yes, even the presidency. Any and all media entities can censor any and all citizens, including the president, whose ability to speak and share his thoughts, plans and platform was shut down, and he lost the critical support of over half of his constituents right in the middle of the election cycle. There was absolutely nothing that could stop the globalist elites and their companies from disenfranchising Americans. That, friends, is one of the worst and scariest outcomes of the globalist takeovers during the COVID-19 pandemic.

Now, it would seem our institutions of higher learning would be exempted from globalist control, but such was not the case before, during, or after the pandemic. Colleges and universities are very literally operating on a global scale. Worldwide systems of knowledge and information flow, because networks and people move between institutions and systems. Most people have long believed that such globalization enlarges global higher education and expands all horizons. The entire education system is the partner of globalization. However, sharing a vast treasure of information on a global scale is worlds apart from what it has become. A great many of our finest institutions now have shockingly deep financial and research ties to the CCP. These institutions were complicit with the globalist intentions for the COVID-19 pandemic, including gain-of-function experimentation in mutual laboratories, development of vaccines, shutdowns, and every other intention of Fauci, Gates, and many other globalist elites. Politicians, educators, scientists, and even prominent Americans in every professional field are extremely protective of the CCP, because they all can make more money selling out to the corrupted dictatorship of China, than they can make within the competition and complexities of a democratic republic and patriotic nation like the U.S.A. So, in a very real sense, many Americans, though they may not have the billions of the globalist elites, have sold America down the river also, just for the LOVE of the almighty dollar. Many of these would answer "globalism is the way of the world today, and we must play the game and stay ahead of it or succumb to the failure that will come if we don't."[10] That's the devil's own lie. Compromising with the world and everything it may have to offer might bring a temporary success, but it will be short-lived. Those who do it will discover too late what they have sold their souls to have, and there will be no turning back.

CHAPTER 6

Characteristics of Top Globalist Wolves

Psychological and Personality Patterns in Common

Dr. Breggin's book says there is a kind of person who could be described as a "predator," meaning they exhibit certain psychological and personality patterns that are recognizable from the majority of people. He called these people predators because as an entity they are merciless in their pursuit of prey. The definition of prey is anything or anyone in the position to be taken advantage of, fleeced, deceived, or robbed, even murdered. "The global 'predators' have made us, humanity, their prey—somewhat akin to a pack of voracious wolves finding a seemingly limitless supply of docile, penned-in game in an unprotected zoo or preserve."[1] In fact, this author uses the word "wolves" throughout this book because of its graphic, apt, and clearest nature.

We might also characterize these "wolves" as perpetrators because they continuously choose to exploit, bully, browbeat, intimidate, terrorize, and abuse other people to achieve their desired goals. There are a number of persistent attitudes and personality traits, even some mental and emotional tendencies that characterize the typical 'wolves' we've already looked at and will see more about as we proceed. Even this list is not exhaustive:

- They regularly deny or at least minimize the harm they are doing to others.

- They rationalize the damage they are doing.
- They blame the victim by disparaging the victim's personality. (eg: "they make it so easy to do")
- They crush any personal feelings of empathy for victims.
- Since they have been victimized by others, it's OK to do the same.
- They will generally react with anger and blame toward anyone who confronts them, based on their own personal history of feeling shame or being humiliated.
- They demean and humiliate their victims, effectively treating them as though they aren't human and have no feelings.
- When they behave in any of these ways, they feel personally more powerful, sometimes even invincible.
- They will almost always try to resolve a conflict with domination, power plays, and abuse of their authority. (e.g. Anthony Fauci)
- They become pompous, pretentious, conceited, prideful, and completely egocentric. As time goes on, they are increasingly narcissistic.
- They actually come to an eventual point of not even understanding their own basic needs ,and are not in touch with reality of what life is even about, just as long as they can keep getting more power and wealth with recognition.[2]

When we view each of the above character points, and there are probably others, it might help answer the perplexing question, "How can these people with so much do such selfish, heartless, and hurtful things to people and still live with themselves?" There are other psychosocial syndromes akin to this such as reactive attachment disorder. It does actually have a known cause, but the upshot is that those diagnosed with this disorder have very little or no conscience. This allows them to do whatever they decide to do with no compunction or remorse. Perhaps some problem in their past has created the "wolves" they've become. Regardless, truth is that the wolves have little real emotion. Their attitudes and personal values are entirely different from most other people which allow wolves to act like wolves instead of humans. Many of them started out hating individuals for perceived affronts and kept right on going. Many of them lived life on the gray edge of the law or worse, but as they get better at being wolves, they also get smarter on how to skirt or just ignore the laws. If you acquire enough of the money and power you yen for, you can run with others like you who do the same things and glean acceptance and protection from one another. Very often, the personal lives of wolves are a train wreck. However, they may actually manage marriages, friendships, and corporate relations, without caring or concern for "normal" humanity. For the most part, wolves are too far above the pack to pay much attention to who they've become. Rather, their acquired skills in manipulation and social analysis tend to alienate 'normal' people anyway.

Political Policies and Attitudes in Common

Those wolves we've been learning about are often individuals who because of their wealth and power have been able to amass large and powerful corporations and institutions also classified as globalist wolves. Most have well-known reputations; often they are notorious reputations, at least far from stellar. In fact many experience their own entanglements with the law. Some have become so exclusive in a certain area of expertise they've had or at least bordered on monopolies and have been sued by the federal government for anti-trust violations. Typically, however, with all their money and clever strategies, owners buy brilliant lawyers, enabling them to walk away with fines and hand slaps. Then get those lawyers to assist them in adjusting their ways and means a bit and keep right on going. Once again, this proves money always talks, and a lot of money can talk over and over! Most of the previous bullet points of wolves are applicable to both the owners/CEOs and to the equally wealthy and powerful corporate entities. There is a plethora of real evidence of the truths above as we look at typical communication and behavior patterns, particularly in the realms of business, education, and politics, as shown below:

- Even if an individual or entity is American, there is no patriotism in word or deed—rather, there is mostly criticism of America, its power, its politics, and its values.
- Globalists have scant interest in American principles of personal liberty, or political liberty, only in their own liberty to do what they want.
- Because of a complete lack of loyalty to any nation, they want nothing to do with democracy or democratic republics. In their minds the ONLY effective way to govern is complete top-down power wielded in either authoritarian or totalitarian government.
- They fully support open borders worldwide but especially in America. The intent is to dilute, divide, then destroy the democratic republics, ultimately unifying all governance into one top-down global union. (New World Order)
- All policies are meant to make the wealthy, wealthier, and desiccate or destroy the poor, the working class, middle class, and upper middle class. The result of course will widen the gap between the ultra-wealthy and all the rest of humanity. They don't seem to be concerned about who will actually do all the work! That is most likely because their system will utterly enslave everyone else.
- In what seems surprising, most wolves have very large, successfully flourishing financial investments in the Communist Chinese Party and China itself, managed

exclusively by the CCP. Their motives are to exponentially increase all their investments without the restraints exercised by Democratic Republics such as America. Meanwhile, they consistently make excuses and apologies for the CCP, its policies, and its abuse of all human rights, even when the CCP is harming their own American countrymen. They simply ignore what isn't right and support whatever CCP does, so they can continue making more money.

- Globalist wolves did everything in their power to oppose and undermine President Trump when he was in office the first time; though we've heard less from the power mongers since President Trump returned to office, their efforts have never stopped, nor will they ever stop. Clearly massive efforts to keep him away from another term in the White House were beyond evident, and they had the full cooperation, efforts and corruption of American liberals.

The major goals of the globalist wolves remain unchanged; they are still more self-promotion of greatness, its associated power, and billions more in wealth. Indeed, after COVID-19, many of the billionaires and their corporate entities became trillionaires, a figure that defies our imaginations. At the same time, they managed to effectively bankrupt a large body of nations with COVID rules and regulations.

With so much international impoverishment, they clearly believe they've 'arrived;' they are truly the elite, superior in every way, and vastly positioned miles above all other people on planet EARTH.

They find no inherent value in individual humans wherever they may be, no matter their sex, age, race, location, or any other consideration. They have no regard for human life while famously touting a completely false concern for world health and humanitarianism. Such a concern couldn't be further from the truth, when their goals include depopulation in their culture of death! Famine, wars, abortion, euthanasia, genocide, etc. all most definitely define their real values in their grand visions of a New World Order.

Except for a few globalist Jihadists and Communists, most wolves have no strong political or religious ideologies or creeds; to increase their own procurement of their personal and corporate goals became their god. American wolves and corporations who because of their full-on support of the CCP, simply abandoned any original moral, ethical, religious, or political priority toward their native origins, beliefs or nationalities.

- Wolves will use whatever unethical or illegal practices necessary to realize their goals, including any illegal political practices, such as election fraud, censorship, deceit, libel and slander against any opposing forces. Like George Soros, they finance illegal activities of other people greedy enough to perform them. This even includes financing terrorist groups with different agendas entirely, who offer valuable distraction from their own goals. Sometimes, they will display a political stance such as 'progressive' or 'capitalist' meaning something entirely different, but the title may work temporarily to their advantage; such was the case of the election of Joseph Biden as President. The 'Progressive' label has succeeded in carving huge slashes into the fiber of American democracy, and striking at its very foundations.
- It is nearly guaranteed, no globalist in today's 'wolf pack' will ever stop to examine the damages, including the millions of lives lost or destroyed. Their collective crimes have caused individuals, families, businesses, schools, and even humankind as a whole to be incurably traumatized for life![3]

Even this list is not exhaustive but it gives the reader a clearer idea of what is meant when we speak in greater depth of all the travesty perpetrated before, during, and after the planned and executed delivery of the COVID-19 Pandemic. These are the criminals truly responsible. This is what they did, and how they did it, along with about a million reasons why they should be arrested, tried, and removed from circulation in the human race. It is a hard and fast guarantee; these wolves are still doing what they've always done at this moment and they have no intention of being stopped.

Globalist Wolves Know Their Common Enemy

Post Pandemic, we have a far better understanding of why wolves who do business on the international plane are unavoidably drawn into partnerships with the CCP; the rewards are too enticing to ignore. We know, for example, that the higher-educational community of the United States is offered enormous incentives to come to China to do scientific work in their labs, instead of the honest rewards they could attain by staying in the States. Offers range from fantastic salaries and benefits to lucrative housing opportunities, and greater upward mobility. The same is true for many of the globalist wolves. China encourages them to believe their best financial and political futures lie in the humongous Chinese market and maybe even that their ultimate safety lies in staying on good terms with the CCP machine which intends to rule the world as soon as possible.

It is yet unknown whether or not global wolves' dependence on the CCP applies also to global criminal enterprises; not nearly enough investigation has been done, nor is it likely to be allowed in China any time soon. We are aware of the criminal offenses of the Biden family and its illegal dealings with the CCP. But, most of the globalist wolves are accepted and operate mostly in the public square, though there is plenty of graft there as well. We do know that much of their gross wealth and information on their various enterprises are made publicly available, as legally required. On the other hand there is known overlap between what is publicly known and what can only be obtained legally in court.

Here is an interesting detail that gives us insight into the size of the globalist network. When Twitter was owned by Jack Dorsey it had a market cap of $50 billion. As the wolfish globalist it is, *Forbes* declared in a February 10, 2021 headline, "Twitter Market Value Surges to $50 Billion Despite Trump Ban, and Shares Could Run Another 25%." Dorsey himself was worth $24 Billion at the time. Millions of Americans were angry when President Trump was not allowed access to Twitter, because globalists hated him. However, this positive response in the stock market to Twitter's 'illegal' suppression of Trump and his supporters completely proved that many wealthy individuals and companies were clearly globalist wolves in their own right. They obviously considered this unlawful action as a plus for their agendas.

Globalist Wolves, including the CCP, internationally know who their biggest common enemy is. They are a mixed and diverse block of American traditionalists, patriots, conservatives, libertarians, constitutionalists and religious people who often own small middle-class businesses. The Wolves, clearly aware of this large segment of people like us, who are determined to support their country and its heritage and defend and protect our personal rights and freedoms guaranteed us by our Constitution, which they disparage.

The fact that thousands of small businesses and religious institutions as well as our massive work force were all either shut down or greatly diminished during COVID19 was not an accident or act of fate! Large corporations and big business, as well as the government remaining open and fully operative was no accident either! Global wolves have intended to destroy the heart and soul of America for at least decades. It has always thrived on its standards and values of personal responsibility, independence, individualism, sound traditions, patriotism, freedom, and God. Working, middle, and upper-class individuals targeted by official Marxism and Progressivism, despise the capitalist classes who own most of society's wealth and means of production. There has always been a conflict of interest between the salt of the earth humanity and the big, self-proclaimed elites.

Unless we can fully grasp the globalists die-hard determination to wreck America and any remaining patriotic and freedom-loving nations, so much of what happened with COVID-19 makes no sense. However, now that we can identify the enemy globally as well as the "prince of the power of the air" and his claim on this Earth, we can begin to gather a unified opposition based on our Constitution and Bill of Rights. We do NOT have to cave to them, nor believe any of the massive lies they tried to use against us. Unfortunately, too many of us didn't know then what we know now. We were not able to protect ourselves from them or from the massively planned and executed pandemic. We unknowingly gave up some ground with the lack of this full understanding, but we have no intention of ever allowing it to happen again.

Some people, especially those who don't like to be recognized as globalist wolves have tried to claim the whole idea of globalist predators is nothing more than a conspiracy theory, but now we know it's not. "It is a highly recognizable, loosely organized coalition of often-competitive centers of money and influence; all of them lacking self-restraint and all of them obsessed with gaining more wealth, self-importance, and influence. Never has there been so many of them operating with so much determination and strength. Globalist wolves are now so dominant in the arena of world politics and governance there is little room, maybe no room, for a more benevolent kind of simply liberal globalism. This notorious globalism is now worldwide, involving many governments and politicians. It brings the United Nations and its World Health Organization together with individual wolves like Bill Gates, Anthony Fauci, Ralph Baric, Peter Daszak, Klaus Schwab (World Economic Forum) and Michael Bloomberg (NEF)."[4]

Almost all large global industries appear to be a part of this wolfish globalism, including Big Tech, Big Pharma, and Global Banking, as well as a plethora of various foundations. Most of the 'foundations' are worth billions and growing as 'non-profits' that are anything but non-profitable! The medical and science establishment and most universities are also deeply involved in it, up to their proverbial eyebrows! Chinese Communists, their CDC and their military, nearly all one and the same, are 'foundational.'

Every one of them is hell-bent on destroying the last bastion or barrier to a complete global victory in the New World Order. That bastion is American patriotism and devotion to freedom and liberty. Our freedoms are at stake, and extremely vulnerable until President Trump and his administration, with our God's help, pulled us back from the brink of the American subjugation, and with us, all humanity. This author believes that Americans, many for the first time, finally understood those impossible stakes and began enlisting the help and protection of our God.

In America, the mainstream media is also a member and key ally in the predatory globalism so abundantly clear, especially during the pandemic. Without it in mid-pandemic, globalists had only a scant chance at winning the election against President Trump, in favor of their weak, mentally debilitated, and ridiculously progressive choice to be their puppet. Here is a glaring and revealing headline of the day, showing exactly how globalists and liberals won the election: "*The Wall Street Journal*, *The Washington Post*, Among Newspapers Paid Millions by Beijing-Controlled News Outlets to Publish Propaganda this Year."[5]

The massive global spread of this news was so universal in scope, it couldn't even be calculated how far and wide it went. Certainly coast-to-coast in America (the *LA Times and The NY Times)* and from Canada to Great Britain. Remember the "Russia, Russia, Russia!" and the baseless, concocted accusations against President Trump? It wasn't "China, China, China!" Why? "Because the CCP is one of the most active participants in predatory globalism, with economic ties to the Democratic Party and mainstream media as well as American education, science, and corporate life."[6]

CHAPTER 7

Globalist Goals for the New World Order

The New World Order is Considered a Conspiracy Theory

An amazing phenomenon too big to miss today is the idea of the New World Order. Most of Big Tech still considers the idea a conspiracy theory, but the irony is globalists are increasingly calling what they imagine to be a one world government presented as totalitarian in nature—the New World Order (NWO). "The provocative title of the panel that lead off the ambitiously named *World Government Summit* here (Dubai) last week (March, 2022) was framed to suggest that a new global order is emerging 'A New World Order is emerging—and the world is not ready for it.'"[1] However, Big Tech in general still wants to label the concept of a New World Order a conspiracy theory. Wikipedia says it is a term used in several conspiracy theories which "hypothesize a secretly emerging totalitarian world government. The common theme in these theories about a New World Order is that a secretive power elite with a globalist agenda is conspiring to eventually achieve world domination and rule the world through an authoritarian one-world government—which will replace sovereign nation-states— and an all-encompassing propaganda whose ideology hails the establishment of the New World Order as the culmination of history's progress."[2]

Even in this attempted description of the difference, whether simply using the term as a true concept or saying it's a mere conspiracy theory; one can see very little difference. What is described a conspiracy theory is no theory at all. We already have seen five chapters of evidence showing a New World Order is not a theory at all, but a set of proven facts describing the whole system of globalist predators and what they want to accomplish to make this New World Order come to fruition. To prove that there is no such conspiracy we will look at their stated goals and how hard they are working to bring it to completion sooner rather than later.

Many different supposed theorists have been accused of conspiracy-based thinking, all the way from fundamentalist, Bible-believing Christians who believe and trust Scripture's prophecies, to Freemasonry, to the Illuminati, to the Elders of Zion, to Britain's Round Table movement, to H. G. Wells' Open Conspiracy, to the New Age, to the Fourth Reich, to Alien Invasions, and finally to the "Brave New World."[3] In reviewing each one of these, even to points of extremism, many of the projected elements are similar to others, and none of these entities believed they supported a conspiracy. It behooves us to look at some of these projected elements and compare them to the lunacies of today's globalist elites who fully believe their ideas are equally plausible and they will see each goal they have fulfilled as well. We've already tracked the planning and execution of a global pandemic. Now, globalists are planning for the New World Order as their next great achievement!

The 2030 Agenda for Sustainable Development goals was originally outlined and approved unanimously by the United Nations. The very first page of an article, asking the question about their progress, has a large poster cover with a black flag showing the blue and green globe and the words, "ONE WORLD!" It's being reported by the World Economic Forum (WEF) and starts with a quote, "A slowdown in progress on key areas is putting the 2030 Sustainable Development Goals 'in peril'!" The article was first published in September 2022 and has been updated. Its 2023 update shows a significant reversal of progress in key areas such as child vaccination rates and income inequality between countries.

The 2030 Agenda for Sustainable Development was adopted by ALL United Nations' member states in 2015. "A shared blueprint for peace and prosperity for people and the planet, now and into the future," it was based on 17 Sustainable Development Goals

(SDGs), which the UN described as an urgent call for action. It said ending global poverty would require focusing on strategies that reduce inequality and spur economic growth, while also tackling climate change. The report of 2022 painted a worrisome picture of expected progress in almost all areas, but the 2023 update delivered an even more solemn warning: "The promises enshrined in the SDGs are in peril," said the UN stats. "Halfway to the 2030 Agenda deadline, the SDGs are disappearing in the rearview mirror, as are the hopes and rights of current and future generations. A fundamental shift is needed—in commitment, solidarity, financing, and action—to put the world on a better path, and it's needed now."[4] This definitely increased the global urgency to ignite progress. However, no matter the promises, history has shown that United Nations promises are seldom worth the paper they are written on.

The gap is widening economically, between developed and developing nations, along with the uneven impacts of the climate crisis thus causing special concern. The decline in progress is pretty much universal, but poorer countries are being disproportionately affected by the consequences, largely due to a lack of representation on the global stage. The number of people in extreme poverty is rising for the first time in a generation and will probably reach 575 million by 2030, if not sooner.

Global narratives say greenhouse gas emissions continue to rise, with expectations that global temperatures will surpass the critical tipping point of 1.5 degrees C above industrial levels in a little more than a decade. Extreme weather events are becoming more common as a result, along with rising sea levels, and vulnerable communities are being hit disproportionately hard, despite having contributed least to climate change. However, just as many climate scientists report that climate shifts and temperature fluctuation have been happening all along for millennia. This is not new and we were never shaken up about it until globalists chose to use it as a reason for depopulation. The last few years have shown extremes in temperatures on both ends of the spectrum, hot and cold. In addition, many other occurrences of 'man-made weather manipulation' have been proven far more detrimental to both climate and the ultimate intensity of severe weather. Some extremely critical devastation has taken place in America since the end of COVID! It's called geoengineering, and has been increasing exponentially. Poisonous fog has been used to alter weather patterns in the forms of cloud seeding, adding chemicals to chem trails, and graphene rain. Our own military did biowarfare in like manner with influenza viruses. Climate engineering researcher Dane Wigington stated, "Extreme drought conditions that have plagued the Western U.S. are being turned around by more climate engineering. California has been in the bullseye. It's not good news because it goes from one destructive extreme to another. We know the technology exists and is being used to steer upper-level wind currents and, thus, steer moisture currents, directing moisture into areas they already engineered back-to-back snow storms! There is no question about this; it's hard science. Testing snow yields the same things listed in climate engineering patents— aluminum, barium, manganese, polymer fibers, graphene and surfactants. These are creating mass flooding now as we speak. (Study the atrocious flooding that happened in N.C. and Texas.) Can there be ANY legitimate discussion about climate change without addressing climate engineering first? The answer is patently 'NO'! We have to stop climate engineering statistically and mathematically or we are done in the very near term. These operations only serve the Masters by masking the true damage done to the climate while using weather as a weapon at the same time."[5]

Some gains have been made since 2015—including decreased childhood mortality, access to electricity, and improved treatments against certain diseases, but the report's overall takeaway is stark. "Unless we act now, the 2030 Agenda will become an epitaph for a world that might have been," says António Guterres, UN Secretary General.[6] However, closing the years 2024 and 2025, the above slight decreases in childhood mortality went out the proverbial window. It is impossible to guesstimate the exponential increase in infant and childhood mortality incurred due to the globally-driven exponential increase in COVID-19 vaccination. It is a case of globalist domination, which includes all the United Nations activities collectively. Its another perfect example of the globalists speaking from both corners of their mouths! No one can continually tout goals for global progress, while destroying them with different goals and actions!

THE 17 SUSTAINABLE DEVELOPMENTAL GOALS REPORT

1. NO Poverty—four years of progress in reducing poverty was erased by the COVID-19 Pandemic. Rising inflation and Ukraine's war caused further setback,; the number of people living in extreme poverty is still rising overall.

2. Zero Hunger—hunger and food insecurity have increased exponentially since 2015, further intensified by the compounded effects of the pandemic, conflict, climate change, and widening inequalities. The UN estimates 9.2% of the world population faced chronic hunger in 2022. 735 million people—up by 122 million from 2019. The 2024 Global Hunger Index score is 18.3, only a 0.5 decrease from 2016, It is highly unlikely it can meet the 2030 goal.
3. Good Health and Well-Being—Impacts of pandemic and other crises continue to take a toll on global health; some progress in early childhood mortality rates was made before the pandemic, but reducing maternal and childhood mortality and expanding universal (read global) health coverage is critically needed. (Again, childhood mortality rates have risen exponentially with the use of COVID-19 vaccines).

4. Quality Education—the pandemic caused severe disruption in 80% of the 104 countries studied. Without action, 84 million children and young people remained out of school and about 300 million students lack essential literacy and numeracy skills. There is still an average annual financing gap of $97 billion for low-and lower-middle-income countries.

5. Gender Equality—Only 15.4% of data indicators are on track. Progress in unpaid care and domestic work is falling behind. Almost 50% of married women lack the power to make decisions over their own sexual and reproductive health. Violence against women remains endemic.

6. Clean Water and Sanitation—water demand is rising due to rapid population growth, increasing pressure from agriculture and industry, and threats to wetland ecosystems. Concerns over water stress and water scarcity are growing. Current rates of progress need to increase 3-to-6 fold. In 2022, 2.2 billion people lacked safely-managed drinking water.

7. Affordable and Clean Energy— about 660 million people will live without electricity in 2030 if nothing changes. Slow progress toward clean cooking solutions means the health of over 2 billion people is also at risk That is approximately 25% of the world population.

8. Decent Work and Economic Growth—global economy is currently threatened by multiple crises—persistent inflation, increasing interest rates, and heightened uncertainties. Global real GDP per capita growth slowed in 2023, leading to decline in global employment, esp. among the young. (Gross Domestic Product is a monetary measure of total market value of all goods and services and produced and rendered in a specific time period by a country or countries—Wiki).

9. 9Industry, Innovation, and Infrastructure—growth in global manufacturing slid to 3.3% from 7.4% in 2021 amid a slow and uneven recovery from the pandemic and the least developed countries are not on track to double their share. Despite the presence of 3G broadband in most countries, the cost of devices and lack of literacy and digital skills remain steep barriers to internet adoption.

10. Reduced Inequalities—Income inequality was narrowing worldwide pre-COVID19, but the pandemic "may have reversed some of this progress." It has also intensified structural and systematic discrimination, leading to the worst between-country inequality in 3 decades. The number of refugees globally hit its highest on record in 2022, at 34.6 million.

11. Sustainable Cities and Communities—more than 50% of world population lives in cities—a rate that could rise to 70% by 2050. Over 1 billion people live in slums or informal settlements, with 2 billion more expected to be in this situation in the next 30 years. In 2022, only half of the world's population had easy access to public transportation.

12. Responsible Consumption and Production—increasing reliance on natural resources has set the Earth on an unsustainable course. It's causing the triple crises of climate change, biodiversity loss and pollution. High-income countries have a material footprint per capita 10 times higher than low-income countries.

13. Climate Action—the world is on the brink of a climate catastrophe and the window to avert it is rapidly closing. To limit warming to 1.5 degrees C, global greenhouse gas emissions need to be almost halved by 2030, but only a 0.3% decrease is predicted in this time. (This author doesn't believe this global warming/climate change narrative having studied trends exhaustively. It's far more dangerous in men's engineering hands than in God's hands!)

14. Life Below Water—continuing ocean acidification, plastic pollution and rising sea temperatures are threatening marine ecosystems. Some progress, but 17 million metric tons of plastic entered the ocean in 2021, while satellite imagery reveals elevated coastal eutrophication—the over-enrichment of water by excessive nutrients. Ocean health is still declining. (Once again, the largest area of problem is man-made!)

15. Life on Land—forest loss, land degradation and species extinction remain major threats to the planet and people, despite positive developments in forest management, environmental policy and accounting. Global forest coverage has decreased annually and extinction risk across mammal, bird, amphibian, and coral species has accelerated by 11% since 1993.

16. Peace, Justice, and Strong Institutions—conflict-related civilian deaths rose by 50% in 2022, largely due to the war in Ukraine. At the end of the year, a record 108.4 million people had been forcibly displaced worldwide—an increase of 19 million compared with end of 2021. Global homicides are at a 20-year high. Civilian deaths have also risen for the first time since the 2030 agenda was adopted. It jumped by 53% between 2021 and 2022 alone!

17. Partnerships for the Goals—record inflation, rising interest rates and growing debt burdens mean many developing countries are finding it harder than ever to thrive economically after the pandemic. Global trade increased after the pandemic restrictions were lifted, but the 2023 outlook is 'subdued.'

"GEOPOLITICAL TENSIONS AND NATIONALISM ARE HINDERING

INTERNATIONAL COORDINATION ON IMPORTANT GLOBAL ISSUES.[7]

The upshot of this particular document originating from the United Nations but being clearly supported by the World Economic Forum is very nearly worthless. We are being told in this report the majority of these goals set in 2015 have realized very little fulfillment and some have gone backward. The majority of the goals that haven't been met seem to have been slowed or stopped in any progress by the advent of the COVID-19 pandemic. The irony of this development is simple and abundantly clear. The United Nations, the World Economic

Forum, and other globalist entities are the groups touting the goals, yet these same globalists were most instrumental in planning and executing the pandemic. This dichotomy of purpose makes no sense unless we understand the reasons why. Staging a pandemic accomplished an entire passel of other goals, based on the real desire to have more recognition per power and money. However, they must maintain the global goals listed to show support for the pie-in-the-sky goals that will bring the unified global benefits they believe are also necessary. There was no mention made of one goal set canceling out the other, or why it actually did. Instead, for each of the 17 UN goals, there are simple but impossible suggestions made in the report that could make it happen in theory but not reality. The clear result is that goals are altruistic and humanitarian but will never be realistic or attainable under the best utopian dreams.

A second irony also surfaces over the term, NEW WORLD ORDER. Globalists want this to go both ways also. They tout the concept openly as if the whole idea is completely plausible and expected in the way they perceive it. However, a NEW WORLD ORDER under any other set of circumstances is a mere pie-in-the-sky theory. No one can have their cake and eat it too! Given the concept of a new world order being one that multiple groups of people have spoken of and planned for in their various belief systems, begs the conclusion there must be some basis for believing it! Naturally, believers of Scripture are very clear about the coming New World Order predicted by our Father, God. That new world order is known as the Tribulation and will be instituted and completed exactly as He has stated it, in His perfect time.

THE NEW WORLD ORDER PREDICTIONS

As it happens, a large group of people spread all over the globe do believe there is a New World Coming and possibly sooner than later. The same book that has been read for millennia, known as the Bible, is the #1 best-selling book of all time (about 1500 years). "According to the Guinness World Records…the Bible is the best-selling book of all time with an estimated 5-7 billion copies sold and distributed."[8] That figure is cited by multiple authoritative sources. The really wonderful news also cited here—in 2024, the US saw a 22% surge in Bible sales believed driven by demand for more printed editions, aesthetic redesigns such as journalling Bibles, and cultural shifts toward faith! Believers of the Bible who live by its inspired words, are very clear about the New World Order coming on this Earth as part of Almighty God's historical timeline. From the very beginning of man on earth, there has been a plan for all the ages, whereby one day, man will have done whatever he pleased for so long, he began to believe the idea "If there is a God who has a plan and actually cares what I do or don't do, I have no proof of it and no reason to believe it, so I'll just continue to live my life the way I want to." That idea has been promoted for millennia; however, it's never been true. What is true is that man sinned against his creator, and was separated from Him forever unless God intervened, which He did. He sent his perfect Son, Jesus, to this Earth, as the God-Man who would pay the price for our sin and make the way open to resume fellowship with God by choosing to accept his Son's sacrifice in our place. It seems like such a simple solution, and it is, so that no one would be excluded unless they chose to be forever separated from Him. Unfortunately, too many people still want to choose their own way instead. There is soon coming a day, when God will judge all those who rejected His Son.

That will be the day when the New World Order starts for a period of seven years. Satan, the enemy of God and His creation will be allowed to set up his reign with a chief ruler named Anti-Christ, so designated in scripture. It will encompass the entire globe, and he will be the most horrible despot the world has ever seen. He will make Xi Jinping look innocent!The Scriptures give us great detail about this New World Order, and all of the really abominable things that will happen at that time. The globalists think they will run the world with their billions or trillions and set it up along the lines of their plans, but that will not happen in the way they imagine. We will look at more of those details later in the book. In the meantime, to any who may now be reading this, please find a copy of the Holy Scriptures, and start reading about the real New World Order, lest you find yourself one day relegated to it.

> "And you will hear of wars and rumors of wars. See that you are NOT troubled; for all these things must come to pass, but the end is not yet. For nation will rise against nation, and kingdom against kingdom. And there will be famines, pestilences, and earthquakes in various places. All these are the beginning of sorrows...And because lawlessness will abound, the love of many will grow cold. And this gospel of the Kingdom will be preached in all the world as a witness to all the nations, and then the end will come. WATCH therefore, for you do not know what hour your Lord is coming. If those days had not been cut short, no one would survive..." Matthew 24:6-8;12;14; 22; 42 NIV

> "...there shall be a time of trouble, such as never was since there was a nation, even to that time. And at that time, your people shall be delivered, every one who is found written in the book, (*Lamb's Book of Life*)." Daniel 12:1 NIV

> "There will be signs in the sun, in the moon, and in the stars; and on the earth distress of nations, with perplexity, the sea and the waves roaring; men's hearts failing them from fear and the expectation of those things which are coming on the earth, for the powers of the heavens will be shaken." Luke 21:25-26 NIV

"Little children, it IS the last hour; and as you have heard that the Antichrist is coming, even now many antichrists have come, by which we know that it IS the last hour."

I John 2:18 NIV

"Let no man in any way deceive you, for this time will not come unless the apostasy comes first, and the man of lawlessness (Antichrist) is revealed, the son of destruction, who opposes and exalts himself above every so-called god or object of worship, so that he takes his seat in the temple of God, displaying himself as being God...Then that lawless one will be revealed whom the Lord will slay with the breath of His mouth and bring to an end by the appearance of HIS COMING" 2 Thessalonians 2:3-4; 8 NIV

"Then the kings of the earth, the princes, the generals, the rich (*including all globalists)*, the mighty, and everyone else, both slave and free, hid in caves and among the rocks of the mountains. They called to the mountains and rocks, 'Fall on us and hide us from the face of Him who sits on the throne (of heaven) and from the wrath of the Lamb! For the great day of Their wrath (judgment) has come, and who can withstand it?" Revelation 6:15 NIV

CHAPTER 8

A Timeline of the COVID-19 Pandemic

Earliest Events Making It All Possible

There are many people, places, and events for which it is necessary to have some understanding, before we can begin to understand how this disaster could have been so timely and well-orchestrated. The reader has already become acquainted with most of the major players and their agendas, but now it is important to see the intentional planning and execution of the major events that brought the pandemic to its expected delivery. The biggest facilitator of this hellacious debacle was clearly Anthony Fauci, so we'll begin with him in the year 1984. Ronald Reagan was President and continued as President in that election, walloping Walter Mondale. The cause of AIDS was identified as HIV. Michael Jackson caught his hair on fire! Crack cocaine showed up in Los Angeles. Alex Trebek gave his first answer on Jeopardy. Astronauts made their first untethered spacewalk. The deadliest mass shooting of the day happened at a McDonald's. Indira Gandhi was assassinated. But one of the worst things that could happen, though no one suspected it...happened.

1. **1984**—Anthony Fauci became the Director of the National Institute of Allergy and Infectious Diseases (NIAID), an Institute within the National Institutes of Health (NIH). These institutes are an agency of the U.S. Department of Health and Human Services (HHS). The NIH is the Federal focal point for health research and the caretaker of medical and behavioral

research for the Nation. For the record, that made Fauci a government employee and certainly in no way the final authority on health in our country! Because of the role he more or less usurped throughout the pandemic, it was assumed he had enormous power, but that was not the case. His decades as Director were NOT due to his expertise as an objective scientist. They were due strictly to his willingness to serve the wolves running the show, and then use and abuse anyone necessary to get the job done. Had he not taken orders, he wouldn't have lasted so long.

2. **March 1997**—At the Department of Microbiology and Immunology of the University of North Carolina at Chapel Hill, Ralph S. Baric engineered a mouse hepatitis coronavirus to cross species and infect baby hamster cells.[1] NIH funded this gain-of-function research. Once again, Dr. Breggin suggested it should be termed "gain-of-lethal-function" research more accurately! This study was a huge step toward infecting humans with animal coronaviruses.

3. **February 2000**—Researchers from the New York State Department of Health in Albany and the Institute of Virology in the Netherlands described the nature of the coronaviruses as having a narrow and specific host range due to host cell-receptors and showed the unlikelihood of Fauci's concern about an animal coronavirus jumping to humans. It could be made to happen in the lab but was extremely rare in nature. Coronaviruses were fairly easily manipulated in the lab but were NOT a major threat to humans unless humans made them into disease organisms.

4. **June 22-23, 2001**—"The Dark Winter Exercise was a simulated scenario involving an initial localized smallpox attack on Oklahoma City with additional smallpox cases in Georgia and Pennsylvania designed to spiral out of control and be an unwinnable bio-attack. Held at Andrews Air Force Base in

Washington D.C. over 2 weeks, it was an extensive war game of the National Security Council in which Johns Hopkins University, (first of many such with JHU), that eventually showed specific foreknowledge of the coming coronavirus pandemic. Such Pandemic Planning and Globalist Promotion began multiplying by 2017.

5. **2002-04—**SARS-CoV-1 (precursor to SARS-CoV-2, agent of COVID-19) appeared in southern China in late 2002 and spread around the world. It was very deadly and killed 10% of infected people but was contained before cases reached the U.S.[2] After it was contained, China promptly began engineering the virus in its labs—demonstrating it might have been able to engineer it originally from benign bat viruses—but the origin of SARS-CoV-1 was still unknown. By 2004, China's Beijing lab started having multiple accidental releases of other SARS-CoVs but with limited deaths. This led to infected persons with variants of SARS-CoV carrying them from labs, sometimes infecting others. Four of these happened in Beijing's Virus Institute. Later, investigators were able to get through the massive misinformation campaign produced by Fauci, Gates, WHO, the CCP, and a large number of other globalist wolves. Some key observations came from this:

    - No SARS-CoV has ever been found in nature—the obvious conclusion—it almost certainly originated in a lab.
    - Some "SARS-like" CoVs had been found in bats in caves, however it took monumental scientific manipulation to convert them into viruses capable of infecting animal or human cells. Consequently, changing "SARS-like" CoV into pandemic SARS-CoV-2 was a ginormous bioengineering feat that took decades of work and billions of dollars, most of which were funneled to labs from American tax-payers largely by Fauci.

- Any risk of SARS-CoV emergence from nature was almost non-existent. But there was a very high risk of accidental or deliberate release, especially considering it had happened several (at least 6) times previously.

6. **April 17, 2003**—Globally, laboratories quickly became able to study and to work with the virus, and a team of scientists submitted the complete genome for a strain of SARS-CoV-1 to the CDC.[3] (Seventeen years before the pandemic)

7. **November 2003**—There are now multiple lab studies supporting the potential use of chloroquine and its derivative hydroxychloroquine for the treatment of SARS-CoV, including in The Lancet, which provided numerous citations.[4] Papers demonstrated their mechanisms of action for prevention and treatment in both cell cultures and in animals. The safety of this already long-term use of this drug IS emphasized. Note: this was also seventeen years before there was any necessity for coronavirus treatment. However, when Big Pharma wanted to apply the Emergency Use Authorization to COVID-19 to fund vaccine and drug research and push them out rapidly without the usual FDA approval, there was a very big hitch. The EUA could not be used by law if there were any other effective drugs available. Therefore, the prior extensive research confirming hydroxychloroquine as effective treatment for COVID-19 infections was both ignored and suppressed while doctors were informed there were no safe treatments available, so that experimental vaccines and toxic remdesivir could be rushed out without adequate testing or completion of clinical trials. This completely fraudulent suppression of effective, safe, and inexpensive treatments clearly made Big Pharma and its investors wealthier and more powerful, but resulted in millions of totally unnecessary deaths and the crushing of economies throughout the Western world during COVID-19.

8. **2006a**—Research proved that when impaired or elderly VACCINATED mice were exposed to SARS-CoV, they had potentially deadly reactions to the 'N' protein within the virus.[5] Additional research found the same problem presented with the spike(S) protein. Animal research continued to establish this deadly 'S' protein risk right up to the time the COVID-19 vaccines were being rushed through the FDA authorization process in Operation Warp Speed.

9. **2006b—Pandemic Planning and Globalist Promotion.** The International Finance Facility for Immunization (IFFIm) was established. Its purpose was to enable poorer nations to obtain guaranteed, inexpensive loans for buying vaccines through novel loan arrangements with the Bank of America and other funding sources. However those loans were connected to two globalist 'wolf' organizations—the Coalition for Epidemic Preparedness Innovations (CEPI) and the Vaccine Alliance (GAVI) and in cooperation with UNICEF, WHO and COVAX. All are globalist wolves who found ways to increase the MARKETS of Big Pharma. Bottom line: the loans cycled back into Big Pharma and its investors.

10. **December 2008**—Vanderbilt University and the University of North Carolina under Ralph Baric developed a "bat SARS-like coronavirus" a "SARS-CoV," that infected live mice and "human ciliated airway epithelial cells" in the lab.[6] This was considered a major breakthrough because it was a turning point, but didn't get much coverage in the media. In other words, they started with a harmless bat virus and an added spike protein, and they made a SARS-CoV that could infect both live mice and human lung cells! Human antibodies would attack this virus in the living mice and the human lung epithelium. This was news to excite global wolves who could make trillions of dollars on vaccines while mandating them for everyone under total authoritarian governance. All that remained was to wait for a COVID-19 pandemic to come along, still 14 years away.

11. **2009—**Moderna, a new pharmaceutical company, was founded with the primary goal of making mRNA vaccines.[7] It had neither products, nor income, but the globalist wolves invested their really big money. This was already known to be a dangerous and highly experimental product Moderna would produce, at best. Following are two quotes that show these facts very clearly:

12. **In 2012, a scientific report in PLOS ONE stated:** "These SARS-CoV vaccines ALL induced antibody protection against infection with SARSCoV. However, a challenge of mice given any of the vaccines led to the occurrence of the-type [sic] immunopathology suggesting hypersensitivity to SARS-CoV components was induced. Caution in proceeding to application of a SARS-CoV vaccine in humans is indicated."[8]

13. **A financial analysis in April 2021 noted retrospectively:** Moderna's technology platform inserted synthetic nucleoside-modified mRNA (modRNA) into human cells using a coating of lipid nanoparticles. This mRNA then reprogramed the cells to prompt immune responses. It was a novel technique, abandoned by other manufacturers due to concerns about the toxicity of lipid nanoparticles at high or frequent doses."[9]

14. **January 2010—Pandemic Planning and Globalist Promotion.** Bill and Melinda Gates called for the next ten years to be the "Decade of Vaccines."[10] Note: The COVID-19 vaccinations were already being made Ten Years before the COVID-19 pandemic started.

15. **May 2010—Pandemic Planning and Globalist Promotion.** Just about one decade before COVID-19, the Rockefeller Foundation published a future pandemic scenario in a business investment-oriented, 53-page booklet, "Scenarios for the Future of Technology and International Development."[11] The first "Scenario Narrative" in the booklet was called "Lock Step: A World of Tighter Top-down Governmental Control and More

Authoritarian Leadership, With Limited Innovation and Growing Citizen Pushbacks." The OPENING LINE was, "In 2012, the pandemic that the world has been anticipating for years finally hit!" The only regret voiced about the pandemic in this imaginary scenario was the lack of investment opportunity! Interestingly, even though dozens of "what if" scientific articles showed up, especially as early as 2008, the idea of a coronavirus pandemic and expensive vaccines with unlimited profit opportunities had supposedly not been imagined by these money-hungry globalist investors. Nevertheless, the ideas presented for this type of governance looked very advantageous and was seen as a permanent fixture after the next coming pandemic.

16. **December 2, 2010—Pandemic Planning and Globalist Promotion**—from the Bill and Melinda Gates Foundation: "New York: The WHO, UNICEF, NIAID, and the Bill and Melinda Gates Foundation announced a collaboration to increase coordination across the international vaccine community to create a Global Vaccine Action Plan."[12] Its Leadership Council was reintroduced with Dr. Margaret Chan (Hong Kong) as Director General of WHO at the top, then Anthony Fauci of NIAID among five elite internationals. This document confirmed Fauci was working with Bill Gates all the way back to December of 2010, making the overall plans for the coming pandemic and the criminal mandating of toxic vaccines on the world. The audacity of it all was/is utterly appalling.

Intensified & Multiplied Events-One Decade Before COVID-19

17. **September 2011—Pandemic Planning and Globalist Promotion.** The U.N. passed Resolution 2030, and declared all governments and international corporations would collaborate under the U.N. to accomplish a huge number of goals for the world by 2030, and became the MODEL for the Great Reset but without U.N. governance. With all its "pie-in-the-sky" aims

there was no mention made of fighting authoritarian governance, and certainly no idea of personal freedoms or political liberty. It mentioned vaccines three separate times. Before the start of the Great Reset, the U.N. called for making vaccines free for everyone, while protecting corporations (i.e. Big Pharma) from "financial risk" or losses: "Achieve universal health coverage, including financial risk protection, access to quality essential health-care services, and access to safe, effective, quality, and affordable, essential medicines and vaccines for all."[13]

18. **September 21,2011—**"A research article by Fauci's NIAID and the University of North Carolina, with Baric's name on it, reconfirmed and illustrated important problems associated with gain-of-function research with coronaviruses:") It began by repeating the lie; there were many SARS-CoV viruses in animal reservoirs waiting to emerge, making it necessary to do more research: "Severe Acute Respiratory Syndrome CoronaVirus (SARS-CoV) was an important emerging virus that was highly pathogenic in aged populations and was maintained with great diversity in zoonotic reservoirs"; B) Further, it made clear they had already created many other pathogenic variations on the original SARSCoV-1, since they were using them in their experiments. It also verified two other serious problems with SARS-CoV vaccines: Vaccines made for one variant of SARS-CoV were not effective for others AND aged vaccinated mice exposed to SARS-Co-V were not protected and instead were vulnerable to human-like severe immune reactions. The spike protein was the source of the problem: "Importantly, aged animals displayed increased eosinophilic immune pathology in the lungs and were NOT protected against significant virus replication" AND "When challenged with zoonotic and human chimeric (a genetic chimera is a single organism composed of cells with more than one distinct genotype) SARSCoV incorporated variant spike glycoproteins; the aged-mouse model reproduced severe lung damage

associated with human disease, including diffuse alveolar damage, hyaline membrane formation, and death." A huge takeaway from all this was the COVID-19 disease itself and deaths from the vaccines, especially in the elderly vaccinated people challenged with SARS-CoV-2 virus, were predicted and seemingly planned from the very beginning. The deadly capacity was built into the spike protein for all mRNA and DNA vaccines to force the cells of the human body to make innumerable exact copies of the SARSCoV-2 spike protein, poisoning the body from the inside out. The research on animals continued confirming this deadly effect even after the vaccines went into production with Operation Warp Speed.[15]

19. **September 2012**—A review article warned against starting research on humans with mRNA vaccines, in part because animals given the vaccines became more ill than expected and even died when they were later exposed to a SARS-CoV lab-engineered virus.

20. **September 2013—Pandemic Planning and Globalist Promotion.** NIH awarded $10,000,000 to Baric and UNC to study and manipulate "highly pathogenic human respiratory and systemic viruses which caused acute and chronic life-threatening disease outcomes. Baric said the "focus" would be on "highly pathogenic coronavirus infections, using SARS-CoV and MERS-CoV as models."[16]

21. **October 2014**—On White House stationery, President Barack Obama called for a moratorium on gain-of-function research that manipulated animal viruses increasing their capacity to infect and harm other species, including humans. Fauci ignored the President's moratorium and worked around this prohibition. In particular, he never stopped funding the single most important and most dangerous gain-of-function research being done by Menachery at the University of North Carolina, which Fauci funds to this very day through EcoHealth Alliance (Peter Daszak).[17]

22. **2015a—**Fauci approved China's first-ever Bio-safety Level-4 (BSL-4) lab at the Wuhan Institute of Virology to facilitate giving money to Wuhan scientists for gain-of-function research.

23. **2015b—Pandemic Planning and Globalist Promotion.** Bill Gates was now investing in the mRNA vaccine industry.[18]

24. **2015c—Pandemic Planning and Globalist Promotion.** Reports in May 2021 confirmed the obvious. In 2015, Chinese Communists discussing among themselves the use of coronaviruses as biological weapons with observations about the acute and permanent fear and disability they would create.[19] Biological warfare experts in the U.S. were likely doing the same thing. The likelihood should be taken for granted, especially since DARPA was openly funding U.S. coronavirus research.

25. **2015d—Pandemic Planning and Globalist Promotion.** Bill Gates conceived of the Coalition for Epidemic Preparedness Innovations (CEPI) in 2015 and funded it through the Bill & Melinda Gates Foundation. Gates organized a worldwide alliance to finance and coordinate the development of new vaccines making a financial killing and reorganizing and basically controlling world governance in the coming pandemic.[20]

    - Klaus Schwab and his WEF was a second founder of CEPI. He worked closely with Gates and in 2020 unveiled his Great Reset, which became the mantra for Bill Gates, Joe Biden, John Kerry, the CCP and all other globalists wanting to suppress all independent, patriotic, freedom-oriented, America-First movements.
    - Wellcome Trust, a British "charitable" trust, another CEPI founder based on Big Pharma funding, focused on the health arena, and was one of the largest charities in the world.

- The government of India, like the CCP is another founder, along with Germany and Japan, completed the fusion between the large corporations, giant "philanthropic" orgs, and very large government.

- WHO joined in 2017 and became the announced scientific arbiter for all CEPI activities and also tied the whole pandemic planning program to both the U.N. and of course to the CCP which controls WHO.
- The CEPI coalition controlled the unfolding of COVID-19 and the Great Reset. Although they were joined by innumerable billionaires, corporations, philanthropic groups, governments and their agencies, Anthony Fauci, a member of Gates' small, elite vaccine Advisory Council, was THE one of Bill Gates' leading implementers most key to the whole program.

26. **January 26-27, 2015—Pandemic Planning and Globalist Promotion.** "At the Berlin Pledging Conference 2015, the Bill and Melinda Gates Foundation announced 1.55 billion USD designated for GAVI's next 2016-2025 strategic period."[21] GAVI is the Global Alliance for Vaccines and Immunization, and, like so many of the Gates' daring ventures, had been roundly criticized for representing the interests of Big Pharma, which he regularly did.[22] It's a corporate/ government fusion which bypassed the decision-making process of a democratic republic such as the U.S. in favor of globalist wolves' plans. It has since been the Great Reset. These large, organized investments in vaccines took place five years before COVID-19!

27. **April 2015—**Pandemic Planning and Globalist Promotion. Bill Gates gave a famous TED Talk explaining that if anything was going to kill 10 million people worldwide, it would be a virus. His usual affect held a touch of grim humor that many people found shocking.[23] All people should find it shocking and diabolical!

28. **December 2015—Menachery and Baric at the University of North Carolina made a major breakthrough.** They transformed benign bat coronaviruses into epidemic SARS-CoV pathogens capable of infecting live mice and human lung tissue preparations. However, a bigger threat was also disclosed by the publication. With Fauci-funding, U.S. researchers collaborated with top CCP scientists from the Wuhan Institute of Virology (WIV), a CCP facility directed by their military's leading biological warfare specialist. Despite President Obama's moratorium on gain-of-function research, Fauci continued to fund both American and CCP researchers in this extremely dangerous type of experimentation. "Those collaborations created at least two nightmare scenarios: a major risk of the poorly managed WIV accidentally leaking one of its many manmade SARS-Co-V pathogens and the certain step of advancing the biological warfare capacity of the CCP and its military."[24]

29. **January-November 2016—Pandemic Planning and Globalist Promotion. CEPI: Preliminary Business Plan & the Big Master Plan.** Actual planning began at least as early as January 2016 and was published in November 2016. It brought global "wolves" together in one organization created by Bill Gates and Klaus Schwab, called CEPI: The Coalition for Epidemic Preparedness Innovations. This fulfilled Gates' ambition to run the financing of the coming pandemic within his partner Klaus Schwab's concept of the Great Reset, effectively fusing corporate/government funding under the control of elite billionaires and other hand-picked entities led by Gates. "The sole purpose was to develop expensive new vaccines at rapid speed with government support, while bypassing FDA requirements—everything Gates and CEPI got abundantly four years later during COVID-19, including all drug company costs fully reimbursed.[25] The corporate/government fusion was clearly seen in the establishment of the Biomedical

Advanced Research and Development Authority (BARDA) and its director Rick Bright who was on both the Task Team for Science and Regulation and the CEPI Scientific Advisory Committee. In 2020, he helped prevent President Trump from spoiling their plans by releasing federal stockpiles of hydroxychloroquine. Other CEPI "partners" included FDA, NIH, NIAID, and WHO. Big Pharma and other elites are the CEPI backbone. Gates and partners led a global governance over all sovereign nations—except Communist China, to which all others deferred.

30. **February 2016—Pandemic Planning and Globalist Promotion.** The Wuhan Institute and other Chinese Communist sponsors announced an international conference to be held on October 21-23, 2016, in Wuhan: "Nature Conference: Viral Infection and Immune Response."[26] Many speakers were from the U.S. including two from NIAID! The conference brochure boasted outrageously about the Wuhan Institute, "Pathogenic study of emerging infectious diseases has become one of the major research fields. Great achievements have been made in animal origin studies of SARS-CoV and avian influenza viruses."[27] The Director of the WIV and two of her four deputies had extensive training in the United States in fields such as gain-of-function and biological warfare. One of the WIV's top three officials was Changcai HE, Deputy Secretary of the Party at the Wuhan Branch, held a high-ranking position in the Communist Party. When the pandemic surfaced in January 2020, the Wuhan Institute of Virology was directly taken over by the military.[28]

31. **March 14, 2016—Pandemic Planning and Globalist Promotion.** The prediction of a COVID-19 scenario gained scientific approval (but NOT validity) from a follow-up article by Menachery et al. in the Proceedings of the National Academy of Sciences (PNAS) The article declared the risk of the spontaneous emergence of a SARS-CoV pandemic pathogen was now more likely because researchers had been able to

make pathogens out of harmless bat viruses in the lab. This was now the preposterous lie: "I was able to construct a plague from an innocent virus, so now I can expect nature to do it!!!"

32. **May 2016—Pandemic Planning and Globalist Promotion.** The governing body of the World Health Organization (WHO) approved the CEPI/Bill Gates' master plan for collaborating with WHO to control the profits, organization, and governance of the coming pandemic, none of which was the designated business of WHO. WHO's primary allegiance was/is to Communist China.

33. **January 2017a—**This is the year Pandemic Planning and Globalist Promotions exploded in anticipation of a coming pandemic, often identified as caused by a SARS-coronavirus.

34. **January 2017b—Pandemic Planning and Globalist Promotion.** "Homeland Security published a 135-page grand plan for an interagency response to "biological incidents"[29] The plan included the application of the Emergency Use Authorization (EUA)!

35. **January 9, 2017—Pandemic Planning and Globalist Promotion.** President Obama's administration officially recommended lifting the moratorium on gain-of-function (GOF) research and provided the necessary steps to be taken.[29] "The recommendation was made by the Director of the Office of Science and Technology Policy (OSTP), also known then as the Science Czar, John Holdren. The American Report identified him as an advocate of "massive-scale human population reduction measures such as adding reproductive sterilization agents to food and water supplies and enacting forced abortions in the U.S."[30] President Obama's HHS Director, responsible for authorizing and lifting the memorandum was "Sylvia Burwell, former President of the Global Development Program and COO of the Bill and Melinda Gates Foundation,"[31] "President Obama took action on this 11 days before Donald Trump took office, and President Trump was kept completely in the dark

about it."[32] However, "on the eve of the Obama-Biden departure, they provided all the authorizations needed for the eventual re-funding of GOF research by the U.S., enabling NIH to finalize the details at the end of 2017."[33] With this information, we know certainly that President Trump had absolutely nothing to do with resurrecting the GOF research. We also now know that lifting the ban was a part of the January 2017 Gates-led resurgence in developing vaccines, still 3 years ahead of the COVID19 onset.

36. **January 10, 2017—Pandemic Planning and Globalist Promotion.** Ten days before President Trump's inauguration, the primary speaker at a Georgetown University Conference on "Pandemic Preparedness in the Next Administration," Fauci unequivocally declared President Trump would "definitely" face a pandemic during his first term. He expressed his certainty several times during his speech. Naturally, Fauci also urged the immediate development of the corporate/government collaborations, part of the coming Great Reset. The Harvard School of Public Health, boasting of being co-founders in tight collaboration with the Chinese Communist Party (CCP), was represented at the conference by Ashish K. Jha, M.D. He gave a speech about his anticipation of the coming pandemic and also advocated for a global response resembling the same ideas of the Global Reset and Operation Warp Speed and urged the complete cooperation of government and business.[34]

37. **Janûary 13, 2017a—Pandemic Planning and Globalist Promotion.** The FDA announced new guidelines for its Emergency Use Authorization (EUA), originally passed by Congress after 9/11.[35] The new regulations strengthened the highly- accelerated development and production of medications and vaccines in an epidemic (which was already planned), completely bypassing the FDA's usual safeguards, and creating extravagantly useless, billion-dollar products for Big Pharma and its investors.

38. **January 13, 2017b—Pandemic Planning and Globalist Promotion.** A White House planning meeting was held when Obama Administration officials briefed the Trump Administration on preparations for a global pandemic. Following is the description given by the leader of said exercise:[36] "January 13, 2017, national security officials assembled in the White House to chart a response to a global pandemic. A new virus **is** spreading with alarming speed, causing global transportation stoppages, supply-chain disruptions, and plunging stock prices. With a vaccine many months away, U.S. health-care infrastructure **is** severely strained."

39. **"No, I didn't get that date wrong! This happened!** It was part of a transition exercise that outgoing officials from the administration of President Barack Obama convened for the benefit of the incoming team of President Donald Trump. As Homeland Security and Counter-terrorism Adviser to President Obama, I led the exercise, in which my colleagues and I sat side by side with the incoming national security team to discuss the most pressing Homeland Security concerns they would face." (Dr. Peter Breggin)[36]

40. **January 20-24, 2017**—Klaus Schwab held his annual World Economic Forum (WEF) at Davos, Switzerland. There was much concern over the U.S. government's America First (MAGA) populist mandate under President Donald Trump. They understood the Trump administration would NOT be docile or subservient with the CCP regime. In direct and deliberate defiance of Trump, **Schwab invited the CCP's despot dictator, Xi Jinping, to give the keynote speech and criticize America.** Later conferences run by Schwab and Bloomberg became more and more antagonistic toward Trump's nationalistic policies and fawned more and more over CCP's leaders.

41. **January 18, 2017—Pandemic Planning and Globalist Promotion. CEPI was officially unveiled** in a press release from Schwab's Davos site *as a* "Global partnership launched to prevent epidemics with new vaccines. New sources of international support were added: CEPI is supported by several leading pharmaceutical companies with strength in vaccines—GSK, Merck, J & J, Pfizer, Sanofi, and Takeda, plus the Biotechnology Innovation Organization (BIO). From the earliest beginning, all this planning had been about making more money from vaccines, along with imposing on governments, philanthropic and corporate governance called the Great Reset. Clearly, the prevailing agenda had a fully 'progressive' face since just a little more than one year previously, 193 nations adopted the U.N.'s "Sustainable Development Goals—the roadmap for the future we want."[37]

42. **January 23 and March 2017—Pandemic Planning and Globalist Promotion.** At Schwab's Davos Conference and then later in Schwab's office at the WEF, Bill Gates described his preparations for an inevitable, forthcoming pandemic. That was when he unveiled the new fund called the Coalition for Epidemic Preparedness Innovations (CEPI). Again it was co-founded by Gates and Schwab. It clearly confirmed the vaccine scam was very closely linked to what was becoming Schwab's totalitarian Great Reset. (Still 3 years from pandemic onset.) CEPI became the multi-billion-dollar collaboration between large private donors and corporations, the U.N., and national governments to research and make vaccines for the much-planned for pandemic. Empowered by the FDA guidelines for EUA, Gates avidly promoted the NEED for bypassing federal regulations to produce the vaccines in a process that normally required years; with EUA it would take 'less than one year. He mentioned Moderna as one of the "key" corporations already working on new platforms for "novel" vaccines, based on either "mRNA" or "DNA." In other, quicker words, Bill Gates showed

he had already invented, invested in, and started the project process identical to what was three years later "unveiled" as *Operation Warp Speed* by Fauci and President Trump. Gates said his plans were for a superspeed vaccine project handled in the context of the new corporate/governmental capitalism SCHWAB WAS ALREADY PROMOTING AS THE GREAT RESET. GATES AND SCHWAB WERE NOT "lone" wolves—they had plenty of powerful, financial support. ALL the top American corporations were obsessed with growing their wealth and power through **unrestricted business with the CCP**, who were then conducting their own unrestricted warfare against America.

43. **February 18, 2017—Pandemic Planning and Globalist Promotion.** At the Munich Security Conference, Bill Gates made the following predictions: "The next epidemic could originate on the computer screen of a terrorist intent on using genetic engineering to create a synthetic version of the smallpox virus...or a super contagious and deadly strain of the flu. Whether it occurs by a quirk of nature or at the hand of a terrorist, epidemiologists say a fast-moving airborne pathogen could kill more than 30 million people in less than a year. And they say there is a reasonable probability the world will experience such an outbreak in the next 10 to 15 years." He again spoke of the need for vaccines, "Most of the things we need to do to protect against a naturally occurring pandemic are the same things we must prepare, for an intentional biological attack."[38] In March 2017, The Lancet- Infectious Diseases (UK) positioned CEPI as the central funding and organizing center for pandemic preparation.

44. **July 21, 2017—Pandemic Planning and Globalist Promotion. In June,2021, (one year into the planned pandemic)**, the actual "master plan" for CEPI was discovered, leading to the discovery of the original CEPI: Preliminary Business Plan. Interim CEO of CEPI, John-Arne Røttingen, presented an amazing 21page

PowerPoint presentation to the WHO Association. That document confirmed and strengthened all the points made in the book about advanced planning, including the enormous profits assigned to Bill Gates. The table gave a broad description of the global predators, only omitting the CCP which worked through WHO. CEPI described how it would divide up the world with WHO during the coming pandemic. Among the more than 20 large global entities described, only one was mentioned by name, "Gates" who would participate in "Development/Licensure." CEPI took control over everything except setting healthcare and scientific standards, the newly designated task of WHO. Clearly, the whole plan sprung primarily from Gates' inspiration and determination—with no regard whatsoever to plans being made for all humanity by people with no elected or appointed status to do so. It also continues to be clear—it was all about making a fortune and increasing power and control through vaccines.[39]

45. **October 2017— Pandemic Planning and Globalist Promotion** The Johns Hopkins University (JHU) Bloomberg School of Public Health released an indepth projection on how to deal with a coming "coronavirus" pandemic with vaccines. The title of said forecast, a play-on-words, was *SARS: The SPARS Pandemic, 2025-2028.* The fictional vaccine was, Corovax, after coronavirus. This was NOT the famous Event 201, conducted live two years later in October, 2019 as a wargame against the coronavirus. The SPARS Pandemic placed more emphasis on pushing the vaccines for the coronavirus—***3 years ahead of COVID-19.***

46. **December 8, 2017**—Dr. Tal Zaks, Moderna's Chief Medical Officer, compared mRNA to a "line of code" in a computer program and declared that with the new mRNA vaccines being used experimentally for cancer treatment, "we are actually hacking the software of life."[40] Transhumanism and vaccine technology united!

47. **March 20, 2018**—A scientific review described a huge upsurge in mRNA vaccine research, "ringing in a new era in vaccinology."[41] A table revealed Moderna, a 2010 upstart company, was funded by the Gates' Foundation, by Defense Advanced Research Project Agency (DARPA), and BARDA (the governmental agency that implemented Operation Warp Speed and the giveaway of billions of dollars to Big Pharma in the style of the Great Reset). The table also revealed Gates was involved with CureVac AG, and supported by the CEPI investment fund, Gates' brainchild. With many other corporations, he created an enormous tangle of complex business interests, all involving vaccines. The scientific review cited a warning that moving from animal to human infections had been stymied by two problems. The first issue involved "rare cases of severe injection site or systemic reactions" from mRNA, requiring further preclinical and clinical studies into "systemic inflammation." The second issue was ineffectiveness in generating immunological responses in humans. Individual scientific reports gave an even worse picture. Evidence mounted that the billionaires, Big Pharma, and government agencies had made an enormously bad bet on mRNA vaccines, but the commitment to it and the momentum for marketing these toxic, experimental vaccines left no room for turning back.[42]

48. **April 27, 2018—Pandemic Planning and Globalist Promotion—** Bill Gates gave an address sponsored by the Massachusetts Medical Society and the New England Journal of Medicine entitled: "Ring the Alarm: The next epidemic is coming. Here's how we can make sure we're ready."[43] Gates described the assembling of forces he, Fauci, and others were already executing while predicting the seemingly inevitable pandemic: "The world must prepare for pandemics in the same manner the military prepares for war. This includes simulations and other preparedness exercises so we can better understand how

diseases will spread and how to deal with things like quarantine and communications to minimize panic."[43] (like that was EVER a concern! The goal was always to incite panic!)

49. **October 2018—Pandemic Planning and Globalist Promotion—** The Johns Hopkins Bloomberg School of Public Health, Division of Public Security, is the source of all JHU pandemic planning events. A nightmarish book entitled, *Technologies to Address Global Catastrophic Biological Risks*, described creating projects for handling any upcoming pandemic threats, specifically including, "SARS and MERS coronaviruses. It was an actual blueprint for how to take complete control of society and mandate vaccines despite public opposition."[44]

The Bloomberg School of Public Health book chilled the reader to the bone when it went on to promote potential solutions previously ridiculed as conspiracy theories that never were such: "Self-Spreading Vaccines: Self-spreading vaccines were genetically engineered to permeate through whole populations exactly like communicable diseases, but instead of causing disease, they conferred protection. The general idea was a small number of people in a target population could be vaccinated like this, and that vaccine strain would then circulate in that population like a pathogenic virus does, causing rapid, widespread immunity."[45]

Worse still, the Hopkins report understood this technology posed lethal potential risks, but the only concern they voiced had nothing to do with the risks; it was only a concern of possibly alienating public opinion due to the risk of vaccine-induced disease.[46]

"As Ginger Breggin said, 'Yesterday's conspiracy theories keep becoming today's headlines!'"[47]

COVID-19 Emerges 2019 Through August, 2021

50. **2019—Pandemic Planning and Globalist Promotion—Fauci's NIAID**, primarily through Peter Daszak's EcoHealth Alliance, was awarded four more years of coronavirus research, including gain-of-function studies. Funding to date went through 2021 and the project itself through 2025.[48]

51. **January 2019—Pandemic Planning and Globalist Promotion—** Klaus Schwab's World Economic Forum (WEF) teamed up with the Harvard Global Health Institute and published an informational document entitled, "Outbreak Readiness and Business Impact—Protecting Lives and Livelihoods Across the Global Economy."[49] The Harvard Global Health Institute (HGHI) was led by Ashish K. Jha, who joined Fauci on January 10, 2019, to predict the pandemic would ensue during the upcoming administration of Donald Trump. The document, one year before the "official" start of COVID-19, mentioned 'coronaviruses' twice and 'SARS' seven times. The focus of the document was to iterate 'The societal threat posed by epidemics provides a compelling platform for engagement across the public and private sectors.' However, in Schwab's and the Globalist wolves' view, pandemics were the perfect way of enforcing the Great Reset doctrine of corporate-government fusion.[48] The goal was to establish totalitarian control to bypass, and crush the legal protection and liberties of the United States' patriotic democratic republic.

52. **May 1, 2019—Pandemic Planning and Globalist Promotion—** More than six months prior to the pandemic breakout in China, a bill was introduced in the U.S. House of Representatives proposing a $100 billion program to FORCE Epidemic Tracking on Americans.[50] The bill was "COVID-19 Testing, Reaching, And Contacting Everyone (TRACE) Act," and its highly interesting number was HR6666!![51] It was heavily criticized as a dangerous step toward totalitarianism and was NOT passed.[52]

Even though there is evidence Gates influenced the creation of the bill, there is no evidence the bill would finance his activities. This insane bill contributed to the mounting evidence of active continued preparation for the coming pandemic.

53. **September 2019—Pandemic Planning and Globalist Promotion—**A World at Risk: Annual Report on Global Preparedness for Health Emergencies by the Global Preparedness Monitoring Board **(GPMB)** is a book sponsored by the World Health Organization (WHO) and the World Bank with acknowledgments to familiar globalist organizations like the Johns Hopkins University Center for Health Security and Wellness Trust. Its emphasis was focused on rapid, innovative vaccine development, and included "surge manufacturing" of "nucleic acid types" which would be "pre-tested and approved for them within mere weeks. Once again, it anticipated the planned Operation Warp Speed. Members of this board included Fauci, Chris Elias, president of Global Development Program (GDP), Gates Foundation-USA, George F. Gao, Director-general of the Chinese CDC-PRC, and MANY other high-ranking global officials. This first annual report surfaced just before the pandemic broke out in China.[53]

54. **October 2019—Pandemic Planning and Globalist Promotion—** The Johns Hopkins Bloomberg School of Public Health—which had published The SPARS Pandemic, 2025-2028, just two years prior, held the greatly publicized pandemic simulation called Event 201. It literally brought together representatives of governments, corporations, and investors exactly as planned for the near future to collaborate in wargame style against a "pandemic" caused by a SARS-CoV virus. It was sponsored by Bill Gates, Klaus Schwab, and Michael Bloomberg for whom the School of Public Health was named, along with many other globalist participants. It magnified and strengthened connections between pandemic prep, the Great Reset, and Gates' Warp Speed-like program. Once again, the chronic

theme was "Governments, international organizations, and businesses planning ahead for how essential corporate capabilities would be utilized during a large-scale pandemic.'"[54]

55. **November 2019**—Michael Bloomberg directly assaulted President Trump's policies and diplomacy when he held his second New Economy Forum in Beijing, China, where the CCP's despot Xi Jinping made a smiling appearance. His conference was co-sponsored by the CCP and its theme was "recoupling with China." Funding partners included 3M, Exxon Mobile, FedEx, HSBC, Hyundai, and Master Card. Right after the conference, Bloomberg announced his candidacy for President of the U.S., THE nation he was deliberately sacrificing for the additional wealth he could attain with the CCP. He did not glean the nomination, but what we got wasn't any better.[55]

56. **December 1, 2019**—Cases of "viral pneumonia" began showing up in China, although in retrospect, there were cases in November and probably sooner. The pandemic was exactly the boon to all the globalists and CCP they expected. At least 400 billionaires grew their already sickening wealth by an average of 60% in the first year of COVID.

57. **January 2020—Pandemic Planning and Globalist Promotions**—Using the same title as the 2017 book by Johns Hopkins, The SPARS Pandemic was republished as a one-subject work in the Journal of International Crisis and Risk, with a new subtitle and focus: "A Futurist Scenario to Facilitate Medical Countermeasure Communication."[56] Like the original book, the star vaccine was named Corovax. Naturally, the emphasis was on communication with the public to overcome criticism of the vaccines and gain their compliance with vaccinations. It takes time to publish a journal article and since the original was published in 2019 or sooner, this 'reprint' looked like a prediction when it was planned all along.

58. **January 2020a**—The Wuhan Institute was openly seized by the CCP's Peoples' Liberation Army under General Chen Wei, a leading expert in biochemical weapons and bioterrorism.[57] However, the truth was that the CCP policy of military-civil fusion (MCF), and the WIV and its work had already been inseparable from the military for several decades.[58] A U.S. State Department memo defined military-civil fusion as follows: "As the name suggests, a key part of MCF is the elimination of barriers between China's civilian research and commercial sectors, and its military and defense industrial sectors. The CCP implemented this strategy, not just through its own research and development efforts, but also by acquiring and diverting the world's cutting-edge technologies—including through theft—in order to achieve military dominance."[59] 57. January 2020b—"Multiple scientific sources within China concluded SARS-CoV2 was a chimeric or man-made virus based on, among other things, the artificially tailored spike protein inserted into the virus which enables it to attack humans and is NOT found in nature. Then China began censoring, punishing, and "disappearing" doctors, scientists, and journalists who described the pandemic or identified its source as the Wuhan Institute."[60] As a result, one researcher rejected his original conclusions, at least one physician died, and another disappeared. Another courageous scientist fled to America to tell the truth. The WHO generously covered up for the CCP, and retold their lies. From this time on, the entire wolf pack of globalists who dominated Western governments, media, educational institutions, medicine, and science declared adamantly that the Wuhan Institute of Virology (WIV) was NOT the origin of the virus and it came from nature! Social media started deleting or censoring comments calling the SARS-CoV-2 virus, the 'China virus' or attributing it to the WIV. It was labeled a baseless conspiracy theory. This process continued from the Big Tech industry for the duration of the pandemic and even now has changed little; Big Tech remains

in the hip pockets of the globalist wolves for all intent and purposes. It was / is, however, essential to remember these CCP labs, especially Wuhan, had been creating virulent SARS coronaviruses since BEFORE 2015, often in collaboration with U.S. scientists and even more on its own. Fauci's NIAID and Francis Collins' NIH funded the collaborative research with the CCP, including certain individuals within the Wuhan Institute. EVERY CCP researcher works under the control of the CCP and its army, and the Wuhan lab was / is essentially a military facility. In addition to all of this, the WIV had been notoriously insecure, and Chinese research facilities had numerous leaks of SARS-CoV and other viruses in the past.

59. **January 21, 2020**—The Chinese Communists belatedly admitted human-to-human transmission of the new coronavirus, and the U.S. CDC confirmed the first case in America. Note: There are many who believe they had all the symptoms of COVID-19 before this date, but weren't tested much before this date.

60. **January 23, 2020—Years of Planning Took Off Much Faster Than the Actual Pandemic!**

61. **January 23, 2020a—Pandemic Planning and Globalist Promotion—CEPI** made a shocking announcement from its Norway office, expressing how fully prepared the globalist wolves had become, never mentioning the three+ years of documented preparation for the arrival of the planned pandemic. The virus had not even been named SARS-CoV-2 and no one had yet confirmed a serious worldwide pandemic. Further, the program would not be able to get the necessary EUA funding unless there were no effective treatment options available. But, the **CEPI** hurtled ahead with the aid of Moderna and Fauci's NIAID: CEPI announced the start of three programs to develop vaccines against the novel coronavirus, nCoV-2019. These programs utilized rapid response platforms already supported by CEPI as well as a new partnership. The goal was

to push nCoV-2019 vaccine candidates into clinical testing as rapidly as possible...that same day CEPI announced their new partnership with Moderna, Inc., (Nasdaq: MRNA) and the U.S. NIAID. Bill Gates and Klaus Schwab as CEPI founders were now official partners with Anthony Fauci!

62. **January 23, 2020b**—Moderna announced a collaborative effort with the NIH to use its genetic drug development platform to fast-track an experimental vaccine in less than a year.[62] (A recent approval for an Ebola vaccine had taken two decades!)[63] In summary, CEPI now had partnerships with Moderna and NIAID. Moderna was already in partnership with NIAID and NIH, so NIH owned and profited from a large percentage of Moderna's patents for the vaccine.[64] Bill Gates basically told them all what to do, including CEPI, Moderna, NIH, and Fauci's NIAID.

63. **January 23, 2020c**—an article in JAMA coauthored by **Anthony Fauci** pushed the false narrative of an emergence of a dangerous coronavirus from nature, even though his NIAID-funded research showed pathogenic CoVs were created near the site of the so-called emergence.[65] He also advanced the unproven "suspicion" the original SARS epidemic of 2002-2004 emerged from nature. That article concluded, "The emergence of yet another outbreak of human disease caused by a pathogen from a viral family formerly thought to be relatively benign underscores the perpetual challenge of emerging infectious diseases and the importance of sustained preparedness"[65] Actually, NO SARS-CoV viruses have EVER been found in nature or proven to have emerged from nature to cause an epidemic.

64. **January 30, 2020**—WHO reported 7,818 total confirmed SARS-CoV-2 cases worldwide with a risk assessment of very high for China and high at the global level.

65. **January 31**, **2020**—Against Fauci's resistance, President Trump banned all traffic from China except returning U.S. citizens.

66. **Early February 2020—Pandemic Planning and Globalist Promotion**—The NIH once again described how fully prepared their establishment was for the coronavirus pandemic:[66] Many years before the COVID-19 pandemic began, experts at the NIH Vaccine Research Center (VRC) studied coronaviruses to figure out how to protect against them. Scientists chose to focus on one "prototype" coronavirus and created a vaccine for it… The VCR worked with Moderna (Bill Gates), using this information to quickly customize their prototype approach to the SARS-CoV-2 spike protein. By early February, a COVID-19 vaccine candidate had been designed and manufactured!! This vaccine was named mRNA-1273. By March 16, 2020 (roughly 6 weeks), this vaccine had entered the first phase of clinical trials. Other vaccines, including a similar one from Pfizer and BioNTech SE (China), entered trials shortly after. ' "NOTE: The "design" and "manufacture" of a specific coronavirus vaccine within days after the I.D. of the pandemic in early February was either the luckiest guess ever made by mankind, a miracle, or the product of huge investments made with enormous planning and specific foreknowledge of when the SARS-Co-V would be released!!"[67]

67. **February 4, 2020**—The CDC sent out its test kits for COVID-19 and independent labs found out they DID NOT WORK! CDC bumbling delayed America's response to the pandemic by several weeks as public health officials flew blindly, unable to confirm hot spots. This was only one of multiple CDC mess-ups which came regularly.[68]

68. **February 19**, **2020**—The previously, highly-esteemed, British journal, The Lancet, published a letter organized by **Peter** Daszak from more than two dozen professionals fawning over China and rejecting any criticism of the CCP regime. It also

rejected the "conspiratorial" accusations that SARS-Co-V-2 leaked from the Wuhan Institute. This piece clearly showed how the global wolves in the medical and scientific communities deliberately organized to put the CCP's image over scientific truth and the well-being of both America and all humanity.

69. **March 2020a—The Trusted News Initiative** (TNI) was launched in December 2019 by the BBC to "protect audiences and users from disinformation, particularly around moments of jeopardy, such as elections." Its stated goal was to censor anything positive about President Trump or European populism in the upcoming elections. Very soon, however, it took on COVID-19 'disinformation.' One year later, the partners of Big Tech included "BBC, Facebook, Google / You Tube, Twitter, Microsoft, AFP (a news agency), Reuters, European Broadcasting Union (EBU), Financial Times, The Wall Street Journal, The Hindu, CBC / Radio Canada, First Draft (a left-wing disinformation group), and Reuters Institute for the Study of Journalism." Their agenda and goals were: "An industry collaboration of major news and tech organizations would all work together to rapidly identify and stop the spread of harmful Coronavirus disinformation."[69] In August 2020, these entities were all joined by projects with the AP, the New York Times, and the Washington Post to specifically work against President Trump's re-election.[70] Their motto should have been, "Global predators of the world unite!"

70. **March 2020b—**The health bureaucracy worldwide took action to suppress and later ban the use of hydroxychloroquine or any other safe, effective, and inexpensive drugs for treating COVID-19 patients, including early, at-home treatment which had often prevented hospitalization. The suppression was most harsh in wealthier Western nations (who could and would pay for the development and use of very expensive medications.) This was just one of the many areas of fraud conducted by the globalist wolves to make more money. The active and

intentional suppression of good, lifesaving treatments by so many trusted authorities to increase their wealth and control was/is still beyond either imagination or belief. Deliberately, they allowed patients to die; in fact, they facilitated the deaths of thousands for a lack of good available treatment, while mortally overdosing others to prove the good available treatments weren't any good. That is premeditated murder in the first degree and still punishable by death in many places. Even death would be far too good for the likes of these criminals! Following is a brief analysis of what truly occurred:

- **January 2020**, the EUA act enabled Operation Warp Speed but the related escalation toward the Great Reset had a catch to it.
- **The catch**—the hideously enormous amount of taxpayer money going to Big Pharma and its investors under that Act, could not go into effect if there were already existing safe, effective treatments. If there were; no money. If at any time those were available, all money mongers would lose the legal right to receive money for new vaccines or drugs.
- **Another reason** for stopping all effective medical treatments was to induce people to believe they MUST take the vaccines. If most people recovered with effective treatments, there was no hurry to take toxic, experimental, and expensive vaccines.
- **A third reason** for making COVID seem untreatable was to enable globalists to keep Americans completely panicked and willing to do what they were told. The fear factor justified the totalitarian lockdown of all America, the one great nation standing in the way of the globalist wolves. Klaus knew a strong America thwarted all his ambitions for the Great Reset.

71. **March 2020c—Family physician Vladimir Zelenko M.D.**, the author of one of the introductions to the Breggins' book, searched the scientific literature and contacted physicians worldwide, concluding hydroxychloroquine with additional medications and therapeutics was proven a very safe and effective treatment for COVID-19. He successfully treated thousands of patients in his office just north of New York City, (the pandemic's epicenter). He communicated with President Trump and became friends with Rudy Giuliani; but he met with so much opposition from New York City officials and fearful people in his community, he was forced to leave his clinic and his hometown.

72. **March 11, 2020a**—WHO declared the pandemic![71] On the same day, Anthony Fauci testified before Congress seeking even more funding. He also declared COVID-19 was TEN times more lethal than the 'seasonal influenza'.[72] Since the mortality rate for the flu was 0.1%, the mortality rate for COVID-19 would be 1.0%, meaning one in ten people could die. Fauci claimed this was the reason he emphasized the need to "stay ahead of the game in preventing this."[73] Interestingly, each time Fauci spouted figures on severity and mortality, they got worse, sometimes in mere days. Fauci always spoke politically to serve his globalist masters, and never used real science to serve the truth. The truth was—COVID-19 was much LESS dangerous than the flu for people under age 55, and was negligible or absent for children, teens, and young adults. Most deaths occurred in patients over 80 who already suffered from secondary medical diagnoses. However with adequate medical treatment which Fauci completely opposed—deaths in older people could be and usually were greatly reduced.

73. **March 11, 2020b**—"Dr. Anthony Fauci shared a [virtual] platform with a CCP 'health expert,' and it was largely unreported by ANY Western media outlets. However, Chinese state media could not get enough of it, because Fauci gave a whopping propaganda coup for the Communist regime in Beijing."[74]

74. **March 13, 2020**—-With much resistance from the globalists who wanted to grow international commerce and weaken America, President Trump banned travel from Europe except for U.S. citizens returning home.

75. **March 19, 2020a—California became the first state to order a lockdown.** This marked the beginning of the travesty of increasing top-down governmental control in the U.S., weakening America and acclimating its citizens to greater docility and subservience, while the global wolves increased their own wealth, grandiosity, and power.

76. **March 19, 2020b**—During a press conference on COVID-19, President Trump reported positive news from other countries, including China, proving the effectiveness of hydroxychloroquine against COVID-19. His avid personal support of HCQ led the globalist and 'progressive' anti-Trump media to further mock it as "Trump's drug." One Big Tech commentator on Fox News, Neil Cavuto, hysterically accused President Trump of killing people, warning anyone who was even taking hydroxychloroquine as prophylaxis like the President, "it will kill you; I cannot stress it enough, it will kill you."[75]

77. **March 23-24, 2020**—Hydroxychloroquine was urgently needed throughout the country as a prophylactic measure for vulnerable people, to save individual lives of people infected with COVID-19, to reduce hospital admissions and deaths, and

to shorten and stop the pandemic. President Trump's Secretary of HHS, Alex Azar, directed his deputy, Rick Bright, to make Hydroxychloroquine available from the U.S. National Stockpile.[76] However, Deputy Bright didn't comply with orders, and instead colluded with the FDA's Janet Woodcock to sabotage the HCQ by restricting its use to hospitalized patients, when its proven worth was specifically in early treatment. Trump was repeatedly stymied by the embedded globalist bureaucracy at the cost of thousands of American lives and a violent lockdown that wrecked individual lives, family life, society, and the economy.

78. **March 25, 2020**—New York Governor Andrew Cuomo signed an order requiring unprepared and ill-equipped nursing homes to accept COVID-19 patients discharged from the hospital, turning those facilities into death traps for thousands of elderly citizens. One year later, Cuomo was accused by his own Attorney General of suppressing the actual number of deaths, when the actual number doubled, going from 5000 to 10,000 or more deliberate and heinous fatalities. In addition, Cuomo issued one of the most restrictive orders in the U.S. to prevent access to hydroxychloroquine for treating early COVID-19 patients; then influenced many other Democrat governors to repeat his nonsense orders, resulting in multiple thousands of unnecessary deaths.[77] "While an impeachment inquiry was launched against him almost a full year later, with formal accusations of sexual harassment …reignited calls for impeachment, his nursing home scandals continued to go unmentioned."[78] Judging by the reactions, it would appear many viewed sexual harassment as more repugnant than negligent homicide!

79. **April 3, 2020**—The CDC reversed its policy and recommended wearing face masks in public spaces and indoor gatherings. There was no scientific basis for these requirements, but wearing masks was an effective way to frighten and demoralize

people, while also isolating them and creating a greater degree of submission. Fauci reversed his original March 8, 2020 statement, "there's no reason to be walking around with a mask."[79] At no time did Fauci or the CDC produce any scientific documentation for their stances on face masks, and scientific reviews showed they do more harm than good outside of healthcare facilities.[80]

80. **April 7, 2020—Dr. Deborah Birx** confirmed the CDC was counting deaths of people with coronavirus, as caused by coronavirus regardless of other co-morbid, underlying, or primary causes: "So, I think in this country we've taken a very liberal approach to mortality…the intent right now is if someone dies with COVID-19, we are counting it as a COVID-19 death."[81]

81. **April 8, 2020**—New Jersey became the first state to require customers and employees to wear face masks at essential businesses and construction sites.

82. **April 11, 2020**—The Journal of the American Medical Association (JAMA) rushes to put a study from Brazil online supposedly showing chloroquine (earlier version of hydroxychloroquine) had killed many COVID-19 patients. However, an "examination of the pre-publication paper AND the published paper showed victims were consistently killed by systematic, substantial overdoses of the drug until an oversight committee stopped the murderous experiment."[82] JAMA NEVER retracted the criminal study, so many American doctors were terrified to give the HCQ to their patients.

83. **April 14, 2020**—President Trump announced the U.S. had withdrawn funding from WHO for covering up China's lies early in COVID-19 and for other Chinese actions. Naturally, Bill Gates roundly criticized Trump and quickly made himself the second largest contributor to WHO after the CCP.

84. **April 14-15, 2020**—The Breggins discovered the 2015 scientific paper by Menachery proving Fauci-funded U.S. scientists in 2015 collaborated with top Wuhan Institute scientists to make the lethal SARS-Co-Vs in both American and Wuhan labs.[83] They published a blog and a video and sent them to the media and to close allies of President Trump. Two days later, President Trump stopped the Fauci-funded collaborative research with the CCP. The Breggins pointed out in their blog and video just how closely related the SARS-Co-V of 2015 was to the SARS-CoV-2 in its clinical characteristics. They also warned that the 2015 version resisted treatment in mice. The warning included the fact that some of the elderly vaccinated mice became severely ill and died when exposed to the SARS-Co-V virus; a warning which was NOT heeded, then or since, by the NIAID, the FDA, or the CDC. They reminded all entities the Wuhan Institute continued to be run by the CCP's military, a fact that MUST STAY in the forefront of our minds. There is little doubt the SARS-Co-V pathogen from the 2015 collaboration of U.S./ CCP labs was the forerunner of the SARS-Co-V-2.

85. **April 16, 2020**—The U.S. government through BARDA (in HHS) under Rick Bright, awarded Moderna $483 million "to Accelerate Development of mRNA Vaccine (mRNA-1273) Against the Novel Coronavirus."[84]The U.S. taxpayers paid for Moderna's clinical trials before they had ever begun.

86. **May 15, 2020**—President Trump, with Fauci hanging over his shoulder, announced Operation Warp Speed. The program aped everything Bill Gates had announced in January 2017 and was completely consistent with all Schwab called the Great Reset with its corporate-government fusions. There was no indication President Trump knew the whole idea of Operation Warp Speed had been planned and organized years earlier by Bill Gates with Moderna and other investors, confident of the coming vaccine boon from the planned pandemic.

87. **June 3, 2020**—Schwab designated John Kerry and then Prince, Charles to announce the Great Reset.

88. **July 2020**—A team of Chinese researchers with the aid of Ralph Baric from North Carolina, published a scientific paper about engineering a SARS-Co-V-2 into one that caused an unusually high death rate in mice due to encephalitis.[85] Baric continued making even more highly dangerous SARS-Co-V pathogens with the CCP.

89. **July 14, 2020**—Klaus Schwab released his book, *COVID-19 and the Great Reset.* He touted it as exploring "the far-reaching and dramatic implications of COVID-19 on tomorrow's world, and advocated for a 'Great Reset' in the economy and society."[86] Note the direct use of COVID-19 to promote the New World Order of the Global Reset—the goal the globalists have been aiming at for decades. Schwab described how globalism is making great strides under COVID-19, but has been greatly threatened by American populism and similar trends in Europe. He warned the success of globalism depends on the stifling of America's democratic, patriotic revival under President Trump.

90. **July 15, 2020**—Moderna became the first drug company to begin clinical trials and announced supposedly successful results in its initial trials. But remember, Moderna was already being heavily promoted by Bill Gates in Jan-March, 2017 as a drug company preparing novel vaccines on rush platforms for the coming great pandemic. The many years of investment, scientific research, and organizational planning by Bill Gates, Klaus Schwab, Michael Bloomberg, Moderna, Fauci, and many other globalists were just coming to fruition.

91. **July 22, 2020**—In a $1.95 billion deal, the United States bought 100 million doses of Pfizer's vaccine with an option for 500 million MORE—five months BEFORE it was even approved for use! [87-88]

92. **July-August 20, 2020**—Attorney Tom Renz asked Dr. Peter Breggin to write a medical-legal document in support of an injunction to stop the oppressive, unending emergency measures in Ohio and other states. Renz succeeded in getting his lawsuit accepted by the court, the start of a nationwide series of legal actions, and the Breggins began their book, COVID-19 and the Global Predators: We Are the Prey. The injunction caused the governor of Ohio to halt his emergency edict, but he never stopped his oppressive activities.

93. **August 7, 2020**—Peter A. McCullough, MD led a large team of physicians and researchers to publish an article in the American Journal of Medicine (AJM) presenting a pathophysiological basis for understanding the existing, safe, and effective early treatment options for COVID-19.[89] The study carefully outlined a treatment approach including hydroxychloroquine in combination with other antiviral medications including zinc, prednisone, and anti-clotting drugs when necessary. However, the government and the medical and scientific establishment continued to withhold from doctors and patients ANY adequate form of lifesaving, early treatment!

94. **Late August 2020**—The CDC admitted only 6% of COVID-19 death certificates had just one cause of death listed and for the other 94% there were an average of 2.5 co-morbidities per patient, many of which could have been the primary cause of death.[90] The inflation of death rates was always to frighten people into taking vaccines. The obscure and uniquely inadequate process of counting also made accurate accounting impossible.

95. **September 2020**—There were continued warnings about the lethality of the COVID-19 vaccines. In the middle of Operation Warp Speed, another major review warned the vaccines were "being expedited through preclinical and clinical development and could easily exacerbate COVID-19 through antibody-

dependent enhancement (ADE),[91] which meant being vaccinated and then exposed to COVID-19 could produce unusually severe respiratory disease related to the cytokine storms of severe COVID-19. Fauci, Gates, Moderna, Pfizer—everyone knowingly putting any of the vaccines through Operation Warp Speed—were acting recklessly and their actions would certainly lead to thousands of deaths in the U.S. and around the world.

96. **September 14, 2020**—An interview with Bill Gates described him as not a "fan" of President Trump but closer to Fauci.[92]

97. **September 14, 2020**—Li-Meng Yan MD, PhD—who had escaped from China— along with three colleagues, published a paper linking SARS-CoV-2 to a chain of Chinese and American research going back to 2013 and to the Wuhan Institute from which it was released.[93]

98. **October 2020**—Peter A. McCullough MD, Jane Orient MD, and Elizabeth Lee Vliet MD (writer of the document) jointly authored, A Guide to Home-Based COVID Treatment: Step-by-Step Doctors' P*lan That Could Save Your Life.* The free, regularly updated booklet was distributed by the Association of American Physicians and Surgeons (AAPS), but it was suppressed by the mainstream media, social media, and the medical and scientific establishment, and every other global predatory institution in America and the world.

99. **October 8, 2020**—Li-Meng Yan MD, PhD and her colleagues put a second paper onto the internet, "SARS-CoV-2 IS an Unrestricted Bioweapon: A Truth Revealed Through Uncovering a Large-Scale, Organized Scientific Fraud."[94]

100. **November 12, 2020**—JAMA Network issued a preliminary analysis that fluvoxamine vs. placebo is helpful for outpatient early treatment of COVID-19. Fluvoxamine is an SSRI antidepressant with an especially strong profile of adverse

events including mania, hypomania, and violence.[95] It also went out of favor in the U.S. since Eric Harris, the Columbine High School shooter, was taking fluvoxamine at the time he perpetrated the mass murders. Breggin's medical/legal analysis of Harris' medical records—made available to Dr Breggin as a medical expert—found Harris deteriorated while taking the antidepressant for months leading up to the day of the mass murders, with an increase in dosage not long beforehand. On the day of the shootings, he no doubt continued taking the medication. In the autopsy after his death by suicide at the scene of the murders, Harris had an effective concentration of fluvoxamine in his bloodstream. The coroner ironically described it as a "therapeutic" level. Note: For those who find it hard to believe that the media and Big Pharma worked together to deceive the public during COVID-19, the press uniformly ignored the story or falsely reported Harris was NOT taking antidepressants at the time of the shootings. That was all an issue a full two decades before that current information.

101. **November 16-19, 2020**—Michael Bloomberg's annual New Economic Forum (NEF) was held virtually. The CCP cosponsored it once again. The theme was defiance of President Trump's policies and the necessity of recoupling China with the world's billionaires and giant corporations. Top global corporate executives lent their support, including McDonald's, IBM, MasterCard, FedEx, Prudential, Goldman Sachs, Honeywell, and numerous huge banks. The Clintons and Bill Gates were all present.

102. **November 19 and December 8,2020**—the U.S. Senate Oversight Committee for Homeland Security and Government Affairs under Senator Ron Johnson held two hearings with extremely well-qualified medical experts who testified under oath about the effective, early, home-based treatment of COVID-19 to save lives. Videos of the Senate expert testimonies were censored by You Tube, Facebook, and Twitter, and the hearings were NOT

covered by the mainstream media. Democrats boycotted and attacked both the hearings and the participants. Every effort was made to continue keeping Americans in the dark, about the safe, inexpensive, and effective treatments for COVID-19.

103. **November 20, 2021 (*one year later*)**—"WHO gave a "conditional recommendation' against the use of Remdesivir." This drug was the toxic, deadly, non-effective, and hyper-expensive drug pushed out without adequate trials to replace the safe, effective, and inexpensive ones they banned. It could only be given by IV administration and many diagnosed COVID-19 patients who were not critical were treated with remdesivir in the hospital and died of the treatment instead of the disease. A conditional recommendation simply means there isn't enough evidence to support its use. The undermining of another treatment drug was almost certainly aimed at increasing the necessity of the vaccines. The global wolves were now putting all emphasis on vaccines to glean their enormous profits and enforce more fear with greater top-down government, especially in America.

104. **November 24, 2020**—After the "election" of Joe Biden, an absolute necessity for the triumph of the global wolves, the Great Reset became U.S. policy. At Schwab's 2020 World Economic Forum, John Kerry—Biden's special consultant, cabinet member, and Climate Envoy—made the final connection. He declared, "In effect, the citizens of the United States have just done a Great Reset. We've done a Great Reset."[96]

105. **December 3, 2020**—John Ratcliffe, Director of National Intelligence for the United States, declared: "If I could communicate one thing to the American people from this unique vantage point, it is that the People's Republic of China poses the greatest threat to America today, and the greatest threat to democracy and freedom worldwide since WWII. The intelligence is clear: Beijing intends to dominate the U.S. and the rest of the planet economically, militarily, and

technologically. Many of China's major public initiatives and prominent companies offer only a layer of camouflage to the activities of the CCP. I call its approach of economic espionage 'rob, replicate, and replace.' China robs U.S. companies of their intellectual property, replicates the technology, and then replaces the U.S. firms in the global marketplace."[97]

106. **December 11, 2020**—The Pfizer-BioNTech vaccine was authorized by an Emergency Use Authorization (EUA) by the FDA. The Chinese were also beneficiaries through their corporate partnership with Germany's BioNTech.[98]

107. **December 18, 2020**—Moderna's vaccine was authorized for use by an Emergency Use Authorization (EUA) by the FDA. NIH claims "joint ownership" of the vaccines making it a perfect corporate-government fusion.[99]

108. **Late December 2020**—Two scientific articles were posted online and then published in journals showing the spike protein (S protein) ALONE can cause inflammation and damage to the endothelial cells in blood vessels in the body and brain in both animals and humans. They documented that the mRNA vaccines are causing recipient's bodies to produce spike proteins which are in themselves potentially harmful to the body.100-101

109. **December 30, 2020**—Peter A. McCullogh MD, MPH and 32 other physicians and researchers—including Elizabeth Lee Vliet MD and Vladimir Zelenko MD—published the most extensive review of the benefits of early treatment of COVID-19.[102]

110. **January 14, 2021**—The Vaccine Credential Initiative (VCI) was unveiled as a coalition of Big Tech and Big Healthcare corporations, as well as WHO and others. It claimed a "Trustworthy, traceable, verifiable, and universally recognized digital record of vaccination status is urgently needed

worldwide to safely enable people to return to work, school, events, and travel.[103] It was closely involved with the Commons Project,"[104] which was supported by the Rockefeller Foundation and Schwab's WEF, and aimed to develop a Common Pass, a vaccine and medical record passport, working with Apple Health for iOS and Common Health for Android. Every global wolf could end up having a piece of this project, and along with it, a piece of each of us as well.

111. **January 19, 2021—** "BioNTech-Pfizer and Moderna COVID-19 vaccine sales were expected to generate $14.7 billion in revenue by 2023."[105]

112. **February 2021—**Israel experienced an escalating death rate in association with Pfizer vaccine—a controversy that continues to this day. Surprisingly, the Israeli government remained adamant about vaccinating its entire population.[106]

113. **February 8, 2021—**South Africa suspended the use of AstraZeneca's COVID-19 shot after data showed it only gave protection against mild to moderate infection caused by the country's dominant coronavirus variant.[107]

114. **March 2021—**Dr. Li-Meng Yan and her colleagues published a third paper further emphasizing SARS-CoV-2 was released as a bioweapon in China's unrestricted warfare against the West. They described the collusion to cover this up and answered globalist critics.[108] Note: By the time the Breggins completed their book, they were in complete agreement with Dr. Yan. The lengthy, costly, intensive, and worldwide preparation and planning they/we have seen showed clear intention by the globalist wolves, including the CCP, to create a coronavirus pandemic. The time of the pandemic directly corresponds with the perceived 'desperate need' of the globalists and governmental policies to hinder their power, control, and increase of their wealth. Worse still, globalist wolves, led by the CCP, systematically took full advantage of the pandemic and

deliberately spread it worldwide, especially into America with their strategy of unrestricted warfare. The pandemic benefited globalists tremendously and it vastly enriched their billions. It helped the CCP reduce its burdensome and aged population, and gain tighter control over its own hordes. Of course it weakened America in many ways; and gave the CCP a biological weapon for current and future use. The CCP used the pandemic to strengthen its own economy in relation to the rest of the world. With its principle of 'unrestricted warfare' the CCP deliberately spread SARS-CoV-2 throughout an unsuspecting world by continuing all international flights. Hundreds of thousands of potentially infected Chinese were flown from Wuhan, Beijing, and other Chinese cities into the United States and the rest of the world. This assault continued until President Trump, on his own, and completely against Fauci's expressed orders, stopped the traffic from China.

115. **March 8, 2021**—The Breggins decided to place their book *COVID-19 and the Global Predators* on advanced sale with a unique bonus: Everyone who bought the book immediately received the working manuscript by email. Within weeks, many thousands of people began reading and learning, especially about the particulars against Anthony Fauci. Copies were also sent to the media and to critics of COVID-19 policies. Criticism of Fauci certainly began heating up in May and June, surrounding issues they fully documented.

116. **March 9, 2021**—Fauci met "side-by-side" with the CCP medical leader Dr. Zhong Nanshan on a virtual panel sponsored by the University of Edinburgh.[109] Nanshan had been awarded the Medal of the Republic—the highest honor bestowed by the CCP. Fauci declared the U.S. had been "hurt" more than any other country by COVID-19, citing falsified CDC data to prove his point. He accused the past administration of "divisiveness." Both men were critical of President Trump. They praised President Biden and called for global solidarity.[110] Zhong ended

his presentation by "urging other countries NOT to open their economies just yet, and to perhaps wait until the entire world was vaccinated, which would take a few years." Meanwhile, China's economy had been largely opened for a year with a very low per capita vaccination rate! More deliberate globalist deception to perpetuate the damaging lockdown and hurting economies.

117. **March 19, 2021**—"The PREP Act and COVID-19—Limiting Liability for Medical Countermeasures Updated March 19, 2021. To be sure there would be expeditious development and initiation of medical countermeasures during a public health emergency, the Public Readiness and Emergency Preparedness Act (PREP Act) gave authority to the Secretary of Health and Human Services (HHS) to determine limits on legal liability for any losses related to the administration of medical countermeasures such as diagnostics, treatments, and vaccines."[111] Under earlier legislation, Big Pharma was already immune to vaccine lawsuits, but this Act gave almost complete immunity to healthcare providers as well. In this instance, individual and patient rights (i.e. the right to sue healthcare providers for injuries and deaths—continued to be trampled on.)

118. **March 26, 2021**—Former CDC Director Robert Redfield stated in an interview he believed coronavirus escaped from a Wuhan lab,[112] a FACT demonstrated by the Breggins a full year before.

119. **April 2021a**—As the death grip of COVID-19 propaganda on Americans began to ease up a bit, the Biden Administration and the CCP ramped up their collaboration in turning greater attention to the Global Warming or Climate Change as it's come to be called since there is still considerable debate on the truth of real global warming. This campaign is an integral part of weakening America and increasing the spread of totalitarian control worldwide. John Kerry went on a world tour to warn the nations they MUST restrict their economies to diminish this

'global warming,' purported to be of dire need by all globalist wolves.[113]

120. **April 2021b**—Bill Gates was heavily criticized after he spontaneously stated he was against giving India, which was struggling with a resurgence of COVID-19, the legal rights or the know-how to manufacture the Oxford AstraZeneca vaccine. Gates gave reasons, but the clearly biggest one was not wanting to share profits from his intellectual property.[114] Note: Behind the conflict between Bill Gates and India there are three less noticed, but very dangerous facts. 1) One man, Bill Gates is deeply invested in and has control of three out of four of the world's COVID-19 vaccines—Moderna, Pfizer, and Oxford AstraZeneca, and also invested in BioNTech, the German vaccine maker who is partnered with Pfizer and CCP. 2) This same single man fully believes his financial investments and corporate influence give him the unrestricted right to make all life-and-death decisions for the multi-millions of people in the second largest nation in the world, India. 3) Previous documentation shows Bill Gates is fully aligned with the CCP and WHO, and India is an adversary of the CCP. The fact that Bill Gates feels free and can casually express his cavalier life-and-death decisions on a TV interview is horrifying and eerie at the least.

121. **April 15, 2021**—WHO announced it would begin storing and sharing dangerous pathogens internationally. It declared, "This will pave the way towards a system which will promote the rapid and timely sharing of biological materials with epidemic or pandemic potential, facilitate rapid access to pathogens, and promote equitable access to countermeasures."[115] The Scientist raised alarms about this![116] This is definitely globalism at its most irrational and terrifying. The audacity of such a declaration is stunning in its magnitude. Before long at this rate, the United Nations could begin worldwide sharing of the designs for nuclear weapons, which many experts consider far less

dangerous than biological warfare with pathogens. It would be impossible for WHO or any other body to fully secure pathogen storage. That scenario would be human annihilation at the ready.

122. **April 24, 2021**—The Biden Administration added to India's COVID-19 crisis by refusing to lift its ban on sending India raw materials for the Oxford AstraZeneca vaccine. Biden claimed to be putting America's needs first, but he had NOT done that since taking office—claim has no proof![117] The truth is clear. The CCP is and has been in constant conflict with India at every level, including militarily. Weakening India is exactly what the CCP desires while aiding its own empirical plans. None of the globalist entities will cross or thwart the CCP.

123. **April 25, 2021a**—The headline in the Financial Times praised the sinister declaration of the CCP's dictator despot at an international trade conference: "Xi warns against economic decoupling and calls for a new world order."[118] Xi Jinping, Klaus Schwab, Bill Gates, Michael Bloomberg, Big Tech, Big Banking, and all the other globalist wolves know the only roadblock to their ambitions for world domination is the populist, freedom-loving, patriotic, and democratic republic of the United States of America, and the former President Donald Trump.

124. **April 25, 2021b**— "On NBC's Meet the Press, National Institutes of Health (NIH) Director Francis Collins stated Moderna's and Pfizer's vaccines cannot receive actual permanent FDA approval because more follow-up is needed "to look at any possible late safety signals. There have NOT been any for Pfizer and Moderna."[119] This was an attempt to sound responsible about vaccines, but was a bold-faced lie. There have ALWAYS been significant safety signals with all COVID-19 "vaccines!" Vaccine Adverse Event Report(s) (VAERS) is the system used to report any/all adverse events from vaccines including deaths. In the first four months only of COVID-19 vaccinations, the deaths reported to VAERS had reached 3,489. VAERS reports are

notoriously under-reported and adverse events other than death were NOT included.[120] Current data on the number of deaths from vaccine associated adverse effects since the beginning of vaccinations are exponential, but once again accurate information is NOT available from the CDC or other sources, because they claim they cannot be proven. However, it's abundantly clear that VAERs are woefully lacking and few of us there are who do NOT know someone who died in direct association with having received the jabs. The number for only four months is extremely high even barring under-reporting. Prior to COVID-19, ANY other medicine or vaccine would have been permanently removed from the market. Naturally, the CDC's claim that none of these cases were actually related to the vaccines is absurd, unconscionable, and extremely irresponsible. Such shenanigans can only be explained by the tremendous pressure of globalists and Big Pharma on the agency.

125. **April 30, 2021a**—"CDC transitioned to reporting only patients with COVID19 vaccine breakthrough-infection who were hospitalized or died."[121] Once again, information was being removed or edited before any of us could see it to protect the vaccines.

126. **April 30, 2021b**—Patrick Coffin, a courageous fighter for liberty, had his You Tube channel taken down shortly before his virtual "Truth Over Fear Summit was scheduled. Though he managed to have nearly 50,000 signups, his summit was shut down by its Australian platform after barely getting started. One week later, with volunteer help from a conservative platform, he resumed his conference. Speakers at the 3-day celebration of freedom and truth in science included Dr. Peter Breggin and three other outstanding physicians who wrote intros for his book. Patrick stood for all Americans being canceled for such things as opposition to election fraud or criticism of COVID-19 policies, and most importantly he stood for resilience as a Re-founder of America.[122]

127. May 2021—Six German researchers from Goethe-University of Frankfurt and Ulm University posted an online report based on the concept of "Vaccine-induced COVID-19 Mimicry."[123] That is, the vaccination alone can produce similar syndromes to SARS-CoV-2. They focused on vaccine-induced thromboses (clots in blood vessels). Clots often formed in the brain (chief cause of strokes) and elsewhere in the body. They said, "This type of adverse event has not been observed in the clinical studies of AstraZeneca, but it led to the immediate halting of vaccinations in several European countries. These events were mostly associated with thrombocytopenia, or low blood platelets."[123] The findings confirmed the SARS-CoV-2 spike protein created in the body as a result of vaccination is in itself toxic and can mimic the effects of COVID19.

128. May 2, 2021—Michael Bloomberg's newsletter editorial set the record straight on how much the global wolves love the violent CCP dictatorship and how much they hate the spirit of freedom in America. In one of the most sickeningly dismal displays of American self-loathing, Bloomberg's editor declared, "Only one year ago, the world stood dumbfounded as the richest nation on earth, under the leadership of a COVID-denying president, botched its response to the pandemic, sacrificing hundreds of thousands of lives to a deadly combination of incompetence, hubris, and political partisanship. Meanwhile, it was equally obvious Xi's swift decision to contain the virus with draconian lockdowns, blanket surveillance, and Mao-style social controls delivered stunning results. China flattened the curve—while Republicans swore off face masks and social distancing as America perished..."[124] Just think about this travesty: A former NYC mayor, now a leading globalist wolf, unashamedly declares, "Mao good!" "Trump bad!"—preferring the Communist nightmare to the American Dream. Everything we Americans hold dearest is under attack and threatened by the globalist wolves!

129. May 07, 2021—Dr. Peter McCullough was interviewed at length by Tucker Carlson on Fox Nation, followed by an excerpt that evening on his show on the Fox News Channel. Carlson was openly dismayed to learn about the innumerable deaths caused by the unprecedented and inexcusable suppression of safe and effective treatments for COVID-19. Tucker was seen asking Dr. McCullough "WHY?" and "WHO's behind it?" multiple times. The Breggins sent their book manuscript to Tucker hoping he would use it to answer these essential questions, which would have been an enormous media breakthrough in broadcasting truth for a change!

130. May 10, 2021—Research that should have been required reading for all concerned was published in the International Journal of Vaccine Theory, Practice, and Research,[125] and described the unparalleled circumstances surrounding the Moderna vaccine, and made it such a radical, dangerous experiment on humanity:[126] UNPRECEDENTED— Many aspects of COVID-19 and subsequent vaccine development are unprecedented for a vaccine deployed for use in the general population. Some of these include the following:

- First to use PEG (polyethylene glycol) in an injection
- First to use mRNA vaccine technology against an infectious agent
- First time Moderna had brought ANY product to market
- First to have public health officials telling those receiving the vaccination to expect an adverse reaction
- First to be implemented publicly with nothing more than preliminary efficacy data
- First vaccine to make no clear claims about reducing infections, transmissibility, or deaths

- First coronavirus vaccine ever attempted in humans
- First injection of genetically modified polynucleotides in the general population.

131. May 11, 2021—Fauci lied to Senator Rand Paul under oath at a Senate hearing when he declared that neither his NIAID nor the NIH had funded gain-of-function research with the Wuhan Institute of Virology in China. Afterward he continued lying to the press as well.[127]

132. May 13, 2021—Now the CDC had received a total of 4,434 reports of deaths associated with vaccination in the U.S.[128] By any standard, this was catastrophic. Once again, because underreporting is always true in these systems, the actual number of deaths could have easily been ten times greater or more. In years past, a vaccine would have been withdrawn after just 100 reports of deaths. Many physicians and nations were calling for an end to this heinous vaccine slaughter. However, a striking pattern emerged. The CDC and other authorities had been vastly exaggerating the number of deaths caused by COVID-19 all along, so now they were simply ignoring the multitude of deaths caused by the vaccines. It's always been all about the billions being made by the globalist wolves from vaccines. Clearly, they continued to weaken America's resistance to their globalism while enforcing submission among citizens and politicians alike.

133. May 19, 2021—"The COVID-19 pandemic brought into sharp focus two main issues: the human right to access a life-saving drug and a physician's right to exercise his/her Hippocratic Oath. Therefore, the Front Line COVID-19 Critical Care Alliance (FLCCC) called for the 'Immediate and Global Use of Ivermectin to End the COVID-19 Pandemic.'"[129]

134. May 21, 2021—An article published in Clinical Infectious Diseases demonstrated patients recently vaccinated with mRNA have SARS-CoV-2 spike protein remnants circulating in their blood stream. This confirmed the spike protein distribution is not contained within the injection site, as was claimed by advocates, and therefore makes all cells in the body vulnerable to attack.

135. **June 9, 2021**—Dr. Tess Lawrie, Director, Evidence-based Medicine Consultancy Ltd., sent an "urgent" report to the British drug monitoring agency (MHRA) based on a preliminary analysis of adverse vaccine reports to the agency from January through May 26, 2021. Here is her warning: "We are sharing this preliminary report due to the urgent need to communicate information that should lead to cessation of the vaccination rollout while a full investigation is conducted.[130] The three vaccines used in Great Britain are made by AstraZeneca, Pfizer, and Moderna (spanning DNA and RNA). The adverse reactions are not limited to any particular vaccine brand or type. The report counts 1,253 deaths and 256,224 individual adverse event reports in what is called the Yellow Card system. Drawing on Seneff and Nigh (previously cited),[131] Dr. Lawrie categorized the types of adverse events reported:

- Pathogenic priming, multi-system inflammatory disease, and autoimmunity
- Allergic reactions and anaphylaxis
- Antibody dependent enhancement
- Activation of latent viral infections
- Neurodegeneration and prion diseases
- Emergence of novel variants of SARS-CoV-2
- Integration of the spike protein gene into the human DNA Dr. Lawrie also observed that spike proteins which are produced by the vaccines in the body are also "toxic to the human body."[131] She summarized the

reports to the British government as including all of the above events. These horrible outcomes have already been documented in animals under laboratory conditions, and that in itself should have prevented the vaccines from ever being even tested in humans as too dangerous.

136. June 10, 2021—The CDC announced an upcoming emergency meeting.[132] As of May 31, the CDC had received 275 preliminary reports of myocarditis and pericarditis in fully vaccinated 16-to-24-year-olds—a number much higher than what scientists expected to see, which means they KNEW there would be serious heart issues in young adults who were vaccinated.[133]

137. June 11, 2021a—BMJ's *Journal of Medical Ethics* published "Voluntary COVID-19 vaccination of children: a social responsibility."[134] In other words, these authors say children should be vaccinated to benefit society, and even their parents should do so voluntarily for that reason. The article also revealed that "Israel, which is a world pioneer in the vaccination of its adult population, signed a contract with Pfizer for sharing data on vaccinated citizens."[135]

138. June 11, 2021b—VAERS data released today showed 329,021 reports of adverse events following COVID-19 vaccines, including 5,888 deaths and 28,441 serious injuries between December 14, 2020 and June 4, 2021.[136] Giving vaccines to younger and younger children is no doubt the single greatest example of mass child abuse in human history. A medical storm of potential harm like this has NEVER before been unleashed on humanity.

139. June 22, 2021—Pandemic Planning and Globalist Promotion—A new report in SCIENCE led by Ralph Baric's team (University of North Carolina) defines the future of humanity for what he termed the 'endless assault on vaccines.'

It was entitled, "Chimeric spike mRNA vaccines protect against Sarbecovirus challenge in mice." He continued to falsely claim SARS-CoV-2 emerged from nature, and are now claiming to have developed new mRNA vaccines: "multiplexed-chimeric spikes" that "can prevent SARS-like zoonotic coronavirus infections with pandemic potential." They also continue to perpetuate the lie that SARS-CoV viruses are lurking about in nature ready to emerge. They MUST perpetuate the lie to justify their continued humanity-endangering gain-of-function experiments, and creating multiple new pandemic-worthy CoVs in their labs. This whole vaccine scheme can then continue to engorge the massive wealth of the globalist wolves, while demanding totalitarian control, and it will never go away on its own. This same research also exposes all of Anthony Fauci's lies about NIAID and NIH NOT funding gain-of-function research with Ralph Baric. The continued creation of "chimeric" pandemic viruses is still being supported by several grants from the NIAID and NIH, as well as by Big Pharma-based Burroughs-Wellcome Funding and by Facebook's Zuckerberg Fund.[137]

140. July 20, 2021—Reports of vaccine-related deaths in COVID-19 have now exceeded 10,000. A detailed CDC report published in 2015 found that "multiple studies and scientific reviews have found no association between vaccination and deaths except in rare cases."[138] The study noted a polio vaccine was withdrawn after five deaths among recipients and five among contact persons. It was called "one of the worst pharmaceutical disasters to U.S. history." The CDC further explained that swine flu vaccine was withdrawn after a Guillain-Barré syndrome (paralysis, often followed by death) resulted in 53 deaths. "In comparison to stopping the use of vaccine-related deaths after 10 to 53 reported deaths previously, as of July 9, 2021, there had been 10,991 COVID-19 vaccine-related reported deaths to the CDC.[139] Nothing in the history of American medicine has ever come remotely near the size of the

> COVID-19 vaccine catastrophe with many thousands of deaths from COVID-19 in a vaccination program that still has not been stopped to date."(January, 2026-almost 6 years!)

In addition, we must also consider these reports of vaccine-related deaths to the CDC are only a fraction of the actual number of deaths that have occurred. According to all the studies evaluated by the Breggins in their book, only 1% to 10% of serious adverse events are even reported to the CDC's reporting system. The actual number of vaccine-related deaths is certainly many, many multiples higher than the already horrifying number of 10,991 deaths reported by early July 2021.

Dr. Peter McCullough MD, MPH provided the Breggins with the following updated stats. All COVID-19 vaccines are causing record safety reports. In 1990, the VAERS reporting system was established as a national early warning system to detect possible safety issues in U.S. licensed vaccines.[140] Comparing this to previous rates of reporting of adverse vaccine events to the CDC, the current reporting for COVID-19 is a catastrophic avalanche. The total number of safety reports in VAERS for COVID vaccines ALONE through July 7, 2021, was 438,440.[141]

Dr. McCullough also observed people were dying and being hospitalized in record numbers in the days right after COVID-19 vaccination. Based on VAERS as of June 25, 2021, there were 9,048 COVID-19 vaccine deaths reported and over 26,818 hospitalizations reported for the COVID-19 vaccines (Pfizer, Moderna, and J&J). By historical comparison, from 1999 until December 31, 2019, VAERS received only 3,167 (158 per year) adult death reports for all vaccines combined. Thus, the COVID-19 mass vaccination program is associated with at least a 57-fold annualized increase in vaccine deaths reported to VAERS. COVID-19 vaccine adverse events account for 99% of ALL vaccine-related events from December 2020 through the present in VAERS.

The Breggins and any other reader of these stats can only agree with Dr. McCullough that COVID-19 deaths should have been taken seriously and investigated thoroughly, then analyzed for the public, when cases were far less than 150 total. After exceeding 200, ALL the vaccines should have been withdrawn. Now they have far exceeded 10,000 and rapidly counting. Unlike ALL other large clinical investigations, the U.S. COVID-19 mass vaccination program has NO critical event committee, data safety and monitoring board, and no human ethics committee. In a nutshell, there is nothing in the program to protect Americans from safety problems that have arisen with the vaccines, and apparently, there continues to be very little concern shown for this slaughter.[142] This planned and deliberate mass murder of innocent people, many of whom were coerced to take it, is a federal and international war crime in the truest sense of the word. We are now well into 2025, and the vaccination war is still being waged at many levels and globalist wolves have no intention of stopping it.

141. **August 4, 2021**—Final Entry of Pandemic Planning and Globalist Promotion Timeline. There was a private communication to the Breggins on August 2, 2021, from Dr. Elizabeth Lee Vliet. She confirmed President Trump's adviser, Peter Navarro, and the President himself were aware of the importance and availability of safe, effective treatments but failed to follow through. Senator Ron Johnson also communicated directly with the President about the need for allowing American physicians and their patients access to these medications. Her observations were well-documented.

Dr. Vliet had been working with Senator Johnson as far back as early April, 2020 on organizing a letter from American physicians to President Trump urging him to "give patients the right to try this drug (hydroxychloroquine) early in the course of their COVID-19 diagnosis."[143] *On June 2, 2020*, The Association of American Physicians and Surgeons (AAPS) announced a lawsuit against the FDA to release the national stockpile of hydroxychloroquine for use by American citizens in the early and effective treatment of COVID19.[144] On June 22, 2020, the

AAPS filed its motion for a preliminary injunction to compel release to the public of hydroxychloroquine by the FDA and the Department of Health and Human Services. "Nearly 100 million doses of hydroxychloroquine were "DONATED" to the health agencies, but none had been released to the public."[145] The president's adviser, Peter Navarro denounced the obstruction by officials of the FDA to making this medication available to the public, and President Trump had already endorsed it. But at least another 18-24 months passed and the effective medications for early treatment of COVID-19 remained unavailable and multiple thousands would have been spared weeks to months of painful hospitalization treatments, including the toxic remdesivir that literally killed thousands of hospitalized patients who were barely diagnosed with COVID-19.

Many analysts believe President Trump had the ability to stop the globalist wolves in their tracks, but didn't do it. They maintain he succumbed to the globalist wolves by shutting down the American economy and society and endorsing Gate's Operation Warp Speed. Perhaps his actions or lack of them also contributed to the untold numbers of deaths. Perhaps, he actually had as little control of globalist perpetrators as the rest of us did. It is certainly true that he was under constant attack no matter what he did. Several things are takeaways we need to examine carefully if we would be able to disrupt globalist plans in our future.

A large portion of our American citizenry became completely demoralized by all the globalist plans and tactics. After all, they had been making their plans for decades, and they had the money and power to carry them out. Time was on their side. They have profoundly compromised America's individual and political freedoms. They also used every fraudulent trick in the book to put a hand-picked globalist defender in the White House for four long years to perpetrate their Great Reset. Our country very literally hung in the balance for its survival when President Trump returned to office. Now, we MUST look at what has been done to us as a nation and understand it's up to conservative grass-roots Americans to sit up, pay attention, understand the crimes perpetrated against us, and work with everything in us to be prepared for the next assault. Much progress has been made but, Make no mistake! Globalism, the Great Reset, and what they mean to our potential destruction have NOT gone away, nor have they even slowed down in their driven quest for victory in this WAR! We dare not ever let down our guard again.

God described in His Word exactly WHO and WHAT these Globalist Wolves are so that any of us may easily recognize them and assess them correctly. By it, they have identified themselves clearly and we can KNOW what God already knows. Their future is settled.

"None is righteous, NO, NOT ONE; All have turned aside; together they have become WORTHLESS; NO ONE does good, not even one. Their throats are open graves; they use their tongues to DECEIVE. The VENOM of ASPS is literally under their lips. Their mouths are full of curses and bitterness. Their feet are SWIFT to SHED BLOOD; in their paths are ruin and misery, the way of peace they have not known. There is NO FEAR OF GOD before their eyes." Romans 3:12-18 ESV

"They will suffer the punishment of eternal destruction, away from the presence of the Lord"...(as they chose to do). 2 Thessalonians 1:9 ESV

However, we can also clearly see how our Father tells us to respond:

"So whoever knows the right thing to do and fails to do it, for him it is sin." James 4:17 ESV

"Do you not know that the unrighteous will not inherit the kingdom of God? Do not be deceived; neither the sexually immoral, nor idolators, nor adulterers, nor men who practice homosexuality, nor thieves, nor the greedy, nor drunkards, nor revilers, nor swindlers will inherit the kingdom of God. Such were some of you. But you were washed, you were sanctified, and you were justified in the name of the Lord Jesus Christ by the Spirit of our God." I Corinthians 6: 9-11

"But those who desire to be rich fall into temptation, into a snare, into many senseless and harmful desires that plunge people into ruin and destruction." I Timothy 6:9 ESV

"Watch and pray that you may not enter into temptation. The spirit indeed is willing, but the flesh is weak." Matthew26:41 ESV

"You are the salt of the earth, but if salt has lost its taste, how shall its saltiness be restored? It is no longer good for anything except to be thrown out and trampled under people's feet. You are the light of the world. A city set on a hill cannot be hidden. Nor do people light a lamp and put it under a basket, but on a stand, and it gives light to all in the house. In the same way, let your light shine before others, so that they may see your good works and give glory to your Father Who is in heaven." Matthew 5:13-16 ESV

"He has told you, O man, what is good; and what does the LORD require of you but to do justice, and to love kindness, and to walk humbly with your God?" Micah 6:8 ESV

"For by wise guidance you can wage your war, and in abundance of counselors there is victory." Proverbs 24:6 ESV

"Be on your guard; stand firm in the faith; be courageous; be strong." I Corinthians 16:13 NIV

"For the Lord loves the just and will not forsake His faithful ones. Wrongdoers will be completely destroyed; the offspring of the wicked will perish." Psalm 37:28 NIV

"I have told you these things, so that you may have peace. In this world you WILL HAVE TROUBLE. But take heart! I (Jesus Christ) have overcome the world." John 16:33 NIV

Part II

Pandemic's Event Chronology

CHAPTER 9

Pandemia—The First Six Months

Planned Progression of Global Insanity

When a large, very elite, commonly-driven cabal of individuals, with a chosen agenda and plenty of wealth with which to achieve it, use all the resources at their disposal and their carefully laid plans to change the world, they can and did make it happen. In a nutshell, that endeavor has become known to the world as the COVID-19 Pandemic. However, all the details and intricacies of their plan require a great deal of learning and examination to understand the enormity of what this cabal perpetrated on our entire global society. Thanks to a minority of brilliant, tenacious, and truth-seeking individuals, we can come to know what happened, starting decades ago, to bring about the catastrophe we all experienced. For at least two to three years this debacle brought mammoth changes to fruition in all our lives, which for many of us were irreversible.

Many of these sage individuals have written widely, but most of them were also heavily censored and banned from free participation in the morass of social media. Big Tech was not in the habit of allowing the truth to be exposed if it could be stopped. Any news or information not meshing with the global narrative was not given a voice. Consequently, much of the truth was collected, written, edited, and published by private individuals and companies operating outside the reach of Big Tech and the globalist wolves. However, as is evident in this book, the truth IS available and provable, and can be accessed by all who care enough to find it.

One of those courageous and conscientious individuals is also an award-winning author and journalist, a Yale alumnus, and brilliant at writing both fiction and non-fiction reporting. Alex Berenson wrote an excellent treatise about the COVID-19 era and its truth-telling and easily understood premises are eye-opening. We will look at many of his facts and observations through the remainder of this book. One book in particular will give us clarity and understanding with the ability to refute the ever-present lies and propaganda still circulating throughout the media today. *Pandemia: How Coronavirus Hysteria Took Over Our Government, Rights, and Lives* is a message you, the reader, will want to grab hold of, and hold tight to, if you have the chance to peruse it. Pandemic panic took hold very quickly, corrupted real science, jeopardized our Constitutional liberties, and ignored ethics, truth, and of course all morality. If we Americans and other peoples value our foundations, it is essential to understand what happened in order to take back our nation, based on reason, honesty, freedom, and liberty for all. While faith-based individuals and groups continue to believe all of this proves Scripture and its predictions of end-times events, it still behooves us to stand for those institutions that honor God, country, truth and justice.

First, a note on Mr. Alex Berenson will let the reader know how hard individuals have worked and persevered to bring and preserve the truth for us. Regardless of what his personal faith-walk may or may not look like, he is an honorable man, presenting us with sober, factual information under considerable pushback. The Twitter platform regularly censored him. The main-stream media also tried to discredit and cancel him. However, as a gifted journalist, he pored over the best medical data we had. He exposed so-called 'conventional wisdom', while keeping a sharp eye strictly on the facts. Through all of this chaos, Alex was so consistently right, the globalist 'guardians' of the 'official' narrative dubbed him, "the pandemic's wrongest man!" In this case, it should be considered his "badge of honor!"

Pandemia tells the highly alarming, but true story of the thoughts, intents, plans, agendas, and appalling evil of the globalist wolves we've already seen at a bit of distance. Now, however, we see them in all their abominable characters of power-hungry, greed-driven, and ultra-controlling actions. Many of them actually changed their minds on the how-tos of their plans so many times, they botched a good many of them and even revealed how heinously they behaved through it all. As they joined forces and aims with Big Tech, Big Business, Big Pharma, and Big Government to frighten and control the people, they exploited and magnified the purported crisis. It was all to gain unprecedented control over our very bodies, our lives, and even what we were allowed to say.

In the early days and weeks of the 'Plague', with the plethora of dire predictions and warnings, a panicked mentality for the masses seemed to make some sense; after all, it was a 'novel' disease, supposedly of unknown origin, spreading like wildfire, and the ramifications were still relatively unknown for most of us. However, after a few weeks, so many conflicting pieces of information had been disseminated and lockdowns were beginning globally. However, after denying their necessity, they were being rapidly demanded. Too many things were NOT making good sense. MOST of us should have been far more suspicious of the nonsense being perpetrated, and many of us were asking a lot of questions which were NOT being satisfactorily answered! Worse, even our leadership, which at first did not succumb to the fear-mongering, ultimately bowed to it. Perhaps, as leaders, with the responsibility for the welfare of millions, they finally surrendered to it, rather than be responsible for the constantly-pandered disaster they might later be able to prevent. Ultimately, the "CURE" was exponentially more costly and damaging than ANY virus had ever been, but it was already too late for reason and common sense.

So, there really is a clear, true story of how media fear-mongering, bad politics, over-reliance on unproven technology, and scientific illiteracy nearly brought the United States and the world to the brink of irretrievable destruction. It's the true story of how even our leaders either ignored or trashed our civil liberties and values, treasured since our nation's birth. We denied our children proper education in ALL its aspects, we annihilated small businesses and we locked down and hid our faces from one another on the scantest possible evidences. At the same time, this so-called public-health emergency became a mega-business almost overnight. Our already bankrupted government spent trillions to fight a coronavirus most of us had never heard of and which couldn't even be proven. While the unnecessary lockdowns destroyed small businesses, they massively enriched the already filthy-rich globalist wolves, salivating for more. It forced the masses off of paid jobs and independent living, to receive governmental stimulus checks and dependent living.

In a very few months (though it had never happened before), and through the idiocy of earlier legislation and revision use of Emergency Use Authorization, the magical COVID-19 vaccinations appeared, many months to years before they should have been allowed out of the labs. The heavy risks, ultra-toxicity, and totally experimental nature of the vaccines were hidden and instead were highly overrated, supposedly to bring a certain end to the pandemic. But they were not only experimental, new, biotechnology, but actual Chinese bio-weaponry that several United States scientists happily helped the Chinese produce. Then, insult to injury, these vaccines were mandated for millions of unwilling Americans, while anyone raising legitimate questions about them was quickly censored. Ultimately, the vaccines maimed and will continue to cripple tens of millions of people and kill millions more. Meanwhile, the "proper" public-health agencies continued to deny it, and the globalist billionaire wolves increased their wealth into the trillions selling the toxic vaccines. Supposedly, improved vaccines have been upgraded to non-experimental status per all internet information, but if you dig deep enough, you can find they are still experimental. Though nearly every informational site on the web claims the vaccines are new and improved, the lists of their ingredients have changed very little. They are still deemed "safe and effective," even though the evidence of adverse effects and deaths continues to rise exponentially.

This extremely brief overview shows what occurred in response to a so-called "virus," now known to be far less virulent than the historically-deadly 'Spanish flu', and far less dangerous to infants, healthy children, and young adults than any influenza has ever been. Just like other 'viral' influenza, most illness happened to older adults, many of whom had a plethora of other potential underlying or secondary health issues (called co-morbidities), and many were already nearing end of life. This virus actually killed only slightly more people globally than either diarrhea or Alzheimer's disease in 2020. The FACTS reported since March, 2020, are readily available in government documents, hospital records, and "reliable" scientific papers. Note: There are now many papers from education and science journals once highly regarded for truth and quality that sold out to the globalist elite wolves, and are no longer reliable. More on that later. But the legal facts are not secrets, though there is arguably some mystery in them due to perspective and perception. However, though figures are accurate when accurately reported, it is still true that numbers can always be made by interpretation and presentation to say whatever the reporter wants them to say. Stats are manipulated constantly in all aspects of our lives, e.g. the advertising and marketing industries. "Consumers, beware of the reporter!"

It is most unfortunate, but the American mainstream media was committed, with the help and cooperation of the globalist wolves running the entire farce, to showing the coronavirus as far more dangerous and virulent than it was. Therefore, the only real help for it was getting the vaccine; NO other options were conceivable!. Large, globalist-driven newspapers such as the New York Times wrote for the express purpose of continuously striking the panic button and ignoring the many positive views always available for the looking, providing individuals had motivation to look. There were still physicians and scientists who showed their integrity and ability to write truth even when they were threatened with every attempt to do so. There were still many such professionals producing accurate scientific studies with objective, provable, factual information available for the serious seeker.

Earlier globalist-produced models and pandemic drills promised dire outcomes but all proved to be doomsday-oriented and fear-mongering. Just a handful of hospitals or cities experienced a small number of difficult days, especially where really poor public policies regarding elders existed. However, the lion's share of American hospitals was NEVER inundated or rendered helpless or hopeless, and fully able to function adequately. This author is a veteran RN, and experienced the ever, ongoing disaster-training and regular drills within American hospitals, in order to be adequately prepared for unexpected events of any kind. Many back-up arrangements were made for additional space and treatment if the need arose, but those arrangements were scarcely ever utilized. Today, Disaster Drills remain a constant. The FACT is: in the spring of 2020, just a few months into the pandemic, many hospitals actually had space to spare and laid-off workers. One possible exception was in New York City, where there was more need present than in most other places in the US. Yet, the facts indicate some badly mismanaged efforts and stupid decisions were made, particularly by Governor Cuomo himself. Preparations for medical ships and field hospitals were made, but even in New York City were mostly unused and removed shortly thereafter. However, with continuous media misrepresentation of the facts and some carefully selected photos, people believed the lies and renewed their panic. After all, few of us could go there to check reality for ourselves!

The pandemic focus was not on the total number of COVID-19 cases that survived; that enormous number was far too many to count, even if there was an accurate number of positive tests calculated. The majority of COVID-19 cases quarantined at home. There is no way to get accurate counts of those. It would be interesting to add a few questions to the next census! Naturally the mainstream media was programmed to obsess on the total number of Americans who died, purportedly of COVID-19. The progressive number was constantly tracked and flashed before the public eye, lest the panic and fear be diminished, but those numbers were never truly legitimate. The methods used for reporting deaths weren't legitimate either. Consequently, numbers were grossly skewed, since anyone with a positive COVID-19 diagnosis who died, was counted as a COVID-19 death, regardless of any other existing diagnoses, even accidental injury! Despite the aggressive manipulation of statistics, the COVID death rate only represented just over 10% of ALL deaths in 2020.

Normally, reporters see themselves as governmental watchdogs looking for both errors and overreach for ALL government. However, since globalist wolves had clearly programmed liberals and mainstream media with their narrative, the hatred for President Trump and his supporters knew no bounds. Big Tech was totally oblivious to whatever state governors, and unelected scientific and medical advisors were powerfully able to accomplish as the pandemic went on. When the pandemic was announced, governors in many states usurped unprecedented and unlawful control over the citizens of their states. Many of these controls went far beyond the already overdone national standard. Some states were fortunate to have some thinking leaders who refused to follow the crowd. Journalists and many of the people NEVER questioned these extreme intrusions in their lives. Most people complied, no matter their disgust, but paid scant attention to real scientific and medical authorities who actually challenged the "official" rules. In fact, social media and tech giants went even further, blocking and censoring videos, books, groups, or individuals who dared to question the rules or have differing thoughts. Those who questioned the value of lockdowns were heavily censored since each and every corporation under globalist influence made enormous amounts of money because of those lockdowns and no intention of shutting down its rapid flow!

Giant globalist elites such as WHO used the highly cooperative mainstream media to suppress honest dissent and debate. This was particularly egregious because it set such a dangerous precedent of ignoring our First Amendment right of free speech. This is exactly the way dictatorships maintain control over their subjects; they deny the free exchange of ideas which speak against the words and actions of the regime. Besides that, the suppression led to the rise of even wilder conspiracy theories. Thankfully, the globalist leadership was NOT able to silence everyone! Much to the surprise of Alex Berenson, who became a strong voice of truth and reason to several hundred thousand Americans, yet was also considered a villain, who didn't care how many people might die of COVID because they heeded his words. However, many Americans were looking specifically for the truth and reason which was difficult to find elsewhere. When he cited his factual sources, they followed him. His tone and somewhat satirical style engaged them, piquing their interest with his approach, "Against hysteria—satire. Against storytelling—data. Against group think— reporting. Against authoritarianism—bravery. Most of all: against millennialism—realism, and hope."[1]

His obsession for truth did cost Alex a lot but he could NOT and would NOT stop fighting. He was fully aware the American response to COVID-19 was the MOST horrific public policy debacle in over a century; since before the start of WWI. At that time European leaders sent millions of young men to die for ridiculous reasons no one could even explain. Over a century later, few will ever understand the depth of that senseless slaughter, or for that matter, the depth of this one.

Now, the people perpetrating the panic had NO intention of stopping it. They clearly didn't want a "back to normal" any time soon! Once we were through with the lockdowns, but there was no guarantee they wouldn't be reinstituted should circumstances change and globalists start pushing them again. At the whim of powerful authority figures, they could theoretically be resumed for nothing more than when they had first begun. Even now, we could be returned to its influence and the change made permanent! We still encounter vestiges of mask-wearing, social-distancing, school closings, bans on indoor dining, endless testing, travel restrictions, quarantines without symptoms, and vaccination mandates in 2025, should it all be beneficial to policy makers and globalists, especially in the event of another so-called novel-virus outbreak. None of these, despite their enormous intrusion on our lives, have EVER been shown to slow the spread of COVID or any other pathogen. Our children and teens will forever bear the scars and carry the influence of the denial of their normal schooling and lack of normal social interaction. "In August 2020, 25% of young adults, aged 18-24 years, said they had seriously considered suicide,"[2] per CDC figures. This number doubled from two years previously. While these same young adults faced no serious risk from COVID, they had become terrified for their futures and while locked up, had to deal with many of their emotional issues alone! The data also revealed a surge of anxiety and substance abuse with more than 40% of those surveyed reporting they experienced a mental or behavioral health condition associated with the COVID-19 'emergency.' The numbers fell heaviest among young adults, caregivers, essential workers, and minorities. More than another 13% of respondents said they had turned to substance abuse, including alcohol and prescription or illicit drugs, to cope with the stress of the pandemic.

According to Alex, the COVID-19 debacle was only one part pandemic and five parts hysteria! In his opinion, the COVID crisis could NOT have happened one generation ago, maybe not even one decade ago, but it wasn't because of the virus. A large part of what we were told simply WAS NOT TRUE! The fact is: NO part of the predicted crisis was even fractionally as bad as the predictions. That being the case, why was the response to this 'ordinary' virus so much more exaggerated than the reaction to any other disease in humanity's history? The answer is: BECAUSE IT COULD BE! Today's society is always on continuous information overload ad nauseam, yet it demands more information every minute of every hour. It has become increasingly close to information addiction. Most of us know we should stop and regain some balance, but are seemingly either unable or unwilling to do so.

Our citizens tested for the virus endlessly—Because We Could! Testing for the novel coronavirus was done by machines which counted the number of "polymerase chain reactions (PCRs) by magnifying a single fragment of the 'virus' a trillion times. Vaccines were created, developed, and rolled out for worldwide distribution in far less than one year—faster than any other 'vaccine' in history, just the latest example of our supposed scientific brilliance. Sadly, we mostly accepted the magic tricks being played on us while forgetting or ignoring many crucial facts. Such medical 'wonders' came at the highest possible cost! When a viral fragment is multiplied a trillion times, it was easy to show positive test results in thousands who weren't even sick, likely had no symptoms and possibly never would be actively ill. But we told these healthy people they were ill, and made them and the people around them stay home, causing a "medical cascade" of over-tested, healthy people.[3]

The coronavirus itself did not disrupt the food chain, although the totally unnecessary lockdowns did cause various disruptions. That same virus did not overrun our hospitals as was frequently reported, also proven wrong. However, the vaccination requirements for highly-reluctant nurses put the whole system under enormous stress for want of needed and qualified medical personnel. The virus killed far fewer American children than "drowning, cancer, abuse, accidents, and a dozen other potential causes, but globalist wolves and governmental leadership "panicked" and led us all to believe this virus was so much more deadly than these known causes. After all, it was planned that way. COVID-19 did only a small fraction of the damage feared when it first left China, however, the dangers it revealed are still here to stay. The total medicalization of society will never go away now, nor will our reliance on supposedly advanced technology. In spite of that, there is an entire camp of professional scientists and medical personnel who maintain the SARS-CoV-2 was NOT a virus, because viruses themselves have never been seen or proven, and are often considered a wild theory, making no sense, but keeping at least half an army of 'professional virologists busy working with them!

Starting a New Year with a New Pandemic

Right after the holidays of 2019, rumors began flying about a strange outbreak of a respiratory disease in China. By January 14, 2020, the World Health Organization (WHO) tweeted an announcement, "Preliminary investigations conducted by Chinese (CCP) authorities have found NO clear evidence of human-to-human transmission of the novel coronavirus, (2019-nCoV) identified in Wuhan, China."[4] In truth, this was one of only a few statements the WHO has actually ever been correct about, since contagion from person-to-person or person-to-anything else is also still just a theory.

From the very beginning of the "leak" in China, the CCP was very busy with denial of having a problem at all. When it became well known, the research at Wuhan was just doing exactly what CCP's military had ordered it to do. Since the biotechnology was all a part of the military's bioweapons preparation, the military wanted the so-called virus well disseminated as planned, with less chance of containment, and greater escalation of fear and panic from the start. The United States had already made several offers of help with investigation which were categorically refused. In fact, no one was allowed to investigate anything reported as dire first-hand. WHO was finally allowed to take a team in by mid-February, but that was an expected concession for a globalist partner. Meanwhile, the CCP sent thousands of its own infected people internationally through multiple airlines to multiple destinations to further disseminate the virus. Then President Trump banned all Chinese flights to the United States. In addition to the deliberate infection of possibly millions globally, the CCP officials instructed Chinese companies to buy up all the gloves, masks, and ventilators they could locate worldwide, to horde all available medical supplies and short the rest of the world of the same needed supplies as demand increased, which massively inflated prices.

Meanwhile, social media continued performing its designated role; fanning the flames of panic and fear, a task already done regularly, for which they were uniquely qualified and skilled to do. Today we know and can prove the majority of news, contrived videos, and propaganda were being posted constantly. All the "what-ifs" of speculation ran the gamut of the media's imaginations. When President Trump announced the travel ban, the first media and political wars ensued. Liberal Democrats and the media criticized the President, and the ban, while the WHO claimed it was not necessary. Strangely, all the hype made it look very necessary! No one wanted the President to act on the hype, but continued to criticize him for not doing more. By March, however, most countries had closed their borders.

Some of the historical elements of epidemic-type diseases were brought up for comparison with the COVID-19 pandemic, however, they definitely required further examination, and a good deal of closer scrutiny. The 'Spanish Flu' was a well-known respiratory disease that happened globally for a variety of reasons during the WWI era. Similar to today, the illness was often cyclic and seasonal in nature. The horrors observed at that time provoked a global scientific and medical response. The ideas of public health and epidemiology emerged, due to two, mid-nineteenth century British scientists, John Snow and William Farr. Snow was famous for mapping a cholera epidemic and tracing it back to a public water pump. He was able to persuade the city to remove the offending pump handle and that outbreak quickly ended.

Farr demonstrated that "epidemics" often rose and fell in remarkably symmetrical patterns which could be approximated statistically by a normal bell curve. The data closely fit a normal distribution of cresting and declining, no matter what the actual underlying disease was. "Illnesses spreading quickly tended to burn out equally fast." (Farr's Law) Also, they often seemed more deadly at first, then they tended to become less virulent in time. Farr offered many common-sense ideas to reduce the number of outbreaks. Some examples were: No burying decaying bodies near crowded areas and dwellings, nor near public water sources, nor those of sewage disposal. Animals should not be crowded into small spaces. Apartment buildings needed indoor plumbing. Cities must be cleaner and healthier. Following these ideas, people began to live much longer. During the Spanish Flu, local public health departments did some temporary closing of public places and some cities recommended or required masks, but the epidemic waxed and waned on its own. That's exactly what COVID-19 would have done, had it lacked all the unnecessary manipulations used.

Shortly after the epidemic ended in 1919, Dr. W.H. Kellogg, the Executive Officer of the California State Board of Health published a *Summary of Conclusions Reached as a Result of the Study of the Control Measures Adopted.* He said, "When I compared the course of the epidemic in different cities, I found that most regulations had made very little difference, and was particularly dismissive of masks. The very complete records at the disposal of the California State Board of Health indicated conclusively that the compulsory wearing of masks did NOT affect the progress of the epidemic. Three Eastern cities that had no mask rules had seen the same course of the epidemic as that of the masked San Francisco." Nor did mass closings seem to matter. Kellogg wrote, "Instead, he argued that self-isolation of sick people appeared to be the most effective tactic against the flu."[5]

In the late 19th Century the famous German physician, Robert Koch, did studies of so-called 'infectious diseases.' Physicians believed bacteria might be a cause, but some(bacteria) might be too small to see and coined the term "viruses" for those. This idea was nothing but a theory which has yet to be proven today with the true scientific method. A "virus" has NEVER been isolated without the use of electro-magnetic microscopes. Due to the highly-destructive nature of the preparation of a slide for this microscope, it is extremely unlikely the final results seen on that slide bear any resemblance to a living organism. Dr. Thomas Rivers postulated, "viruses could NOT reproduce on their own," yet by law, all living creatures reproduce. It is known that ALL life depends on genetic foundations, found in long strands of amino acids. Small fragments of these strands can be seen, but there are no guarantees that the fragments belong to 'viruses' with a plethora of other protein possibilities on the 'dressed-up' slide culture. There are a few things virologists "suppose" or "theorize" about 'viruses' but there is simply "NO Proof" available scientifically because there are no control studies showing scientific evidence that "viruses" even exist."[5]

Though modern death tolls may shock us, they have actually changed very little from their norms—within COVID-19. Though the CDC would have us believe COVID has caused more deaths; interestingly, flu deaths almost disappeared. Truth is, death numbers year-to-year as a whole changed very little. As we view the Spanish Flu pandemic, fortunately, even without lockdowns, vaccinations, or year-long school closures, it passed and was forgotten surprisingly quickly. Sociologists would tell us people over a century ago were undoubtedly far more accustomed to facing their mortality. After all, women still routinely died in childbirth. Political leadership was also far more ruthless. European governments had just sacrificed millions of their citizens lives for a pointless war—with little protest, even from those men who were being sent to the slaughter. The numbers for war and for the flu were comparable.

Still, the 'flu' NEVER disappeared. Several other supposed varieties surfaced (at least they were given different names) and killed hundreds; The Hong Kong flu of 1968 produced at least 100,000 deaths. Diagnosed cases received little extra attention, and did NOT require masks, much less school closings, quarantines, or lockdowns. In fact, we can examine Woodstock, the massive concert where 100's of thousands of people gathered for days at a farm in upstate New York during the Hong Kong flu. So what in the world caused the total hysteria and overblown public health measures for another respiratory illness that differed little from and replicated influenza? Epidemic focus had ceased for almost an entire generation. In that era, the majority of people were far more interested in wellness. It was an outstanding way to live, but of course, anyone in the health-care industry wasn't making much money. Then in 1976, just slightly more than two decades later, The "swine flu" surfaced and so did the panic. Predictions said it might become another Spanish Flu, but they proved to be wildly wrong and in fact, backfired. "Big Pharma very hastily prepared a vaccination which was later blamed for hundreds of cases of Guillain-Barre syndrome, a neurological ailment that often leads to muscle weakness, paralysis, and even death."[6]

About a decade after the flu vaccine debacle, Dr. Anthony Fauci became the Director of the National Institute of Allergies and Infectious Diseases, during the HIV/AIDS era and his rise to influence was meteoric, though his actual contribution to the problem was anything but heroic. There was an extreme political and medical demand for appropriate life-saving treatments. Fauci did have the ability to get the needed financial backing. By 1996, there were some effective drug treatments, and he was given credit for helping many affected people. Sadly, the truth was that HIV killed nearly everyone it affected. It was actually a totally dismal failure for Fauci, but when other illnesses, including COVID-19 later appeared, far too many people ignored his previous failures.

In 2005, President George Bush ordered the Federal Government to update its plans for an epidemic, whether natural or by bioterror attack. CDC scientists began working on a report to guide federal response. It focused on "non-pharmaceutical interventions (NPIs), a catch-all term for ways to 'slow the spread of disease besides actual medical treatments.' These could be as basic as encouraging simple handwashing or as aggressive as shutting down whole countries. Dr. Robert Gleason, following the lead of his own 14-year-old daughter's simple science model, suggested school and business closures might slow the flu. He created a simulation "proving lockdowns could reduce a hypothetical epidemic spread. He and his wife wrote about the simulation in a CDC journal showing this "mitigation strategy worked."

Of course it is crucial to know these model simulations were NOT based on realworld data. There was little if any available data on the subject to simulate. Models relied on small singular studies on hand-washing and other simple interventions. They also used reports about masks and quarantines used during the 1918 Spanish Flu epidemic. But more importantly they admitted later they were just guessing! A 2007 paper in the *Proceedings of the National Academy of Sciences* acknowledged, "A recent review concluded that the evidence base for recommending such interventions is extremely limited, consisting primarily of historical and contemporary observations, RATHER THAN Controlled Studies."[7]

The modelers gained ground as the debate progressed and the CDC released its report in February 2007. The report divided epidemics into five categories by size. Steps such as school closures of up to 12 weeks were recommended ONLY for the most serious outbreaks. The report didn't even mention the possibility of complete societal lockdowns! Still, an official government document had now recommended restricting public gatherings. In 2017, the CDC revised its planning forecast and removed the five categories of epidemics, but the die was cast, and this change definitely gave lawmakers (no one else) more flexibility to impose strict measures, should a NEED arise. In 2019, even the WHO did not discuss broad lockdowns. Even prior to that, scientists with expertise in epidemiology worried hyper-interventions wouldn't work and might very well backfire.

In 2006, Henderson, et al. stated, "We must ask whether any or all of the proposed measures are epidemiologically sound...and consider possible secondary social and economic impacts. The writers declared similar previous efforts to slow the spread of flu in past epidemics had largely failed. They pinpointed quarantines, travel bans, and school closings of more than two weeks as likely counterproductive, and didn't even mention full lockdowns." Near the end of their paper, they pled with leadership to simply focus on the best support to medical systems and "let life go on as normal. Experience has shown communities faced with epidemics or other adverse events respond best and with the least anxiety when the normal social functioning of the community is least disrupted."[7] The authors finally added models and simulations should be viewed as aids to decision-making. Unfortunately, in the midst of a crisis, there is always pressure for government to employ public health interventions, "*even in the absence of proven benefits.*" That's exactly what happened a mere 14 years later!

As the case numbers rose, official panic set in. There was a huge demand for cleaning supplies and masks. The cost of a box of 100 dust masks rose from $8 to $200 in just a few days. Public health experts discouraged civilians from buying masks, stating there was "NO ROLE for these masks in the community," per Dr. Robert Redfield, director of the CDC. Further, three days later, Dr. Jerome Adams, surgeon general said, "You can increase your risk of getting sick by wearing a mask if you are not a healthcare provider. There are things people can do to stay safe. There are things they shouldn't be doing and one of those things is going out and buying masks in the general public."[9] My goodness, even professionals changed their minds on the efficacy of wearing masks, creating even more fear and confusion.

The 'run' on masks both reflected and amplified the global spread of sheer panic. However, the world at large seemed to continue functioning normally. Then on March 6, 2020, a huge tweet from Italy told people globally this COVID thing was so much worse than anyone thought and Italy locked down completely. For the first time since WWII, an advanced democracy had "asserted the right to interfere" in the most basic of its citizens' lives, without any discussion or debate. With Italy's aging population and harsh northern winters, it regularly suffered severe winter flu epidemics. In 2016-2017 alone, the flu and other respiratory illnesses had killed more than 40,000 Italians, a full 80 times more than had yet died of COVID when it locked down. Yet, no one globally questioned whether Italy had overreacted. Meanwhile, Anthony Fauci continued declaring it would get far worse on March 11, 2020. By that time, Fauci had become the FACE of COVID response in the U.S. and globally, exactly as planned by the globalist wolves.

Remember, Fauci was just a member of the federal COVID-19 task force, but he did not head it up. He was NOT the most senior doctor or scientist in American government. He also was NOT the head of the NIH or the CDC. He was NOT the surgeon general or secretary of the U.S. Department of Health and Human Services. Robert Redfield, the CDC Director, should naturally have been the face of the Federal response, but he lacked Fauci's dignity, presence, and solemnity of manner! Long before this Fauci had become more powerful than his relatively modest title suggested. However, Fauci had a long history of unregulated power in his NIAID, and was always able to procure big money from people and groups for research with barely a question. Besides all of that, he had a highly-elevated opinion of himself and more than anyone else, he had a place of power with the global wolves and their multi-billions. President George W. Bush respected him so much he awarded Fauci with the Presidential Medal of Freedom—one of the two highest awards given to civilians in the U.S.

Democratic liberals and progressives wanted desperately to remove President Trump from office at ANY cost. Anthony Fauci was more than willing to work with them on this agenda. He was not only a willing player, but was very clear on the importance of the media. He had spent decades cultivating relationships with all those who covered science and medicine regularly and was always available to these people. Even after President Trump put Vice President Pence in charge of the COVID Task Force on February 25, 2020, Fauci was still considered the "go-to guy," for decisions.

He used that power to make sure the United States responded to the COVID-19 as aggressively as possible, no matter the cost.

New Mantra: "Flatten the Curve in 15 Days"

The World Health Organization declared COVID-19 a Pandemic, not just an epidemic! Soon, Big Tech made a laughing stock of anyone in the public eye who showed or spoke about NOT taking the pandemic seriously enough, especially anyone young. The NBA suspended its season. The NHL and college basketball followed suit. Suspensions of regular sports venues fanned the public panic. Someone came up with a new mantra, "Flatten the Curve" which meant to slow the spread of the virus to reduce peak numbers. It was supposed to take 15 days to do this 'flattening.' This seemingly looked like an attainable goal everyone could get behind and a plausible reason to temporarily lockdown everything to attain it. The stock markets and S & P plunged. About two million firearms were sold in March of 2020, reflecting the level of panic. A massive decline in travel to go anywhere occurred. By mid-March, school districts had begun to close. Researchers at Imperial College-London had used an entire week to make terrifying predictions to British, European, and American leaders.[10]

Meanwhile, a physicist-turned epidemiologist named Neil Ferguson who had failed miserably to crunch the prediction numbers earlier, had been able to influence French President Emmanuel Macron. Just like Fauci with his scientific/medical jargon, he changed it regularly to fit the narrative, Ferguson became even more important when he went to work for the World Health Organization. With no evidence of efficiency seen, he was in a uniquely influential position in the UK to drive public health policies in Europe and the U.S. as well. China kept spouting their figures on quelling the virus with extreme lockdown measures, and Ferguson believed ALL countries should do the same, but he didn't believe Western nations would "tolerate" lockdowns. However, they just might comply if sufficiently terrified! Therefore, horrific numbers were posited along with dire threats of breaking hospital systems. Instead of mere mitigation, their report called for full "suppression," defined as "social distancing of the entire population," including household quarantines and school closures. Even more extreme, it determined the suppression would be necessary until a vaccination became available. At that time, it might well be another 18 months. ONLY indefinite closures would work, so suppression was the "preferred policy option." Social media stepped up the panic. Ferguson's report was considered perfect for Twitter as it had "academic authority." It made no difference that these world-changing recommendations were made on the very weakest possible evidence and really bad mathematics. It went absolutely viral-thousands of times more viral than the virus![11]

Consequently, the Imperial College report basically guaranteed the full-on lockdowns, a step of intentional and irresponsible nonsense which was not debated or delayed. There were already hints of the potential catastrophe being greatly over-projected. One of those was the news from the Diamond Princess Cruise ship. Three thousand, six hundred, and fifty passengers plus crew members had been quarantined. Despite confined quarters and a fully-shared ventilation system, only 712 people got sick, which was less than 20% of the total. Only 14 died, a rate of only 2% with the majority of the cruising people being over 60 years old. Early Italian data showed very similar figures.

While Fauci got much closer to accurate figures. He did say it was clear the overwhelming numbers of serious disease cases and mortality were found in the elderly and in those with other serious underlying disease entities. He didn't seriously expect to see much mortality among the young and healthy and he was right. However, Fauci and other so-called "experts then changed course and deliberately obscured the fact that COVID posed no serious risk to healthy people under 50 years of age. The question is, "Why?" The answer is because pretending the virus posed a significant risk to everyone, was the only way for the government to ensure the public would accept the lockdowns. In Ferguson's report, *Options for Increasing Adherence to Social Distancing Measures*, his committee clearly laid out the issues, "Perceived Threats: A substantial number of people still do not feel sufficiently personally threatened; it could be they are reassured by the low death rate in their demographic group…the perceived level of personal threat needs to be increased among those who are complacent, using hard-hitting emotional messaging. Communication strategies should provide social approval for desired behaviors…social disapproval from one's community can play an important role in preventing anti-social behavior…consideration should be given to the use of social disapproval, but with a strong caveat around unwanted negative consequences."[12] Does the reader feel the anger at being psychologically discussed and manipulated like a theater of puppets? This one surely did!

It's true governments and public health agencies have long discouraged certain behaviors and encouraged others—-drunk driving, smoking cigarettes and marijuana, healthy nutrition, medical screening, etc. However this campaign of promoting complete social distancing and lockdowns became the world's MOST aggressive propaganda campaign democracies anywhere had conducted since WWI, if not ever. A few skeptical scientists and in fact many well-informed individuals tried to push back the rabid frenzy—but the lockdowns spread. At first the push backs were simply ignored. But many refused to give up and began posting protests on social media. They were quickly and continuously shut down with deliberate censoring of anything that defied the propaganda of the globalist elite agenda. On March 19, 2020, California's Governor Newsom, announced the stay-at-home order for the entire state of California. Its population of 40 million had fewer than 2000 cases of COVID and fewer than 20 deaths. Clearly this policy was pure overkill and its enforcement bordered on the brutal and asinine.

During the HIV epidemic decades earlier, newspapers questioned public health pronouncements and WARNED against government overreach. As early as June of 1983, the New York Times published an opinion piece entitled, "AIDS and Civil Liberties," citing the "danger that the judicial and political systems would fall prey to the irrational demands of a frightened public and impose groundless and onerous regulation resulting in the widespread loss of freedom. The response to COVID was entirely reversed![13]

"Following the Science" That Wasn't Really Science

All the science demanded the same degree of sophistication to determine if people were infected with SARS-CoV-2, as it supposedly took to create it in the first place. Kary Mullis won the 1993 Nobel Prize in chemistry for inventing the PCR technology that was used to test for COVID-19. "Polymerase Chain Reaction, or PCR is the basis of the most common, gold standard tests for the SARS-CoV-2 coronavirus and was used in almost any form of DNA study. To test DNA strands, very small sequences of the DNA chain are copied exponentially so tests can detect them. The PCR test is a multi-faceted process that duplicates the viral DNA in a continuing cycle of at least 30 times in order to detect the presence of the virus."[14] This is an extremely simplified description of the process, but it's important to understand pros and cons of using it as a COVID test, rather than just the process it was invented for.

This PCR test for COVID-19 looked for specific chains of mRNA nucleotides supposedly unique to SARS-CoV-2, then used this complex chemical process to multiply those chains hundreds of times until they could easily be detected. In theory, the test is both specific and sensitive. Supposedly it was capable of identifying ALL SARS-CoV-2 disease without being fooled by any other similar viruses. Originally, the discovery of such an accurate test was seen as a really big breakthrough. ONLY LATER did it become clear that basing everything on this untried sequence for diagnostic purposes was not only risky, but highly misleading. However, the PCR became the global standard, regardless of its major flaws, and in fact was really BAD Science!!

Next, there was an enormous controversy over the drugs used for treating COVID-19. As previously discussed, hydroxychloroquine was being used very effectively along with ivermectin and was clearly saving lives. The major problem was with the globalist elites who weren't making big money on these standard medications which were readily available and inexpensive. After saving hundreds of thousands of lives and preventing hospitalizations, the FDA conducted some bogus trials on them, exaggerating dosages to prove they didn't work, then banned their use in deference to their new drug, remdesivir, which was truly toxic, ineffective, expensive, and had to be administered by I.V. It was touted as the only drug needed to treat COVID patients, especially if they were hospitalized. Remdesivir wasn't even approved by the FDA in early 2020, but was rapidly pushed through the EUA process to get it. This lethal drug, approved by the FDA, CDC, WHO, etc., caused

100s of thousands of deaths in hospitals before it was stopped. Patients who entered the hospital with COVID who often weren't even seriously ill, could quickly deteriorate and die on remdesivir. There had been only one very bad and abbreviated clinical trial done with no control group and it was aborted before finished. Anthony Fauci did the major pushing, announcing, and over-estimating the drug's value. The drug company, Gilead, made over $4 billion on it in just 9 months of use. IT WAS EXTREMELY BAD SCIENCE!! In fact, it was one of the worst, most heinous crimes ever perpetrated on the American people, and wasn't done for or because of science at all. It was pure, unadulterated greed for an enormous amount of money. Aborting the one and only partial clinical trial and pushing it out for use when they knew its track record proves once again that it was premeditated murder.

Most of the patients placed on remdesivir wound up on ventilators before dying. There was significant protest among healthcare staffers who watched this process happen time and again. Yet, medical staff also knew that using ventilators could also help protect patients. While intubated they did not cough nor have need of treatment with nebulizing masks that delivered more virus-filled droplets into the air. Ventilators could also introduce doses of other drugs. At the same time, some felt a sense of panic that there might not be enough ventilators to go around. Unfortunately, the overly aggressive use of ventilators also backfired. The intubation of patients should always be an absolute last-resort procedure. Ventilated patients are also at high risk for additional bacterial lung infections. Most ventilated patients must also be sedated with powerful opioids because ventilation is uncomfortable and often painful. Sedated patients can't/don't move much—another risk for increased pneumonia, and bedsores. The high lung pressures can also destroy the lungs of many patients, even if they live through it.

In April of 2020, only 38 patients out of 1,151 in a New York City hospital who had all been on ventilators during the earlier COVID wave had been discharged and 282 died. The remainder of the patients were still hospitalized with grim prognoses. These figures were taken from the Hopewell Health COVID-19 Research Consortium with support from the Feinstein Institutes for Medical Research. It was the largest such to date from the U.S. over a 35-day period, and published in the Journal of the American Medical Association (JAMA). Of the patients studied, co-morbidities were also determined. 57 % had hypertension, 41% had obesity, and 34% had diabetes, and the most common underlying problems seen. Patients with diabetes were more likely to have received invasive mechanical ventilation, treatment in the ICU, and development of acute kidney disease. The majority of patients were male and median age was 63 years old. Mortality rates were also higher for male patients in each 10-year age interval. This was an early landmark COVID-19 study that provided a great deal of early insight into front line response. It also helped speed the end of overly-aggressive ventilation tactics.[15] For almost the whole first year of the pandemic, there were only two main treatment advances. One was the use of a 60-year-old steroid (Prednisone) and the second was the "proning"(lying on stomach) of patients because it appeared to make patients breathe easier. Medicine is never easy—the human body is wondrous and very complicated. Truly rapid advances are exceedingly rare.

> "For You formed my inmost being. You knit me together in my mother's womb. I will give thanks to You, for I am fearfully and wonderfully made." Psalm 139:13-14 NLT

Panic Reigned in Citizens, AND in the Globalist Wolves

Everything and every perpetrator in this chapter had what appeared to be one main goal—to keep the fear factor running high and wide. At the epicenter of COVID-19 of the U.S., was a New York City reprobate named Andrew Cuomo, governor of New York state and right-hand man to the grim reaper. He NEVER appeared to care for the people of his state, nor even humanity in general. Despite a rather unsavory reputation, his popularity grew rapidly as the pandemic grew increasingly dismal, thanks to mainstream media efforts. COVID-19 had smashed NYC and its environs like a typhoon early in 2020 along with its 20 million residents, but it was also the largest global media capital in the U.S., if not the world.

In the very beginning, Governor Cuomo had fought against a lockdown in NYC, saying it couldn't happen legally and he wouldn't do it, but the very next day it happened just the same. An enormous number of new COVID cases had forced his hand; the number of positive COVID tests went from 700 to 8,000 in one week. By Sunday, March 22, 2020, the number of patients hospitalized in the state had doubled over the weekend to more than 2000. Panic also increased exponentially, and dire predictions of hospitals being overwhelmed and supplies being exhausted scared New Yorkers badly. Such possibilities along with a need for triage tents were actually the norm for public health planners, but few normal citizens were aware this was already covered. In fact, the headlines in previous influenza epidemics of 2018 and 2000 were actually very similar.[16]

Soon, however, people began to notice a very large difference between the horrendous reports of the press and what was really happening in hospitals. They started posting pictures and videos of hospitals with empty parking lots and almost empty emergency rooms on social media. When this went viral, it forced the so-called media fact-checkers to clarify reality. They stressed that although some hospital beds might be temporarily empty, the COVID-19 crisis was still very real and far from being over. Patients were dying—in fact a Times reporter wrote of a former colleague who had died, saying it could have been any one of us and it could have been YOU! That was definitely the kind of news that increased the fear factor. Another attempt at skewing the facts to perpetrate fear was the reporting of an 81- year-old former spokesman for gay life and HIV who supposedly died of complications of COVID-19, causing some rage over his loss. However, much later, it was revealed the man had also been suffering from lung cancer and COPD before incurring COVID-19. He was the epitome of the typical kind of COVID death.

Like most influenza outbreaks, the numbers of cases rose, then the rate of increase slowed sharply; the usual pattern for so-called infectious diseases is hills and valleys, often lasting for an average of two years. COVID-19 was no different. Unfortunately, many health care workers, in the midst of an infectious onslaught also have to deal with fear and panic. They work in the midst of the infected first-hand; some incur the disease, maybe take it home to their family, and then recover. A few don't recover, which was also what happened to many medical personnel forced to take the vax jabs by mandate, and never recovered. Reporters often seek out staff who are minority nay-sayers for interviews about their circumstances and fears, instead of asking those who stay objective in the reality. More fear-mongering was constantly being delivered to all those focused on hearing it. A very large amount of the same was daily coming out of NYC, full of the worst possible predictions. The other reason for all the negative propaganda was to gain more compliance with all the public-health demands. Here again, do NOT be deceived—Mandates are NOT Laws and should NEVER be treated as Laws!

When all the negative hype and heinous predictions reached an all-time high, Governor Cuomo began talking of "rationing ventilators." Anyone listening to the social media were not only panicked, but verbal about it, which increased the believability of how bad it really was. It seemed like almost everyone was scared, which of course was exactly the goal of Big Tech globalists. In late March, one Brooklyn writer made a totally unfounded prediction that from 2 to 7% of Americans (about 23 million people) would ultimately die of the "virus." Later, that writer deleted her post! Don't we all wonder how much she was paid to write that!

Naturally, ALL of the mainstream media and Big Tech knew exactly who should be blamed for this whole disaster—President Donald Trump. Just 3 months into the pandemic, circa late March, there was just as much fear and anger focused on the President, as on the virus itself. He had somehow failed us according to Democrat leftists and progressives, as well as the whole of the Globalist Elite camp. Almost all end-of-civilization predictions were produced by leftists. They didn't just attack his COVID response, but his moral/ ethical integrity as well. This was NO accident to be sure. It had all been planned by globalist elite wolves intentionally because President Trump did not fit their agenda and he had to go. President Trump would always fight for the freedoms and opportunities of Americans FIRST, and they would do whatever it took to keep him far from the oval office in any upcoming elections.

President Trump had no reason to know any more about COVID-19 than literally ANYONE else, but he was never prone to panic or to act irrationally in crisis. To his credit, he tried to stabilize the fear-mongering and offer solutions, but most of the time was either beaten down, misquoted, or ignored by the media. In the beginning of COVID-19, he predicted and stuck to his statement that it would go away more than a dozen times and he was eventually right. "He was right on the most important point of all points. Trump was right from the beginning and ultimately right!" He had done his homework also and he didn't believe the worst of predictions. He said the death rate from COVID would be only a fraction of 1% of cases as opposed to the 3-4% then being reported. He could see we'd had hundreds of thousands of people who got COVID and recovered in a few days when no one else seemed to see it—they preferred the dire predictions of the hospitalized. Naturally, that statement was trounced on like a bunch of ravenous wolves on dead prey. But President Trump's optimism was correct. The COVID-19 death rate turned out to be well below the 1% he'd said. "Trump was not just right, but he was right for all the right reasons."[17] Main-steam media reporters NEVER acknowledged it when President Trump was right, only when they claimed he wasn't right or if his statements failed to promote their whole global agenda. To this day, they would have us and the world believe Trump was an utter failure and accomplished nothing in his administration. That couldn't be farther from the truth.

In spite of the above nauseating scenario, President Trump's numbers and supporters were excellent. He had accomplished some superior things in his first term. He had managed to keep almost every pre-election promise he made. America was Great Again in spite of COVID-19. The stock market was at an all-time high, and unemployment had dropped to its lowest level in 50 years. But his stellar record would never do for leftists or globalists. He MUST NOT be re-elected under any circumstances. Therefore, the coronavirus and its handlers destroyed the U.S. economy almost overnight! The idiotic and unnecessary lockdowns were announced. It was no surprise to the globalists—THEY planned it all. Once again, unemployment soared to the worst level since the Depression. President Trump was attacked constantly while Anthony Fauci became the pandemic icon, even though he NEVER had anything good to say and continuously touted, supported, and extended all the mandates he'd promoted from the beginning.

Within just a few weeks, it became abundantly clear there were no ventilator shortages. Actually, by mid-April, New York was shipping ventilators to other states. One week later, the Northwell Health study showed conclusively that ventilator use had been highly overrated for saving lives and had in fact been shown to have likely killed some patients. The media ignored the facts completely. Trump bashing continued, even to accusations he had caused many preventable deaths, but almost all the anti-Trump rhetoric was categorically false. The truth remains—the whole coronavirus narrative was intended to destroy President Trump. His power to handle many decisions was already out of his hands and very limited, but American federalism remained strong. The truth is that unless President Trump had declared martial law, he personally could NOT have locked down the entire country, even had he wanted to. That power is given to the individual states. A similar issue was also true in the debate first on schools closing and then re-opening. President Trump was fully aware of the horrific damage it was doing and wanted all schools re-opened, but that was NOT up to his discretion either.

In addition to all of the above issues, all the critics who had so much to say about the President, should have been offering constructive solutions for Trump's supposed failures, but nothing positive ever came from any of them. A good number of the critics didn't even like the travel ban that the President wisely put into place to stop the deliberate global movement of infected Chinese—way too many of them were in cahoots with the CCP and its globalist plans. Even before the ban happened later studies of blood donors have shown the coronavirus had already reached the U.S. by December 2019, long BEFORE the CCP had allowed news of it to go public. Interestingly, European countries where lockdowns began sooner, and were actually more stringent, had even more deaths than the United States did in Spring, 2020.

Of greater importance, President Trump's instincts had been right all along. The majority of deaths were of people over 75 years-old and severely ill or both. Finding healthy people who had died of COVID-19 was rare. Anyone dying under the age of thirty, especially if they were NOT vaccinated, were nearly nil. Most strains of influenza are more dangerous! In reality, the supposed lethal virus posed only minor risks for most people, and therefore was NOT a risk to society. Hence, all of the ridiculous and ineffective measures forced on individuals and society ILLEGALLY, were essentially worthless, yet caused so much personal and societal damage, it can NEVER be adequately assessed or prosecuted. In all likelihood, few of the powerful globalist wolves will see trials or jail, though every crime in the books was committed. If it can be proven that American globalists committed treason and other acts that threatened United States sovereignty, the military tribunals can get involved and perhaps convict and prosecute them—a definitely hopeful thought! Regardless, horrendous losses remain lost, and our Great Judge will one day make all wrongs right again. An important purpose of this book is to help readers understand what wrongs happened without restitution, and make us all wiser and more vigilant, should such actions be tried again. Why? Because the criminals are still out there and they will try this again; of that we may be sure! None have been known to relent on their hell-bent courses.

Far Too Many Things Make NO Sense

How is it that globalist Big Investors of very Big Money never seem to be sincerely concerned about the state of the globe when utter confusion and chaos reign everywhere? Preppers heard all the news of empty grocery store shelves and broken supply chains and started stocking up on essential supplies, including masks, long before mandates existed. The lives of many people were beginning to fray as their jobs were no longer available and schools closed. Many wondered, even if only briefly, how it made any sense to close down the entire economy. Families became concerned for loved ones and friends living in confined spaces. Older people in the United States could still remember other hard times and epidemic illnesses where none of this nonsense happened and most people survived. There was just as much skepticism as there was fear. A vast majority of seasoned adults knew how to think and read the reports which viewed all sides of the problem logically and could still reason with healthy common sense. As we talked and discussed the issues with others, many of us could see very clearly what was happening to our nation. Why was there no real concern shown for elder adults with greater risk factors who needed additional care, information, and help when quarantining? Instead they were just controlled and locked into situations that challenged their health and well-being. Whose idea was it to lock down all our children, jeopardizing their education, health, and social development which could NEVER be fully restored? Was it true this 'novel' virus was really a worldwide menace? We had already learned some time ago that the main-stream media was NOT even a little trustworthy and was always skewed to the left and towards the globalist agenda. COVID-19 coverage wasn't worth listening to because it changed courses so regularly. False data could be proven, but proving it was NOT allowed. Because the whole reason for planning the pandemic was based on the continued exploitation of Big Pharma, backed 100% by the globalist wolves' agenda, contriving to make billions more money on vaccines and drugs for treatment. On that basis, the calls for a vaccine were constant.

Before the global pandemic, not many people had an understanding of all the real reasons for making vaccines. Granted, Big Pharma and its controlling business of getting new drugs and vaccines to consumers was still a somewhat gray area. Even today, after all the vaccine hoopla, many folks simply do not understand the degree of criminal activity involved in Big Pharma. Of course, making and promoting vaccines has NEVER really been about developing a reliable preventive measure to keep people from getting sick with various diseases. Now we know for certain that many microbiologists the world over are focused on making more infectious pathogens, and making them more capable of sickening more people, more critically. This will ensure that new vaccines are considered forever mandatory for humanity's existence. They will continue promoting globalists and Big Pharma's greed-infested, money-making. By it they can control and maintain the New World Order with their ungodly trillions. All of the crimes committed to make this happen and keep happening are NOT prosecuted because the criminals generally have the power and money to prevent it. This is the simplest description of reality in today's world. There is additional detail later.

As we recently discussed, a so-called "expert," Neil Ferguson, of the Imperial College in London had just produced a major report on ALL the health-based measures necessary to treat and contain this heinous disaster, however, a couple weeks later, this blowhard "expert" did a total reversal on the previous report and redacted it. Now, the problem became greater as thousands of people either missed the redaction or just refused to believe it. After all, who can you believe? Consequently, the political and scientific wars over the coronavirus, lockdowns, etc., began escalating over all our heads. Why was there so much opposing information? Because the so-called "expert's" report was the only one the globalists wanted taken seriously, and promoting the lockdowns brought the necessary governmental control into focus.

It turned out the idiot "expert" and later, many other self-appointed "experts" with long histories of failed predictions as well as journalists were NOT going to report the nonsense of what he said in redaction. Naturally, the media and Big Tech worked hand-in-hand with government agencies to stoke the COVID hysteria, even if they had to lie continuously to do so. Anyone who dared to think and act rationally, had their thoughts and words censored regularly, especially when they didn't fit the globalist narrative. If we persisted in promoting the truth, we could be banned from social media platforms permanently. The promise and directive law of our Constitution was vigorously ignored and denied. Freedom of Speech was robbed from any American who dared to point that out. Globalists have no time for or inclination toward patriotism, freedoms, or federal government with democracy.

In April 2020, the grim reality of lockdowns set in with vengeance, grinding most of the globe to a screeching halt. Businesses and schools were closed. Hospitals remained open but no elective procedures or surgeries were scheduled, causing thousands of hurting people to put off needed procedures because they weren't an emergency. All normal activities stopped. There were no professional sports, few restaurants, no movies or regular entertainments, and no haircuts! It was abundantly clear with the TV ads that even extended families were NOT to visit with one another, not even for a holiday. Some people were able to take pleasure in the quiet joys of everyday life within their immediate family circles, but statistics proved that any/all addictions got worse. "Alcohol consumption increased more during COVID-19 than in the last 50 years. Risky alcohol use became an epidemic inside the COVID-19 epidemic. With stresses at an all-time high, many people turned to alcohol despite other risks of alcohol-related problems. Alcohol-related illness and deaths also rose during the pandemic. The biggest stress for most was the isolation from their fellow human beings. About 25% of people drank more than their usual, and this type of change in habit can last for years. The number of death certificates listing alcohol as a contributing factor increased by nearly 38%."[18]

Whether due to fear, sheer boredom, or some urge to become virtuous, many Americans were overcome with the urge to "rat" on their neighbors. They would actually call 911 to report simple backyard parties where people weren't wearing masks! Worse still, politicians and media encouraged this trend to call the cops. Some cities and states actually set up "tip" lines and websites, asking people to inform on one another and on businesses that tried to stay open. "Los Angeles mayor Garcetti told his city "Snitches get rewards" while encouraging his city to report businesses violating the 'Safer at Home' order, (*CBS News*, March 24, 2020)."[19] Think of it—turning in a neighbor in the presence of your children, and trying to explain it to them. It may not have been so bad in the United States with our Constitutional freedoms and protections, but who knows to what level some people might stoop to look better than their neighbors! Then, if you did get stopped or reported, you could always say you were an essential worker or you needed groceries!

American governors focused on closing retailers, schools, bars, restaurants, and public places like parks and libraries. The goal was to keep everyone at home by giving them no place to go. Exceptions were made for groceries, gas, and large-box stores who had the advantage, mostly because many of them were tied to globalist profits. Initially, the first big lockdown was essentially effective because it had been presented as temporary. Once the first lockdown was lifted, many churches resumed regular worship with some precautions, but far more churches did not reopen and some never reopened to this day. Closing churches was a glaring breach of Constitutional rights. The decline of movement in the U.S. was guesstimated at around 60%, but it was still unprecedented. Governments also self-appointed the rules (NOT legislation) were a big part of people staying at home, but the media outlets at every level did all in their power to elevate and maintain that fear factor. The perfect example of this was the addition of even more sanitation rules. You could get your groceries, but before storing them at home, they should all be disinfected. It was shocking to hear the numbers of people who followed this idiotic advice just like a bunch of sheep. Then people were warned that "even if you and your family or friends are all having no symptoms, they should not be visiting them. People should not gather in groups of more than two, even when outside, and continue to keep the distance of six feet away from them.

Next, the New York Times decided to "memorialize COVID victims to "convey the human toll of COVID-19 in a way it had never been done for any other illness or cause of death. They began running obituaries of people who had died of COVID continually, and indefinitely making the pandemic "feel" far worse than it really was. 13,365 people in the United States died of heart disease every week in 2021, (That is 1 in every 5 deaths) per the CDC.[20] If the media were to report these incessantly, the same way they did with COVID deaths, the fear of cardiac death would also increase exponentially! The media's insistence on hiding real facts simply meant almost no one could ever perceive their real odds of illness or death. The handful of states in the U.S. that didn't lockdown received a monsoon of criticism from the media, all of which had Republican governors. The truth, when all was said and done—they were absolutely right in standing their ground. In that treacherous time, for example, New York City might be quiet at 4 AM, but never ever silent. But during the lockdown, it was silent. It was also so eerie to the single person outside, it was like seeing end-of-the-world scenes playing. Can anyone imagine a city of multi-millions empty and deserted?

Yet, globalists with their agenda of depopulation thought Time Square had never looked better!

People from the leftist, progressive camp, shouting for socialist changes, began pressing for broader societal changes, and would happily allow the COVID-19 to get the job done if they could. This was being touted by globalists as well, all the way from the beginning of the crisis. It was just evidence that their destructive plans for a global reset and new world order were running along well. The globalist agenda and supporters of it made many such disparaging comments. Michael Hiltzik, a leftist columnist for the L.A. Times, wrote, "...the coronavirus could boost our plans for universal basic income— government-provided welfare payments for all."[21] That is a major tenet of the whole global reset agenda. In October, actress and liberal activist Jane Fonda made an even more blunt statement, "I just think COVID is God's gift to the left," (because it could help Biden defeat Trump). A statement of that ilk is nothing short of blasphemy which she probably intended it to be! For the threat of COVID to justify the entire remaking of American society, COVID simply had to be construed as both dangerous and deadly. Similarly, the WOKE leftists by then had placed themselves in the unbelievable position of actually rooting for disaster. Along with them were the globalists—the extremely wealthy and powerful heads of the world's largest and most profitable companies also wanted the lockdowns to continue. Giant chains like Walmart made enormous profits from government-mandated lockdowns over nearly all of their competitors. Beyond that, the massive profits of Big Tech, social media companies, and Big Pharma cannot even be imagined. When COVID arrived, it gave an absolutely unthinkable advantage to each of them that could never be measured.

Finally, in May 2020, the Democratic governor of Michigan over-extended Michigan's lockdowns. This move was completely illogical and bordering on rabid obstruction of Constitutional law. This severe governmental overreach finally inspired many residents of Michigan to pushback and organize against the lockdowns. Several thousand held a peaceful protest in Lansing. They stayed calm and orderly in their cars. The government loosened the stringent restrictions only slightly. The next protest was more forceful and citizens entered their Capitol, some of them openly carrying firearms. Similar efforts in New York and Illinois basically fizzled and their lockdowns remained.

Lockdowns—Pointless, Useless, and Counterproductive

Looking specifically at COVID-19 data as early as April 30, 2020, two crucial facts became clearly apparent: 1) The coronavirus was far less threatening than it had initially appeared. It would definitely NOT overwhelm the medical system, much less society. 2) Lockdowns, at least in the U.S. and Europe, were pointless, useless, and counterproductive! Thinkers and proponents of reality knew these facts were true, but it was still next to impossible with the mountain of false information in the narrative to get them stopped. By any reasonable thought process, if the hospitals weren't overwhelmed, there was no sound reason for lockdowns. There is a huge difference between lockdowns and quarantines, which normally would have and should have been instituted first. Lockdowns are and should have been the absolute last resort. However, that would NOT help achieve globalist goals. In this case lockdowns were needed not only to instill fear in the masses but keep them fearing endlessly. Then, it wasn't just lockdown, but additional restrictions of movement, assembly, and commerce. These restrictions permitted the massive transfer of wealth from the many to the few— the "Brazen Mass Theft of 2020-2022."

Gradually, citizens began to realize that the true reason for lockdowns had absolutely nothing to do with health. The real reason was that the globalist wolves' war was primarily against the West and restrictions were their weapons of choice. The reason—because historically, "restrictions" work amazingly well to remove power from those who are restricted, leaving them open to the theft of their lands and assets. The ruling class has all the power and ordinary people have very little power. By presenting "restrictions" as a " public heath necessity," they could forcefully implement them with far less resistance, especially in the beginning. It took some time for people in free lands to recognize all they had lost and why. It was so unfamiliar to our way of life and with the constant fear-mongering, it left many of us confused and disoriented. Material and cultural wealth are a constant result of a free people and we had become not only accustomed to it, but far too complacent about it. However, for those two years, all of our basic rights were systematically suspended, dissolved, ignored, and trampled over. By February of 2021, 47 of our 50 states were under emergency law.

It had transpired without any military involvement and not a shot was fired. Let it be clearly understood, the ENEMY had first used stealth, and then total deception. Throughout the Biden regime, globalists were still wielding power over us to a slightly lesser degree, as much of the ground they gained was still deemed safe. With the constant support of the Biden admin, every dirty trick in the book was wielded in an attempt to keep former President Trump out of the White House and out of their hair. Thankfully, all their conniving schemes didn't work, a majority of Americans saw the unfolding of sure disaster, and put a wiser and more experienced President Trump back into the White House, which has already brought much of the globalist agenda to nearly grinding stop. Unfortunately, this setback will NOT stop them entirely, but much of the damage they created during COVID-19 has or will be rectified.

Globalist imprisonment per lockdowns was deceptively labeled as a "quarantine," but the emergency orders that restricted movement, assembly, and commerce showed no resemblance to traditional quarantines. Historically, quarantines were always limited in time and location, and they only kept the sick or newly arrived travelers away from everyone else. Note: such lockdowns frequently occur in totalitarian states, but NEVER in free countries. Isolation of disease-infected members within the community is an ancient practice, going back to the earliest civilizations, and is treated at length in the Bible. God gave those restrictions on health concerns for the protection of the entire community. When a sick person was examined and found healthy, he could be returned to his family and clan. When used correctly, in the intended manner of separating the ill from the well, it was highly effective in controlling infectious disease. NEVER, EVER was it used on the entire population or for an indefinite time. It also NEVER included a mass economic shutdown of society. Their mostly agrarian societies would have all died out without the needed dependence on one another.

COVID-19's highly exaggerated lethality was always the answer to explain away any realistic expectations of personal privacy or autonomy. The very last thing globalists wanted was personal privacy or autonomy for anyone! Now it was similar to the opposite of the old adage, "Innocent until proven guilty." Even if it wasn't said, it became "everyone is sick, until proven healthy." We had all become "hypothetically" ill. What circumstances laid the groundwork for the easy-win takeover of our liberties? It was the peace and contentment we usually felt; Most of us lived reasonably comfortably in our normal day-to-day endeavors. Many of us, as citizens of the USA were woefully ignorant of the structure of our Democratic Republic. Many took no notice that our rights and freedoms were literally being pulled out from under us. We have an essential tendency to think all things will continue as they've always been. For most of the last 75 years we had freedom of movement and access to almost anything we wanted; we were completely accustomed to an unprecedented and unchallenged level of freedom and human rights. We freely gathered in all public places, often in mammoth venues, and traveled freely. It would be foolish to say it was heaven on earth, but it was certainly one of the best lifestyles to be had on Earth. Why else would half the world work so hard to get here to have the opportunity we enjoy? Maybe, we did sometimes appreciate our freedoms, but didn't really understand just how important they are. At any rate, we certainly didn't realize just how fast evil economic predators could break it all down and take it away.

A very strong and apt example of this same idea can be seen on a bit smaller scale by looking at the European Union. On its public face it appeared to be ideal. Travel barriers between countries were dropped. Having a single monetary currency greatly facilitated commerce. But a far too many Europeans missed the attached caveat. In order to have a 'Union', each country needed to surrender its own national sovereignty to Brussels, the head of the one central EU government. It was humane and very civilized, but it came at a heavy cost. There would be no more national or personal autonomy. Britain said it wasn't interested and stayed out of it. But most of the European nations didn't really understand what it was about. Many thought it would be a federation of states, akin to the United States.

This was not surprising because great effort had been made to keep the true governance of it hidden, secret, and buried in confusion, obscuring the real intent. It was next to impossible for any nation to get hold of founding documents. Does it start to seem as fishy as it truly was? Our friend Naomi Wolf told a personal story illustrating exactly what the European Union was really about.

It's a story revealing how individual citizens of a national state were victimized when the involved nations signed away their sovereignty and their people. With their various cultures and heritage virtually gone, they truly lost so much more than they could ever have gained in the EU power grab. Most of details were orchestrated by European globalists and the WEF.[22]

Ultimately, COVID-19 was relatively predictable, and very similar to the patterns already well known for influenza. Many people who tested positive NEVER had any symptoms. Those who did have symptoms usually got sicker within the next 4-5 days and recovered completely soon after. A few got worse and wound up in the hospital, also like influenza. The unlucky few who died usually did so in 7-10 days past the hospitalization. Cases differed, but the very elderly or very frail people tended to die more quickly, some without even being hospitalized at all. Rising death rates from those hospitalized in March, 2020 led to a new wave of media hysteria, but in reality, the peak of the pandemic in New York had already passed. Florida didn't lockdown until April 1, 2020 amidst dire predictions of what this delay could mean; they expected a huge surge of new patients, but the surge never came.

By mid-April, hospitals had even more space available, indicating infection had NOT spread after mid-March. The false predictors had to turn their stories around again and lie to cover their major errors. Truth was, Florida's late lockdown had no effect on the numbers at all. Other than a few states in the Northeast, hospitals' patient counts were well below normal for April. Some hospitals even laid off workers and a few actually closed down. News outlets in New York and Washington were completely clueless about this turn of events. Ultimately, even though New

York's numbers and issues lasted a bit longer, the takeaway was the same. In all likelihood, New York's lockdowns mattered very little either, and in all cases they did far more harm than good. The proof showed in the failures of all projected models. Forecasters completely overestimated the impact lockdowns would have on transmission. Also, according to model predictions, after the lockdowns, new hospitalizations and deaths should have dropped dramatically, as quickly as they rose. Instead, they all lingered into May, especially in New York. Later, in New York, another COVID-19 surge brought in 3.000 patients in 3 days. A survey found 66% of those patients had sickened at home in lockdown but 84% of them stayed home every day! Nosocomial infections are those that occur while patients are hospitalized. Lockdowns did nothing to slow those rates either.

The worst news/or best news of all (depending on your outlook), which stood to reason and common sense all along; by early April 2020, there was strong evidence the coronavirus did not spread outdoors. Consequently, making people stay inside was NOT just pointless; it was totally counterproductive as well. Tragically, there were no suggestions of causal outdoor interactions available, yet the efforts to shame people continuously into staying home continued through 2020 and well into 2021 in many places. The lockdowns went on and on, and though most people were sick to death of them, many still complied unnecessarily. Idiotic mandates were still being complied with, primarily because open rebellion was too much work! This is a key concept—globalists were fairly certain people acted habitually would probably continue to do so—part of the plan. The slightly increased flexibility and a few new loopholes acted as pacifiers. Had the media ever taken a hard look at the lockdown data, public opinion could have shifted sooner, however, hard looks at facts rarely happened either. Depending on the state you lived in, many people had already returned to their mostly normal lives as much as possible, only complying with rules and regs when forced to do so.

The prize for the biggest idiot reprobate in government leadership goes to Governor Andrew Cuomo. He almost single-handedly decided there was benefit to moving recovering COVID-19 patients to nursing homes to finish their recovery, freeing up additional hospital space. Everyone knows, except Cuomo apparently, that nursing homes contain residents already at the highest risk for contracting COVID and potentially dying from it. Naturally, a large number of elder-care people were exposed to COVID and died without concern or appropriate care. Eventually, Cuomo realized how dumb his decision had been and reversed the order, but unfathomable damage was done. In all, almost 8,000 nursing home residents died in New York—the worst per capita death rate anywhere. To add insult to injury, New York's many critical errors definitely fueled the lockdown fires, and no end was in sight. The outcries from the families of these residents were primarily ignored, and the globalist agenda for depopulating got a shot in the arm.

Weighing the Benefits and Costs of Lockdowns

Meanwhile, an enormous moral and ethical debate raged on whether legitimate benefit came out of the lockdowns. A large number of analyses have been done in the attempt to answer these questions. Policymakers and the public often vehemently disagreed on the pros and cons of lockdowns and other restrictions. "Proponents of restrictions argued they saved lives; opponents say they destroyed livelihoods. Amid these nasty debates, researchers churned out *benefit-cost analyses*, aiming to shed light on which restrictions were "worth it" and which were not."[23]

Lisa Robinson, senior research scientist and deputy director of the Center for Health Decision Science at Harvard T.H. Chan School of Public Health, said it all became an enormous undertaking. For her part, Robinson explored the complexities involved in valuing deaths averted by COVID-19 policies, using a well-established but widely-misunderstood metric called the "value per statistical life," or VSL. In the big picture, policies needed to take into account how many lives they could potentially save. But they also needed to consider the potential downsides, such as how many people could lose their jobs if a state puts a lockdown into effect? What educational losses will occur among kids who missed months of in-person school? If restrictions on restaurants were lifted, how do we weigh the economic benefits against the potential increase in COVID-19 cases—and the deaths that could result?

Benefit-cost analysis required people to carefully and rigorously explore the impacts of a policy. Digging more deeply into the real-world effects often unearthed unexpected consequences. It also highlighted the trade-offs implied when making decisions about how to allocate resources. How, then, can we assign a money value to a life? Faith-based people would immediately say it can't be done, since no one can value a life more than the God of the Universe does and He doesn't use money to value it! A metric commonly used was known as "the value per statistical life," which then and still suggests the government, or someone else somehow placed a value on someone's life, but that wasn't it. "Rather, economists start by investigating how much of their own income individuals are willing to exchange to reduce their own chance of dying by a small amount—such as by buying a safer car or choosing a less risky job for lower pay. Then these estimates are converted into estimates of value of reducing expected deaths, or into a VSL."[24] U.S. regulatory agencies currently use a VSL estimate at around $10 million. That means roughly that an average age person was/is willing to pay $1,000 to reduce his/her chance of dying, within a given year by 1 in 10,000.

Naturally, the figure would change based on other factors such as age, years of opportunity of future earnings, how much people would pay to avoid the pain and suffering caused by severe illness, etc. People might place a higher value on avoiding risks they view as "dreaded, uncertain, catastrophic, or ambiguous—like COVID. However, the real problem with scientific analysis of this issue was that it was totally after the fact for COVID-19 lockdowns. No one was given the opportunity to discuss or debate the advisability of lockdowns with or without the risk perspective. Any decision to initiate lockdowns was once again top-down, and authoritarian, exactly as globalist wolves planned it to be. They can say it was done to save lives every day of the year, but given all we know about their agenda, we can also see that saving lives was NOT a part of the decision at all. The agenda then and now is still depopulation, wanting fewer dissenters, and fewer people to control. Consequently, to say plainly that it was either saving lives or saving economies is a bold-faced lie, since neither mattered to the globalists. We've already shown the lockdowns made very little difference to the number of lives saved.

By contrast, the negative effects of the lockdowns were so profound, this book can barely address the subject. We can only name the most prominent effects briefly, including acute stress disorders at all ages, anxiety, irritability, poor concentration, indecisiveness, deteriorating work performance, PTSDs, high psychological distress such as feelings of loneliness, loss, sadness, stress, anger, depression, and insomnia, all of which are personal, mental and emotional effects. Extended physical effects of social isolation initiated serious health implications, from heart disease to dementia, and depression to death. Use of extraneous 'helpers' like overeating, alcohol, and all kinds of drugs both by prescription and illegally, increased exponentially. During the pandemic, our diets and lifestyles deteriorated generally, increasing our individual vulnerability to the very illness that isolation was supposed to be addressing. Negative economic effects included reduced incomes, rising unemployment rates, worker layoffs, increased household debt, and overall economic recession.

Studies abound, along with the concerns of a multitude of concerned parents, on both current and long-range effects the lockdowns had on students and their education. Math, reading, and history scores from those three pandemic years show students experienced a significant decline in learning. At the two-year mark of pandemic-induced school shutdowns, academic normalcy remained out of reach for many students, educators, and parents. Severe staff shortages, absenteeism, quarantines, and rolling school closures all came to challenge the whole system. Students and teachers still struggled with mental health challenges, higher rates of violence and misbehavior, and much concern about the lost instructional time. "The cumulative effect on students' academic achievement was staggering. In January, 2022, a research study reported changes in math and reading test scores across two years using data from 5.4 million U.S. students, grades 3-8. Scores were markedly lower. Test score gaps between students in poverty level elementary schools grew 20% in math and 15% in reading, indicating disruptions to learning continue to negatively impact students well past the lockdowns."[25] No blame was placed, no statements of disparity or giving up hope were dwelt on, but the numbers are significant and we still have a monumental task to rectify the damage done.

In addition to the educational impact of lockdowns on our students, we can't discount the social effects. Children at all ages experienced extended periods of social isolation. The profound and long-term effects and mental health risks of social isolation include anxiety, depression, and suicidal tendencies. Physical health risks of high blood pressure, high cholesterol and adult obesity also increased. Traumatic stress scores were as much as four times higher than normally-socialized peers. Many had sharp spikes in levels of depression. When schools closed, students often lost the structure and routine they developed from educational expectations for behavioral and academic performance. Most were sent home with packets of assignments to complete, but that responsibility became theirs, to decide when and in what order they would complete their assignments. "Consequently, actual learning was jeopardized in time spent; effectiveness of self-learning was poor to nil for many students. Little or no feedback from educators, especially if students were not self-driven learners, contributed to the losses, and much more. Many students could not rely on parental help if they too were working from home. The impacts of lags in education continued. Children who resumed learning at the same pace as before the pandemic made progress but did not rebound or catch up what was lost. There are too many difficult concepts children can't learn hurriedly, but school leaders MUST expand recovery efforts today. This is unlikely to happen without a major increase in instructional time. In recent years, the average amount of dedicated instructional time had decreased, even before COVID. Since COVID, that amount of time has not increased even with the known necessity. Inequity in educational systems has been a key problem for decades and wasn't well addressed after COVID either."[26] Education's "Long COVID" continued but much of America's educational system has been broken or jeopardized by socialist indoctrination and misdirected leadership. We all hope for sound educational reform in this administration —it's desperately needed.

How Deadly Was COVID-19 Really?

The entire world was subjected to the travesty of a major pandemic, and people's lives changed immeasurably in a relatively short space of time. Except for the faraway bio-pathologists in China, very little was known about this 'novel' virus, nor were experts inclined to pass out information. If they made us believe the virus was deadly, it would keep everyone more panicked. Researchers around the globe were busy attacking the virus, but there were no brilliant breakthroughs on its 'secrets.' Early on, no one was known to have a drug combination for treating it. A vaccine was (or should have been) a long way from development. The media repeated the same old information with equal or greater insistence and we heard from celebrities who, as usual, knew absolutely nothing more about it than the rest of us. However, because of their self-proclaimed status they thought they knew more, or at least the media thought they did! The huge focus on the overall death toll from COVID-19 was constantly and publicly displayed, like the ticker tapes on Wall Street. The numbers inched higher every hour of every day because they were cumulative and never reset, a powerful ploy for increasing panic. But for the globalists, even the ever-escalating number wasn't quite scary enough, so the CDC decided medical examiners and physicians should "loosen the criteria" by labeling deaths as 'COVID-related'. A new International Classification of Diseases (ICD) code was created for COVID deaths. This system is a mostly standardized global code for classifying diseases, and is basically the universal language of medicine which all of healthcare understands. Now the CDC specifically encouraged (ordered) people, coding death certificates, to use the new code in ANY case where COVID-19 was suspected.

A confirmed COVID-19 lab result wasn't even necessary! The rules for coding and selection of the underlying cause were expected to name COVID-19 more often than not. The CDC alert made it clear that deaths of people who did NOT have a positive PCR test for SARS-CoV-2 could still be reported as COVID-related. "COVID-19 should be reported on the death certificate for ALL decedents where the disease caused, or was 'assumed' to have caused, or contributed to death."[27] At the same time, a positive PCR test for SARS-CoV-2 meant a death would be counted as COVID related, even if the death certificate didn't mention COVID. In this manner, the CDC created a double standard for death coding (for COVID). It was the best way to skew the numbers and make them appear far more significant than they really were. Not all states did it the exact same way due to testing figures such as how long a positive test was valid, etc., so clearly there were definite absurdities and inconsistencies in the numbers.

Another issue in the coding of COVID deaths was larger and even more difficult to fix. The obvious reality no one ever talked about in the media was the vast majority of COVID victims who were elderly, often obese, and very unhealthy, or all three, long BEFORE COVID surfaced. In the U.S. about 35% of all COVID-19 victims lived in nursing-care residences and other long-term care facilities. "In September 2020, Service Corp International, the largest American funeral home operator, reported about one-third of all the funerals of people who died of COVID, would have died in 2020 anyway. The second third or more would have passed in the next year, 2021. COVID victims with dementia, Alzheimer's, or cancer accounted for over 100,000 deaths in the U.S. alone. For 1000's of those deaths, it would likely be impossible to distinguish between dying FROM COVID, and dying WITH COVID. But they were all counted as COVID deaths!"[28] Further, part of the 2020 increased total of deaths came because of lockdowns. Deaths of despair surged; a sharp increase in overdosing was the most obvious example. COVID killed nearly one of every 30 people globally in 2020. Yet, COVID was still far from the world's leading killer. Despite all the skewed death figures, heart disease was still the #1 killer at 9 million people, and strokes were second at 6 million people.

A fair conclusion on the incidence and severity of COVID-19 (the disease) as compared with influenza, is actually not complicated. While there are a few differences, they are relatively insignificant on the whole. Influenza symptoms could be mild, moderate, severe, and even fatal, as were COVID-19 symptoms. The CDC claimed COVID-19 was more likely to become severe or critical than the various influenzae, but much of the medical establishment would disagree with that assessment. 80% of COVID cases were either mild or asymptomatic. The other 20% of COVID cases would require oxygen support and if critical might require mechanical ventilation. In past epidemics of influenzae these percentages were very similar. In fact, when the COVID19 cases increased in the US, influenza cases diminished almost to non-existence, because almost everything infectious was deemed COVID, and testing for influenza strains also diminished. More groups of people were at higher risk for influenza than for COVID-19, including children, infants, pregnant women, and young adults. If we had as much focus on ALL people who developed flu-like symptoms and tested for it, rather than just COVID-19, it was strongly believed each case would be as manageable and non-problematic as the others. In general, most of us would call the COVID-19 hype, "making mountains out of molehills." Deaths from complicated influenza or complicated COVID-19 looked exactly the same! How do believers in Jesus Christ respond to illness and even to the dying process?

"Is anyone among you suffering? Let him pray…Is anyone among you sick? Let him call for the elders of the church, and let them pray over him, anointing him with oil in the name of the Lord. The prayer of faith will save the one who is sick, and the Lord will raise him up…the prayer of a righteous person has great power as it is working." James 5:13-16 ESV

"Peace I leave with you; My peace I give to you. Not as the world gives do I give to you. Let not your hearts be troubled, neither let them be afraid." John 14:27 ESV

"Jesus said, 'I AM the resurrection and the life. Whoever believes in Me, though he be dead, yet shall he live, and everyone who lives and believes in Me shall never die. Do you believe this?" John11:25-26 ESV

"Bless the LORD, O my soul, and forget not all His benefits, Who forgives all your iniquity, WHO HEALS ALL YOUR DISEASES." Psalm 103:2-3 ESV

"Precious in the sight of the LORD is the death of His saints." Psalm116:15 ESV

"The Lord is close to the brokenhearted and saves those who are crushed in spirit." Psalm 34:18

CHAPTER 10

Pandemia-2 The Second Year and More

A Stunning Storm to our Economy

COVID-19's effect on government was as monstrous as everything else it caused. By May of 2020, the Feds had spent hundreds of millions every week on just the PCR testing alone. Extra federal payments going to hospitals alone came to more than $3 billion every week for more than a year; that's easily a minimum of $200 billion or more. Those figures were all dwarfed by the expense of mitigating the economic costs of the extensive lockdowns.

Unemployment claims rose to $6.9 billion the last week of March, 2020, alone. By the end of April, 30 million Americans had filed for unemployment. Food and energy supply chains were at significant risk of disruption and long delays. Grocery store shelves were often empty of certain necessary commodities. Fresh fruits, staple goods, and meats, were in especially short supply. The financial system had also become highly stressed. Markets were volatile. Banks were endangered with unpaid mortgages of the unemployed. The Federal Reserve had to step in with its support. Near the end of March, Congress passed a $2 TRILLION economic aid package—more than $6,000, in new spending for each American family via stimulus payments. Many people wound up being paid more money to stay home and do nothing than they were paid when they worked!

Airlines, hotels, and travel agencies received $25 billion in cash, and another $25 billion in loans. State and local governments were given $150 billion in cash. The largest borrowing binge in our history paid for all of this. Such frivolous spending in the name of "help" for COVID victims raised the national debt to almost $25

Trillion dollars by September of 2020. "Here is the irony! When private firms conspire to raise prices on consumers, it's called collusion and is a violation of federal anti-trust laws. But when the federal government seeks an international conspiracy to extract more taxes from our nation's largest employers, it is called 'once-in-a-generation investment in America.'"[1] Furthermore, record budget deficits from overambitious spending causes the federal government to borrow historically large sums to balance its books. So, many economists estimated the COVID relief acts alone increased total federal debt by 40% over the next decade. As of February, 2024, the public debt of the U.S. was nearly $34.47 Trillion U.S. dollars, up from $32.6 trillion in July, 2023.

"If the economy cannot grow sufficiently under significant tax rate increases to pay this huge tax bill in the future, the only other means to avoid default is to pursue the go-to strategy of poorly-run third-world countries: inflate your way out of debt. Expanding the money supply and letting the overall price level rise over time made payment promises today much easier to pay off in the future—at the expense of those people who lent the government their hard-earned money. For American investors, this was primarily older folks living on a fixed income, with a portfolio heavily invested in U.S. bonds. What price should we pay for economic stimulus?"[2]

However, interestingly, the effects on our economy were almost immediate. Within months, our economy had not only stabilized, but turned upward. The extra unemployment payments saved millions of Americans from poverty. Over the summer, American recovery continued rapidly, regaining strength almost as quickly as it had lost it in the spring. Unemployment rates fell. This all sounds extraordinarily great, however, by blunting the economic hardships of lockdowns, policymakers also reduced the pressure to end them quickly. March 2020 was rock bottom, and stocks had already begun rising, even before the lockdowns began. Hedge funds and big investors already knew the media hysteria was portrayed wrongly (they planned it), and the United States would weather COVID-19.

By May, the pandemic's first wave had waned nationally. Led by Georgia and Florida, large Republican-run states eased their lockdowns to the chagrin of media forecasters who had boldly proclaimed their dire predictions of a COVID rebound in those same states. Accusations flew about constantly, but Georgia saw NO increase in the COVID case rates for an entire month after lifting its lockdown. Enter the national main-stream media fanning the panic and fear of another wave of COVID. One article predicted daily deaths would rise more than 50% in May, but they actually declined by 50%. Yet, the New York Times NEVER updated their predictions nor did they EVER admit their erroneous predictions. The more reporters treated President Trump with contempt, the more they fawned over Fauci. The White House was trying desperately to wind down its Coronavirus Task Force in a clear attempt to lower Fauci's profile in public-health policymaking. However, within just a few hours, President Trump was forced to reverse course.

Throughout the Spring and Summer of 2020, President Trump and the White House could NOT find a way to counter all the globalist elite-driven, media narratives blasting the airwaves and cyberspace with their news that the President and the United States had failed. There was massive, all-out effort to make very sure President Trump and his supporters would not stay in the White House come election day in America. The 'media ignored the fact that United States figures were clearly functioning along the same lines as the Western European countries per capita.' When our government corrected one supposed problem or failure, the main-stream media moved on to another. We always needed something more. There was a viable excitement which could be felt on the part of the main-stream media when the death counts approached 100,000! One might say that sounds like an accusation from the White House itself, but it wasn't so—it's just the only way to describe the whole tone and atmosphere of what sounded celebratory on their part.

On Saturday, May 23, 2020, the New York Times prematurely announced figures not yet reached, adding its editorial propaganda… "it's an INCALCULABLE LOSS!" Naturally the words were meant to be emotionally hard-hitting, but they were also completely illogical on so many levels. That article NEVER mentioned the more than ONE Million Americans who had died of other causes in January-May of 2020. Their deaths simply held NO significance to the globalist agenda and its Big Tech wolves.

Returning to the subject of economic losses more generally, there are so many ways the United States and its citizens lost more than can ever be accurately known. "The risks to the economy from the spread of the virus can be contained—even if the virus cannot."[3] This was the view of the Center for American Progress. They reported COVID-19 would most directly shape economic losses through supply chains, demand, and financial markets and this would require smart, timely, responses from the government. They felt the burden of meeting these economic challenges fell squarely on Congress and the Trump administration. Both groups did utilize many of the ideas posited by this group, but it was impossible to mitigate all the economic risks brought on by COVID-19.

Revenue from air travel, indoor dining, and participation in large in-person gatherings fell by more than 50% during the first 30 months of the COVID-19 pandemic. Changes in the public's behavior, brought about by regulations and personal health concerns, caused the decline. Another team of economists from USC Dornsife used economic modeling to approximate the revenue lost due to mandatory business closures at the beginning of the pandemic. It was also used to assess the economic blows from the many changes in personal behavior that continued long after the lockdown orders were lifted—such as avoiding restaurants, theaters, and other crowded places. Workplace absences, and sales lost due to the cessation of brick-and-mortar retail shopping, air travel, and public gatherings, contributed the most. At the height of the pandemic in spring, 2020, their survey showed international and domestic airline travel fell by nearly 60%, indoor dining by

65%, and in-store shopping by 43%. Losses were somewhat offset by surges in online purchases, a series of large fiscal stimuli and economic relief packages and an unprecedented expansion of the number of Americans working from home—thus being able to keep doing jobs that might otherwise have been cut.[4]

"From 2020 to 2023, the cumulative net economic output of the U.S. would amount to about $103 trillion. Without the pandemic, the total GDP over those four years would have been a projected $117 trillion—nearly 14% higher in inflation-adjusted 2020 dollars, according to our analysis."[5] The direct health expenses, driven by hospitalization costs in four different scenarios, would have totaled $20 billion in a best-case scenario in which 65,000 Americans would have died from January 2020 to June 2022. In the worst-case scenario, about 2 million would have died during the same period, with $365 billion in direct health-related expenses. Based on these findings, they concluded that most economic losses were NOT due to these health care expenditures.

Why does it matter now? "The COVID-19 pandemic's economic consequences were totally unprecedented for the U.S. by any measure. They estimated the toll it took on the nation's gross domestic product (GDP) was twice the size of that of the Great Recession of 2007-2009. It's 20 times greater than the economic costs of the 9/11 terrorist attacks and 40 times greater than the toll of any other disaster to befall the U.S. in the 21st Century to date. In addition, even after the pandemic was declared to be over, the pandemic was still influencing the U.S. economy. The labor force participation rate, which stood at 62.6% in April 2023, has only recently come close to the February 2020 level of 63.3%."[6] No economic loss estimates were made for the huge array of economic costs tied to COVID-19 itself, such as lost years of work after an early death or a severe case of long-COVID-19. They also did not attempt to assess the costs due to the many ways the disease has affected the physical and mental health of the U.S. population or the learning losses experiences by students.

One third of U.S. adults say they or someone in their household was laid off or lost a job (including being furloughed and temporarily laid off) from February 2020 onward. In addition, 31% said they or someone in their household had a cut in pay due to reduced hours or demand for their work. There were enormous disruptions in family routines, employment, and finances. Among households with children, lower-income households experienced higher rates of hardship than higher-income households. Families with an income less than $25,000 clearly were more likely to report economic hardship. Large market income declines of greater than 10% based on their previous year's incomes felt the lack. Estimates stated 120 million people were pushed into extreme poverty in the massive global recession. Obviously, COVID-19 impacted personal living standards and quality of life, though an actual number of those greatly-affected is difficult to estimate. For a family of four, the estimated financial loss over the whole COVID era was nearly $200,000. Even now, the economic inequality is pitifully wrong; in the United States, the top 20% of citizens earn more than 20% of the nation's income, while the bottom 20% earn less than 20% of that income.[7]

Extreme global poverty is beyond our understanding in its depth. The impoverished generally lack access to proper nutrition, clean water, and sanitation facilities already. These lead to an increased susceptibility to diseases. Malnutrition, infant mortality and preventable illnesses remain prevalent issues in such communities. The globalist elite agenda with all their billions tout the fact of their spending billions in charitable giving to aid such countries in improving these travesties. But the truth of that claim is that most of that money came from foundations that profit as much or more than they ever gave. Foundation and trust moneys have huge tax shelters that ultimately make them richer and richer, and global peoples get some meager benefits at best.. However, the fact that so many billions of dollars are "donated" in this manner is something that globalists heavily tout to pat themselves on the back, making them feel less responsible for the travesties they could actually help assuage, if money wasn't their god.

Ironically, as we have seen previously, given the knowledge of the globalist wolves who ran the entire COVID-19 fiasco, there is an underlying agenda to collaborate with each other, accumulating as much power and wealth as they possibly can, turning the entire globe into a communistically centered governance of stakeholders in a New World Order, under an entire Global Reset, in a climate-controlled environment of top-down totalitarianism. There are many parts to their agenda as we have seen previously, but it suffices to say, none of them suffered from the effects of COVID-19, even in their supposed charitable donation of billions. In fact, when you look at each globalist entity's total financial worth today, compared to what those figures were pre-COVID-19, each of them gained billions and some now have personal net worths of trillions. "According to Forbes, roughly 650 billionaires in America saw their net worth increase by more than $1 trillion…and they're now worth more than $4 trillion. That's all true, according to Forbes data—but the numbers are actually a bit richer yet. Total American billionaire wealth stands at $4.6 trillion as of stock market close on April 28, 2021, by our count. That's up 35% from the market opening on January 1, 2020. In other words, U.S. billionaires (alone) got $1.2 trillion richer during the pandemic."[8] After cleaning up all the profits since, with immunizations and inflation, just imagine the totals they have now ending 2024!

Freedom of Speech Trampled On—Often Stolen

The author of the book—*Pandemia: How Coronavirus Hysteria Took Over Our Government, Rights, and Lives*,. During COVID-19, Alex Berenson actively researched, twittered, and wrote about it, but there came a point, he said, when he couldn't fully pay his bills that way. He said he decided to write another booklet entitled, *Unreported Truths About COVID-19 and Lockdowns*, and sent it to Kindle Direct Publishing. The very next morning, Amazon emailed him to say it had rejected his booklet because it "did NOT comply with our guidelines! As a result we are not offering your book for sale. Due to the rapidly changing nature of information around the

COVID-19 virus, we are referring customers to 'official' sources for health information about the virus. Please consider removing references to COVID-19 for this book. Amazon reserves the right to determine what content we offer according to our content guidelines."[9] "Hello!" The book was about COVID-19; what is left of a book about COVID-19 when all mention of COVID-19 is removed? All he needed to do to get his book printed and sold was to remove all references to COVID!

Have you, dear readers, ever been faced with the dilemma of speaking or writing your opinion, based on researched facts, in the United States of America, and been told you can't exercise your Constitutional right to do so? That happened to a multitude of people, even professionals, who did everything in their power to get the truth out to the masses and were thwarted at every turn. As Mr. Berenson reported, there was seemingly no way to appeal Amazon's decision nor even to find out exactly what they found offensive. Alex suspected Amazon, as well as most other social media platforms and Big Tech, were blocking just about everything pertaining to COVID-19 because they weren't allowing anything said in disagreement with the 'official' narrative. Most of these platforms were automated to the extent that any KEY words pertaining to the narrative were automatically blocked.

Amazon was certainly not the only Big Tech entity censoring opinions or even facts about COVID-19. There was an established and 'preferred' public health and governmental narrative that changed constantly, but never in favor of truth! You Tube was at that time already notorious for censoring content, on more things than COVID. Facebook wasn't censoring just videos and posts—it erased entire groups organizing anti-lockdown protests, most notably a Michigan group containing no fewer than 400,000 members![10] With the supposed world population relying on the media for information and virtual communities, tech and social media companies had more than overstepped their assumed power; in some cases, they no doubt violated the boundaries of national anti-trust laws. In fact, the federal laws had not caught up to the assumed power of Big Tech. The censorship was and still is particularly ugly and maddening since Big Tech companies were all benefiting royally from the lockdowns. Naturally, there was NO way they would allow a group of people to stop those benefits from rolling in.

No company or individual gained more than Amazon, or its founder, Jeff Bezos. Under all these circumstances, Mr. Berenson believed that both the founder and the company, had a moral and ethical obligation to allow open debate over COVID-19 and all matters pertaining to it. After all, it was still clearly illegal to ignore or shut down First Amendment rights just because they didn't like the information presented. In the not too distant past, Amazon had generally allowed people to publish whatever they wanted, even Neo-Nazi pamphlets! The bottom line: the tolerance Amazon offered the Neo-Nazis, did not extend to books that could hurt business! Mr. Berenson found out his options for quick publishing were very few and not optimal, so he thought he might try simply confronting Amazon or Jeff Bezos, making a public fuss about what had happened to him and hoping Bezos would relent on his prior decision. Of course, that plan was a long-shot at best, knowing that Amazon is a giant behemoth and does pretty much as it pleases. However, Alex had little to lose, so he posted the email Amazon had sent him on Twitter with three angry sentences. This, too, was censored. Then he responded back with the following post: "THEY CENSORED IT! (The post) is based entirely on published governmental data and scientific papers. It doesn't say coronavirus isn't real or doesn't kill people. In fact, the worst-case death toll is likely to be shocking to people. Amazon wouldn't run it!"[11]

Privately, Berenson mailed fellow journalists he knew and asked them to speak out as well. A few did. One lawyer-turned-journalist named Glen Greenwald wrote he had found Berenson's stance on anti-lockdown "reckless, but book banning by corporate tech giants is a far worse danger than whatever threats his book supposedly presents...if you like their assumed ability to ban a book or author they don't like, a book or author you approve of will be next."[12] Various others followed, including mainstream journalist Brit Hume who offered more support. But all of his former media colleagues at the New York Times remained silent. Berenson worried that Amazon would simply continue to ignore him. However, Elon Musk stepped in, from his own personal race with Bezos for the world's richest person. Musk already had tens of millions of followers on Twitter and a speaking relationship with Bezos. Berenson told Musk what Amazon had done. A few minutes later, Musk tweeted his 30-million-plus followers: "This is INSANE@Jeff Bezos." The @ sign meant Musk was sending the message publicly and directly to Bezos' Twitter account. Then Musk quickly added, "Time to break up Amazon. Monopolies are wrong!" Those two tweets were liked or retweeted almost 60,000 times.

Less than one hour later, Amazon emailed Berenson to say the company would publish his book!

Consequently, that whole story ended well. The publicity from the aborted attempt at censorship by Amazon was like a missile launch for Berenson's book, as well it should have been. The Wall Street Journal published two articles about the whole controversy. Even the Washington Post, owned by Amazon founder, Jeff Bezos, ran an article on the debacle. The next week after that, Berenson appeared on *Fox With Tucker Carlson* to talk about the censorship of his book, and sold 10,000 copies in one hour. By that weekend, his book was briefly the top-selling book on Kindle. That booklet and several follow-up booklets he wrote went on to sell hundreds of thousands of copies. The simple truth of all this is that hundreds of thousands more people than anyone could ever have imagined were almost desperate to get hold of just this kind of information. This author was just one of those who wanted unbiased, well-sourced, and above all, accurate information about COVID-19 and all its surrounding issues. Knowledge is power and it must be the source of right actions. Without it, the fear and panic will continue to be stoked. Americans have longed for truth, and justice more and more since well before COVID, and hopefully having access to them, will remind us they are commodities we do NOT want to do without or take for granted. Thankfully, Alex Berenson's voice and determination to be heard with that truth enabled many to do the same. Truly, his voice against lockdowns, mask mandates, and many other forms of government overreach were revealed, and will be less likely to be used against us in any future attempts. No one can succeed in shutting down TRUTH indefinitely.

To Mask or Not to Mask, the Big Question

In the late Spring of 2020, amid the global pandemic, and issues of masking and lockdowns, we had a striking convergence of all these with the supposed brutal death of George Floyd in Minneapolis. It was animated by the clearly leftist-promotion of the Black Lives Matter movement. In the thick of pandemic lockdowns, BLM protestors took to the streets to criminally destroy half of downtown Minneapolis. To show the significance of this unfortunate convergence, a landmark study was done by collecting about 20,000 tweets joining George Floyd with COVID-19 as dual hashtags. This was no accident! It showed contested discourses of race, virality, mobilization, and national identity, where all of them hung on four symbolic word hooks: death, breath, masks, and voice. The question: how did these all intersect so closely? Obviously, there is no intrinsic tie between a prolonged global pandemic that kills millions and a single police encounter that kills one. The BLM dates back to 2013, but through a series of deaths of black men, some of whom were totally innocent, the movement picked up steam nationally, and was vastly fueled by the forces of the leftist, socialist movement, including financial backing. As the lockdowns became prolonged, tensions mounted. Most cities and states enacted a range of measures to enforce physical distancing that were very politically divisive, and general compliance or resistance also tended to fall along party lines.

Ironically, many who advocated for and adhered to physical distancing practices, also supported and/or participated in racial justice protests which had people pressed together in the streets. At the same time, many who contested shutdown measures now cast the protests as public health hazards and the protestors as hypocritical actors. This dichotomy became at once a signal of the protests' power and also, a means for conservative critics to undermine both the protests themselves and the progressive position on public health mandates. 'Sociology said the George Floyd protests and COVID-19 came together as part of a socially transformative moment, marked by ideological shifts and deep social divisions.' The data revealed complex narratives about justice and injustice, systemic inequality, degrading trust in institutions, and the changing identity of a nation. While such analysis might be helpful to the studies of sociologists and psychologists, it seemed to the student of Scripture as wasted effort to try to understand such complexity. Scripture is very clear about how humanity will continue to degrade and demean itself without the presence of the Holy Spirit in each life. All of these four, word hooks will take on entirely different meanings of association when viewed through the eyes of Holy Scripture. In the final analysis of these added geopolitical issues, we can say the stressors of the COVID-19 pandemic more than contributed to the eruption of secondary issues, but globalists did their very best to fan the flames of disturbance, financially bought those who would keep them burning, and did nothing to rectify the damage.

On another note, while George Floyd's "I can't breathe" protest sparked antipolice rhetoric, anti-law enforcement protests, and rioters who destroyed whole cities EVEN in the midst of lockdowns, for some 'unknown reason elements of this lawlessness were suddenly no longer an issue! Now the same epidemiologists who had decried all the anti-lockdown protestors just one month before, argued that the Floyd protestors had every right to crowd into city streets, ten abreast, and it should NOT be considered as risky behavior for COVID transmission. Physicians and public health "experts" wrote in an open letter that these protests were vital to NATIONAL public health! Now, when the "experts" change direction in their arguments by 180 degrees in a month, it raises a plethora of questions and significant confusion. First, it smacks of utter hypocrisy. Many people had taken the 'need' for lockdowns very seriously, and this policy flip screamed of political shenanigans more than public health concern. To tolerate this public display of trouble-makers and rabble-rousers packed together in the streets, destroying everything in sight while their businesses collapsed, did NOT sit well with most American citizens. Immediately following the mass destruction, the media's obsession with coronavirus roared back into the picture with vengeance. It was a constant case of playing both ends to the middle to prolong the debacle of pandemic under some newer rules. The media had no reason to continue screaming about ventilators and testing, so wearing masks became the media's newest and most irritating obsession yet. It was just like watching a drama played out and drug out to prolong the suspense.

Now reporters spent endless hours and more energy talking about "the raging necessity of masks and mandates use." They belittled and abused anyone who didn't want to wear one. In truth, by all normal standards, wearing surgical masks does absolutely nothing to control the spread of respiratory viruses. This fact was supported by Anthony Fauci, and the CDC in the beginning stages of COVID-19 for all the right reasons, but as the need to prolong the benefits of the pandemic for the globalist wolves, their stories changed in another about-face, and became absolutely the most important deterrent to the spread of the virus. (not one iota of truth there). Cloth masks and bandanas were even more useless, and in fact were shown to be counterproductive and unhealthy in a variety of ways. Studies were conducted on mask efficiency but obviously, a double-blind clinical trial doesn't work for wearing masks, since people are very clear as to whether they are wearing a mask or not! A compilation of ten studies found NO benefit from masks. Even health-care workers should NOT wear cloth masks.

So-called 'scientific' evidence said to support a mask mandate on safety grounds is insufficient proof—show me. If it can't be proven (and it hasn't been), forget masking for the healthy, general public. They are highly uncomfortable, get wet and become germ-breeding grounds. They often cause skin irritations, acne, and in some cases impetigo (staphylococcus-based) rashes. In the confused public mind after much programmed deception, masks were assumed to prevent infection. This gives rise to a second problem. "The widespread misconception about the use of surgical masks—that wearing a mask protects against the transmission of virus—is a problem that was theorized by German sociologist Ulrich Beck. *The surgical mask communicates RISK.* For most, risk is perceived as the potential loss of something of value…people living in the present moment conceive of risk in terms of the physical tools used to mitigate risk while still 'maintaining the source of the filth.' Therefore risk measures that aren't truly preventive act rather as a symbolic measure to eliminate the increase in risk."[13] In the 1919 flu pandemic, masks were available and were dispensed, but they had no impact on the epidemic curve. "As recently as 2010, the US National Academy of Sciences declared in the community setting, 'face masks are not designed or certified to protect the wearer from exposure to respiratory hazards.' A number of studies have shown the inefficiency of the surgical mask in household settings to prevent transmission of the flu virus."[13] In addition to all this, wearing a mask reinforces fear. It should be noted in this citation that its base is the corrupted National Institutes of Health (Fauci base) and that the information was documented at least 3 years before the onset of COVID-19.

In a Sept 6, 2018 decision, after considerable refusal of nurses to wear masks and a couple of court cases, James Hayes and William Kaplan called the evidence for mask mandates "insufficient, inadequate, and completely unpersuasive. The preponderance of the ruling of the masking evidence is compelling—surgical and procedural masks are extremely limited in terms of source control; they do not prevent the transmission of the influenza virus."[14] Further, the reason that standard cloth and surgical masks do not stop transmission of either flu or the coronavirus is that even when worn correctly, they simply cannot block enough of the microscopic particles that account for viral transmission. They fail entirely, both when people inhale particles that infect them, and again when they exhale and spread them. In 2009, four researchers examined how well surgical masks filtered small particles, those of one micron or less. A micron is a tiny unit of measurement, far too small to be seen. (One million microns equal one meter or 1,000 microns equal one millimeter.) Note: a micron is actually about 10 times larger than a single SARS-CoV-2 viral particle. Scientists tested five different surgical mask brands. Two of the masks allowed more than half of the particles through, others were only slightly better, confirming again that surgical masks should not be used for respiratory protection. They are a farce and false crutch to lean on.

Today, the public health sector recognizes the complete limitations of the use of regular surgical mask wearing, but insists that even with all of the above notes, the wearing may prevent some transmission of particles and should still be worn. However, this author, a medical professional as well, believes it should never be mandated for a wide range of reasons we will explore. However, "You may be surprised that the CDC does NOT recommend routine use of ANY type of respirator or medical mask by the general public outside of the healthcare setting to prevent the spread of any viruses— even those which may be airborne. Instead, the CDC recommends Americans wear cloth or disposable face coverings in public settings where social distancing is difficult. Masks should be tightly woven but breathable, fit snugly around your face, and include more than one layer."[15]

Few people actually wore the masks appropriately, because they simply cannot breathe well and are most uncomfortable for anything more than short-term use. The only reliable alternative in the case of must use was the N95 mask. While it is much more effective and reliable, it is more uncomfortable and more expensive. It simply is not practical for masses of people or any length of wearing time. Throughout the mask mandate era, fewer and fewer people chose to wear a mask unless someone else decided to play the role of mask patrol and demand it! This happened frequently and when it did, most would comply only long enough to leave the patrol area. Most would simply pull the mask down off their noses to get fresh air. Those of us with chronic respiratory challenges such as asthma, allergies, COPD, etc., simply needed the additional oxygen to feel well. Imagine a person who was already on oxygen trying to get the needed percentage of it with a mask over the nose and mouth. This author understands that well since her spouse was trying to do just that! We saw parents attempting to keep masks on the faces of small children who had no understanding of the need and no compunction to do so. The elderly were often challenged enough already with other underlying medical conditions for which they, too, struggled to get the oxygen they needed, without knowing why. These are just a few examples of the problems caused by mandating masks.

Even before the Spring of 2020, when the first wave of the pandemic was all but over, the World Health Organization officials announced, "There is no specific evidence to suggest that the wearing of masks by the mass population has any potential benefit. In fact, there's some evidence to suggest the opposite in the misuse of wearing a mask properly or fitting it properly…in the community, we do NOT recommend the use of masks unless you yourself ARE SICK and as a measure to help prevent onward spread from YOU if YOU are ill."[16]

When the pandemic started, public health and Antony Fauci himself adhered to the research. He said, "There's no reason to be walking around with a mask"; and reported the above research which he supported! Fauci even said, "There are often unintended consequences because people keep 'fiddling' with the mask, then touch their face."[17] This statement has been thoroughly documented across the web, and is easily located. Further, Fauci made similar statements in various interviews early in the pandemic. "Critics did note at the time that the implication that face masks protect health care workers from COVID-19 but somehow DON'T protect the general public was scientifically implausible."[18] Defenders of Fauci argued he had to change his mind because other public health officials had changed theirs—that is that since they had found out there was more significant risk of carriers with no symptoms transmitting the disease. This was the explanation given for changing recommendations, however "this was NOT a newly discovered fact. It had been known for months that the mean COVID19 incubation period was five or six days, and there were several reports indicating that a substantial share of people infected by the virus NEVER develop symptoms, meaning carriers who did not feel sick could still spread the virus."[19]

In a July 2020 interview with the Washington Post, Fauci explained his change of mind this way, "Back then, the critical issue was to save the masks for the people who really needed them, because it was felt that there was a shortage of masks. Also, we didn't realize the extent of asymptomatic spread…as the weeks and months went by, federal health officials realized there wasn't a shortage of masks, especially given the availability of plain cloth coverings and there were a lot of asymptomatic people spreading infection."[20] Both of his explanations were highly suspect. Based on Fauci's former statements, as quoted, neither explanation is fully satisfactory in truth. Therefore, many people since that time with additional reasons have NOT fully trusted what Fauci offers because there are nearly always contradictions or mind-changes that should not be present in someone who is always completely dogmatic about his facts and figures, nor from fact-checkers, who come prominently from Big Tech and mainstream media sources. The thing most reporters fail to understand is the general public is simply not as gullible and trusting as it once may have been. In summary, the reader will begin to wonder as we proceed, how much of the "need" for masks was determined by real desire to lessen the spread of COVID-19, and how much was determined by the 'desire' of the globalist wolves to extend the highly profitable pandemic to their advantage?*

As late as April 1, 2020, physicians writing in the New England Journal of Medicine (NEJM), the most prestigious health-care publication in the US, explained, "We know that wearing a mask outside health-care facilities offers little, if any, protection from infection…in many cases the *desire* for widespread masking is a reflexive reaction to anxiety over the pandemic."[21] However, a few days later, Fauci and other top public health officials totally reversed course! Now, masks were no longer useless for the general public—the complete opposite stance in days! Fauci promoted universal masking even in people with NO symptoms. "If everyone does it, we're each protecting each other," he told PBS.

President Trump did NOT drive the new revised policy. Instead he grudgingly gave out the new mask recommendation, making it very clear he wasn't convinced. It all started out as a voluntary recommendation; "you don't have to do it, but…" For a short time, the "science did not drive the change." Denmark did a randomized controlled trial of 6,000 people late that Spring and found that MASKS DID NOT WORK! However, once again, false reports of totally uncontrolled "studies" and heavy propaganda from the main-stream media kicked in. Consequently, if there were any possible reason for all the quickly-instigated 'back-pedaling' and mask mandates later, it could only be purely psychological manipulation. Masks were useless as protection, but they were necessary as "signifiers." Seeing them constantly on other people reinforced the message of danger and increased the fear factor.

One year later, by May 2021, the manipulation continued. The CDC, and other public health officials stated unequivocally that masks could now be dropped for all those who had been vaccinated, incentivizing the vaccines. If this were not so ridiculous, it would be humorous, because this new guidance totally backfired. Within a few weeks, very few people continued wearing masks; after all, who would know if you were vaxxed or not?!! Since it was now true that no one really knew who was vaxxed and who was not, the vaccination rates plunged even further!

In the summer of 2020, however, most people had been convinced they were truly 'following the science.' Not wearing a mask was considered selfish and a sign of it. People were told exactly how they should be treating those MONSTERS who had the unmitigated gall to refuse to wear their mask. Rulebreakers could actually be narcissists or sociopaths, according to media. The propaganda had worked like a charm. Pseudo-science and panic had driven EVERY aspect of the pandemic response. Still, voluntary compliance should have been the order of the day; far different than mandates, Americans, at least, should ALWAYS have had the freedom of personal choice by the law of the land, which was NOT the case, resulting in the removal of freedoms given to us by the Constitution of the United States. Globalists, however, with the help of leftist government and public health officials drove their agenda right past our federal laws because too many Americans refused to rise up and say "NO!" Because, psychologically, the globalist agenda wanted people to hide their faces from one another to discourage them from socializing and possibly unifying in groups that could rebel against their chosen system. So, the masses wore their "face diapers" obediently. Since we know how much Big Tech resents the human advantage and seeks to destroy it, we can understand more of why the mask mandates became so essential to the globalist agenda. As a medical professional, it was immediately clear to this author that constant mask-wearing was a huge threat to physical health, but in addition to that, it became increasingly clear that masks had an even more detrimental effect on our emotional health.

Author Megan Mansell wrote a great book entitled, *Accommodating Chaos* and spoke at length about the plethora of ways masking was not only counterproductive, but also very damaging. In an above paragraph we looked at the size factor of so-called viruses, compared to the enormity of the size of the mesh weave in the masks. Clearly, masks were totally unable to do the job, amounting to disastrous results, especially with all the problems they create. Further they weren't just dangerous, especially to children, but illegally dangerous. Because the "science" facts changed so many times, there have been numerous misconceptions, here corrected:

- A COVID particle is 0.06-0.14 microns in size when a person forces exhalation. By wearing a mask, you can induce any single droplet, force-filtered, to be aerosolized and many other aerosols are generated within a single respiratory outburst such as a cough, sneeze, or even a scream, as well as just a normal exhalation.

- All aerosolized particles can be force-filtered through the mask or whenever the mesh or weave of the mask is larger than the particles.
- In general, when NOT wearing a mask, all particulate would fall in a predictable six-foot arc. However, with a mask aerosolizing it you will send it in an 18-20-foot trajectory where it remains aloft within respiratory range for hours.
- In the world outside, airflow is not restricted, making it pointless to wear a mask outside for the benefit of others, and reduces oxygenation and increases carbon dioxide to the mask wearer.
- Wearing a mask for COVID would be like building a chain-link fence to keep the mosquitos out!
- According to the Americans with Disabilities Act, individuals cannot be discriminated against because they can't or won't wear masks.
- Along with mask mandates, vaccine passports have also been proposed. According to HIPPA rules and the ADA, no one is allowed to know what is wrong with someone else. Also under the Individuals with Disabilities Education Act (IDEA), all children within American school districts have a right to the least restrictive educational environment. Many disabled students cannot tolerate mask-wearing. Medical consent is required to use any kind of mitigating apparatus, in addition to medical clearance within workplaces, under OSHA. BY LAW, no one can force someone else to wear a mask. Why was this not brought to the attention of those mandating? The laws are very clear! Here's the recap on this legal matter: "It's against the ADA law to discriminate in

any way between mask-wearing people and non-mask-wearing people. It's also against the law in terms of medical consent to ask anyone if they've been vaccinated or allow them in or out of settings based on that status."[22]

- When masking in schools, a major problem with special-needs children is that not all of them have a known diagnosis. They might have hearing disabilities, be somewhere on the autism spectrum; children having any kind of learning disability or hearing challenge will NOT learn. Other social-emotional learning is also impaired and brain development is impaired when a child cannot see others' faces. Early infant/childhood development in social, emotional, and language areas involve teeth, lips, and tongue placement. Children develop expression and social understanding by seeing and mimicking caregivers' expressions.
- Children mandated to wear masks is violation of IDEA law.
- Remember, exhalation is one of our body's cleaning mechanisms. The air we breathe out is being rejected by our bodies. If we don't need or want it, we certainly don't want to rebreathe it into our bodies.
- There is also a higher rate of miscarriage and stillbirth in mothers who wore masks. Good oxygenation is already essential for an expectant mom who is providing oxygen to her unborn infant as well as herself. We are very clear that in the process of birthing a baby, if oxygen to the infant is depleted even for a minute, there could be a lifetime disability. No one would be clearer on this than the obstetrician, yet many still masked the mother through her labor and delivery and tried to compensate by giving her additional oxygen, which only increased the carbon dioxide load!
- Many people function every day with an "oxygen deficit,"

even much less than they should have, and may not even be aware of it. Such a person who is aware of their oxygen deficit, and a breathing challenge has only to say, " I can NOT wear a mask due to medical issues." By HIPPA, no one has the right to challenge that or attempt to force the issue!

- Currently, there are instances of patients requiring needed surgery or other medical care, who have been DENIED that care if they are NOT vaccinated! Some have died. That would be premeditated murder.

During the pandemic, masks became fetishes. If you adjusted it in a public place, or God forbid, pulled it off your nose to get a breath of fresh air, someone might start gesturing wildly and acting like the mask gestapo with their orders to get the mask back up over your nose! This actually happened in many retail establishments. In better times, Americans were kinder to others because free people usually are, but in the pandemic, many became self-appointed mask cops. Yes, it was definitely authoritarian, many times cruel and insensitive, and nearly always anger-inducing to be accosted by peers with a Nazi attitude. Managers instructed employees to "remind' customers, (not OK) but the reminders often bordered on the insane.

The bottom line—the whole point of it all had nothing to do with a virus or the vaccines. The goal was always to transform our free countries into totalitarian regimes. We had been persons who respected others' rights to privacy. Now, we had become people who monitored others' behaviors like the Soviets and Chinese do. We had been people of greater kindness and generosity, usually living with at least a measure of ethics and morality. Now, we had become intolerant people who supported social cruelty and injustice. After all, misery loves company!

The whole 'masking of the masses' was at once unnecessary, uncomfortable, and very unhealthy. While it was very bad for adults, it was heinous for developing children of all ages. The children often looked lethargic and expressionless. It became increasingly difficult to hear or be heard behind them. It also reached levels of abuse in the classroom. Some parents received notes from their children's teacher, "If Johnny cannot remember to wear his mask properly, there would be a punishment of 'double-masking!' Truly, that was more abusive than the proverbial paddle and, of course, that teacher had no right to address it at all. Schools already take far too many liberties with children's issues when they should be determined by parents, whose rights have been badly trampled in today's educational system. Neurologists know the extraordinary communication gifts of the human face. Our faces have 43 muscles and most of us, even small children, can mirror the expressions of others. Further, the non-verbal gestures and signs are just as important as the spoken ones. More and more, parents are teaching infants simple sign language to enable them to communicate before their verbal skills are developed. Kudos to those perceptive parents.

However, it seems few educators, or child psychologists at that point, had even tried to analyze the effects of forcing children to wear masks, anywhere in the country. It was the least of their concerns to be denying them access to others' expressions, squelching free breathing for 6-8 hours/day—trying to get more oxygen, and not understanding why the whole world had gone mad and they were being punished. In general, people and children are pretty good at adapting to their environments, but it doesn't mean there were no ill effects, or even long-term developmental effects. We may never know enough about the depth of damage to effectively mitigate it. In our world today, the mental and emotional effects of just doing life have already exponentially increased mental health issues. Astute educators are already aware of these challenges, but many had no compunction about exacerbating them with masks.

It has been said that if one is faint or hungry, he cannot write or argue well— cognitive and communication skills are harmed. A mask is like a corset—you can't be brave, or fight, or debate, or track a delicate thought if you can't breathe, freely and easily. The mask era was literally one of humans struggling for the breath of life—survival. There was a plethora of completely nonsensical ironies, all happening so quickly, even the best medical professionals working in fields where respiratory function was of enormous importance, were simply swept along in the tide. Perhaps the most revealing point of all the dastardly lies is the real reasons why. By forcing the people, especially children, to live with restricted breathing, the world was prepared for the domination of humans by machines, Big Tech, the CCP, and ultimately totalitarianism. Once we've lost the human advantage of human faces and freely-breathing, human imagination, you have a world with no empathy for one another. Masking was the tool the globalist wolves used to literally remove real life, by making it frustrating and intolerable. It made most of us hurry with outside tasks and hurry to get back home, where even if you were alone, at least you could breathe freely.

Education/Socialization of Our Kids Ignored For the Agenda

The entire agenda of closing down our educational system, for prevention of the spread of the COVID-19, was probably one of the worst debacles of the entire pandemic era. In addition, it no doubt created the most detrimental long-range results for the future of our next generation's children and young people. As parents and grandparents, we have already seen the more immediate damage that was done, and which still has a long way to go in terms of remediation. On the surface alone, it is difficult to understand the motivations of globalist wolves for having perpetrated such a disastrous outcome, but it becomes increasingly obvious, the more we understand all of their agenda for the future; those motivations are beyond selfish and smack of evil.

The 2007 CDC future pandemic guidelines supported possible short-term (a week or two at the most) school closings during influenza outbreaks. Certainly no one ever anticipated permanent and semi-permanent closings. In the case of a severe epidemic, a rare possibility of a twelve-week closure term might have to be considered. But the pro-closings agenda had a name and face in the person of Dr. Carter Mecher who, from the beginning of the pandemic, vigorously campaigned for school closings to all ranking officials and anyone who would listen. "Mecher had a personal agenda he wanted to test. As a disciple of computer modeling, he had a closure/lockdown/social-distance model on which he'd been working for 14 years, and this whole COVID situation was ideal. He sent out hundreds of messages increasing alarm over the predicted 5 million Americans expected to die of COVID. He was also an avid pusher of the 'cooties theory' of viruses in which running and hiding is always the answer."[23] He demanded closures and amassed an unprecedented set of frantic propaganda to convince officials he was right. That set off the entire lockdown.

The first problem with this agenda was that scientists already knew early in March, 2020, that children and young adults were at very low risk of infection by SARSCoV-2. Some educational leaders were concerned about collateral damage to the children, especially those already challenged by poverty and subsequent developmental and educational delays. In addition, about 30 million children rely on their schools for free or low-cost meals and snacks to augment their necessary nutritional needs. It has always been true that malnourishment is a huge factor in the proper development and education of children. That lack alone, in many cases has caused irreparable damage in the past, and it certainly did the same thing during school lockdowns.

Children at high risk of abuse and neglect were another crucial worry. New York City Mayor DeBlasio advocated for open schools. More than 100,000 of the city's million students (10%) were already homeless and living in various shelters. However, once again, the intense pressure from Big Tech, media, and teachers' unions forced his hand. Many parents had less than 24 hours-notice that their children would not be going to school the next day. By the end of March, schools almost everywhere globally were closed, except in Sweden. 1.5 billion students, 20% of the total global population were out of school. Desperate parents, working to support their families, needed immediate child care that wasn't available. This required so many challenging adjustments within families which were neither good for the children or their parents. Struggles of every kind ensued and before anything more could even be readjusted, weeks, months, and a whole other school year had passed in complete frustration on the part of every family member caught in the throes of this terrible decision, which simply was never necessary.

Parents tried to balance at-home work and teaching children which was exhausting and mostly unmanageable. They were grateful for teachers still working hard to crank out lessons and maintain a semblance of help for their online students, but so many students didn't learn well alone and more of them couldn't keep up by themselves. Most children (even teens) do not have the maturity to manage the complexities of their own education alone. The education received by a large percentage of the children was a mere fraction of what they would have received in school. So many families in this scenario were stressed to the max. For essential workers with their children at home, it was often worse. Latch-key kids were at even higher risk. Some parents were forced to quit jobs and use unemployment because childcare was either unavailable or not affordable.

Closures weighed most heavily on the children. Few schools had prior experience in remote learning. This required setting up virtual classrooms and devising workable curriculums on the fly. In many cases that first Spring, education slowly ground to a halt, with the profound hope that the fall would put everything back to rights. At its best, virtual learning did NOT work well for a majority of students. Many parents and grandparents worked hard to do their best, but felt totally inadequate and helpless to make much headway. Children were lonely for social contact and missing their friends— even physical activity outside had been sorely diminished. Kids with little supervision are NOT normally doing necessary schoolwork. Leadership in government simply refused to carefully and seriously view the problems, and ran completely empty defenses of virtual education. Globally, many countries did respond to the problems and reopened quickly, but not the US! In countries like the Netherlands, sophisticated contact tracing showed children were NOT passing the virus. If a child did become infected, it was almost always because of their pre-existing illnesses or chronic disease; only about one child in 2 million might die!

As usual, media disinformation, distortion or exaggeration of the real facts painted a much more dismal picture of COVID-19 in children. Scant truth, constant false propaganda, and refusal to give out the truth of global studies, all contributed to the nonsense, drama, and bipartisan politics controlling the educational stagnation of our children. All the international re-openings of schools had no effect on United States politics or the utter lack of concern toward the dilemmas of its own young citizens and their families. Parents mostly believed the constant hype and official arguments and kept their children home anyway. Some parents even bragged about having kept their children home indefinitely. The left-driven teachers' unions exaggerated the risk to their teachers, ignoring the facts and reality. President Trump was rightly pressing for school re-openings in the fall—he seemed 100% certain of it, but he had no idea of the strength of the globalist and union forces. It didn't help that socialist teachers' unions were even MORE opposed to re-opening, and were calling for randomized testing of students to afford further delays. Naturally, they already had contrived political positives and had a pre-planned set of motives for remaining closed. Union demands became completely unrealistic and intentional, a planned setup to ensure schools could NOT reopen. Journalists aided and abetted their agenda. Anyone taking a stand for children and their educational rights were effectively demonized. Worse, many of those who spoke out against re-opening HAD NO CHILDREN—no dog in the fight!

Teachers' unions had simpler and baser motives for fighting against re-opening. Their teachers could work from home, and they were part of the anti-Trump globalist crowd working night and day to remove him from office in the upcoming election. Unions then started calling for massively expensive retrofitting of schools with new ventilation systems. They said publicly-funded charter schools should be closed on the theory that they shared spaces with existing schools, hence worsening the crowding. They argued there was no way there could be full-time schools for all students and all teachers the way it used to be. They even advocated for de-funding police, another leftist demand, so that money could be re-allocated to educational and other essential needs. Retrofitting schools would take months to years to get accomplished which they were certain would indefinitely delay school re-openings. Meanwhile, the level of negative propaganda for re-opening schools had escalated so much, the fears of American parents having their children in school also escalated. Union pressure was NOT relenting. Local teachers' unions threatened strikes and even encouraged teachers to seek disability leaves. Attempts to stand up to the unions with truth generated more blowback, name-calling, and considerable evil rebuke. It became truly ugly and base. They might even be able to convince the public the epidemic had remained uncontrolled because of President Trump's failures. Ultimately, by that fall, the unions had won and the children had lost; virtual learning would continue. The utter absurdity of the situation was proven by a plan that "some schools would still offer "supervised learning centers" in the School! What?

By the end of the 2021 school year, the full extent of the damage from virtual learning became ABUNDANTLY CLEAR! Standardized testing showed enormous gaps between in-person and virtual education. Math and reading benchmarks had plummeted. Minority groups of children were even harder hit. By that time, virtual schooling had become so unpopular, the unions were denying their prominent role in driving it, even saying they had tried to re-open, but… Tens of millions of American children had lost more than a year of schooling they would NEVER get back. One thing that parents and grandparents noted sadly, in addition to educational losses, was the apathy of many children toward their education, and considerable discouragement in even trying to jump back in, knowing themselves how far behind they had fallen. For many students, even renewing friendships at school could barely interest them to return.

The whole process of re-inventing education by no means stopped with high school graduations, most of which occurred sporadically in outdoor venues that minimized the herculean efforts of some students to get their education no matter what was thrown at them, making their celebrations far less than their normal importance due to circumstances. Colleges and universities raced to implement some of the most impossible restrictions against their students, while supposedly keeping them safe. Online classes were a mere first step. Many didn't allow their students to return to campus at all and barred all visitors. They forced students to wear masks even when alone outside. They banned gatherings of greater than six people which precluded almost all clubs, and activities crucial to the college experience. Some had to have permission to leave campus, and travel restrictions were beyond asinine. Some were not even able to exercise outside even by February, 2021, even with proven very-low risk factors. At Boston's Northwestern, eleven students were dismissed for having an off-campus party in a downtown hotel room and their tuition was NOT refunded! Most of the administrations demanded students be vaccinated to return to in-class learning. This was no different than the mandatory vaccinations for healthcare, military, and large business. The insanity was completely unnecessary for any of these groups and in many cases, vaccines cost these coerced individuals their very lives, no matter that even now, globalists and their "official healthcare agencies" refuse to admit it. Refusal to admit it doesn't remove it, or bring back all of the innocent victims who would still be doing the important jobs they were doing, and alive with their loved ones, had they NOT been forced to take the toxic vaccines. It is an American travesty that can never be justified or rectified in this life.

Schools declared "Cooperation and compliance with public health guidelines is absolutely essential." There is absolutely no way that such tight restrictions without any statistical need for them, was not purely political. Soon, the ugly habit of "snitching" also spread on campuses. Students were encouraged by memos from schools across the country to do this! In fact, the University of Miami paid students to walk around their campus and report on people who refused to comply with masking and social distancing. "As college students began policing each other, campuses became places of paranoia, finger pointing, and mistrust. Some students got into social media battles about social distancing infractions. Life on campus was transformed by the pandemic. For those students remaining on campus, new safety measures limited social interaction and students missed out on staying up late in dorm lounges, sitting next to classmates, making new friends, tailgating at football games, and many other such traditions."[24] In light of these and other realities, about 23% of those college students took their Spring 2021 semesters off, and many did not return the following Fall. How many students' lifetime careers were jeopardized by all the COVID agenda nonsense?

Others pushed back. Students and their parents all over the country complained about their situations—stupid, unreasonable rules and regulations while schools continued charging full tuition for an inferior college experience. Worse, the rules didn't apply to their faculties! Sports programs were very close to vanishing entirely. Different schools—different rules! There were dire predictions that athletes who contracted COVID-19 would be in danger also of getting myocarditis and potentially dying. Those predictions were unfounded—the truth was that those who took the jab were in the greatest danger of getting myocarditis. Though the CDC refused to admit it, many young athletes globally who took the jab, did experience myocarditis, and other life-threatening conditions. Many of those simply dropped and died during or after participation in competitive or strenuous sports activities. It began happening almost every day with the mandated vaccinations which most schools required. Multiple media sources and public health agencies denied this truth but several studies have confirmed its truth. Among those, was a study conducted by the Journal of the American Medical Association (JAMA). The primary data used were VAERS reports, which we already know get only a small percentage of the actual numbers of cases reported in that system. "Based on passive surveillance reporting in the US, the risk of myocarditis after receiving mRNA-based COVID-19 vaccines, was increased across multiple age and sex strata and was highest after the second vaccination dose in adolescent males and young men. This risk should be considered in the context of the benefits of COVID-19 vaccination."[25] That quote implies that the risk of getting COVID-19 is greater than the risk of myocarditis, which is NOT true. Young adults have little risk of getting a serious case of COVID-19 with no later sequelae, while the chance of contracting myocarditis from taking the vaccine is a serious life-changing risk. Therefore, that quote is extremely misleading, and of no benefit in the decision. Tragically, this knowledge has still not concerned 'health-care officials enough to stop pushing the poison on our infants, children, and young adults! That is the biggest travesty of all! The death rate for newborns (of vaxxed mothers), infants, and small children has risen exponentially, another FACT still being vehemently denied.

A general policy of 'safety-ism' became prominent on most college campuses and elsewhere since. In the 2018 book, The *Coddling of the American Mind: How Good Intentions and Bad Ideas Are Setting Up a Generation for Failure*, the authors defined 'Safetyism' as "a culture or belief system in which safety has become a sacred value, meaning people are unwilling to make tradeoffs demanded by other practical and moral concerns."[26] We see it often in many families with 'helicopter parenting' where every effort is made to maintain tight control on children. The children then become fearful and unable to make good decisions for themselves. Such parenting almost always backfires. Hence, the similar obsession of governments mainly, to minimize COVID's effects. This produced a lack of confidence; anxiety among teens and young adults sky-rocketed. The CDC reported suicide attempts especially of young adolescent girls in February and March of 2021 were up 50% from the same time period in 2020. Many rules tightened even more as the Fall of 2020 semester came. Many switched to online learning only. Colleges continued to punish students who were caught breaking their impossible rules. There was a huge pushback. Off campus parties continued quietly. Roommates promised each other they would NOT get COVID-tested or report cases. Still, despite anger and frustration, the majority of students mostly complied. The vast majority of them had little choice. Not many wanted to postpone their plans to finish or risk being expelled, so once again, the bureaucracy and lawyers prevailed.

Meanwhile, life for young people off-campus was probably worse. Preventable deaths soared. Suicides—deaths from drug overdoses rose 30% and mandatory lockdowns played a far larger role in those than COVID-19 ever could. Restaurant, bar, and retail closings disproportionately took their jobs, leaving them stuck at home. Fentanyl, a Chinese-manufactured synthetic opioid, became another epidemic of overdosing, primarily because it is cheap, easy to buy, and represents an enormously increased risk of overdosing in its massive toxicity. Far too many young lives were lost in this epidemic, before they started dying from COVID vaccinations. This drug is still one of the worst plagues ever visited on our nation, and still killing large numbers of unsuspecting teens and young adults, thanks to globalism and the socialist liberals' obsession with the CCP. Don't think it an accident, Chinese Fentanyl has been readily available to help depopulate our American youth for many years.

Homicides also soared in 2020 by 25% across the US. Philadelphia's homicides increased by 40%, second only to Chicago. There were increased deaths from alcohol abuse, by an estimated 20,000 from previous years' figures. All of these preventable deaths were frequently called "deaths of despair." In all, more than 250,000 Americans died from preventable deaths in 2020, an increase of over 50,000, primarily occurring in young people. More staggering than all of that, increases in the numbers from 2019-2020 were exponentially larger than the total number of COVID deaths of those in the same age range. Most tragic of all, none of these horrific preventable deaths were even mentioned in the hour-by-hour death tallies! Those figures weren't even available until the middle of 2021. The media sources were only interested in presenting figures that promoted their COVID narrative. The naked truth is that lockdowns across our nation and globe Saved NO Lives! Figures only reported assets, not liabilities— only the lives quarantines might save and NEVER any of those that were lost. It was indeed an impossibly high price we all paid. Still, there was NO effort made to halt the deadly lockdowns.

Not the Virus, but the Agenda that Wouldn't Quit

At this point in the Pandemic, all the possibly sound reasons for continuing the rigid structure established had truly run their course. Most people had learned the SARS-CoV-2 was far less dangerous than it had been touted to be. Children, in particular proved to be at very low risk of even getting sick, much less dying. Contrary to the facts, the doomsayers and the public-health rogues had once again gone ballistic instead of backing off the stringent measures. Any thinking person could find no good reason for this, except to continue browbeating and blaming President Trump and promoting continued extension of the virus to prolong the moneymaking for globalists. Whenever a localized surge of the virus first occurred and then began to burn out, media quickly jumped on the propaganda to stir up more panic. The idea was always to use everything at their disposal to keep the momentum of the pandemic going for as long as possible and 'milk it' ad nauseum.

The waxing and waning of COVID cases seen in the Sunbelt matched that of Every Other Major COVID-19 wave in 2020, EVERYWHERE IN THE WORLD. On the few occasions when reports proclaimed the end of the Sunbelt wave, the media simply credited the lockdown and mask restrictions. However, lockdowns clearly did NOT deserve any credit for the rapid turnaround since the lockdowns were NOT in force during the majority of the surge. President Trump, followed by Governor DeSantis in Florida had expressed the importance of keeping the economy open and that strategy paid off in spades throughout the summer and fall of 2020.

By September, Florida and some other southern states had approached their pre-pandemic employment levels. This PROVED the lockdowns were far more detrimental to the economy and many other societal areas, then was the virus.

However, just to add insult to injury, contact tracing programs were instituted. For the remainder of 2020, the touted PCR testing became even less reliable, in fact it was truly bogus. The increase in contact tracing and rules on quarantining people for as much as two weeks at a time, whether they exhibited any symptoms or not, started another huge debacle. Massive amounts of funding were earmarked to pay all the people doing the tracing, but none of this was even a tiny bit beneficial in slowing the virus. The extra funds, about $700 billion, were an utter waste in every way because the majority of citizens had no desire to talk to tracers and potentially be further quarantined, much less help perpetrate that on others. The backlash got nasty, and the lack of cooperation even worse. It became clearly useless to even try tracing something spread on a potentially global level, not to mention the extremely intensive labor involved in it. If a COVID surge did occur, tracers couldn't begin to keep up. The system failed miserably. Next, when travelers left home for another state, many were ordered to isolate for two weeks upon their return. Who had an extra two weeks for traveling? Topping all of that, most people were just plain sick to death of all the lectures and general inconvenience the virus caused them, possibly one of the best things that could happen. Americans had been compliant to a fault, but enough was finally and rapidly becoming more than enough.

Similar unrest and frustration were also bubbling up in Europe. Tens of thousands of protests broke out, but they did NOT keep governments from mandating new lockdown rules. In some countries such as Colombia, extreme lockdowns simply increased crime rates and economic misery. In fact, massive violence and protests were becoming worse and happening in cities all over the globe, including Bogota, Colombia, Bangalore, India, Bangkok, Thailand, and Buenos Aires, Argentina. The greatest surprise is that there were NOT dozens more brewing at all times.

Another huge bone of contention in all things mandatory became the dreaded PCR tests. Those letters stand for "polymerase chain-reaction." First and foremost, the PCR process was never designed by its creator to FIND SARS-CoV-2! They were simply a means to look for ANY type of genetic material in a sample. An example is using it to detect DNA in crime labs. The early test process was mechanically brutal, time consuming, and technically not necessary. Most people found them painful; at the least very uncomfortable, describing it as trying to scratch your brain from the back of the nasal sinuses! Samples would be sent to a lab where a chemical was added to isolate any genetic material (RNA). Then an enzyme was added to that genetic material (RNA) to transform it into the double-stranded DNA, because this complicated process of amplification ONLY worked on DNA. The newly created DNA was heated to break up the two strands. More chemicals and enzymes were added to the newly 'fractured' DNA. The newly added material then fused with the broken halves of the DNA strand, ending with two identical strands where only one existed previously. That process was repeated over and over and over. After multiplying the DNA strands exponentially, millions of copies now existed. When the test was "READ," a glowing vial of material equaled a "POSITIVE" test that MEANT ABSOLUTELY NOTHING! The risks of failure were high. The more cycles that were run, the more likely the test would be positive. After 10 cycles, a single piece of DNA became1,024 pieces; after 20 cycles, it became more than a million. If the cycles were over-multiplied, the greater was the chance of a false positive test due to lab contamination by microscopic traces of genetic material remaining from previous tests.

Consequently, any PCR test that required more than 30 cycles to become positive showed that the original sample contained minimal amounts of genetic material with no guarantee that the material found was identifiable as SARS-CoV-2 virus. Remember, there are many good scientists who do not even believe viruses exist! The "virus" we tested for, may never have existed at all! When samples turn positive at lower levels of 20 or less, patients may have high viral loads, and may even get much sicker, but there is still NO certainty of identifying it as COVID, by current knowledge of the tests SINCE most COVID ended. High cycle positives were extremely likely to be useless, especially when the person tested had NO COVID symptoms. Therefore, to test people with no apparent symptoms for the sole purpose of surveillance/tracking was very highly likely to produce worthless false positives that helped no one, and clearly wasted people's lives and work days, wasted huge amounts of money and were an enormously worthless exercise in futility!

The worst issue of all PCR testing—-it simply made NO difference whether the results were at the high threshold (false positives likely) or the low threshold (possibly positive but not differentiated from other possible viral organisms). They meant two completely different things, but were treated exactly the same by health-care providers. Fauci clearly knew this nonsense and understood the dichotomy. He even acknowledged the truth of it, but NOTHING CHANGED. The majority of public citizenry didn't understand it at all. It suffices to say, PCR tests were NOT a simple positive or negative indicator of COVID-19. It did not help providers make good decisions on treatment modalities or the lack of them, much less the degree of contagion or length of quarantines. Barring ALL of these issues, it is clear the number of cases diagnosed as positive for COVID-19 is at best highly debatable for real cases and naturally the statistics reported were greatly inflated. Tested persons were rarely EVER told anything more than a simple positive or negative, a probable guesstimate at best. They had no idea what their test result really meant, and no one else did either.

High-cycle positives extended already lengthy hospital stays when those patients could have been home. They also forced many folks into contact-tracing protocols requiring totally unnecessary quarantine from their entire social circles, often for weeks. Rates of real contagion appeared to be only about 10% of reported cases in reality. Further, case counts along with death counts were ridiculously skewed and exaggerated, so the fear of becoming infected with SARS-CoV-2 was also exponentially increased. In fact, of all truly positive cases, only about 50% had any symptoms, while an additional 25% had only early mild symptoms. In other words, 75% of people weren't any worse off than they would have been with a common cold! Considering that the PCR testing for COVID-19 was initially considered the "Gold Standard" for testing, the reality was it really was mostly useless since so many cases were without symptoms. PCRs are still considered highly sensitive, and valid for that reason. Officials continue to call it the ultimate "Gold Standard" over home-testing which was considered 96% accurate. Given the evidence discussed, that evaluation remains highly suspect. So, here was the real question: When at-home tests were approved as early as November and December of 2020 and considered 96% accurate, why did they continue to use PCRs? There doesn't seem to be any sound answer to this question and many others, however, there were some interesting observations. By mid-July, the US was doing about 20 million tests per month at a cost of $3 billion/month on tests alone. It seems the testing insanity continued mainly because public health officials needed to do something, whether it made any sense or not.

In the Fall of 2020, media sources began reporting on yet another health crisis called Long COVID or Long-haul COVID. In October 2020, UK researchers examined brain function in 84,000 post-Covid patients and found diminished IQs in those who had succumbed to COVID-19. Researchers concluded that having COVID-19 likely increased the chances for some cognitive dysfunction that might persist. The media took off with that information. The London Times warned, "Coronavirus could age the brain by ten years or cause the IQ to fall."[27] However, with such a vast number of subjects, only 60 of the 84,000 (0.7%), all of whom had been on ventilators, showed a mental decline of 8.5 IQ points. Reasonably, it seemed those results should have been very reassuring for anyone concerned that COVID might have damaged their mental acumen indefinitely, but few were reassured. In February of 2021, the National Institutes of Health (NIH) announced a $1.5 billion grant program to research Long-COVID; the official name given was "post-acute sequelae of SARS-CoV-2" infection (PASC). Within just a few months, the AMA called for additional funds. The AMA also required new ICD codes to enable the billing to insurance companies.

Just shortly, many other groups climbed on the Long-Haul bandwagon. This new COVID-related 'concern' actually fit into the whole picture like a piece in a puzzle, since one of the globalist wolves most burning desires was to use COVID for the total remaking of society. It would bring increased governmental intervention in both the government and in medical care. Just think!! If COVID-19 ever went away, the Long-haul COVID might just be sustainable forever. Anthony Fauci lost no time promoting this globalist rhetoric. He wrote, "international travel and other living improvements achieved in recent centuries came at a high cost that we pay for in deadly disease emergencies." He and his co-author ended their paper by adding, "Our human activities represent aggressive, damaging, and unbalanced interaction with nature and we will increasingly provoke new disease emergencies… COVID should force us to begin thinking in earnest collectively about living in more thoughtful and creative harmony with nature," (see the agenda of the World Economic Forum) [28] Never mind that Fauci is one of the biggest perpetrators of gain-of-function research which seeks to make disease organisms more virulent and transmissible! This has no conceivable relationship to 'thoughtful and creative harmony with nature!

Having said all that, Long-COVID is a real illness and can result in chronic conditions requiring comprehensive care. There are many resources available. It may also be called Post-COVID and is broadly defined as signs, symptoms, and conditions that continue or develop after acute COVID-19 infection. It may also become Chronic COVID. Long-COVID can include a wide range of ongoing health problems lasting weeks, months, or years. It tends to occur more often in people who had severe COVID-19 illness, but anyone who was infected can still experience it. People have contracted COVID-19 more than once, even multiple times, but the reality is that most people who have incurred COVID-19 repeatedly actually took the jab. Many qualified physicians believe if a person has had a moderate documented case of COVID-19, he has natural immunity and will not get it again. This author and her spouse were very ill with COVID-19 and hospitalized in June of 2021 with the Delta Variant. Neither of us have had it again, though the author had Long Covid. It's also believed each time a person is infected or re-infected with the virus, there is risk of developing Long-COVID. It is even possible to have not been tested as positive or known they were infected with the virus and still develop a Long-COVID illness. In July of 2021, Long-COVID was added as a recognized condition that could result in a disability under the Americans with Disabilities Act (ADA).

"Long-COVID is a wide range of new, returning, or ongoing health problems people experience after being infected with the virus that causes COVID-19. Most infected people get better within a few days to a few weeks after infection, therefore about four weeks after infection is the probable soonest time to suspect Long-COVID or begin to identify it. Anyone who was infected can experience it. There is no test to determine if your symptoms or condition is due to COVID-19, because Long-COVID is not one illness. A health-care provider considers a diagnosis of Long-COVID based on the person's health history including history of COVID infection with severity and the presence of pre-existing medical problems."[29] People with Long-COVID most commonly report symptoms such as tiredness/fatigue, fever, feeling worse after physical or mental exertion, shortness of breath, cough, chest pain, rapid heart rate, brain fog, headaches, sleep problems, dizziness, changes in taste and smell, depression/anxiety, diarrhea, stomach pain, joint/muscle/nerve pain, rash, and changes in menstrual pattern. Many patients have symptoms unexplained by tests and are not easy to manage. Considerably more study is indicated for the treatment of Long-COVID.

Another concept talked about incessantly with respect to the pandemic, and ever since vaccinations, was that of herd-immunity. In August 2020, Dr. Scott Atlas joined President Trump's Coronavirus Task Force. Almost overnight he became Trump's right-hand man for COVID medical advice. He was not a part of the public health or infectious disease camp, but had an expert knowledge and understanding of the science and data regarding COVID. His medical credentials were second to none. He argued for reducing restrictions because of his personal skepticism of their value and efficacy. He said, "The impact of prolonging the lockdown was worse than the impact of the disease...so many people were already immune to the disease, the virus was no longer capable of causing widespread outbreaks."[30] Naturally, Fauci, and other public health minions pushed back immediately, and Dr. Atlas became associated with the concept of herd-immunity.

People can only become immune in two ways—either natural recovery from the disease that produced antibodies or by inoculation with an effective vaccine, also 'intended' to produce antibodies. Therein is the rub when we speak of the COVID "vaccines" and the fact they aren't truly vaccines, when they fail to produce the needed antibodies. Since there was no effective vaccine (nor is there one now), the only way to achieve 'herd immunity' was to allow enough people to get the infection itself and recover from it, producing natural antibodies. The object was never to have everyone get sick for that reason and it would most definitely be time-consuming and potentially kill more people in such a process. No one would even entertain a discussion on that. However the flak about it became so egregious by September, Atlas denied ever suggesting the idea to the President. CDC's director Robert Redfield was heard bashing Dr. Atlas on a flight to Washington. Fauci attacked Atlas that same day on CNN. Meanwhile, COVID-19 cases and deaths had dropped by almost 50% in the US from July through late September!

The herd immunity concept was discredited by every leftist liberal and globalist on the planet and Dr. Atlas was totally disregarded in everything else he said because he was in cahoots with the President who supposedly embraced it, and of course because it didn't fit the globalist narrative. Dr. Atlas called for protecting the most vulnerable, primarily the elderly, but allow the virus to spread through the rest of the population creating natural immunity. It discouraged masks, lockdowns and mass testing. The doctor's discrediting even by other members of the President's Task Force brought a fairly quick end to the discussion at that time, but the subject of herd-immunity as a goal of "vaccine pushing" was, of course, perfectly acceptable to the globalists because it meant the vast majority of people would have received the vaccine in order to attain herd-immunity. That plan was neither appropriate nor effective, and many people decried it, but the push for herd-immunity via the toxic vaccines was never discredited as it should have been, given the millions of people with vaccine injuries and death that ensued with them.

On September 25, Governor DeSantis of Florida removed all remaining restrictions in his state and led the way for other Red states to return to business as usual. Fauci was extremely vocal about this development, but DeSantis paid no attention to him and moved ahead. About a week later a panel of renowned epidemiologists produced a paper entitled, *The Great Barrington Declaration* that declared, "Coming from both the left and right, and around the world, we have devoted our careers to protecting people. Current lockdown policies are producing devastating effects…we have grave concerns about the damaging physical and mental health impacts of the prevailing COVID-19 policies, and recommend an approach we call 'Focused Protection'."[31] Having read the document in its entirety, this health professional fully agreed with this group of highly esteemed professionals.

Once again this massively signed declaration drew immediate counterattack calling it, "an effort to rebrand herd immunity." Fauci said it was dangerous nonsense, which in truth was Fauci nonsense! In his egregious arrogance, he refused to entertain any discussion on it. It was nothing new for Fauci—he always became odiously snooty and unwilling to speak whenever he was challenged. The words, "Quite frankly…" became his forever "go to" phrase! Ultimately, the global signatures reached almost one million when it was released. Undoubtedly, the numbers would have soared higher, but Big Tech censored it. Globally, as people searched for the Declaration on Google, invariably, it returned denouncements of it and buried all links to it. Just two days before its release, President Trump became the world's MOST famous COVID patient.

President Trump Had COVID; Globalists and Media Joyful

It was abundantly clear that President Trump had no intention of playing the panic game over COVID-19. Naturally that brought continuous criticism from the mainstream media who, first, were looking for anything they could jump on, and second, it gave opportunity to build the fear factor. Visiting the President and the White House did not require a Pentagon assessment of risk; neither testing nor masking were necessary there. In the midst of a presidential campaign, the President refused to eliminate the necessary rallies and appearances and wasn't all that concerned about his personal risk. By contrast, Joe Biden hid out in his basement most of the time. All the criticism of the press and public health officials seemed to just roll off the President, because he was nearly immune to it by that time and had no intention of changing his plans. Then Trump's aide, Hope Hicks, tested positive for COVID, and rumors flew, speculating about his possible infection. On October 2, nine months past the beginning of the pandemic, President Trump announced that he and his wife had both tested positive for COVID-19 and would begin their quarantine and recovery process immediately. He never displayed fear, panic, or doubt of their complete recovery.

While it was true the President had some mild co-morbidity issues due to age and moderate overweight, and he had displayed symptoms fairly rapidly, he was not overly concerned. That afternoon, Trump boarded a helicopter taking him to the Walter Reed National Medical Center for treatment. The mainstream media fell over itself almost gleefully announcing this development.

Immediately, there ensued heavy discussions on Presidential succession, and the Washington Who's Who! While hospitalized, the President was treated with medications known to work well at that time and a bit of additional oxygen, but he had no fever and only mild symptoms per his personal physician. Later he was not on oxygen and had no difficulty breathing or walking per his pulmonologist, who readily stated that Trump was in exceptionally good spirits. Oddly, Trump's own chief-of-staff undercut his doctors' statements. Trump did receive some Remdesivir and did very well despite the normal responses to it. He also received monoclonal antibodies to augment his recovery. Barely 48 hours later, the President had already returned to the White House. President Trump and his doctors were right on, while all the naysayers were dead wrong. "As he exited the medical center, Trump gave his signature fist pump in the air, and upon his arrival home, walked up the staircase entrance, took off his mask, gave reporters a thumbs-up, and saluted Marine One!"[32]

Critics couldn't wait to credit the President's rapid recovery to his aggressive care, implying anyone else would not have received such special treatment. Really folks! Why in the world would we NOT give the best of care to our President, the head of the free world? However, as Fauci himself would say when he had no other appropriate comeback, "Quite frankly…," even with anything lesser by way of treatments, Trump would probably have recovered fairly well without much treatment— the majority of people in relatively decent health did not require hospitalization. Yes, the President was overweight, but he was and always has been physically robust and energetic, an avid golfer, and not easily tiring while on the campaign trail. The virus was always much harder on older folks who were mostly unhealthy with multiple risk factors. Trump was healthy faster than most patients and after several negative tests, he went on campaigning a week later. Having had the virus, he had no real need to wear a mask, choosing rather to show his face to his supporters without apology. That was the way it always should have been, and he was bold enough to represent the truth. Of course the press continued to bad-mouth him due to his irresponsible lack of mask-wearing, and he most certainly had NOT given the virus its proper respect!

President Trump openly assured people and told them NOT to be afraid of the virus nor allow it to dominate their lives, reminding them of his own personal example. Author Alex Berenson tweeted, "It may be the smartest comment Trump has ever made…For too long we allowed this virus and the media hysteria surrounding it—to dominate us. We need to take back our lives, our schools, and our whole world."[33] However, the media always chose to believe or at least perpetuate the opposite. The backlash was immediate in their accusations. They accused the President of undermining public health messages. The "experts" were incensed by the President's comments, while journalists claimed his words were hurtful to Americans whose relatives had died of COVID. That would be exactly like saying we shouldn't say anything helpful or hopeful about cancer for fear of offending the relatives and friends of those who had succumbed to it. But those false narratives continued and no one dared to speak up in opposition for fear of being censored or canceled altogether.

The media narrative continued even after the fraudulent election with president-elect Joe Biden gloating over his 'win'. The Washington Post brought a scathing report on the pandemic situation from the globalist-driven narrative that squarely placed all blame for everything imaginable on President Trump. The spurned four public-health specialists, Fauci, Birx, Hahn, and Redfield, whose dire warnings had gone largely unheeded for months by the White House, sounded alarms far and wide about the coming winter with COVID. Chief-of-Staff, Mark Meadows told them he did NOT believe their troublesome data assessment and basically accused them of outlining problems without prescribing any solutions. In response they said the solutions were still clear, and should be heeded more than ever. They accused the President of abdicating his responsibility to manage the public health crisis and instead "used his megaphone to spread misinformation." Then they touted the "miraculous arrival of the coronavirus vaccines, marking the first glimmer of hope...yet the virus had caused more infections and deaths in the US than in most other developed nations—a result, experts said, of a dysfunctional federal response led by a president perpetually in denial. We could have done better...with more adherence to masks. The idea that we had this national debate on the question of whether masks infringed on your liberty was deeply unfortunate and put us in a bad position...The catastrophe began with Trump's initial refusal to take seriously the threat of a once-in-a-century pandemic."[34]

This was an example of the continuous tripe broadcast far and wide with 'the real misinformation', and the continuous politically stringent efforts of the globalists with their skewed 'Big Tech blaming President Trump for everything they, themselves, had planned, perpetrated, and executed. In the manner of a full-on totalitarian agenda they focused, not on the pandemic, but on removing our freedom-loving President from a position of influence that flew in their globalist faces. This is the unmitigated truth of what was really happening. Removing our President and putting their Biden pawn in his place would be their best shot at perpetrating their New World Order, and Global Reset. As of April of 2024, that agenda had not changed.

By now, of course, most people understood that regardless of all denials, and efforts to thwart the truth, Donald Trump was cheated out of his second term in office as the President BECAUSE of his America First/MAGA policies and his focus on our own freedoms, liberty, and sovereignty. The globalist wolves with access to multiple billions of dollars to spend, made sure his leadership would NOT continue. That money, the criminal cooperation of their pawn, Joe Biden, and the leftist socialists illegally stole that election. That kind of money can buy anything, including a fraudulent election. With their complicit Big Tech, they censored and even arrested anyone who dared to suggest exactly what they had done. Americans en masse knew and understood what really happened as was clearly reflected by the next election bid. Leftist media, Hollywood, academia, and most of the enormous, globalist, corporate America did NOT want Trump to continue as President, even at the expense of an orchestrated failure in leadership. All of these groups in cooperation with the globalist wolves openly and tirelessly, as well as criminally, strove to defeat him. Billions can buy a whole lot of fraud in some fairly high places. Wolves run in packs and stick together against their prey!

As had been the case for all of 2020, the pandemic continued, both regionalized and seasonalized. A fresh wave arrived near the end of 2020, very much like the influenza does every year, and about one year after its onset. Stay at home orders ramped up for the holidays—you can't have people gathering in a pandemic to discuss the insanity. Most outdoor venues were closed, even though transmission there didn't even exist. Absolutely NOTHING was learned from 2020's mistakes. Statistics continued to soar with the help of number manipulation. Public health "experts" and media refused to see reality, much less admit to it. The stories didn't change much either. Hospitals were overflowing. Oxygen and supplies were running out—but they never did. Extra field hospitals remained empty. The media NEVER learned to adjust their dire predictions or expectations. When bad-news predictions proved wrong they were simply forgotten; never corrected. But, glory—hallelujah, the COVID vaccines had arrived!! The very shortly-awaited and planned solution for advancing the entire globalist agenda would whip COVID-19 and 'normal' could return.

COVID Vaccines—Ultimate Panacea or Tragic Curse

Vaccines were the total panacea—they would fix everything, slow and stop the pandemic, and enable FREEDOM from the mandates at last! Pfizer announced in November 2020, the vaccines were coming and were greater than 90% effective! The touted effectiveness was the first massive lie told, but certainly not the last. In fact, to this day, 'officials' are still telling it! Fauci claimed the pandemic would soon be over because the vaccine would turn it all around. In the same month, Moderna announced its vaccine that was 94% effective, another lie! Then Pfizer posted its "more complete results" and now its vaccine actually jumped to 95% effectiveness. Hogwash! Sound a bit optimistic to anyone? It should, since these were experimental vaccines, that weren't 'vaccines.' They had incomplete clinical trials before they were rolled out, and previous laboratory results weren't even close to those percentages of effectiveness, nor could it be proven. Worse, both companies stated that NO SERIOUS concerns had been observed and were generally well tolerated. All lies! You only have to get hold of Pfizer's and Moderna's patent papers to see the real facts, even today! After all those COVID months, the vaccines looked like the sure fix from science and medicine. They offered a chance to 'get back to normal soon!' Of course, now we ALL know the vaccine optimism was extremely short-lived in reality. No one seemed able to hear what Big Pharma wasn't saying about the 'vaccines!'

1. Anyone in the medical profession, researchers, and experienced journalists who had not bought into this narrative, knew full-well and many first-hand that these big drug companies (Big Pharma) simply were NOT trustworthy! They never disclosed side effects, problems, costs, etc. with their products unless legally forced to do so. These companies know far more about their products than anyone else, including regulators. However, they are NOT interested in protecting the public from their products and do not routinely disclose information to that end. They have long histories of hiding negative clinical trial results, marketing their drugs for unapproved uses, and paying physicians handsome incentives to promote their products to patients with written prescriptions. Anyone in the medical professions knows how the system operates just by being observant. In addition, the mandatory clinical trials can be and usually are manipulated in all kinds of ways to get the new products approved by the FDA, who must qualify them as safe and effective. A major problem is the FDA does NOT conduct its own clinical trials so it must rely on the data given to it by

said pharmaceutical companies. Naturally, this is a wide-open invitation to fraudulent or incomplete data and conflict of interests. Companies will most certainly structure their clinical trials to maximize the benefits of their products while minimizing the side effects and problems. Absolutely everyone who spends any time around Big Pharma is clear and well aware of exactly how this whole game is played.

2. Alex Berenson is one of the journalists that looked hard and long at the clinical trials Pfizer and Moderna had conducted, along with other data and research on mRNA vaccines, and had history of association with the issues. The more he looked, the more serious the flaws he found and wound up writing a booklet about the vaccines. Based on his research and analysis of the vaccines, he made a number of statements that were challenged by the drug companies. The State of Texas, Lubbock County, filed a petition against Pfizer, Inc. clearly stating the claims Pfizer made about its vaccine, and how in most cases they were false. The petition was 54 pages in length and listed a number of factual allegations against Pfizer. It listed a plethora of "Unreported Truths" that Pfizer failed to ever mention and other major problems with the ethical and moral ramifications violated by Pfizer. It gave recommendations for appropriate restitution for all the wrongs committed and grief caused.
3. The booklet Alex wrote about the vaccines at the time was a must-read, but subsequently there is so much more information on the vaccines today. All the politics surrounding their continued push will involve a dedicated chapter or two for vaccines alone. For now, it suffices to say potential problems with the vaccines were abundantly obvious long before regulators and the White House acknowledged them. Even then, there were summarily at least four major and crucial problems with the vaccines as follows:[35]
   - The vaccines were scarcely tested on elderly people who were obviously at the highest risk of death from COVID.

- There was intense pressure on regulators for speedy approval.
- There was a total lack of preclinical work done to ensure safety and efficacy of the vaccines.
- There was scarcely anything said concerning side effects, which showed up almost immediately and escalated exponentially.

The booklet gave some basic facts of things everyone should know about potential problems with the vaccines. Following are a few excerpt summaries of the above four crucial problems:[35]

1. Vaccines were scarcely tested on elderly people at highest risk of death from COVID. On March 5, a team of German researchers tested how well people over 80 responded to Pfizer's vaccine when compared to people under 60. The vaccine produced a much weaker immune response in the elders. After 2 doses, 1/3 of the elders had NO detectable antibodies in their blood. Other studies showed whatever protection was received peaked between one and four weeks after dose number 2 and slowly declined after that. In reality, rates of infection in vaccinated and unvaccinated were very little different. Given the size of trials, that scant difference offered no evidence to suggest the vaccines either saved or cost lives. Both companies did their vaccine testing on mostly younger, healthy people.
2. Regulators who approved vaccines did so under pressure. Both companies knew they wouldn't be required to say whether vaccines reduced deaths. As long as the top-line data looked impressive, the pressure for approval was at maximum. No one would look too hard at what the trials had actually proven—that the vaccine might reduce moderate illness in essentially already healthy people at low risk of COVID already. Pfizer and Moderna were right. The LACK of data did not stop regulators from rushing the vaccines forward.

3. Preclinical work to ensure safety was inadequate. In early COVID days, the risks of rushing a vaccine seemed small compared to the virus. The US government called its multi-billion-dollar effort to jump-start vaccine development Operation Warp Speed (Meriam-Webster dictionary defines that as "the highest possible speed"). Even though we knew by this time that COVID was far less dangerous than what was feared, governments rushed ahead with vaccine development anyway. Normally the process requires years of study and testing on animals in order to choose the best possible candidate long before it can ever be tried on willing, healthy volunteers. More months / years are spent reviewing trials to be sure of any possible problems or side effects or contraindications. Only then, do they even start the approval process. However, Pfizer and Moderna compressed that 5-10-year timeline into a few months. Moderna didn't even finish its pre-clinical study for its vaccine. European regulators called the companies' work "inadequate for evaluating the repeated dose toxicity of MRNA-1273," but gave the company a pass anyway on seriously dubious grounds.
4. Significant side effects showed up almost immediately. In the rush, nearly everyone just ignored some very sobering data on side effects. The trials made it clear neither company had fully addressed the concerns that had already slowed development of the mRNA vaccines for an entire previous decade or more! Their vaccines caused very serious side effects in many people, even young people, including deaths after jab #2. Pfizer reported almost 80% of people who received the vaccine had pain and / or swelling. About 30% had moderate to severe pain. Rates of systemic adverse events like fever, nausea, or diarrhea were also far higher in the vaxxed. The fact that people in the trials had so many severe adverse events shows the vaccine can cause strong immune reaction. From earlier studies, warning signs included potential blood and cardiovascular problems. Vaccines

reduced disease-fighting WBCs called lymphocytes and increased inflammation. They also caused some pre-cancerous bone marrow changes. These and other potential problems clearly indicated they should have been investigated much longer.

Reporting of adverse events in both the US and Europe has designated systems to use. Both systems received far more reports of side effects after COVID vaccines were given than any other previous vaccine. In just over three months of vaccinations, VAERS had received more than 30,000 reports of adverse events from COVID vaccines—as many as all other vaccines combined during the whole year before them. More than 800 of these were deaths. An even bigger issue to remember is that these systems are laborious and time-consuming for caregivers, especially and it is estimated the VAERS system only receives about 10% of the reports that needed to be filed. However, many people continued to laud vaccines. When you research on the web, the lack of truth in reporting problems is glaringly visible and disheartening to truth-lovers. However, in the long run, it became increasingly difficult to hide the growing montage of serious and even deadly long-term effects that would continue devastating our health. By the time we knew the full extent of damages caused by vaccines, it was far too late to rectify the problems for most people, and fatal for many more. Even now, as a medical bystander, people report the ongoing health issues and deaths they and their family members and friends have experienced as a result of the jabs. The reports mount daily, while the CDC refused to acknowledge the clear associations between the documented times, circumstances, and doses with rampant deaths even in newborn babies and older infants, due mostly to vaccinating pregnant women.

The Psychology of Succumbing to Vaccines/Boosters

So, COVID vaccines were then available to any and all, much like those created theoretically for preventing influenza. But, as prominent as influenza has been in some years, there were never gigantic pushes to get them or else. Public health officials used the usual techniques to encourage their use, but generally, most people never felt threatened if they chose not to take them annually. Contrary to tradition, Big Tech and social media plugged COVID vaccination continually, in all our faces. If someone had good reasons for NOT getting the jabs, they weren't allowed to say so. You couldn't ask good, intelligent questions, and you certainly could not say anything negative about the vaccines, especially on social media. It wasn't OK to think critically for yourself anymore. People had been told what they could and could not do for well over a year, and yet a small majority did what they were told to do. They had followed all the rules and had resigned themselves to this one with apathy or fear of potential consequences. They were also sick to death of hiding out in isolation from other people, and thought if they complied with the jabs, maybe, just maybe, they could get their lives back and feel 'normal' again. Vaccination fanatics simply couldn't wait to spread the great news! Almost everyone was still skeptical of the rushed vaccine when President Trump was in office, but when Sleepy Joe took the office, leftist libs completely reversed that notion. The media giant and so-called public health officials began a massive vaccination campaign.

Amazingly, legislators on both sides of the aisle simply didn't understand vaccines might actually be dangerous and harmful, or at best ineffective. There were clinical trials, right? Wrong, they weren't real, scientifically sound trials. The FDA and CDC had signed off on them—under much duress. After all, entire medical and scientific communities couldn't ALL be wrong—but they could be, they were and continued to be wrong if they bought the narrative! Even many conservatives had a strange naiveté. History records some really awful stories of drugs and vaccines gone wrong, but people lined up to get them anyway. Today, it all sounds so foolhardy, but at that point in the travesty, to even question the advisability of getting the jab was programmed to look like insanity. Many more people made wild and undocumented claims about the vaccine 'miracle' that were anything but true. If any of these had been wise enough to check the facts, they could have looked at the UK or Israel, both of which had initiated the jab much sooner than the US. As their mass vaccination campaigns ramped up, so did infections and deaths. By late January of 2021, the UK was averaging more than 1200 deaths per day in vaccinated people! British physicians began to notice the obvious connection. Denmark did a study in March and confirmed the connection. Leaders reported the vaccines actually had negative effectiveness at only 2 weeks after the first shot That meant those people who received the jab were MORE APT to become infected than those who hadn't. Health care workers with greater exposure, thinking they were protected, were more than twice as likely to get COVID and home residents were about 40% more likely due to closer proximity. This same phenomenon hit country after country. "Immunogenicity data indicated that antibody titers waned relatively rapidly after the receipt of TWO doses of vaccine, suggesting that waning would be an important factor in reported decreases in vaccine effectiveness over time..."[36] Questions about overall effectiveness of the vaccines became more crucial, and less answered.

Instead of more answers, there was more backward thinking from media. The continuing increases in deaths from COVID simply increased the media and public health push to get the vaccine. Ironically, just as soon as the first COVID vaccines were offered, VAERS reports started flooding in. By January of 2021, COVID VAERS reports outpaced the number of reports for all other vaccines. Many adverse events were moderate, but thousands of reports of serious injuries and deaths also came in. Six weeks later, by mid-February, 934 deaths from COVID vaccines were reported, but guess what?—Public health officials were still in complete denial. They were not about to acknowledge this huge rise in report numbers might actually indicate there were clear safety issues with the vaccines. Media simply attacked the database and anyone who mentioned the troublesome stats. After decades of less than adequate VAERS reporting, media responded that VAERS reports couldn't really be trusted since they did not prove all the nasty adverse events were actually caused by the COVID vaccines. Interesting, since the real problem with VAERS reports is that they don't report but about 10% of the cases of adverse events! After all, anyone could submit a report to the system—except that those who should be reporting most, often didn't get the tedious job done, partly because they became so stressed and busy with the adverse events! Reality was that pretending all those reports did NOT represent an extremely disturbing picture was bizarre beyond belief.

By April 2021, cases of myocarditis after COVID-19 vaccination, particularly among male vaccine recipients, were reported to the VAERS system. An 18-month study in Oregon of death records in young men did not prove conclusively with just three cases, that the deaths were caused by COVID vaccines. However NO attempt was made to investigate the actual VAERS reports of myocarditis and sudden deaths in the associated young men. Instead of looking at specifics, the CDC simply made a blanket statement that these cases were not caused by the vaccine. To this day, the CDC refuses to admit these literal hundreds of cases globally, especially in young athletes, simply could NOT be caused in these numbers by anything else. By Spring 2024, the same risks existed with the vaccines, even though the original vaccines were ordered to be updated in 2023. All of the health care "experts" continued to insist they were safe and effective, even for infants 6 months and older. The CDC and the Mayo Clinic still reported, "The risk of myocarditis or pericarditis after a COVID-19 vaccine is RARE. Most cases have been reported in males ages 12 to 39. Of the cases reported, the problem happened more often after the second dose of the COVID-19 vaccine and typically within one week of getting it."[37] Seeing this choice bit of stonewalling is supposed to assure us we can trust the safety of the COVID-19 vaccines. The claim was that the incidence of heart problems and potential death is RARE, but that simply can't be true when we see reported evidence almost daily! Would you still want to rush right to the doctor with your 6-month-old infant or small child for this miracle 'vaccine' based on this bogus assurance? Just because the powers that be have set the law to require 6-month infants get COVID-19 vaccination, then continuing them on the child immunization schedule, was certainly NOT enough for this parent to comply, permanently endangering my children's lives!

By Spring, there were still many people unwilling to think about potential problems with the vaccines, but they were moving into the minority. There was a newer group of anti-vaxxers like Robert F. Kennedy Jr and Naomi Wolf who became increasingly vocal about the hazards of the vaccines. Fortunately there were still a few public figures like Tucker Carlson and Joe Rogan who continued to raise the important vaccine questions no one would answer. They naturally distrusted all bureaucracies, and Big Pharma was chief among them. They weren't often heard over the screeching of the powerful media, as well as the corporate and governmental bigwigs who vehemently pushed the COVID vaccines. Governments at every level spent literally billions of dollars advertising the vaccines with enticing and clever marketing. They continued promising the vaccines were "safe and effective, and side effects rare." However, when those claims became clearly false, the side effects then became "mild and expected." The greatest lie of all, and easily proven so, was that the vaccines had NOT been "rushed," when everyone knew they had only been tested on a few hundred healthy people before they were rolled out. There were NO drugs or vaccines even remotely close to being given to humans globally when the pandemic began, and they had already been working on them secretly for MANY years. Only the title of "EMERGENCY" and the planned introduction of these drugs and vaccines under the "Emergency Use Authorization Act" could allow them the needed rush of experimental products which then could NOT be argued, and the big bucks could flow like rivers.

Another sticky vaccine issue came to the public eye on June 11, 2021. The World Health Organization (WHO) website recommended that children under age 18 NOT receive the COVID-19 vaccine. That statement contradicted the US CDC policy advising that children 12-17 years be vaccinated. But WHO stated there was not yet enough evidence for using vaccines against COVID-19 in children, to make any recommendations. Children and adolescents tended to have either no disease or a very mild disease when compared to adults. The very next day, WHO wrote another less specific version of their previous announcement; (they hadn't received the previous CDC memo). As Spring progressed, the media constantly reported the "truth" about how well the vaccines were working, though it was crystal clear they were NOT convincing the numbers of people they hoped to convince. However, many people were optimistic about the vaccine, such that real facts and concerns were unable to burst their proverbial bubble. The truth was, much of the optimism was short-lived and lasted about as long as the abbreviated clinical trials had run. Once again, the summer was coming, and that was the more probable reason for the decline in positive COVID tests, new cases, and deaths, much as would normally be seen with seasonal influenza decline. The declining started about mid-March when fewer than one in eight Americans had been vaxxed, so it was very unlikely the vaccines had made the difference. Naturally vaccine promoters still gave all the credit for declines to the vaccines, but they couldn't convince the majority. Vaccination numbers dropped like a boulder in a pond!

There was an apparent irony of at least two factors. The people who had wanted the vaccines the most were already vaccinated by this time. On April 13, the Johnson & Johnson vaccine was suspended when a number of young women suffered from a rare blood-clotting condition after receiving that vaccine. As well it should, this new wrinkle increased concerns over all vaccine side effects. In May, safety regulators announced the mRNA vaccines appeared to cause heart problems in young men. "Duh!—Surprise, Surprise!" Consequently, the jab numbers fell from 4 million/day in April to under one million/day in late June. In spite of this, vaccine promoters pushed harder and Big Pharma was ecstatic. Pfizer's CEO claimed European countries would certainly reach "herd immunity" by August. Vaccine advocates continuously touted the "miracle" vaccines. Something closer to every-day 'normalcy' had been achieved. However, vaccine fanatics were still not satisfied with their purported successes. The fact that more than 100 million American adults still refused to be jabbed was a bitter pill to swallow. They needed more coaxing; maybe even some kind of incentives could convince them. One noteworthy newspaper in Vancouver, British Columbia, Canada published an article entitled, "The 'Vaccine Hesitant' Are a Threat to Society; But We Must Show Them Compassion."[38] Though this was loaded with sarcasm, they would see the error of their ways for the benefit of all society.

The plunging numbers of hospitalizations and deaths definitely didn't encourage a greater need for vaccination. After all, if the vaccines worked so well, the unvaccinated could only hurt themselves. The argument that unvaccinated adults posed a danger to children was a mammoth, bold-faced lie. Then the unscientific 'medical scientist' Fauci posited the whopper of the century when he erroneously claimed, "Vaccinations would aid in keeping coronavirus variants from surfacing, because coronaviruses naturally tend to evolve in ways that increase contagion, but are less dangerous when contracted!"[39] The truth is that the SARS-CoV-2 virus, like any virus can mutate in both vaccinated and unvaccinated people, but vaccinations have the ability to create more mutations, which by definition would render the vaccines less effective. In reality, as with everything else COVID-related, the globalists' insistence on vaccinations was motivated far more by their financial and sociological concerns than by anything science-related. They don't care whether vaccines work or don't work as long as they accomplish their real goals and keep the big bucks rolling in.

By Spring of 2021, states and corporations jumped onto the bandwagon of jab incentives—programs designed to persuade people to get the jab. Every new effort to do so became increasingly demeaning. States offered lotteries with rewards of up to $5 million. Some folks could receive $50 gift cards for simply driving someone else to a vaccination location. Ubers gave free rides. No matter how much prodding and pushing, insulting and incentivizing, the vaccine rates changed very little.

Further, in the almost 6 months of their availability, they had still not approached legal FDA approval. All the bribery of people to take the jab was extremely unethical and immoral at the very least. All the tricky efforts made convinced very few people they needed the vaccines, and the numbers being jabbed continued to decline. By July, it was beyond obvious people had no desire to trade in their personal medical rights, no matter what reward was offered. Leadership of all political persuasions became extremely frustrated with all Americans who refused to succumb to the jabs, but at that time did not plan to use forceful persuasion such as the posited vaccination mandates or passports.

Believe it or not, President Biden had actually ruled out mandates before the vaccines rolled out and House Speaker Pelosi had actually agreed. It seemed the leftist leaders truly believed everyone would eventually see the long-range need for vaccination compliance. Perhaps they also believed the true anti-vaxxers were a small minority. They had been convinced the advent of the "miraculous" vaccine would be the ultimate panacea, and any doubters would hopefully fall off the planet.

However, this plan had a monumental flaw that couldn't be ignored. The vaccines were failing, but worse, the longed-for billions expected by the globalist elites were not quite as enriching as they had hoped. The efficacy of the mRNA vaccine was nowhere near the expectations. The downfall of mRNA vaccines began in Israel where a greater percentage of its people had been vaccinated (approximately 80%). In early June, the numbers of positive COVID-19 tests had almost ended. Within just two weeks, the numbers of positive tests were rising quickly again. Another two weeks brought in 300 positive tests. By July 15, Israel saw 1000 positives, and two weeks later, they approached 3000 positive tests—an increase of 200% in just two months!! The United Kingdom went down the same path, almost exactly. As we clearly could expect, this massive rise in new cases, brought unprecedented rationalization and justification, but every attempt held a pack of more lies. Fauci rose to his self-made throne and brought the world his "illuminated words of assuring brilliance" that there was nothing to worry about and all was well.

However, in spite of that, very soon the hospitalizations and rapidly increasing case numbers of vaccinated people were crystal clear. By early August, death rates also rose. The epidemiological issue of NO randomized, controlled, clinical trials done by real scientific methods, were glaringly missing. Upshot—there was absolutely no legitimate course of action to rightfully determine if a drug or vaccine EVER really worked at all.[40]

COVID-19 deaths continued to increase, both in Israel and the United Kingdom, whether vaccinated or unvaccinated. However, interestingly, the COVID deaths for the same months of August and September were higher in 2021 than they had been in 2020, when vaccines didn't even exist. No matter how many protests, explanations, and excuses were offered, it was abundantly clear vaccine failure was real. Nearly 70% of the dead victims had been fully vaccinated; another 5% had at least one dose of vaccine (75%.) This author attempted to find documentation of the quandary in epidemiologists scrambling about for explanations of why the vaccines had so quickly lost their efficacy. However, the global, science, education, and medical communities closed ranks very quickly and what little information was available at the time was either absent by that time or badly skewed and polished up to make it seem plausible. Regardless, whatever 'antibodies' which aren't really antibodies the vaccines had produced, they had declined severely and hastily. Israel's stats showed the decline had risen up to 40% per month. Today, most researchers would say it's all a moot point, since all previous vaccines have been discontinued and updated. No one could prove it now, as the incidences of new cases are relatively few, and are not monitored as they were.

Another significantly large study of August 25, 2021 in Israel demonstrated the "reality of 'naïve,' vaccinated people being over 13 times more likely to be infected with the SARS-CoV-2 than those who had developed natural immunity after being infected previously. From June 1 through August 15, 2021 (2.5 months), only

19 of 16,000 people with natural immunity were reinfected. The increased risk was significant for symptomatic disease as well... vaccinees were also at a greater risk for COVID-19 related hospitalizations compared to those that were previously infected. The study proved that natural immunity confers longer lasting and stronger protection against infection, symptomatic disease, and hospitalization, even in the Delta variant, when compared to those that were previously vaccinated."[41] This study was textbook proof that natural immunity was/is truly superior to vaccination.

In July, 2021, the fourth wave of American coronavirus began. Cases rose exponentially. 15,000 positive tests on July 5, leaped to 165,000 in early September. The death rate rose from 300 per day in July, to 1600 per day by mid-September. It could easily be predicted—vaccine pushers blamed the vaccination failures on the unvaccinated population, no matter how little sense that made. Clearly the lying increased as fast as the new cases and death rate. Anthony Fauci and the US Surgeon General Dr. Vivek Murthy both pretended 97-99% of all these rises were in unvaccinated people, but it was proven completely false more than once. Alex Berenson remarked, "As much as the figures may be skewed, they don't lie!" No truer words were ever spoken.

Most of this data was, at best, difficult to prove absolutely without real-time figures, since the CDC had previously stopped counting infections in non-hospitalized, vaccinated people in May, a ridiculously unexplained decision for people who live by their statistics! Fortunately, however, we had all the international data which proved conclusively the reality of vaccine failure was clearly undeniable. One might say this large summer surge of COVID-19 was the "pandemic of the vaccinated!" All of this effort to deny reality led to a myriad of bizarre statements. 'Suddenly', vaccinated people were having "breakthrough infections." Endless lies and exaggerations of political and media sources did have a seriously ugly real-world effect. There arose "the great divide" between the vaccinated and the unvaccinated, or the haves and havenots! The vaccinated were far less sure of their decisions to be jabbed.

Frightened, unsure people need something or someone to blame, which conveniently became the unvaccinated. The blame game was false and ugly, and the illustrious administration encouraged this divisive shame and blame attitude. President Biden blamed the unvaccinated for every self-inflicted, deep-state problem in America, including slowed job growth, inflation, stagnant economy, fossil fuel, climate change, etc. He actually declared, "the unvaccinated are prolonging the epidemic and contributing to anxieties that impact the economy!"[42]

One can't even count the number of ironies in this psychotically-sick attitude. The idea of unvaccinated folks being used as a scapegoat, ran opposite to the scientific facts and of course to common sense (a commodity sadly either missing or rare in his administration.) The fact is leftist Democrats and 'progressives' proudly proclaimed on a regular basis that they were society's MOST tolerant people, and then they lead an intolerance drive against a large group of people who seemed to retain at least some common sense in their decisions. For whole generations, public health officials called for tolerance—such as tolerance for gay men with AIDS, tolerance for smokers, drug addicts, alcoholics, and even the morbidly obese. After all, they should not be denied acceptance without judgment and the best of healthcare. Ironically, this tolerance should NOT be extended to perfectly normal healthy people who wanted to stay that way by refusing to accept an experimental, ultra-toxic, and highly questionable foreign substance in their bodies!

In July, the total idiocy developing became even more insane with the badgering of a New York Times writer who demanded that unvaccinated people be segregated from the lawfully vaccinated folks in restaurants, bars, movie theaters, sports arenas, entertainment venues, and other public places. This was then "lawfully" established in New York City by Mayor Bill de Blasio by August 1, the nation's largest effort yet to exclude the unvaccinated from public places. Signs warned patrons they must present proof of COVID-19 immunization in order to stay (a glaring violation of citizen rights). Obviously, the Mayor aimed to persuade more people to get vaccinated Or miss out on city amenities. Even now, the audacity of this mandate and others infuriated the writer and her reader! The employees of said venues were under the threat of losing their jobs if they had not been jabbed. Once again, the notion that anyone could remove personal freedoms for any reason is absolutely galling. Consider the absurdity of DeBlasio's own pious explanation, "We do not want to go back to restrictions, (what, this isn't a restriction?)—the key to our progress is vaccination."[43]

San Francisco, New Orleans, Las Vegas, and Los Angeles all adopted versions of the same, but all were relatively short-lived by recension. Another suggestion, just as nauseating and irresponsible as the previous one, suggested that if the unvaccinated became ill and needed hospitalization, they should be denied insurance coverage, possibly even denied medical care, beginning in 2023.

As we've already seen, this travesty actually happened on numerous occasions. As wildly unethical as that was, it doesn't touch the inhumanity of the notion or the subsequent usage of it. Fortunately, such a decision was/is "illegal under the Affordable Care Act and other federal law, as reaffirmed in a bulletin from the federal Centers for Medicare and Medicaid Services in October. Plans and issuers may not discriminate in eligibility for benefits or coverage based on whether or not an individual obtains a COVID-19 vaccination."[44] The author was unable to determine if the known instances of this illegality have been appropriately charged. If not, it's probably the main reason similar incidences have been illegally repeated.

The greatest of all governmental overreaches occurred on September 9, 2021. After a full year of promising he would NOT mandate vaccines, Sleepy Joe announced that federal workplace safety rules (think OSHA) would now require businesses with more than 100 employees to mandate vaccines for every employee. He claimed "'Pandemic politics are making people sick. He had no idea how close he finally came to the truth! The president's frustration was NOT that people were getting sick, but that he could not, nor could anyone else, CONTROL the fact of 80 million Americans 'failing' to get the shot, in spite of five months of free vaccines and availability at some 80,000 different locations."[45] He had missed his vaccination goals, and said he was running out of patience waiting for unvaccinated Americans to get their shots. He added, "We've been patient, but our patience is wearing thin, and the refusal has cost all of us. So please do the right thing."[45] That rhetoric could easily be the subject for much debate! He spoke as if getting the jab were unequivocally the right thing to do—one man's opinion as well as others' opinions, but all of those opinions were based in their own variable self-motivations. What's right is a very personal decision he and others had no right to make. He also had no right to mandate vaccinations for all federal employees, including our military, and all those folks engaged in health care. Even if it could have been deemed a national emergency, which it wasn't, he vastly and criminally overstepped his authority, President or no president. This was absolutely unconscionable!

First, there was the absurdity and discrimination of a rule that applied only to large employers. That was clearly beyond Biden's authority and smacked of denying the personal rights given in our American Constitution. There was no science (we were supposed to be following the science) behind the rule. Scientifically speaking, the vaccinated were clearly just as capable of shedding infectious virus as the unvaccinated, and in most cases, more so. But the real bottom line question was: Since the vaccines failed so miserably within just a few months, why in the world would the government decide to illegally force that failure on the yet unvaccinated? Was it necessary that everyone suffer the same highly potential failures and risks of the vaccines just to keep the game even?! There is no question this decision was foolhardy, moronic, unwise, downright dangerous, and of course, illegal, meaning literally criminal. As a matter of fact, two shots were no longer adequate—boosters were now encouraged and pushed in a renewed effort to increase their efficacy. Obviously, the ramped-up speed with which all this was done was proof that Biden, Big Pharma, globalists, and all others with a piece of the proverbial vaccine pie truly understood how quickly their wealth-based goals would be thwarted by the failure of the vaccines. In addition, on the day Biden announced boosters would start, neither the FDA nor the CDC had even begun to recommend the boosters! Biden's insanity was past showing worse than ever.

On August 31, 2021, two prominent, senior FDA regulators in the review office resigned, while the agency was neck-deep in high-profile decisions around COVID-19 vaccine approvals, authorizations for young children, and boosters. They were director, Dr. Marion Gruber, and deputy director Dr. Philip Krause of the FDA's Center for Biologics Evaluation and Research. There were clearly differences of opinion on next steps. The known statistical evidence on COVID-19 vaccines did not appear to support a need for booster shots in the general public at that time, according to an international group of vaccine scientists, including from the US-FDA and the WHO. Drs. Gruber and Krause wrote a paper published in The Lancet, where they noted they reviewed randomized trials and observational studies on COVID-19 vaccines. They consistently found, "vaccine efficacy is substantially greater against severe disease than against any infection; in addition, vaccination appears to be substantially protective against severe disease from all the main viral variants—including the Delta variant."[47] They also made it clear in their opinions that, "the message that boosting might soon be needed, if not justified by robust data and analysis, could adversely affect confidence in vaccines and undermine messaging about the value of primary vaccination."[47] Those views and others did NOT reflect the views of remaining FDA officials!

Meanwhile, the White House continued charging ahead, even in the face of rising scientific opposition. This breech of protocol perpetrated by President Biden and Anthony Fauci on the supposed upcoming of boosters was a MAJOR FAUS PAS for which President Trump would have been crucified, but then pro-globalist Biden always had a different set of rules. This case was definitely actionable, but not enough to be considered scandalous by his 'deep state' cronies. The FDA advisory panel vehemently rejected boosters for the general public on September 17, which marked a public rebuke of Biden and Fauci who had already publicly pushed boosters for EVERYONE. For the very first time in two full years, independent scientists actually stood up and challenged Fauci's gargantuan overreach of authority. However, these efforts and others to push vaccines and boosters on everyone— including healthy children and adults continued to date.

Alex Berenson and many others continued to write, tweet, and post to social media about the vaccines' dangers—especially young people dying of heart failure and myocarditis. He spoke about the multi-billions of dollars Big Pharma, especially the offending vaccine companies were raking in on the vaccines and COVID drugs. These journalists spoke the verified, documentable truth still being denied by Big Pharma, public health officials, and globalists. Unfortunately, the pressure was still on from the White House-down requiring Big Tech media outlets to take action against all anti-vaccine posts. They were actually calling for even tighter censorship, and asking all Big Tech companies to "create robust enforcement strategies. Anything they did not like would automatically be termed 'misinformation'. A massive document was created by the Carter Center entitled "The Big Lie and Big Tech." Initially, it was established in detail to create the ground rules for Big Tech to monitor all information related to election interference, but it worked even better through the pandemic. "It identified the basic need for 'fact checkers'—always a left-leaning joke. More importantly it fully controlled what could or could not be allowed on the media platforms. When information did NOT line up with the accepted narrative it was, by an elaborate system of algorithms, domestic repeat-offenders' listings, and AI, deemed 'misinformation,' and dealt with accordingly. The numbers of techniques used to mitigate the 'misinformation' literally boggles the mind of the citizen who still believed there is any such thing remaining in the US as freedom of speech! Thankfully, even after continuous vilification, these truth-bearing journalists, though censored again and again, were not fully silenced."[47] Many of the facts given, have been substantially accepted as truth by the majority of caring, thinking people, but the battles for speaking out truth continue to date. Unquestionably, the truth still needs to be shared everywhere, particularly when the health and lives of our infants and children desperately need to be protected from the toxic effects of COVID vaccines. It has become a plague rivaling the abortion agenda.

Part III

Part III—Pandemic Aftermath Issues

CHAPTER 11

Fundamental Truths on Pandemic Controversies

Authoritarianism-No More Individual Focus

The definition of the word is the enforcement or advocacy of strict obedience to authority at the expense of personal freedom. Legally, it is the enforcement of obedience to a central authority at the expense of person freedoms, rule of law, and other constitutional values and principles. In its extreme, it is totalitarianism, wherein all socio-political power is held by a dictator, indeed a despot, who also controls the national politics and the people of the nation with continual propaganda campaigns broadcast by state-controlled media. Globally, in 2022, "freedom faces a dire threat. Around the world, the enemies of democracy...are accelerating their attacks. Such regimes have become more adept at co-opting or circumventing the norms and institutions meant to support basic liberties, and providing aid to others who wish to do the same. In countries or republics like ours, with long-established democracies, internal forces have exploited the shortcomings in their systems, and distorted national politics to promote hatred, violence, and unbridled power. Many more countries are leaning toward it—the present threat to democracy is the product of 16 consecutive years of decline in global freedom."[1] At this point, if democracy's defenders do not work together to help guarantee our freedoms, the authoritarian model of government will prevail, exactly as planned and dreamed by Klaus Schwab, and his World Economic Forum with its global reset. That may sound like a scary prediction, but those who know Scripture, will recognize this as the direction

God said the world will ultimately go with the advent of the Antichrist and God's Tribulation Judgment.

"The war against the virus was really a war waged via technologies and their masters, to dissolve human culture and dismember human beings. It was a war on free thought and free speech—a war against our most fundamental beliefs…a war aimed at undoing humanity itself."[2] The people of the world did not vote to abandon 'old systems' and destroy 'our old ways.' During the pandemic we all experienced some form of attack on our religious communities. The Chinese Communist Party (CCP) determined that churches were among the first institutions to be removed in China which of course was not difficult for a nearly totalitarian government. In the case of the US, churches and religious organizations were singled out, and threatened with permanent closures for choosing not to follow imposed COVID rules. Other churches were fined again and again for meeting together weekly as God's Word directs:

> "Not neglecting to meet together as is the habit of some, but encouraging one another; and all the more as you see the Day drawing near." Hebrews 10:25 ESV

It took an act of the United States Supreme Court against the governor of California, Gavin Newsom, a 'died in the wool globalist,' to allow worship at church in person, as our Constitution guarantees. After the initial lockdown, many churches reopened with additional precautions for the remainder of the pandemic, understanding that further closing was against our Constitution. However, with the constant fearmongering and threats, some churches NEVER reopened for public worship and streamed their services to their once large and active congregations. This was a travesty at many levels when the chief reason for church besides corporate worship is fellowship of the family. We are all well aware of the real reason for attacking churches in this manner. The rules and regulations of the pandemic were established primarily to break all bonds between human beings that would in turn break down families and all other institutions unifying our society. Scare tactics such as shame and blame, shunning, tattling on others' behaviors, bribery, harassment, bullying, threatening, fearmongering, and policing by self-appointed do-gooders looked very much like those of Communism. The power-grabbing globalist wolves were calling almost all the shots, and changing the rules at will as they deemed necessary.

Members of the public health community usurped unelected control over hundreds of areas of our public life, then hounded and demanded everyone else to do as they were told. Anthony Fauci's self-assumed powers went far beyond the reach of his position and he got away with it because globalist wolves had given him a basic carte blanche just as long as he played their game. School boards and liberal teachers' unions also wielded unprecedented power to intimidate parents and cheat children out of their educations. Formerly safe schools became hostile and authoritarian, caring little about the total health of the children. Any parent who tried to vocalize their very real concerns were labeled 'domestic terrorists' in a way similar to the method CCP controls every aspect of life in China.

In a land where freedom of speech is protected Constitutionally, US social media outlets were instructed to censor ANY communication which didn't fit the COVID narrative. There was NOTHING free about speech in America. Reader, do not believe any of these events were accidental! These policies were perpetrated upon Americans and had absolutely nothing to do with applying the science; they didn't even resemble traditional science-based thoughts or behaviors. Note: early in the pandemic studies showed 'lockdowns' DID NOT slow or halt the disease; in fact, they were often counterproductive. However, the lockdown nonsense continued to be pushed, and many called for tightening the lockdown guidelines as the pandemic progressed. Social distancing and masking were also proven ineffective as we have already seen, but for at least two years—in some places more—they did not stop or even lessen.

All of the above measures did far more harm to individuals and our society, than good. They were all unnecessary, egregious, and far reaching; the cumulative effects caused remain unknown. We do know there was long-term damage to all people, especially our children as confirmed by most psychologists. The destruction of the pandemic war on humanity was carefully and extensively planned decades before by the globalist wolves whose primary aim was to totally renovate our world to totalitarianism under their complete control. They intended, by every means possible, to divide and conquer anything and anyone who represented traditional human spaces, speech, communication, and Western civilization; including our value systems, liberty, and freedoms. The methods they used to achieve these goals were first modeled by machines, then programmed to command all policies. Ultimately, Western cultures, in particular, would be reprogrammed to accept the CCP-like structures of government.

Much of the world lives in what we know as an analog/humane society. That means we are "biologically able to fit within the natural world. We are flexible and tolerant. We excel at perception, at creativity, at the ability to go beyond the information given, and able to make sense of otherwise chaotic events. We often have to interpret events far beyond the information available. Our ability to do this efficiently and effortlessly, usually without even being aware we are doing so, greatly adds to our ability to function. This ability to put together a sensible, coherent image of the world in the face of limited evidence allows us to anticipate and predict events, to better cope with an ambiguous, ever-changing world."[3] Deliberate, intentional attacks on this society during the pandemic were perpetrated on physical things, such as books, markets, libraries, real money, maps, workplaces, places of real entertainment, pubs/bars, restaurants, classrooms, churches, dinner parties, summer camps, recess and playgrounds, Boy/Girl Scouts, clubs, team sports, real cars, traditional holidays, and rituals.

Globalist wolves detest our representative-based democratic republic, operating live at our national and state capitals, our Congress, and town halls. They hate our museums, historical sites, memorial statues, and anything else that connects us to our common history, our roots, our meaningful lives, and our beliefs and values. Human beings touch and feel; they communicate openly in face-to-face interaction, and all these things make us powerful in our human unity. Therefore, social distancing and masking were/are two of the most effective means of alienation from other people. Humans require closeness, and connection with others. Without it, we humans suffer physical, mental, social, spiritual, and emotional damage. The evidence of those unrequited human needs is abundantly clear to free people who visit places like China, Russia, and Eastern Europe to name a few. These peoples are so depleted in decent human to human contact, it is quite difficult to establish or build connection with them. To create the desired top-down authoritarian governments globalists plan for, they will continue to make any/every attempt possible to destroy all of this; separating and isolating people long enough to produce sheep who will follow the prescribed agenda with little or no questions or pushback.

"Indeed, one reason that solitary confinement has been seen as an ultimate torture by prison policy-makers and networks is because isolation can cause permanent change to the human brain, resulting in madness."[3] We can develop 'touch deprivation' further inducing PTSD symptoms. It has been shown in hundreds of studies—positive events, even moments of human touch calm the nervous system, boost mood, and release endorphins, our 'feel-good' chemicals. They even strengthen our immune systems and improve healing. We know the isolating requirements of the pandemic, supposedly initiated to prevent the spread of COVID-19, DID NOT WORK! Instead, they led many people to debilitating sadness, personal isolation, anxiety, depression, substance abuse, and other physical and psychological problems, even including suicide. As we've seen, this was intentionally planned and cleverly perpetrated on individuals and society alike. Globalist wolves caused a plethora of damaging outcomes to all of society. Since we know one of the ultimate goals of globalists and the WEF is depopulation, we also saw that nothing perpetrated by globalist goals was done in the interest of better health, healing, or diminishing the death toll. As the two+-year extension of these measures continued, it became abundantly clear—health and abundant life were the exact commodities they aimed to destroy.

So, as we have seen and innately know, there is no viable or technological replacement for groups of people interacting with one another—in speaking, smiling, touching, teaching, singing, laughing, dining, and all other interpersonal activities we enjoy and engage in regularly. Big Tech, globalist wolves, and their minions know and understand these concepts, and hate what they represent. They seek to destroy it all, and the stifling of each area was always fully intentional. It was their best and most focused shot at making all of us more manageable and more easily controlled. Consequently, the obvious first step in accomplishing their goals was the complete annihilation of free assembly and community focus. Today, we understand these mandated measures were well-orchestrated offenses by government, in cooperation with Big Tech, Big Pharma, and the mainstream media, all directed by the globalist wolves' vision and plan.

"World-wide, we saw all government levels aligned with the same instructions to deal with anyone who dared to speak up and challenge this plan. They completely bypassed lawmakers and gave power to all healthcare agencies to restrict our rights and liberties as needed illegally! We saw loss of personal autonomy, i.e. the control over our own bodies, also illegal. We witnessed all the aforementioned tactics used to abuse those who refused to lose their personal rights. Failure to comply with the new rules, whether unconstitutional or not, brought additional abuse down on your head in one form or another."[4]

The ultimate goal of the globalist wolves, such as Klaus Schwab (WEF), Bill Gates (Gates Foundation), Jeff Cook (Apple CEO), Jamie Dimon (JPMorgan Chase CEO), David Solomon (Goldman Sachs CEO) and Jeff Bezos (Amazon) just to name a few, is darkly clear. Their agenda was both diabolical and dangerous to all of humanity, yet most people did not understand this fact, and many didn't even suspect it. These current globalists were preceded by many others who had similar goals, but were less vocal or known for their global aspirations, so their ideas are many decades old. True students of history are able to detect such efforts to achieve similar goals which were observable several decades ago. Millionaire moguls such as the Rockefellers, Carnegies, Vanderbilts, J.P. Morgan, and Henry Ford were all highly instrumental in the development of the US, as well as the globe during their "Golden Age" and later to the 'Robber Barons' and 'Captains of Industry.' John D. Rockefeller set today's Big Pharma on a firm foundation that still thrives, but much of the business conducted by such moguls was little different than that of today's globalist wolves. Their money bought whatever they wanted and few dared to argue. Rockefeller deliberately banned the influence and effectiveness of herbal and alternative medical choices, to enable the monopoly of Big Pharma. In succeeding decades, the influence of Big Pharma completely changed the philosophy and focus of our modern medicine to the allopathic form it is today. It was everything but an improvement to the American ideas that often worked better, and still do.

Today's globalist wolves were hoping, even expecting, that our pre-COVID days were gone forever and could never be retrieved. They intended to annihilate all Western and human culture, replace it with totalitarian governance, fully tech-control the culture, and make certain we would all rapidly forget what it meant to be fully-free humans. "An abysmal crime of the largest proportions ever known to man was perpetrated on our country and on our world in 2020-2022. There is 100% commitment to continue perpetrating this crime. It is beyond time for us to wake up and take back control as we know it, and defeat the black tide of globalism with its New World Order."[5]

The New Top-Down, Unquestioned, Order-Following State

Of particular interest to us all is the narrative written by author, Dr. Naomi Wolf, when the planned lockdowns started. All over the world people were being introduced to what this New World Order for the pandemic would look like. Ms. Wolf was in London, England March of 2020, when the first changes were being instituted.

"The Southbank Centre in London represented the finest Western cultural and civic delights to every human in every walk of life without much cost. It held free association and easy sharing. A favored bastion of the United Kingdom." This was where Ms. Wolf was, when lockdowns began. Milan, Italy had just been locked down in what had been a free, modern nation. It meant free citizens could be held in an area against their wishes. Liberty to assemble freely was restricted. "The flower of Europe was being struck at its root."[6]

The location of Ms .Wolf's meeting was full of human crowds. The ideas flowed freely, and were educating, illuminating, and enlightening. It brought energy and communication to the masses. Crowds of people felt elevated and energized after having met in such gatherings and they held their heads a bit higher because they'd been there. They felt confidence that empowered their souls. But that was the very last day of their old world, and old lives. Other countries were also locking or closing down. Ms. Wolf's husband told her she needed to come home (USA) ASAP, as all the flights from Europe were shutting down. From her perspective, after that night, London was effectively destroyed in many ways, and has never been the same since.[6]

Ms. Wolf lived in the South Bronx neighborhood of New York City. The entire area had been experiencing a real renaissance with renewal, rebuilding, and revitalizing. It looked forward to abounding new opportunities. Hundreds of small businesses were thriving and running their enterprises efficiently. Something new or good was happening every place you looked by February of 2020. Hope and anticipation were in the air. However, the downside of the Bronx was its older, more systematic and yet to be improved problems. The people's health suffered disproportionately. Long-term poverty brought many illnesses to many people. Bronx children had the highest rate of childhood asthma in the city. Obesity and poor nutrition were often chronic. Fresh nutritious food was hard to obtain and expensive. There was very little open space available for exercise and children to play. Almost no one had decent medical care and there were high rates of diabetes, obesity, heart disease, asthma, HIV/AIDS, increased infant morbidity and mortality, etc. Respiratory illnesses were especially bad and medicines far too expensive. Shutting the area down certainly was NOT going to help anyone.[6]

On March 11, 2020, all of Broadway closed. Not one venue or theatre was left open. In one gigantic, iconic, and sweeping, Soviet-style, autocratic move, Broadway went black. As Ms. Wolf stated, she and her husband had both lived in closed countries previously, so they knew instinctively whatever was coming was NOT going to be good. Their first thoughts were simply to 'get out of town,' and off the extremely crowded island. Since they owned a small cottage in the Hudson valley, they moved there the very next day, hoping it would be for the short term. "But the South Bronx was never the same again and the small towns they moved to, never recovered either. It felt more like Cuba or even Beijing—and the dictates and new norms looked and felt more like the Republic of China, than the culture and beliefs of the United States of America."[6]

In New York State, Governor Andrew Cuomo declared Emergency Law on March 7, 2020. Ms. Wolf knew about emergency laws from studying about the decline of Democracies, and also recognized that something catastrophic had just happened. Two Years later, New York State remained under Emergency Law! It wasn't even written in the legal language of declarations; just under

> emergency law. Stores and restaurants were ordered closed, but 'essential businesses' could remain open. "It was an order, but like most other orders and mandates, never came from our legislature. It was the first of many 'edicts', 'mandates', and 'orders' perpetrated on citizens. Every one of these were designed to get citizens in the habit of a top-down, unquestioned, 'order-following' lifestyle instead of knowing and following the democratic laws of the land. Everyone in the state went 'on hold' for the 'safety of all'!"[7] Most of the people were literally shocked into submission. Another red flag rose for Ms. Wolf and her husband who had lived in war zones. They knew that COMMERCE is NEVER closed, even in the very worst of crises. People must keep working to make their living and survive the crisis and the economy MUST be sustained for communities to survive. When societies are forbidden to buy and sell, they can't fight back. The death of an economy can only lead to eventual enslavement or occupation. As discussed previously, that is exactly what was planned all along.

The next edict read, "Governor Cuomo Signs the 'New York State on PAUSE' Executive Order."[8] It was touted to 'Assure Uniform Safety for Everyone.' It also banned all non-essential gatherings of individuals of any size for any reason. The governor also announced "Matilda's Law," named for his mother, to better protect the elderly, the most vulnerable population, whereby they were simply to stay home and limit home visitation. Additionally, all PPE products were to be sold back to the state to be certain they would have enough for all care providers. Public transportation, in a city where a large per cent of the workforce relies on it, was prohibited except in an emergency. Everyone, everywhere was to social distance.

Just in case this doesn't sound scary enough, the reader should be aware that even in refugee camps around the world, people can buy and sell as needed. Even while under attack, children can still try to go to school! There was unbelievable usurping of unwarranted authority all over our country and many others. Most of us in America had assumed we were sovereign individuals and could NOT be placed on 'pause' or 'hold' by any leader. It would still be each citizen's responsibility to deal with his/her own decisions with reference to their personal risk, but that wasn't so. Worse still, who was actually deemed "essential?" Walmart, Target, and McDonalds were all open; bookstores, libraries, plays, theaters, concert halls, churches, small restaurants, etc. were all closed and thousands of people were without jobs. Churches were protected by our Constitution and were essential to multitudes of people, but not to the government; it did not want churches open! Large chain-restaurants were 'essential' and illogically deemed "germ-free" while owner-run restaurants must surely be cesspools of disease that must be forcibly closed. Tech companies, telecoms, chain drugstores, liquor stores, pet stores, etc. were all deemed 'essential'. Only groceries and drugs were on sale. There was no discussion or debate about any of these stupid decisions and many others. It was all about top-down control.

Schools were suddenly and systematically "forced" to close. Overnight, "distance learning" appeared and was launched. Such programs would normally require months or years to develop and much longer to implement. However, programs were suddenly present everywhere, ready to go at all levels for all subjects! Even more shocking, no one except parents and students were alarmed at this brand-new prospect of millions of children sitting at home on screens alone as a legitimate replacement for "school." Most teachers, if they felt alarmed, weren't given any other options, just new orders. Teacher unions and other spokespeople FOR the teachers claimed the teachers lived in mortal fear of being infected by students and it was actually the teachers who refused to go to school to teach. As a parent of teachers and friend to dozens of other teachers, this author knew this bunch of drivel simply was not so! Most of them would far rather teach in a classroom and engage active children, than try to do the job most inadequately on a remote basis. No one bothered to poll the teachers and accurately find out what they thought or how they felt. This was the "new normal" for education whether anyone liked it or not (very few liked it), and there was no place anyone could go to debate the subject, or even express how badly it was affecting the children. It never mattered if you had a child suffering alone, and falling far behind in their studies. Most college students were sent home and schools closed indefinitely. Consequently, many college students never returned to resume their education.

We discussed some of these problems before, but we return to them now simply to remind us of the reasons all these things were done so high-handedly and so poorly. Top-down autocrats had their orders from globalist wolves and they exercised their own wills and overgrown egos to bring about the globalist agenda in every area they could get hold of. It was always about control, and teaching people accustomed to democratic processes how to submit to these new rules without questions, speaking out, or rebellion. Playgrounds and parks OUTSIDE were taped off like crime scenes. OUTSIDE trails, state parks, and beaches were closed off by regional stay-at-home orders for over a year. Just like in China with the CCP, people were told what they could do, what they could or could not buy, where they could and could not go and how close they could be to the next person. With constant pandemic fear-mongering, many were scared and confused, especially with constant changes in the 'official rhetoric', but most helplessly complied.

Using the Communist system of 'essential' and 'non-essential', governors CHOSE which businesses were expendable to 'kill', and kept those they deemed would not only survive, but thrive. You see, the new rule-makers ditched our traditional capitalism which allowed reasonably fair competition. "That isn't the kind of capitalism the new rules demanded. Massive national economies, giant corporations, and billionaire globalist owners wanted to run their own kind of capitalism, called stakeholder capitalism. Globalists like to define it in a way that sounds almost palatable;... 'corporations should serve the interests of all their stakeholders, not just their shareholders. Stakeholders can include investors, owners, employees, vendors, customers, and the *public at large*. The focus was on long-term 'value' creation (making more money makes more money), not merely enhancing shareholder values only. What it really is: the rich get richer, and the poor, poorer! Classic communism!"[9] Boards of health are NOT elected by the people, so their pompous operations and decisions bypassed the will of the people and the Congress. Tens of thousands of businesses were forcibly closed, and millions of citizens made subject to mandates that weren't legal, but they were enforced by people who didn't care about their legality or because someone, with higher perceived authority than they had, was breathing down their necks.

In one democracy after another democracy, the COVID-19 "emergency" was USED to create emergency governance to hyper-empower health officials and agencies. This simultaneously drained decision-making powers from Congresses and Parliaments. It was the softest and sneakiest coup in all history. Once again, Ms. Wolf had been a CEO of a website devoted to normal legislation and she followed real laws very closely. She had NEVER BEFORE seen, "bills structured to facilitate the wholesale bribery and promote the corruption of so many individuals and civil institutions. 500 years of ever-developing capitalism gave opportunity to millions of middle-class and working-class investors, entrepreneurs, and landlords. In just TWO YEARS, all of that was replaced with a bleak, coercive, Marxist-style, crony oligarchy. When the dust settled, billions of dollars...were seen to have been essentially stolen from one group (the middle-class and working-class people of the West) and handed to another, the billionaire, globalist, oligarchs (wolves)."[10]

Freedom of choice and personal sovereignty were gone, in the above areas as well as in many others, such as vaccination mandates. We became just like little children who needed large circles and arrows on the supermarket floor to direct the chosen path for us. They decided we were now the powerless. The bright, cheery letters and colors really said, "You can't be trusted to behave sensibly and make your own decisions!" Folks, the circles and arrows on the floor were anything but trivial nonsense to joke about. They symbolically removed our positions in society as adults who could be trusted to make our own decisions. No more dreaming; it might become dangerous. After all, dreaming might lead us in a different direction than those indicated on the floor! This my friend, is what was planned in advance for us, and perfectly executed to do what was planned for us. Since the majority of people laid down and played dead last time, the globalists feel quite confident we would do it all again. Leftist leaders in our nation were completely cooperative with the new rule-makers. Consequently, we must educate ourselves to the ways and means of our nation's real enemies, and commit ourselves to following only the laws of our land with leaders we elect. Globalist wolves will try this again someday soon if they are allowed. Are we ready to defend our lives, children, homes, churches, jobs, and all else that is American? Only then will we stop usurpers from gaining any further ground. It will require every thinking adult to stand in unison with all other thinking adults and declare we will not relinquish any more freedom and liberty to their agenda. May God Almighty guide and direct us, and enable us to fight for the freedom He gave us:

> "If my people who are called by my name will humble themselves, and pray, and seek my face and turn from their wicked ways, then I will hear from heaven and will forgive their sin and heal their land." 2 Chronicles 7:14 ESV

The True Nature of the Crimes Committed

The globalist wolves' plans in 2020-2022 were to crush Western peoples, crush Western economies, and steal all the assets of the working and middle classes. To do so, they used mass vaccination of an incompletely-tested substance as the panacea for a pandemic. They imposed a digital identity system which would enable them to create a CCP-styled surveillance society to generate unbelievable riches in data harvesting. Not only was this personally intrusive in our own nation, but the information was/is always subject to international cyber hackers' usage. The CCP banks a vast collection of genomic and other healthcare data from America in its quest for world dominance. There is high risk to personal privacy and to US economic and national security. Would you want your DNA or other healthcare data going to a rival authoritarian regime with the known record of exploiting DNA for repression and surveillance, and for purposes only the CCP knows and controls? This vast collection of DNAs has enabled the CCP to carry out all kinds of human rights abuses against their own domestic minority groups. A vivid case in point is the "Muslim Uyghurs and other minorities in the Xinjiang region, which have been swept up in a years-long crackdown China says is aimed at counter-terrorism and deradicalization. (LIES). Rights groups argue Beijing's systematic mistreatment of ethnic minorities throughout the country targets cultural and religious erasure. (More than that, it's another fast-track to depopulation of its own 'expendable' people). "Ongoing rights violations in Xinjiang recently included 'the arbitrary imprisonment or other severe deprivation of physical liberties of more than 1 million civilians,' said a report published by the US State Department's Bureau of Democracy, Human Rights, and Labor...Uyghur women were subjected to 'forced sterilization, coerced abortions, and other more restrictive application of the country's birth control policies', as well as rape and other forms of sexual and gender-based violence."[11]

Your DNA is the most valuable thing you own and it cannot be replaced. The loss of your DNA not only affects you, but your relatives and potentially, generations to come. "The CCP views bulk personal data, including healthcare and genomic data, as a strategic commodity to be collected and used for its economic and national security priorities. It has heavily invested in the 'biotech revolution' and enacted national policies prioritizing the collection of healthcare data both at home and abroad to achieve its goal of becoming THE global biotech leader."[12]

The CCP understands the collection and analysis of large genomic data sets from diverse populations helps foster new medical discoveries and cures having substantial commercial value and advances its Artificial Intelligence and precision medicine industries. In 2016, four years before the intentional COVID-19 plans were even imminent, "the CCP announced a $9 billion, 15-year project to collect, analyze, and sequence genomic data to become a global leader in precision medicine—a process designed to provide tailored treatments based on the genetic makeup, environment, and lifestyle of individual patients."[13]

"With the COVID-19 pandemic, the CCP aggressively marketed Chinese COVID-19 testing kits around the world, along with laboratories to support the testing. By August 2020, China's leading genomics company, Beijing Genomics Institute (BGI), said it had sold test kits to 180 countries and established labs in 18 countries in just six months. According to the US-China Economic and Security Review Commission, these same COVID-19 labs provided Chinese researchers with access to healthcare data from around the globe. It is believed there are no Chinese COVID labs in the US, however, for years, the CCP has been able to gain access to US healthcare data, including genomic data, through a variety of channels, both legal and illegal."[14] US healthcare data appears more valuable to China because of the massive ethnic diversity of the US population. In addition, compared to other nations, the US has fewer safeguards on medical and healthcare data, including data for research purposes, because its focus is primarily on privacy, not national security, which creates vulnerability and enables foreign actors to gain access to data on far more people of the US. Over the years, Chinese companies took advantage of this by investing in US firms handling sensitive healthcare and other types of personal data, providing them entry to the US market and access to this data.

The crimes perpetrated on our world, and especially our Western world, are so massive, so intentionally planned over decades, and so detailed in their execution, it is almost impossible for the minds of average, normal, hard-working, and conscientious people to grasp its enormity. The caliber of criminality is so heinous, we simply can't imagine it. It has always been diabolically evil, because it takes NO Account of the well-being of literal billions of people. The majority of us in grassroots America tend to believe other people are at least somewhat like us, and think similarly. In this case, nothing could be further from the truth. "The masterminds of the globalist wolves exercised such brutal tyranny upon our world, our minds cannot comprehend it. Granted, there are thousands of subcultures, tyrants, and ideologies that clearly do not share our core values. However, we must face the facts that these monsters are not just long-dead Nazis or members of the CCP far, far away. Many monsters live very near us. Some monsters wear lovely suits, and can chat amicably about their kids at dinner parties. Some kinds of monstrosities and sociopaths are actively cultivated by the norms and within networks all around us. Though they may be partially hidden at locally elite levels, they are systematized and accepted at very high levels of globalism."[15]

Ironically, after the smoke of World War II cleared, and the carnage buried, various national and international organizations were founded, such as the World Trade Org. (WTO), the United Nations, the Regional Comprehensive Economic Partnership (RCEP), as well as other global corporate and investment communities that birthed the early Global Elites. They too were policymakers, non-profit leaders and bureaucrats. It seemed nothing could stop them from engaging in cruel and oppressive policymaking precisely because they were no longer a part of the communities whose lives would be affected by what they imposed on others. Ironically, like true predators, they talked about encouraging a more harmonious, unified world where no hatred existed between age-old enemies like France and Germany. They claimed such a structure would greatly benefit the lower classes better than individual countries could. At the same time they pontificated about such an entity. Similar current government works for nobody except these wealthy, control-freak predators. Whether nation states are the best idea, or not, for long-term peace and happiness, we who have known democracy, value our freedoms too much to live under the totalitarian government globalists constantly push for.

Tragically, the globalist wolves have rapidly formed super-structured organizations that intend to make all necessary decisions

OVER the heads, hearts, and wishes of the citizens. We witnessed this effect during COVID-19 when life-changing decisions were made for us, and we didn't see anyone who felt peaceful or happy! Another perfect example of this thought process was seen in the unelected decision-makers of the European Union. That body quickly became more important and powerful than the parliaments of any individual country at national levels. It happened to Greece, Portugal, and Spain. Fortunately, the UK was diametrically opposed to that kind of rule and wisely opted out, much to the chagrin of the other countries. Then the citizens of the individual countries were programmed to simply leave any high-level decisions to the unelected bureaucrats of the European Union. The propaganda of these bureaucrats shamed citizens for being proud and loyal to their own nations. They've been scolded, hammered on, and belittled for worrying about their nations' future well-being. But understand this: It is NOT racist to be patriotic; and it is NOT disloyal or uncaring to want safe borders, and the right to vote open only to legal citizens!

Not long ago, nearly one million illegals were given voting rights in New York City; all a part of the globalist strategy. On the surface, rhetoric declared this was anti-racism and equity for all, but in reality, it's every tyrant's dream! The obvious ultimate effect and intent was simply to remove power of the legal citizens. The democratic nation is accountable to its citizens and until recently they had the right to vote out corrupted leaders. Our leaders lately, who have adhered to the dictates of the globalist wolves and their agenda are beyond corrupted, pay no attention to their constituents, and make as many unilateral decisions as they can get by with. There are still a few natural limits to the oppression and yes, tribulation, our leadership can get away with, but America is dangerously close to the brink of authoritarianism!

In a globalist, non-elected bunch of super-egomaniacs, the goal is full control. When leaders act in accordance with their own agendas, nothing can stop the levels of mass cruelty, and constant oppression of all people. There will be no real concern for the welfare of any nation. No one within the nation is as smart, rich, or well-educated as they, therefore ordinary citizens cannot be allowed to make their own decisions. Given an unacceptable and foreign set of circumstances like a pandemic, ordinary people are capable of great cruelty. We saw the best example of this during COVID, when ordinary people took it upon themselves to police others' mask-wearing. How many of us experienced walking through a retail entrance with a mask on, and being told to "get that mask up where it belongs" in front of any number of bystanders! Being told by another patron that you're going the wrong way on a one-way aisle was annoying at best! During that hellish two years, most of us instinctively understood and felt that something had gone horribly wrong. Nothing sounded right or even reasonable, but most people continued to follow the dictates of 'some' authority, that had no real or elected authority to tell us what we could or could not do. It was a global campaign led by globalist wolves who, like Fauci, could sound very sage and worldly, knowledgeable, and maybe even a little bit right, given that no one had been there before. The pseudo-authorities had a lucrative agenda, so they exacted vast cruelties of debilities and death and inflicted morbid carnage with absolutely no compunction or regret.

Some want to know how one author, Ms. Naomi Wolf, knows so much about the ideas, habits, and deeds of these globalist wolves? The answer is, "As a journalist, I've seen them all up close and personal!"[15] As she travels to various places and meetings globally as a writer, she focuses a lot of her attention and conversations on drivers, cleaners, waitstaff, and other service providers, because globalists NEVER "see" these folks or other mere mortals. But these mere mortals tend to see, hear, and know almost everything that is happening. Ms. Wolf said she found they were almost always right!

Then Ms. Wolf recounted a story of one experience she had in the company of the globalists in New York City. "It was hosted by a major hedge-fund manager, an apparently lovely man, educated in the Ivy League. He resided in a fabulous 19th Century mansion. The dining room was fully staffed with beautiful servers, who served a gorgeously perfect dinner. The walls were adorned with impressive portraits and works of art. Every other guest, including other large investors were pleasant, educated, and cultured. Excellent wine flowed freely, and no one was visibly evil in appearance. It was not a clandestine gathering with secret signs or lurking shadows. This group had no need for secrets; they already owned the global milieu in which they operated, and were only somewhat accountable to each other. Discussion centered on the recent BBC flagship meeting that focused on a referendum of Greek people who had the right and will of the people to vote it out of the EU. Naturally, these investors all wanted to keep things the way they were for their mutual benefit. The Greeks voted their wishes in a majority vote, but at the end of the day, though they should have received it, they got what these globalists had already determined they would have. The clincher was that at this table of wolves, no one thought for even an instant there was anything wrong with ignoring and overriding the democratically expressed will of an entire nation of citizens who had legally expressed their will for their nation. The result did not require discussion; it was an already established fait accompli. The silent and agreed upon course of action, should any untoward events occur over this, were already fully understood. So the entire nation of Greece was treated with abject and unrelenting cruelty and these wolves' contempt for the Greek people was palpable. It was all possible because none of these dinner guests would ever have to see, face, or answer to the Greek people."[16]

There was a very beautiful young woman at that dinner who was well-educated, and a favored protégée of the host. Ms. Wolf asked her if she thought her own fellow countrymen and women should have a say in outcomes about their economic future. The young woman calmly explained, "No, the ordinary people of any given country don't have the skills to make the right economic decisions for themselves or their nations, so we should be deciding for them." She had parroted her answer as if she'd been programmed with complete confidence and certainty of a now-privileged twenty-something! The Greeks never had further input in the future of their nation. Many elderly Greek men and women were subjected to abject poverty in their retirement. Many more small and medium-sized businesses were lost. Very much the same as what happened during COVID in the US![16]

"Sometime later at another similar dinner party, among the host and privileged guests was a newcomer, a former Greek politician who had been in agreement with his fellow countrymen on their referendum. He was being introduced all around like a coveted prize," according to Ms. Wolf. "There is no telling what promises had been made to him, or what kind of 'arrangements' had been offered to secure his new alliance with the globalist wolves! One thing is very sure; that man had been introduced to a new level of wealth, power, affluence, and position that massively outweighed any loyalty he might once have felt to his fellow Greeks; that simple, common decency could have afforded him. He, like all of his new comrades had sold his very soul to the Devil!"[16]

In order for us to understand what really happened in 2020-2022, it is first necessary to comprehend the fact—unfathomable evil need not come in looking like a militant soldier, or some kind of armed official knocking at your door. To fathom how COVID-19 policies could be so coordinated, and so evil, and so Fascist, we must get hold of the truth that "evil very often comes in the form of a very well-dressed gentleman, in the latest and most fashionable of clothes, or a sophisticated lady who may even at times wear a crown, far distant from any 'normal human being' having national loyalties and decencies. That evil will enter calmly with great panache, sipping wine. It might be a good idea to remember the entrance of Satan to the Garden of Eden as a beautiful, luminescent and alluring creature that sweet-talked Adam and Eve right out of their perfect home! Beware of the verbal enticements of seemingly good and wise ideas that have no reality, and are really just a bill of bewitching lies."[16]

"The serpent (Satan) was the shrewdest of all the wild animals the Lord God had made. One day he asked the woman (Eve), 'Did

God really say you must not eat the fruit from ANY of the trees in the garden?' 'Of course we may eat fruit from the trees in the garden,' the woman replied. 'It's only the fruit from the tree in the middle of the garden that we are not allowed to eat.' God said, 'You must not eat it OR EVEN TOUCH IT; if you do, you will die.' 'You won't die!' the serpent replied to the woman. 'God knows that your eyes will be opened as soon as you eat it, and you will be like God, knowing both good and evil.' The woman was convinced. She saw that the tree was beautiful and its fruit looked delicious, and she wanted the wisdom it would give her, so she took some of the fruit and ate it. Then she gave some to her husband, who was with her, and he ate it too. At that moment their eyes were opened, and they suddenly felt shame at their nakedness!" Genesis 3:1-7 NLT

Finally, along the above lines, consider who actually committed the heinous pandemic crimes, and how were they perpetrated on an unsuspecting US citizenry. The answer is tied inexplicably to the CCP. Apparently, this concept of true causality is not clearly understood by many Americans. We must know that Communist China is unequivocally the largest globalist entity existing. It has quite easily and systematically infiltrated most of the major institutions of the USA and Western Europe. One who knows and understands China, also knows that China does NOT use its military strength as its best weapon. Its warfare is far bolder, yet subtle, and ideological in nature; it is inexhaustible and unrelenting when targeting other nations, especially its biggest rival, the United States. The United States of America has unarguably been the world's chief super-power, but China's undying goal is to take that position instead. It's strategy, just like Satan himself, is to strike at the enemy's weakest point. Sinologists are 'experts' on all things China; they raised the red flags as they observed a nearly 100-year long drive to overtake the USA with deception as its chief weapon. The CCP generally presents itself to the US as weak and in dire need of Western aid. It's a ruse that has succeeded quite well. Clearly, it's been used quite effectively to entice the US government to freely hand over sensitive information, technology, military know-how, intelligence, and expert advice. What we haven't stupidly given freely, China has stolen. Experts believe the CCP's intent is to become THE WORLD SUPERPOWER by 2049, on its Centennial Anniversary![17] Sinologists have also warned us that thousands of CCP-aligned professors and foreign students in the US are bound by CCP law to report all intelligence back to the CCP. Chinese business associates in every area of commerce are embedded in specifically strategic institutions in US education, culture, law, economics, medicine, and politics. The CCP has categorically denied these facts for decades, but more recently, their goals have been stated openly by the CCP. In 2009, a US Senate hearing began addressing these concerns. Then in 2017, a Senior Research Analyst for East Asia / Freedom House, Sarah Cook, gave Senate testimony to the US / China Economic and Security Review Commission's hearing. The subjects of the hearing included China's information controls, global media influence, and cyber warfare strategies. Her report was updated in January of 2020.

Ms. Cook's "reports showed widespread influence operations aimed by the CCP at affecting staff, content, and messaging in Western and other social media." At the same time, a global influence agenda aimed at worldwide media was found in 2020 by the International Federation of Journalists. Their report was entitled, *The China Story: Reshaping the World's Media.*[18] How does this information relate to the massive crimes of the pandemic? First, China was clearly able to hide or shield the facts of the pandemic's source. Even today, it can still cast doubt on what we all knew from the very beginning. Even if no one believes their denials—it simply wasn't rocket science when the mountain of circumstantial evidence slaps you in the face! There are still no mentions of charges made, or retribution for the mass murders China perpetrated on the world; so much for United Nations' influence! Further, the CCP's global media influence greatly benefited the suppression, even vilification of Western heroes, history, ideals, freedoms, and instincts of spontaneity and individualism. It fanned the warring elements of our culture. This was also well known, but became abundantly clearer during the Biden regime. Its interests align almost perfectly with all the globalists in the World Economic Forum and the drivers of Big Tech. In turn, these groups threw all their weight to globalist China.

Therefore, as we see the assembling of the globalist wolves with their many like interests in common, the New World Order agenda pushed for these same policies, and aimed at intimidating citizens and breaking communities. They surveil citizens in a very lucrative and controlling digital grid regularly. All of them target our freedom of speech and it was crystal clear our words were targeted throughout COVID-19. They have not stopped targeting since COVID, but now they can do it more surreptitiously because fewer Americans are watching as closely as they did during COVID. Now, their highest goal is to keep American children and young people from mastering our treasured values of free thought and expression.

While "policy" determined it was no longer safe for our children and teens to go to school, ask yourself who was really instrumental in that policy formation? We know there are CCP-sent agents in every realm of American society, and the National Teacher's Association is specifically one of those places. Virtual and distance learning was initiated so quickly it almost made our heads spin; barely missing a beat and without any data to prove it was necessary!. With colleges closing down everywhere, the dreams of millions of young people went on hold, and some never got back. There were no new skill acquisitions. Staying at home was enforced passively because the health departments of most states could make all the rules, and those affected had no recourse or alternative. Some did virtual classes, but the joy of a young person, out of the nest, experiencing new things was gone; all the things they looked forward to in going to college were gone. Finally, we have to wonder just how much of that mandatory screen time was used to influence the minds of our kids with subliminal messaging and surveillance. Think how easy it would be to instigate harmful messages to unsuspecting kids and their parents when we know what the number one goal of the CCP and globalists was/is!

The Propaganda, Damage of Masking, and Lost Education

Every kind of messaging available was used to shout out a new 'catch phrase' to anyone with ears, "Mask Up!" Another edgy motto added, "Standing together by Staying Apart!" That advertisement campaign must have made some people independently wealthier than they'd ever been, when it hit global airwaves. It was, of course, created to sound like the best idea anyone ever had and you could positively do your part to keep people safer, while reducing total COVID exposure. There were no caveats of warning about potentially slow suffocation, or the inhibition of speech, or re-breathing the cumulative toxins of carbon dioxide. They didn't bother to tell people they might not feel well breathing CO_2 because it changes the body's blood chemistry and brain function. There were NO stats on the efficacy of masking, nor was there any proof that masks were really needed. That whole campaign smacked of deception and lies from its inception, and the same lies are still being perpetrated today. If you don't believe it, look at the number of people who, at the first mention of new COVID-19 cases or other new viruses are identified, go straight to the store for more masks. There is still a 'knee-jerk' reaction in people, especially already health challenged people, after the many months of COVID mask-wearing established it.

The real facts of this respiratory illness—there was nothing "new" or "novel" about COVID-19 respiratory illness. The message was of severe illness and very possibly death, which could be said for any other infectious respiratory disease. Influenza, the common cold, pneumonia, RSV, MERS, etc. could all display the same degree of illness, especially in the elderly or in folks with many other underlying problems to complicate their cases. Treating it was not different either, and many doctors were very successfully treating their COVID patients at home, keeping them out of hospitals, with mostly minimal effort—until the rules changed. Tuberculosis, for example, has been around for centuries! There are scores of stories in literature where heroes or heroines suffered with it and other respiratory ailments. NEVER, in history, did health managers find it necessary to isolate and mask the Entire Population!

Social distancing, by its very nature, required the majority of people to spend most of their time indoors; the worst possible thing anyone can do is eliminate fresh air and sunshine! Similar health crises throughout history used NONE of these measures. Quarantine was used for the sick folks, not the obviously healthy people. It has NEVER been necessary to diminish commerce and shut down civilization before COVID. In every other crisis Americans faced we remained free according to our Constitution and Rule of Law, after 1776. In fact, both science and common sense told us long ago we need sunlight, Vitamins D and C, good nutrition, exercise, and fresh air—known necessities for both the treatment and prevention of infectious illnesses. But suddenly, for no identifiable reason, healthcare "officials" quit following the science, and mandated all of the exact opposite treatments. There was not one shred of scientific evidence to back their positions. How did we so quickly and thoroughly lose our history, our lifelong knowledge, and yes, our common sense? In addition to all of this, lonely, shut-in, and depressed healthy people became sick by seeking other extremely unhealthy outlets to relieve their emotional pain, fear, and boredom. Many people grew pale, fearful, obsessive, phobic, and sad because of this insane treatment program. We might justifiably ask the question—"how many people got sick and even died because of this insanity foisted upon all of us by unelected "officials.?"

Masking very quickly became a 'sign' and the only acceptable norm for fighting COVID-19. Our society mostly complied, making it standard-operating procedure. Anyone who had the audacity to speak out against masks or masking could easily be shunned by peers, or worse reported to the mask police. Throughout history masks have been used to dehumanize—there is no individual or personal notice. They also represent an entire culture of evil and criminal behavior; used by thieves, executioners, and torturers, and for becoming things representing evil such as ghosts, monsters, devils, witches, demons, and a plethora of evil people. There is ready-made psychology behind the wearing of masks. Isolation, masking, and distancing were all part of a regime of punishment and psychological torture in the Victorian era or in a person from that era. But, in 2020-2022, the globalist agenda turned this thought process completely on its head; with their propaganda, now these measures were not only acceptable, but highly desirable and representative of the "good life." What did that new philosophy do to our psychological equilibrium?

Sigmund Freud called masks "uncanny," a symbol that automatically sparks an unconscious sense of "unease," of being alienated, "not at home," and sensations of creepy and weird. Horror film characters are almost always in masks. It is common knowledge that human beings MUST see faces of fellow human beings in order to feel safe. One survivor of a previous sexual assault described how the masks worn by the perps were both unnerving and also triggered flashbacks when faces could not be seen. She said anyone in a mask seems like a predator! Actually the analogy between a predator and COVID-19 is quite apt! All the repetitive, nonsensical idioms invented to plug the masks were completely demeaning and insulting to anyone's intelligence, but that is exactly how the globalists treat anyone not a part of their hierarchy as we saw in the last section. Everything in each one of us screamed silently from our very souls that this whole mess was pure propaganda, but there were rules, no legal ones, but rules most of us were used to obeying, and not looking for any extra trouble for refusing to wear a mask, we played the stupid game of mask-wearing most of the time. But Freud was on the money in this case! Wearing masks quite effectively dehumanized us and made us wary of others.

However, what about shutting down our schools and punishing children in too many ways to count? In case anyone is too old to remember, schools were NOT just for readin', writin', and rithmetic! Yes, academia is crucial to the development of children's brains, and being equipped to hold a job one day, but it's also a training ground for learning appropriate social behavior and skills. It's problem-solving and key-boarding. So many skills are needed in life, and too many of our children got very little additional education when they were forced to stay home. School helps establish orderly habits, and life skills like thinking, reasoning, memorizing, and comprehension. Relationships are learned and practiced. Important emotional development is done by facial recognition and expression reading. Words are used for affirmation, and correction. Physical development and social skills are learned on the playground; what works and what doesn't work interactively is discerned. Children learn with hands-on projects, material manipulation, field trips, classroom celebrations, and group study. There are literally scores of activities like stories, pictures, chalkboards, learning games, singing, laughing, eating from fun lunch pails, and riding school buses that simply cannot be done alone in front of a computer screen.

Cooperative education in craft projects, drawing pictures, viewing lab results, growing plants, playing recorders, sporting events and good sportsmanship, whether winning or losing, debates, drama, and the list of interactive possibilities are endless, but none can be done alone even on a zoom screen. How can a child explore his emotions or ask necessary questions, from a virtual teacher?—many couldn't! Who would gently correct their mistakes and show them how to fix them? I don't see my teacher smiling at me or calling my name. Will I ever get to play with my friends again? I love to sing, but I can't sing without the others singing along with me. Can we even begin to realize how much learning was seriously robbed from our children, that can NEVER fully be restored or even caught up? Parents everywhere were caught in an untenable situation with juggling virtual jobs and supervising their children's education. They could see their kids missing out on too much, forgetting or missing assignments, or doing them badly because they were unable to focus their attention and had no enthusiasm to try harder. Some just plain couldn't understand alone. Even most adults can't focus for 45 minutes on a person teaching on T.V. without being distracted.

Questions went unanswered, and a child couldn't understand enough to finish assignments on his own. As we said earlier, many children lost as much as 1 ½ years in their education and skill sets. Basic skills testing scores were dismal when they finally returned to their classrooms. Some children didn't even have siblings with which to interact. Many children became almost full-time latch-key kids; left alone to their own imaginations, too young to be unsupervised, far too much and far too long.[19]

Some experts have reported the degree of child abuse and neglect during COVID-19 was indeed the second epidemic of the pandemic. Many children missed meals they received in school, and their nutrition suffered, making them even more vulnerable to illness. "The loss or reduction of jobs and financial stability, health, housing, and child care are all closely associated with an increase in parental stress which in turn was closely associated with increased child abuse and neglect. Families also lost access to social support systems that heightened parental stress and increased mental health issues. All of this adversely impacted parental behaviors and parent-child conflicts. As we noted, children were stressed as well. Add all of that to increased family proximity, increased substance abuse, and significant reduction of reporting due to scant contact with professionals who would detect an abusive situation."[19] In addition, previously at-risk families with previously reported events, were also more vulnerable to repeated abusive behaviors.[20]

Parents everywhere, for a multitude of really good reasons, prayed and hoped their children could go back to school in the fall of 2020. Some survived through the summer with the hope of return to normalcy. Many could clearly see the damage constant isolation was doing, and watched their children struggle with virtual education. Little did they know their views on their children's needs went unheard and uncared about. They had no idea that agenda decisions were already being made over their heads. From that point there simply were no other positive options for most children and teens for another whole year. This was indeed the epitome of tragedy.

Incalculable Losses and Subsequent Grief

The World Economic Forum, home of the globalist wolves, touted depopulation proudly as one of its stated goals. Yet, the WEF weighed in on the inordinate amount of grief people experienced through their entire pandemic process. COVID-19 caused approximately five million deaths worldwide, leaving multitudes of people grieving the loss of one or more loved ones and friends.[21] To quantify just how many people were impacted—there are an estimated nine close family members on average, who were left to grieve following just one COVID-19 death. Add a ton of weight to every one of those survivors who were not allowed to grieve that loss with a last visit, time spent with other grieving family members, or the ability even to bury that loved one properly because of the lockdowns. The support of other relatives and friends was not available for the same reason. This was the very deepest kind of sorrow added to the other existing losses, both psychologically and emotionally. Many said they weren't even allowed to say goodbye or get the necessary closure. Having a belated memorial service two years later or doing a virtual funeral just wasn't adequate and it shouldn't have been that way, but we all had to follow the rules. In 2025, multitudes of people are still trying to finish grieving all of their losses, but it continues evading them indefinitely. As a women's counselor, this author can speak to the ongoing and unresolved grief and trauma that resurfaces and even incapacitated some.[22]

Another consideration altering employment culture markedly—how to navigate grief in the post-pandemic workplace. The WEF wrote a sizable article on the pain and grief of loss in employees. The concern wasn't chiefly for the employees so much as for the impact it's all had on the workplace, because work affects economies, industries, and "global issues!" With collective amounts of grief and pain, and limited opportunities to process it, much of the grief got locked up inside offices, teams and workplaces of every organization across the country, and around the world. The build-up of grief led to burnout, endless fatigue, loss of focus, and changed employee engagement—all of which negatively impacted companies and organizations. Hence, "the Great Resignation" during and after the pandemic. "Employees resigned in large numbers over the years (of pandemic) and after, as a result of burnout, endless stress, and the dramatic blurring of lines separating work and personal life. These factors caused many to deeply contemplate the values they wanted to maintain in their lives, and how they wanted to live and work moving forward. Workplace culture played a crucial role in their choices to resign. Employees operating in toxic work environments, or ones in which they felt uncared for, contributed to these choices."[23]

"In the United States alone, in December 2021, there were circa 157 million workers. Based on the average nine mourners for the 868,000 COVID-19 deaths, we can assume there were approximately 7,812,000 workers grieving or about 4.5% of all employees were grieving the loss of a close loved one, long before the pandemic was over. It was virtually impossible for this grief to not have an impact on productivity. The universally accepted measure of productivity, the GDP, at that time was $20.94 trillion. All things being equal, if 4.5% of the workers had their productivity compromised due to grief, up to $942 billion of productivity and business growth was directly affected by grief." Add to those figures, the exploding numbers of the "Great Resignation," and there was enormous economic loss as well. By nearly three times, a toxic workplace was the leading contributor to this exodus of workers. These are places where employees feel uncared for, harassed, pressured, and discriminated against. Then employers had hefty additional losses, while trying to replace and train new employees. At that time, it became nearly impossible to replace employees, because the labor market was experiencing skills and job shortages rarely seen previously. The fascinating point the writer from WEF made was "employers want to retain their employees who are trained and talented and want to continue growing by implementing a grief-literate and human-first approach within their organization... providing bereavement leave, therapeutic support, and grief training."[24]

Grief and loss researcher Bob Neimeyer and psychologist

Sherman Lee recognized the tidal wave of grief that would be associated with the pandemic. They developed what they called the pandemic grief scale, to help identify cases of dysfunctional grief associated with deaths occurring from the beginning of COVID-19— meaning it impaired someone's ability to work, taking care of children, and maintaining relationships. The symptoms predicting the highest level of dysfunction were:

- Wishing they were dead so they could be with their loved one
- Inability to care about anything
- Inability to access positive memories of their loved one, and instead being preoccupied by the trauma of their loss
- A sense of emptiness and purposelessness
- Substance abuse and dependency
- Increased risk of suicide [25]

"They surveyed more than 800 Americans who lost loved ones during the pandemic—whether from COVID-19 or some other cause—and what they found was that two-thirds of respondents were suffering from dysfunctional grief, or as they called it, 'pandemic grief.' They also discovered people who lost loved ones during the pandemic suffered symptoms on par, or even worse, than people who'd lost loved ones in what we might think of as much more traumatic ways. The severity of their symptoms was on par with those of pre-pandemic people diagnosed with complicated grief and prolonged grief disorder. It was as if the deaths during COVID were violent, leaving people with a sense of shock and horror, along with personal helplessness."[26]

But what made pandemic deaths so traumatic? It didn't have as much to do with the disease itself, but with the era of pandemic. So, if the trauma did not come from the cause of death itself, what made pandemic losses so difficult? These men found the commonality was being separated from their loved one—losing their chance to say goodbye. An enforced emotional distance from their loved one at the end of their life, but for an I-Pad or tablet, was excruciating. All such things as shared memories, photo albums, acts of personal caring, intimate moments of bonding and expression—were denied. It is true that any death feels tragic—it's the end of life on earth. More importantly, it's the end of the living relationship with loved ones. For those who felt like they were going under in the ocean for the third time, grief counseling was needed and definitely recommended. The help of a really excellent book by Kathleen O'Hara, entitled, *A Grief Like No Other; Surviving the Violent Death of Someone You Love* was always a good idea. After all, most of us need some help when we encounter a tough situation, maybe for the first time—take advantage of any and all help you can find. Many of us have a spiritually rich foundation of faith, that enabled us to have hope in the loss. Go to Scripture and receive the hope that Jesus Christ offers us:

"13But I would not have you to be ignorant, brethren; concerning
them which are asleep (have died); that ye sorrow not, even as
others which have no hope. 14For if we believe that Jesus died and
rose again, even so them also which sleep in Jesus will God bring
with Him. 15For this we say unto you by the word of the Lord, that
we which are alive and remain unto the coming of the Lord shall
not precede them which are asleep. 16For the Lord Himself shall
descend from heaven with a shout, with the voice of the archangel,
and with the trump of God; and the dead in Christ shall rise first;
17Then we which are alive and remain shall be caught up together
with them in the clouds, to meet the Lord in the air: and so shall we
ever be with the Lord. 18Wherefore comfort one another with these
words." I Thessalonians 4:13-18 KJV

We have already spoken of many other losses related to COVID-19 and the pandemic, including our autonomy, our life/time, our children's education, finances, jobs, health, safety, several of our freedoms, and of course, loved ones and friends. However, there was one other loss every one of us experienced. That was the loss of our bygone lives as we knew them. The COVID-19 pandemic wasn't just an epidemiological crisis, but a psychological one. The whole situation provoked anxiety, stress, and sadness—it was a collective time of sorrow. We all experienced losses. "Even people who didn't lose anything so concrete as a job or a loved one, were affected—there was a communal grief as we watched our work, health-care, education and economic systems we depended on—completely destabilize! It didn't shake just our faith in systems—it upended our understanding of the world around us…the losses included our senses of predictability, control, justice, and the belief that we can protect our children, and the elderly among us. In many ways, we still mourn what was!"[27]

The nature of a person's attachments has the greatest effect on their grief reactions. We are not only attached to other human beings. We're capable of losing places, projects, possessions, professions, and protections; all things of which we may have strong attachments, even to the routines that make up our days. As the pandemic moved forward, most people had to confront a series of losses such as the sense of safety, social connections, personal freedoms, jobs, and financial security. In some ways, we're experiencing a living loss, one that keeps right on going. We don't grieve just for the things that are missing, but how they affect our individual senses of SELF, causing a loss of identity. An example was losing a job, which we'd definitely miss, however that loss made us see ourselves in a different, possibly NOT kind way. One of the most important things we all need is social connection, which everyone missed during the pandemic. That required some intentionality in a world of social distancing. Remembering the frustration of missing friends and family required making every effort to re-establish those vital connections and building new ones as well. Social support is one of life's greatest gifts, and we now understand what it was to not have it. Many of us can be quite resilient and move on with change fairly quickly, but so many others don't have that ability. Give them some of yours, encouraging and checking up on those you know, who truly needed it badly then, and may still need it today.[27]

The "Unsocial," New Normal!

Now that we are in 2025, we have become somewhat acclimated to the 'New Normal' but it may be beneficial to think back a little bit and remember how our lives used to be before COVID-19. We can easily say that our children's education as they knew it suddenly died. In the workplace, offices also died. Terms used to attempt a concept of normalcy were "remote learning" and "working remotely." Out went 'normalcy', and in came the age of 'Zoom', a concept established almost overnight. A major point of interest was the many parents, whether Moms or Dads, who had asked for remote options for decades to enable them to better care for children at home, to work smarter, to save money, or a variety of other reasons. Businesses generally had thousands of reasons why remote working would never be a manageable option. Suddenly, remote jobs were not just tolerated, but actually pushed and promoted everywhere as THE best option during the pandemic. With the whole family home, each member was on a computer and family time wasn't much different, nor was it really done together. If children weren't watching computer or television screens, and outside time was minimal, while parents worked, who was watching them much of the time?

From the American normal lifestyle of socially and openly shopping for life's necessities, we proceeded to call it in and pick it up. Before COVID, no one had heard of disinfecting all the items we shopped for nor had they been delivered BEFORE, even bringing them inside the house if needed. The "experts" had determined the virus did not spread from surfaces, but if it might happen, we should do it anyway. We were all told the virus needed a live host to survive, but we all needed to hear more lies to focus on and keep us busy while stuck at home!. E-commerce never had it so good. If we could find a restaurant somehow open for business, there were no menus, no salt and pepper shakers, just a few tables to keep social distances, constant cleaning, and few amenities. Meal kits could be picked up or door dashed; any cuisine you wanted could be purchased if you were at least upper middle-class consumers! Everyone else couldn't do so regularly.

In the digital world, every platform and website were thoroughly programmed to continuously remind us we were under global, national, and local restrictions, and the propaganda supporting the pandemic narrative was all about the whys and wherefores of mandates. We were led to believe locking everyone inside and social distancing would be superior for avoiding infection with COVID, and we would find the number of COVID cases dropping rapidly. Subsequently, studies revealed no confirmation of this lie. The Multi-billionaire wolves have no national loyalties, so they played all sides, depending on where they could make the most money. Because of the 'no-contact, locked-down world's reliance on big tech and related companies, many of which were owned and operated by wealthy globalists, they made insanely large sums of money during the pandemic. These wolves loved the post-humane world where nobody could function normally in person.[28]

Very literally, the masses were now relegated to an unlawful form of house arrest, which was barely tolerable at best. It meant a total loss of freedom for people who had always been free to come and go at will. The point of it was to see how long that loss of freedom would be tolerated. Obviously, it was extended again and again by the cooperative socialists of our nation who would play this game with the globalists for as long as they could get by with it, which was way yonder too long. Many folks kept living with it because they were too terrified to go outside or be near anyone else. That was due mostly to the powerful deception of the lying propaganda. If they could keep stoking the fear, most people would comply with their demands. None of this scenario came about accidentally—we must remember the facts—it was all pre-planned for decades. Many procedural changes, like burial of the dead for example, were made macabre for their shock value. "In New York, there was a sudden change where the transfer of dead bodies was no longer an unobtrusive, private matter, but a public display. Bodies were instead rolled outside the hospital, down ramps, and out to city sidewalks where local news reporters awaited to show the public clearly just how many deaths occurred. Normal operating procedures had been replaced by a very public spectacle to demonstrate the magnitude of this heinous COVID tragedy."[28]

After much time elapsed, there were thousands of grieving family members who had loved ones originally buried in mass graves in pine caskets on the notorious Hart Island. Their lives would never be the same. Though New York City has attempted to clean up, sort, mark burial sites, etc., it still requires families of those buried there to go through a lengthy process of registering a visit to a specified person's grave, on one of two days a month, traveling by ferry to the island, and being shuttled to various drop-off points. Park staff guided mourners to the grave-site. Until recently none of that was even possible. It was not an ideal location to start with. Hart Island had a long rather sordid history as a kind of Potter's Field, decades before COVID happened. One person who captured drone footage of the mass grave site actually had his photos confiscated! There is designated money now to improve the island, possibly making it a national park site, but there are no absolute decisions on the fate of Hart Island or those interred there. This scenario points to the global fact of the several million deaths which occurred during the pandemic, that only decades can begin to erase, and the circumstances will never be changed for millions of family members to whom the grief cannot be assuaged at all. It's their 'new normal.'[29]

There will be continued resentment for years to come by people whose loved ones were not treated humanely. Stories still surface and some are reported, though the news media remains reluctant to publish this type of story. Another horrible tragedy also occurred in New York City, under the unmitigated provocation of then Governor Cuomo. As previously mentioned, to acquire more hospital space, Cuomo decided to move still infected COVID patients too sick to return home, to nursing homes. Hundreds of residents in those nursing homes were infected and died as a result of that heinous decision.[30] The asinine irony of that decision was that these residents were not allowed to have healthy family members visit, even with all proper precautions, and many of these elderly folks were isolated completely, while the sick hospital patients were brought in! Who in their right mind would make that kind of decision? Why could well residents, not see family members outside, at the very least? Lonely, sometimes quite elderly citizens spent their last days on earth getting progressively sadder and lonelier, and then ill, for the need of even one beloved family member's face. This was a travesty beyond belief or recovery. The Select Subcommittee on the Coronavirus Pandemic held a hearing titled "Like Fire Through Dry Grass: Mortality & COVID-19 Policies" to gather facts about pandemic-era, nursing home policy decisions— specifically in New York, New Jersey, and Pennsylvania—that led to the deaths of tens of thousands of Americans. The "Hearing Wrap Up 'Must Admit' COVID-19 Nursing Home Mandates were Deadly for Elderly Americans, State Officials Responsible."[31] Further, Governor Cuomo, along with his counterparts in New Jersey and Pennsylvania, engaged in a cover-up to hide the true, nursing-home mortality rates from the public and shift political blame. Over 9,000 coronavirus patients were sent into New York nursing homes alone. However, one statement made from an AP News article truly stands out. "Ethicists said that Cuomo's conduct stands out not because the policy he put in place was especially egregious, but because he obscured public health data for political gain." In other words, ethicists whoever they may be, thought the murders of thousands of people weren't nearly as bad as Cuomo's attempted cover-up to keep him out of political trouble! That idea was just as egregious and appalling as the act itself.[31]

Another thing we must all understand: What is 'New Normal'?; though historically it's never been normal; neither is it new. For those of our citizenry who may never have questioned the ethical and moral deterioration of our laws and legal system, it is now absolutely imperative we look at it with our eyes wide open. There was once a time when a majority of our government leaders at least tried to approximate law-abiding citizens, and who represented us with at least a measure of integrity; we more or less trusted what they said to be 'mostly' true. That is no longer the case; now, the majority of what is represented to us is NOT true or trustworthy. There are still a few politicians trying to be true on the whole, but the vast majority don't even know what is true and what isn't! People who have been entrusted with jobs in various governmental agencies, educational institutions, professionals of all the arts, and even many religious leaders are not ethical or trustworthy either. We watched during the pandemic and listened to those who, even against our laws, usurped positions of authority they weren't elected to hold. All in all, most of us succumbed to at least some of the bold-faced and preposterous lies related to the pandemic narrative. Some would even stand and swear on a stack of Bibles they were telling us the Gospel truth, while lying like rugs. If they weren't lying, they were exaggerating atrociously, skewing the facts and numbers to justify their lies, and spewing unfounded predictions. All of this was done throughout the pandemic to keep fear-mongering alive, and build the web of deceit.

When the next pandemic or crisis arrives, and make no mistake, it will come; its already planned. Citizen, please do everything in your power to verify real facts. Do not swallow the lies of the globalists and their father, Satan himself:

> "For (they) are the children of their father the devil, and they love to do the evil things he does. He was a murderer from the beginning. He has always hated the truth, because there is no truth in him. When he lies, it is consistent with his character; for he is a liar and the father of lies." John 8:44

Given that truth, please do your homework, and make sure that leadership is speaking truth. It may ultimately save your life! If the person talking cannot make eye contact with the camera, has taken on leadership or information that isn't his to take, changes the discourse every time he speaks, and skews the facts you know, beware. He is acting like his father…!

When the mask mandates arrived, for the first time, this "order" was NOT a law passed by our legislative,(law-making) branch of government. It did not come from an elected official, but it was represented as such. For a free people in a Constitutionally free society, this new rule crossed over a very personal boundary line that completely breached our given freedoms. It didn't come as a pleasant request or polite suggestion that might have been OK as long as the person wearing it complied voluntarily, but it was an imperious demand! It was demanded by people who had no authority to do so, therefore it also represented clear and usurped power over every citizen in America.[32]

It was not a temporary emergency measure that would be conscientiously tracked and reviewed for efficacy or efficiency and that would be stopped just as soon as the need expired due to changed conditions. Not one citizen had their personal needs assessed or considered before demanding it. There were thousands of citizens with serious health concerns who were physically and emotionally harmed by wearing masks. There were no concessions for the people who already had significant respiratory challenges who would be most affected by wearing a mask. The personal health and well-being of every single person was jeopardized by wearing a face diaper and re-breathing their own carbon dioxide on a regular, daily basis; CO_2 gas can and will harm a normal person chemically in time. Our own personal autonomies were being forced illegally to do something harmful to our bodies, without any known or proven reason. It was all because some self-imposed autocrat somewhere said we must do it or else! Failure to comply, implied some kind of punishment, even if it only meant personal embarrassment in being accosted for not wearing it.

Even today, hundreds of court cases have been heard re: mandatory mask-wearing. Issues of Constitutionality, including

First Amendment Rights, Due Process Rights, Americans with Disabilities Act, as well as other legal objections have been legally brought to court! There are plenty of people on both sides of the question, but a far lesser number of people supported mask-wearing as necessary and appropriate during the pandemic. There were/are tons of arguments and citizens against them. "There is virtually no case law currently on whether or not mask mandates are constitutional or legal."[33] The obvious other concern was how and what punishment should be exacted and by whom. That was never established, either but one troublesome source of demanding compliance came from the regular, ordinary citizen who self-appointed as the mask-wearing Nazi. It wasn't just wearing one, but wearing it completely correctly over both nose and mouth. Anyone privately or in a business that took on this responsibility was asking for a lot of noncompliance just to prove it could be done! Individual businesses deciding to keep mask Nazis on their premises were really asking for business problems. People do not take kindly to such actions, and they surely could take their shopping elsewhere.

Now that we are this far removed from the pandemic, we can all remember what it was like and still feel the unending frustrations, but we also know life has a way of resuming to some semblance of normalcy. As time passes, we tend to forget the worst of the experience; at least it no longer feels as bothersome. However, it's important not to forget the things we know were not done correctly and determine we will NOT be controlled and used in the manner we were during COVID-19. We still live in a country that values its freedoms, and we must be able to stand our ground when people who want to control us come near. That continues to be the goal of the globalist wolves who want nothing more than to control us, and remove our freedoms and democracy. They have the money and power to accomplish what they want and are not bashful about doing it. Their plans are made and they will keep trying to meet their ungodly goals. We must stand against the tidal wave of aggression but we must also be willing to defend our stand vehemently.

How to Plan and Execute an Emergency

As we are now fully aware of the proven fact, the COVID-19 Pandemic plans began at least two+ decades ago. Because of the presence of wicked, wealthy, and powerful globalist wolves, who wanted to govern and control the New World Order as they call it, they had a master plan to accomplish it in every way possible. Until fairly recently, the majority of Americans had little knowledge of this group, though they were highly- publicized because of their unending multi-billions nobody could even fathom. Few of us really understood their intention to rule the world someday. But anyone with that level of aspirations would obviously be thinking up the how-to for accomplishing such a lofty goal. In a free republic like ours, we would naturally assume any emergency situation would also have readiness plans. Often, we have drills that require all people in jobs affected by such emergencies to practice those readiness plans which enable proficiency should the need arise. We never planned for any actual emergencies to arise for the benefit of a small, select, global group, but they had done just that. Emergency plans allow a need for full social control to reach the intended goals. This enables new emergency policy-making which can become the new full-time policy when the emergency passes.

Policy response to any type of crisis when informing the public would sound like leadership was considering the needs of the masses for that crisis, but it was Not So! In a real emergency, the "inside" policy makers would first consider if a way exists that can be used to the best advantage for the largest number of people first. Behind the scenes, there are scores of corporate lobbyists and globalists who demand to be heard on any emergency legislation or health needs to be met. Many of these same people are NOT even Americans, but even if they were, their personal agendas always come ahead of any national loyalty. Many of them could easily be termed America's enemies. New policies roll out with the appearance of being driven by medical necessity, but it may well be nothing more than a trumped-up lie, as we observed. The goals these wolves have are far more difficult to accomplish under normal circumstances in ordinary times because there are laws controlling the work of lobbyists in the normal legislative process. Therefore, they require production of a perceived Emergency.

In this heavily-planned, 'emergency situation,' however, normal scrutiny is absent, and most debate suspended. Even the mainstream media sources ask less questions and simply do what they are told. Created 'emergencies' are the perfect opportunities for greater benefits of uncharted corruption which escalates the power and money-making capacity for these global wolves. "The truly powerful go to enormous lengths to control the planned narrative and in general achieve great success. What the most powerful people always want is certainty. Randomness and risk are their sworn enemies. What they NEVER want is ANY possibility of a chance effect on their events and outcomes."[34] "Powerful people always seek to control history and markets and limit their risks in a systematic way…they seek to bring about historical outcomes without leaving any written evidence, using nonprofits, cutouts, relatives, lawyers, friends, or friends of friends. They don't use press releases …This high-level aversion to risk and this aim at 'no finger-prints' and 'no paper trail' is NOT conspiracy theory, it's reality."[34]

We previously discussed what happened with COVID-19 early treatment. Doctors were treating most COVID patients as outpatients with medications that had been available for decades. They used their acquired knowledge and skill of practically treating symptoms, and most of the patients were recovering as outpatients with these protocols that were effective and inexpensive, most never needing hospitalization. However, TROUBLE was brewing! Successful treatment of COVID-19 wasn't supposed to happen with the plan for COVID-19. It was to be considered and respected as a highly-dangerous and infectious, novel coronavirus. Effectively treating their virus was destroying all their best-laid plans for a global pandemic, requiring all new emergency-approved drugs and vaccines. The latest drug to be approved on the Emergency Use

Authorization, the use of which had been procured decades prior to this emergency for just such a purpose, was Remdesivir. "The FDA banned the two most effective drugs being used, on the basis of 'skewed" clinical trials, including Ivermectin and Hydroxychloroquine, so the new drug would have to be used instead. People were getting sicker and more of them wound up in the hospital. Fauci had his plans, but his timing was off. They rushed the Remdesivir through the abbreviated clinical trials, and placed it in the hospital because it could only be given by I.V. All the sick people that would have been treated safety and effectively at home, if worsening, went to the hospital for the new drug. We will not repeat the details of the horrid debacle that followed that murderous decision, and the approval of it by the USFDA. It suffices to say the banning of the effective drugs, and the use of the inferior new one was the proven cause of thousands of COVID deaths."[35]

Between the drug ban and the introduction to Remdesivir, patients were simply told to go home from the urgent care or emergency room and only come back if or when their oxygen levels fell dangerously low. These were undoubtedly the most fortunate of COVID patients at that point. People were suffering, but until then had not lost their minds because of the pandemic. However, mainstream media was still reporting every frightful headline possible about ventilators, lung lesions, transplants, permanent lung damage, and continuously dying people. It truly created a culture of death and dying, exactly as planned. For anyone that can locate and read the Remdesivir Papers and/or the Pfizer Papers, that MUST be published by the producing drug company, they will shock you to your deepest core.

Another brilliant campaign came along to further alienate people from one another. The adage, "COVID-19 killed the handshake and the hug!" became the new rallying cry. Enter the fist and elbow-bumping to avoid sharing the virus.[36] One doctor wrote a paper about handshaking as a huge source of spreading pathogens and viruses. Others said that the handshaking "was irreplaceable and people could certainly manage to shake hands AND wash them without spreading disease, thank you very much." But handshakes nearly evaporated during the pandemic—so did hugs, high fives, fist bumps, back pats, shoulder squeezes and pretty much all other little points of contact we made when allowed to stand closer than six feet apart! Even now, much of our original social touching disappeared when the pandemic ended. "I don't think we should ever shake hands again, to be honest with you,"[36] declared Anthony Fauci. There may still be some who are squeamish about such acts of social touch, but thankfully, for most of us, we've resumed it to foster and maintain the relationships we temporarily dumped during COVID.

After the bumping phenomenon came the "bubble" we each lived in and it was most unwise to visit anyone else's bubble. No group or meeting could include more than six people, known as "The Rule of Six." Then the "tiers" of social interaction became so tight, few people even moved about for several months—all because of faulty and errant scientists, sitting somewhere in their respective bubbles with their baseless computer models. In the UK, and in the US, the constantly proclaimed restrictions got increasingly inane and prolonged—it was psychological warfare at its extreme worst. Even policy makers like Anthony Fauci kept changing the rules as often as he changed his underwear, usually negatively. Given the 24/7 propaganda machines many people began to lose their innate sense of independence and ability to make a decision. Without much thought, many just gave up on their rights and freedoms with little or no protest. Normal thinking processes were turned upside down, so that distance was good and keeping a distance became the way to show love, about as upside down as thinking can get. The American way has always been epitomized by connections with family, friends and neighbors who celebrate all holidays together. Ironically, that upside down approach meant embracing distance and separation.[37]

The highly effective ploy of the globalists to attack the mental and emotional well-being of the masses was introduced. The scientific depth of most governmental directives was about like a small mud-puddle! Harsh lockdowns lacked any historical perspective or balance. "Critics of the excesses of lockdown fetishism were attacked as callous. A favorite trope to deflect from lack of scientific justification was to say, 'critics are granny killers.' Anyone having Christmas dinner with Grandma risked burying her in the new year, they warned. Sceptics were challenged 'to look COVID-19 patients in the eyes and tell them the risk isn't real.' The reality was that on January 29, 2021, authorities revealed nearly half the total 220,000 deaths were from non-Covid causes such as canceled operations! A matching shameless emotional manipulation would have been, 'Look her in the eyes and tell her why her Mum's cancer wasn't caught early enough, or why she committed suicide.' Both were equally contemptible."[38]

Consider this: All the while the pandemic dragged on, the manipulative globalist wolves always had one more trick to pull from the magician's hat to continue the illusion of emergency, urgency, danger, risk and control ever deepening to keep the pandemic going, lest it lag and lose its potency. Loving and caring for people was anathema! If you truly loved and cared for them, you would neither touch them nor visit them; instead use your digital screen with Facebook or Skype so they could see a picture of the faces they could barely remember and simply pretend to be hugging them—they would get the idea! With this attack from the media, think about all the little children who have heard these messages regularly because there wasn't much reprieve from the screen and who perhaps lost a beloved grandparent, they felt close with—to COVID-19. Knowing how literally children are apt to think, how many of them may always believe they actually killed grandma or grandpa by hugging them. Rarely do we adults ever know how much trauma our children have internalized in their young lives. Examples of children we know abound with similar lifelong misunderstandings.[38]

Yes, the globalists with cooperation from most governments successfully planned and executed a health crisis. But, bear in mind the definition of an emergency. Merriam-Webster dictionary says an emergency is a serious, unexpected, and often dangerous situation requiring immediate action, or an unforeseen change in circumstances that necessitates immediate action to remedy harm or avert imminent danger to life, health, or property. It is often caused by accident. These situations may allow people to bypass usual procedures. On a normal scale of potential medical emergencies, the possibility of an infection doesn't rank as an emergency. The only things that would make it be one is the magnitude of people involved in it and its perceived danger. These planners were certainly covering all their bases when they planned this "emergency." Not many of the factors defined here were included in this one. However, they planned the one-of-a-kind pathogen and spent years developing its gain-of-function. They clearly plotted with the CCP and its Institutes of Virology to 'accidently' release it to the world. They did all in their power with the Chinese to multiply an unknown infection liberally and intentionally, to infect as many as possible, knowing that was the best way to get an emergency, needing emergency use authorization for new drugs and vaccines. All of this would certainly augment their plans for depopulation of the planet. We could call the COVID pandemic a lot of things, but EMERGENCY was NOT one of them.[38]

Too Much Misinformation and Deceit

From the very beginning of the COVID narrative we were all to "follow the science." The biggest trouble with that statement—there was very little well-defined science to be had. Right away as announcement of the new pathogen called a novel coronavirus was relayed to the global community, there were thousands of questions and very few answers to them. The scientists who supposedly knew what had been transpiring in global labs were seemingly unclear about their vocation and most of the time couldn't even agree with one another. It is impossible to be absolutely sure on anything. Supposedly, this pathogen was brand new, yet all the scientific evidence shows the work on coronaviruses was years in the making, and more years with gain-of-function study to create more transmissibility and virulence in them. In other words, when we get done "fixing" this virus, it will have the ability to be easily given to others and the strength of the disease will be exponentially greater. That was certainly something scientists must do for the good of humanity, as was excusing this work as giving science a higher chance for a specific vaccine that would treat it. Yeah right, even the scientists couldn't follow the science—the only thing we know for sure is that the whole travesty has never even resembled SCIENCE, as most of us learned it in school.[39]

Following the headlines stating this novel coronavirus had probably been "accidentally" leaked from the Chinese Communist Party's (CCP) Institute of Virology in Wuhan, it was and still is the most likely possibility, regardless of how much it's been debated and denied for over 5 years. Other theories were immediately available for distribution, but the SARS-CoV-2 was already spreading wildly in Wuhan. The CCP deliberately sent thousands of Chinese on hundreds of international flights world-wide to be certain the coronavirus was spread globally, and of course it was. Realizing this was happening, President Trump immediately ordered a ban on international flights from China in an attempt to contain the spread to the United States. He got a whole lot of push-back from Washington wolves who knew the plan was unfolding. Naturally, the CCP was horribly insulted at his knowledge and determined attempt to minimize the expected damage. Granted, the effort didn't slow it much, but it did put the CCP on notice that President Trump understood who was to blame. Wild rumors and accusations flew about like a tempest in a teapot. But then, the omnipresent SARS-CoV-2 became a force to be reckoned with.[39]

Soon, COVID-19 maps or dashboards were erected supposedly to show the scary numbers of deaths and the cases of new infections in Panavision and Technicolored detail. Color is one of the easiest visuals to understand and the colors on the dashboards were clearly designed to send the proper subliminal messages to the public. The assumption was that the data it showed revealed 'official' numbers and facts, but this was seldom true. Fauci constantly used the line,

"When you look at the data..." or Walensky of the CDC would repeat, "Follow the science..."; neither 'Doctor' used real data or the scientific publications to validate the dashboard information. Consequently, the statements that Fauci, Walensky, and any other public health officials made were impossible to verify. Why is that? Many of the most frequently used dashboards were created with flawed methods and unverifiable datasets...mere Phantoms! "In the world of digital data, the information when 'translated' by programmers, is fairly simple and easily understood by most people. When the data is available it isn't complicated to create a dashboard. So the data given in real-time from the health department would have to be interfaced with another software application and it might come through garbled and disorganized. Programmers must then 'translate' the original data, and edit and format it into workable datasets. Developers take the datasets and build codes which Media also used these creations to "prove" the horrible outcomes they were seeing. A major problem with this; it allows users to visually look at the data in whatever way developers want them to see it. Technology is like 'too many hands in the kitchen' or data; at the end it doesn't necessarily prove anything. The truth comes from the underlying datasets, but very few news broadcasters can access those. Even fewer would trouble themselves to check the original data for its origins. That has not changed today."[40]

A digital dashboard is not a medical or scientific tool. "It is a simple business intelligence tool with codes that count data inputs and it allows business leaders to track, analyze, and report on key performance indicators and metrics. Modern interactive dashboards made it easy to combine data from multiple sources and deeply explore and analyze the data directly within the dashboard itself. As with the COVID-19 data, it was used for monitoring and decision-making purposes, as well as propaganda, because any tool is only as valuable as the persons using it. The goal is to provide clear, concise, and actionable information at a glance."[41] Developers don't necessarily have backgrounds in science or medicine. The truth is that just about anything could be 'counted' as a 'case', or a 'death' depending on how its programmed.

In other words, if the dashboard has been programmed and developed by certain criteria to count COVID deaths, and someone gives all the parameters of what a COVID death is, including every death where the person had tested positive for COVID, or any death with an unidentified cause, etc. Naturally, the data input must be placed accurately in order to get accurate data back![41]

Another avenue of deliberate deception was the totally fallible PCR tests which relied heavily on subjective reading patterns. Not every positive result was really positive, and not every negative result was truly negative. The limitations of the test were not only too many to depend on the test itself, but the process was never intended to be used as a screening test per its maker. The degree of actual accuracy could not even be accurately determined, so it was essentially improbable if not impossible to know an accurate number of "cases" using these tests. The same type of fallible counting was also used for numbers of "deaths." A standardized definition of what constituted cases or deaths was never devised for everyone counting! Mainstream media reporters made their conclusions based on the dashboards' face values. The reason: Reporters were led by public health officials to believe the dashboards' mere existence represented irrefutable facts. It's a well-established fact that the CDC and other agencies very literally "doctored" the numbers of deaths. When the rates didn't look scary enough, officials changed the rules on what counted as a number one cause of death, and then of course it was necessary to change the International Classification of Diseases (ICD) codes to fit the new rules! Also, a third-party dashboard is NOT verifiable because the data sets used are collected and managed by organizations that don't directly interact with the original source and may be quite different. To be verifiable the dashboard must have no 'middle man' or intermediary system handling the raw data after it leaves the various health sources. Author Naomi Wolf stated, "There is growing evidence that third parties were invited into the handling of the data related to the pandemic in ways degrading its integrity and whether it was intentional or not, it inflated numbers in various ways."[41]

Dr. Henry Ealy and a team of colleagues, along with two Oregon state senators from his home state, called for a grand jury investigation on March 4, 2022, charging the CDC with "willful misconduct" ...in the mishandling and misrepresenting of COVID-19 data. The plaintiffs said government data MUST be dealt with according to the regulations—outsourcing to third parties is one of them.

According to the grand jury petition, that was exactly what Dr. Walensky of the CDC did. The petition was quite lengthy, but later in the document it stated the following:

> "This violation has inevitably resulted in COVID-19 data for cases, hospitalizations, and fatalities being artificially elevated, definitely compromised, prudent decision-making at federal and state executive levels. This includes policy enforcement for a public-health crisis that may not have existed had the CDC abided by the laws that ensure the accuracy of data collection."[42]
>
> Author, Naomi Wolf, herself a deep-thinking journalist and writer extraordinaire, who had suffered many trials, persecution, and the inaccurate title of conspiracy theorist, wanted us all to know how disappointed and sometimes disillusioned she had been in her fellow journalists. She said "some may be naïve, or worse, as they continued assuming the dashboards were absolute truth and verifiable government data. Since they were like the Eveready Batteries, another assumption was that the data was the latest information being constantly updated by the most reliable of engineers, programmers, and developers." However, Naomi iterated that, "in the United States, COVID news was being obtained from only TWO main sources: the Johns Hopkins University's Covid chart, and the New York Times Covid chart." Ms. Wolf said, "When an author checked the actual datasets, they were all deeply flawed."[43] She

learned that much of the data was uploaded by volunteers. It appears there were far too many unknowns and unanswered questions, making the information meaningless without verifiable methodology.[43]

The facts are undeniably incredible, but herein is reality. The Big Tech companies involved with this fully-deliberate deceit, all amassed billions of dollars from the lockdown and the oppressive pandemic policies. They were given the responsibility very literally to present the faulty data which drove, legitimized, and maintained the lockdown and all the pandemic policies placed from the earliest beginning of the pandemic. Some specific media entities can be recognized as the biggest and strongest drivers:

1. The Atlantic—a grantee of the Gates Foundation's $500,222 for at least 2 years, and responsible for the COVID Tracking Project
2. Laurene Jobs—widow of Apple founder, Steve Jobs. Heads "The Emerson Collective" dealing in education reform. One of their scary but unverifiable visuals perpetrated the reasons for full-school closures, giving enormous opportunity for the growth of educational technology. Before COVID, she and other tech heirs bought up other mass-media institutions, dominant in the older information age, such as print media, film and music studios, ad agencies, and radio and television outlets that would be used to keep the public "informed" during the pandemic.
3. Jeff Bezos—2013 Amazon founder who bought the sickly and sinking Washington Post, immediately investing in its journalism and its digital reach very successfully. It became a large player in the game of augmenting mass hysteria day and night for over two years.
4. Steve Ballmer—Microsoft's co-founder, founded "USA Facts.org.
5. Michael Bloomberg Philanthropies—funded the JHS COVID

dashboard.

6. Johns Hopkins Center for Health Security—-in partnership with the World Economic Forum (WEF)and its founder and director, Klaus Schwab and the Bill and Melinda Gates Foundation. Site of "Event 201" in the fall of 2019, just a bit ahead of the COVID-19 onslaught. The reader will remember it was a pandemic exercise on the order of a virtual disaster simulation of the outbreak of a novel, zoonotic coronavirus transmitted from bats to pigs to people, and ultimately transmissible to other people, eventually becoming a severe pandemic. This really wasn't a simulation in the sense that it was already planned as a done deal. Sounds quite recognizable, doesn't it? They were just making sure all planned systems were truly ready for the "accidental" leak to be leaked!!

7. Salesforce—its cofounder, Marc Benioff, sits on the Board of Trustees for the World Economic Forum (WEF), with former globalist director Klaus Schwab. Salesforce and Microsoft (Gates/Ballmer) partnered to build a digital, vaccine passport prototype!

8. Google—proficient in the business of consumer data and directly involved in COVID testing. Project Baseline is owned by Google, whose motto is: "Together, we can invent the future of data-powered healthcare." Google partnered with Rite -Aid Drug for administering COVID tests. As part of the pre-test authorization, individuals had to sign forms for Google and Rite-Aid. In many instances, the testing was compulsory for various reasons like flying or traveling over state lines. They collected data from thousands of people tested at Rite-Aid. In 2019, Google's revenue was $160.4 billion. Just two years later, its revenue increased to $257.64 billion.

By November of 2020, many thinking people were increasingly drawn to a number of outspoken physicians who boldly made a number of claims of misinformation by public health officials. They were adamantly opposed to the lockdown policies, which arguably were creating more health issues than COVID was causing by that time. They proclaimed the damage being done by all the COVID protocols, treatments and drugs were far worse for patients than those these doctors had used effectively until banned by Fauci through the FDA. Fauci's Remdesivir was so toxic, people came to the hospital primarily needing oxygen and often died of the Remdesivir usage. At first people simply thought these doctors were renegade dissidents wanting to rock the COVID boat. However, they were the good guys, attempting to inform people what was going on, and help them in any way they could. Obviously, those driving the COVID narrative did not like being thwarted in their efforts to run a successful pandemic, and really went nuts. As time passed, these doctors and many others formed a general consensus. They were being "policed," banned, persecuted, threatened and squelched constantly in some very "un-American ways, since freedom of speech given by our First Amendment was not to be given during this pandemic. Many were threatened with loss of jobs, appointments, and even loss of their medical licenses. But they went right on contradicting the COVID edicts being reported constantly on the social media platforms and in other media, especially the New York Times. The following is a partial list of these brave professionals:[44]

Dr. Peter McCullough	Dr Robert Malone
Dr. Kulvinda Kaur	Dr. Patrick Phillips
Dr. Paul Alexander	Dr. Andrew Boston
Dr. Harvey Tenenbaum	Dr. Sunetra Gupta
Dr. Martin Kulldorff	Dr. Simon Goddek
Dr. Jay Bhattacharya	Dr. Brian Ardis
Dr. Judy Mikovitz	Dr. Rashad Buttar

Dr. Henry Ealy

Dr. Ryan Cole

Dr. Ben Tapper

Dr. Lee Merritt

Dr. Ben Marble

Dr. David Martin

Dr. Jana Schmidt

Dr. Daniel Nuzom

Dr. Stella Immanuel

Dr. Larry Palevsky

Dr. Paul Barattiero

Dr. Tau Braun

Dr. James Meehan

Dr. Christianne Northrup

Dr. Patrick Quillin

Dr. Carrie Madej

These thirty men and women, along with hundreds of others throughout the healthcare field, including some from cooperative fields such as psychology, nutrition, science, microbiology, law and jurisprudence, chiropractic, natural medicine, and many more were involved and continue to be involved in clearing the real misinformation and disinformation perpetrated during COVID-19. These were not second-rate or pretend professionals like Anthony Fauci, but highly credentialed people from the best institutions of learning—Harvard, Yale, Oxford, Stanford, and others abroad. Experienced epidemiologists, public health experts, statisticians, and medical doctors were all sounding alarms in every way possible. Lockdowns were harmful in dozens of ways, data methodologies were done incorrectly, making them produce false results. PCR tests were misleading if not wrong or unreliable. They had reams of proof of what they were saying even then, but it was nearly impossible to be heard in the chaos of the tyrants screaming their narrative. Reporters attacked them, ran smear campaigns, and, in reality at the end of the pandemic, nearly every one of the media agents should have been legally charged with slander and libel, at the least, for all they had done. Subsequently, the lions' share of these professionals were proven right on everything they said and tried to say.

America's Frontline Doctors, many from the above group, did

everything in their power to protect people from the narrative misinformation, which is still the only kind that is allowed in the media, and those promoting the narrative over every media outlet continue to vilify these good doctors. Despite regular claims by various media moguls that censorship ended, in fact, it has not. This is an ongoing battle that isn't going away any time soon. Globalist wolves have no intention of relenting or admitting wrongs because their plans for further control and other potential pandemics will NOT be thwarted by a group of professionals that have consciences. When you go to the web or any social media, you still cannot find much accurate data, even when you personally know what's right as a medical professional. For a researcher to find real documented facts, it takes an enormous amount of searching.[44]

Another related issue is the lament of the stalwart pandemic controllers, "Why do so many Americans distrust science?" That's a simple question! The simple answer is, "Science that was once trusted for accuracy has been changed by the globalists to agree with their world agenda. Professional medical and science journals, and institutions of higher education, at least taught what could be proven, and reported accurately what most current research showed. Since before COVID, that is no longer true, because these once trusted sources sold out for globalist money, the highest bidders. Science doesn't change—people do. Now, we are each basically on our own to follow our own research and gut instinct to make our own best decisions, because we can no longer trust science that has changed over and over again."[45] Globalists will blame this lack of trust on everything and everyone but themselves, but a good many of us have seen through the charade and like our own brains and instincts better. The truth is that distrust should be expected as a result of all the lies and deception perpetrated on us, because they believed they could get by with it. Most people this author has interviewed have stated they will never blindly trust the science or the media again.

Quarantine and Lockdown Are NOT the Same:

What Restrictions Really Achieved

To understand this, we must first look at the prescribed globalist goal. That goal was and will be again: to fear and fear endlessly. To achieve it, the fear was followed by ever escalating restrictions in movement, assembly, and commerce. Tight restrictions were necessary to allow for the gargantuan transfer of wealth from the masses to the elites. It could have been entitled, "The Brazen Mass Theft of 2020-2022." But why, you ask?

Little by little clarity brought the real reason for restrictions which had absolutely NOTHING to do with medicine or the existence of the Pandemic. The actual reason was and is the global predators' war, waged primarily against the West in general and the United States in particular. They weaponized everything standing between them and their goal. Historically, restrictions have been instrumental in removing the power structures from those who wanted all the power and wealth of the target nations. It strips the targets of their ability to fight invaders, leaving them open and vulnerable to the theft of everything of value, including all assets and real estate. The ruling class, thus stripped, is one that must be stripped as ordinary people have very little already. When the restrictions are a part of public health necessity, they are ramped up forcefully and can be accepted with far less resistance, especially in the beginning. Just as it was at the start of COVID, free people don't recognize or understand what is happening to them immediately. However, when they see the extent of what they have lost, why it's been lost, how long it continues and even grows more restrictive, it's almost too late. But, thinking people start questioning, pushing-back, and become very aware of how wrong this new agenda is, without plausible reasons or explanations. Common sense shouts in their heads that this is not normal or desirable and they want the 'good old days back." The constant fear of a worse case, is confusing and disorienting, but many individuals are NOT prone to 'rock the boat', causing themselves more potential problems.[46]

Oddly, a free people have material and cultural wealth as a consistent by-product of freedom; ironically, they became so accustomed to that lifestyle that they also become complacent and satisfied. However, during the COVID debacle, we lost most ,if not all, of our basic rights; they'd been systematically and indefinitely suspended for "the good of us all." Individual personal rights were simply ignored and trampled on. By February 2021, 47 of 50 states were acting under 'emergency law'. No military was involved and nary a shot fired. Our enemies had used both stealth, then absolute deception against us and, for all practical purposes, had won several campaigns at once.

The new global imprisonment was deliberately termed a 'quarantine', knowing it might be accepted more readily than if it was called a 'lockdown'. For anyone aware of the difference, it was readily clear when the 'emergency' orders restricted our Constitutional rights of Assembly and Commerce. We weren't dealing with a traditional quarantine, which by definition was always limited in time and location, and only separated the sick and newly arrived travelers from all the rest of us. Lockdowns do occur in totalitarian states, but NOT in free countries. Quarantines, requiring simple isolation of disease-infected community members, have been done since the ancient civilizations of the Bible. Used in its purposed manner of isolating the sick, it was very effective in controlling the spread of illness, but was NEVER EVER used on the entire population for an unspecified, lengthy period of time. It also NEVER EVER included massive restrictions on the economic well-being of the globe. The deception of SARS-CoV-2 being more lethal than any other pathogen had ever been was effectively used to make us all certain we could have no expectations of personal autonomy for our individual lives. "It was like the law of 'innocent, until proven guilty' was upended to 'all are potentially ill until proven healthy!"[47] It was like someone had deemed us all immunocompromised, and everyone who became exposed to COVD-19 would automatically become ill, because it was 'novel' and no one had natural immunity to it.

Why was it so easy for these warped and depraved globalists and progressives to victoriously usurp our freedoms and liberty? There was the serenity of reasonably comfortable living for most of us and worse, an ever-growing ignorance on the part of the majority of citizens. The structures of our hard-won Democratic Republic had been and were being systematically destroyed by powerful, money-hungry despots who believe they are more capable of governing us than we are. Unfortunately, free Westerners have always tended to believe all things will continue to be as they now are. Even if our country fell on some difficult times, we have always put our backs to the plow and prevailed over the hard times-it's the pride of our heritage. We could always go where we needed to go and procure whatever we needed—even wanted. Since the end of the World Wars—roughly 75 years—we'd become fully accustomed to our unique levels of freedom and acceptance of all basic human rights. We freely met in public places, often by the thousands; we traveled widely in freedom. Truly we could not say we had 'heaven on earth' but it still seemed like the next best thing. Most of us would say we truly appreciated our freedoms and celebrated patriotism, but just maybe didn't understand the importance of our God-given freedoms, nor just how fast evil predators could execute a near-complete demise.[47]

Once again, a really good example of this same phenomenon can be seen on a smaller scale examining the formation of the now well-known European Union (EU). This governmental group was formed as if it might be like a United States of Europe. It would be a centralized union of individual state governments, billed as bringing a plethora of benefits to the whole of its union. On the face of it, the EU did provide some very popular policies. All barriers to traveling across borders of each country were dropped. A one-unit monetary system (Euros) allowed for better commerce among them. It was humane and civilized, but this came at great cost. Each country was required to surrender its individual, national sovereignty to Brussels to create the single, central EU government.

There would be no further national or personal autonomy. There was a very large snafu with the UK (Great Britain). It said, "Thank you very much, but we simply are NOT interested in this"[48] and it left the EU. Most of the nations didn't really understand what the EU was really about. They thought it would be a simple federation of states retaining their national autonomy, similar to the U.S. This was NOT surprising because the true governance of the EU had been hidden with mostly deliberate confusion and unclear intention. It had been nearly impossible to obtain ANY founding documents in the morass of deceit.

Dr. Naomi Wolf had occasion to be introduced to the Portuguese Island of Madeira and her host explained the EU to her. He said "it was NOT so much a governance entity, but an economic alliance and Germany was, by far, its major influence. Unelected diplomats proposed new laws, but Brussels was loaded with lobbyists. Its real power laid in non-accountable hands with a total façade of democracy.

No matter how great things might appear in Europe on the surface, the powers of the European nation-state had been secretly eliminated from them and they were all rendered vulnerable. All of its people would be totally unable to defend themselves if the EU turned hostile, abusive or even tyrannical! What you see all around you, looking and seeming so lovely is no longer built on a structure belonging to its peoples. Those living under EU governance left continental Europeans especially vulnerable to the COVID tyrants. Just so, the United States also became vulnerable for many similar reasons."[49]

In America's not so distant past, we saw exactly how various restrictions diminished our human capital and weakened our society. Certainly, the future of Native Americans changed as it created victims in the massive re-appropriation of their lands and assets. It was quite easily done by the United States government's 'locking down" tribal peoples in designated reservations on lands scarcely anyone else wanted. They were forbidden to move about freely outside the reservations and subjected to state restrictions on their language, attire, money, and culture. Their once prosperous nations were coerced into defeat and compliance. Shamelessly, this was done by people who had fled their homelands with similar restrictions and lockdowns so they could be free to prosper in America! Later, after our Civil War, African-Americans freed from slavery continued fighting for decades for their God-given rights.[50]

Clearly, the goal of globalist predators as it pertains to our United States, was very similar when they planned and executed the lockdowns and other restrictions on us during the COVID "emergency"! They will do it again in a heartbeat, if American citizens allow them to get by with it again. Restrictions weaken the restricted. Just as they did during COVID-19, globalists and cooperative 'Progressives' will attempt to steal or transfer all of US citizens' assets, dis-empowering them from being able to mount opposition. The globalist's war was waged predominantly by Big Tech moguls who leveraged our culture and its order of technology. Every attempt in the battle was to ultimately defeat all of humanity by striking down every piece of human identity including our speech, touch, creativity, bodies, religion, families, education, and most especially our culture of liberty and freedom.

Restrictions in human history always preceded massive THEFT—theft of the lands, assets, and opportunities of those restricted. In 2020-2022, all of humanity was affected. A perfect example of the tyranny involved in the attempt to ramp up the restrictions even more, was their propaganda on our holidays in November of 2020. It had been a difficult and stressful year for most of us. All predictions were negative with little hope in sight. The media began praising all those folks who planned to forego holiday visits to their families—no traveling. Hosting holiday parties was definitely not tenable. Even if all were well, and your family was doing fine, we were all instructed to NOT be fine! Now this approach, by its very nature was highly suspect. Generally, whenever there is a perceived REAL crisis, media moguls do all in their power to downplay it, and attempt to minimize fear and panic. However, in the case of COVID, never the crisis it was constantly purported to be, fear mongering and panic stoking was especially bad—with the encouragement of the holidays, it was concerning to globalists that many could forget the seriousness of the crisis unless constantly reminded.[51]

"On October 5, 2020, the Great Barrington Declaration was released to the public. It was written from a global public health and humanitarian perspective, with special concerns about how the current COVID-19 strategies were forcing our children, the working class and the poor to carry the heaviest burden. The response to the pandemic in many countries around the world focused on lockdowns, contact tracing and isolation, imposing enormous unnecessary health costs on people. In the long run, it would lead to higher COVID and non-COVID mortality than the focused protection plan we call for in the Declaration. This is an international declaration, written with concerns for the entire world."[52] It was written for the public, fellow scientists, and government officials by Dr. Jay Bhattacharya, Dr. Sunetra Gupta, and Dr. Martin Kulldorff. These doctors met in Massachusetts to record a video outlining an alternative to the then current COVID-19 strategy. Spontaneously they agreed to also write a shorter 'Declaration' to summarize the major points. It was written and signed at the American Institute for Economic Research, located in Great Barrington, MA. After finishing the Declaration, the three authors emailed colleagues asking them to cosign it and most agreed. These original 30+ co-signers are listed on its front page and later thousands of others also signed it online. Less than 1% of signees were scam fakes.

Leading doctors decided to warn the world of the ominous damage to humanity that lockdowns were causing. The harm would be most severe among the poor, the elderly, and children. Physicians and scientists spoke of the economic issues where poor people would soon be starving, possibly by millions globally. They spoke also of physical and emotional "collateral damage," and were100% correct. They believed the lockdowns would not benefit anyone in terms of health goals. Restrictions would do absolutely nothing except harm populations in countless ways, especially in public health. At first, the majority of people responded positively because they were all sick and tired of being sick and tired, as well as horribly disconnected from one another. Dr. Kulldorff spoke of all the normal health concerns of the many people not being treated properly because of their fear of contracting COVID in clinics and hospitals, and of those dying of treatable issues. Closing schools would have serious life-long effects on our children. Mental/emotional health was being strained everywhere. He also declared the collateral damage of the lockdowns had been far more destructive than the virus. Nevertheless, these courageous experts and their Declaration had powerful adversaries. Just as the Declaration was receiving thoughtful and respectful attention, Anthony Fauci and his boss, director of the NIH—Francis Collins, from behind the scenes called for an immediate and lethal take-down of both the Declaration and the good doctors who wrote it.[53] Following that action, for months, the belittling and mud-slinging on these writers was nauseating and beyond disgusting. They were regularly smeared almost to the point of obliteration, while the standard COVID 'narrative' continued unchecked. However, because of the Declaration, far more people were asking a lot more questions than they had dared to ask before.

After the dust settled from the Declaration, Big Tech published a formidable amount of negativity about the epidemiological warnings. Nevertheless, basic epidemiological theory indicates that lockdowns do NOT reduce the total number of cases in the long run and have NEVER in history led to the eradication of a disease. At best, lockdowns delay the increase of cases for a finite period and at Great Cost! The fact is that lockdowns create a great many physical health harms. Medical care plummeted, with people avoiding needed medical care, including a reduction of childhood vaccination rates, less cancer screening, skipped cancer treatment and fewer preventive cardiovascular disease visits, just to name a few.[54]

"Humans have many needs, including the need for community and normal social interactions with each other. Lockdowns severely deteriorated mental health. Emergency departments saw about four times more children and teens in psychiatric crisis than usual. One in four young adults in the US seriously considered suicide. Every extension of the lockdown increased those numbers, especially when it appeared there was no end in sight."[55]In addition, the far-reaching and warned-about damages include a plethora of harms done, including the following:

- Harm to children victimized by interrupted education
- Harm to the working class, higher risks of infection, financial hardship
- Harm to physical and mental health in the developing nations, starvation
- Harm to less-protected elderly exponentially increased
- Harm of constant fear and dread
- Harm of increased isolation for high-risk individuals
- Harm from lying media reports and denials of the Declaration warnings
- Harm from lack of focused protection advocated by the Declaration
- Harm of vaxxing people who already had COVID-19, often recommended

It is still important today to remember the classic totalitarian tactic of the globalists when they use the pronoun "we" to make their dictates slightly more palatable. 'We' Must; in order to stop this pandemic, 'We' must all stay home; 'We' must all sacrifice our holidays to do our part; 'We' must all be vaxxed; 'We' must make sure everyone else gets vaxxed for the common good; etc. When they use the word, "We," they mean "You," since none of the clever recommendations apply to them! Beware of the frequent use of this pronoun! So, like good little boys and girls, "we" followed their orders that weren't even viable orders. CDC "guidance" was plastered on media outlets and parroted by the self-ordained health officials as if they were law, and it wasn't even close to legal. 'Guidance" implies nothing more than suggestion of some course of action recommended for those who can't think for themselves. Fauci told us all every day exactly what we could and could not do, and media parroted that. But his agency, notoriously loaded with fraud and graft, under the auspices of the National Institutes of Health had absolutely NO authority to enforce their orders. Fauci's job description was ONLY to advise the President of the United States on science issues. In addition his track record with his agency was a long way from stellar! We are free people in what remains of a free country. None of these so-called advisors had the authority to control us or our actions…but very few of us, at least for the first year of the pandemic seemed to realize it.[55]

2021—COVID Cult Either More Deceived, Or Abandoned

The virus was becoming the personification of a wicked villain in a horror movie. It had its own theme, signature music, and ominous Satanic personality. It truly required a cult-following. By this point in time, good and responsible science existed and could be found on several platforms if not connected to Big Tech, if the noncult thinker wished to find it, but evil always screamed louder, and longer.

Going back to an encounter that our friend, Dr. Naomi Wolf had, she told of her invitation by Jeffrey Tucker to become a Fellow at the American Institute of Economic Research (AIER). "Under his oversight, AIER was producing the best and most fearless, yet thorough reporting on the pandemic. I spent every day with a thoughtful community of liberty-minded economists, AI theorists, and historians."[55]

When she first walked in the door, it was just like going back to the pre-pandemic days of respect for individuals. About 20 Fellows and staffers were well-dressed, having cocktails and easily chatting with each other—just like 'normal'! Nobody wore masks and they stood close to one another, enjoying the normal conversation of human beings. It was a beautifully appointed center containing plenty of hand sanitizer and baskets of masks sat at hand if any chose to use them, but—just like in the good old days everyone was given choice about what each felt comfortable doing. There was good ventilation. No one had been seriously ill or died, but life continued. While most of the world was still in fear's grip, Ms. Wolf was amongst a community that respected each other, their bodies, and their own personal choices which had once been our norm, but clearly had been taken very much for granted. While working there, she didn't get sick, nor did her husband. It was an intellectually rich time when she enjoyed new friendships and stimulating conversations. Ironically, most of her friends were still locked-down, in the proverbial suspended animation, worried sick about her going to an office every day. Yet she knew of other communities besides AIER that had no serious illness either.

The Amish community near her home did not lockdown, and there were no seriously ill throughout their population. The Orthodox Jewish community to which her relatives belonged had no serious illness either. She wondered why there were no studies by 'science' from these places not locked down. Such places where people clearly chose their own level of risk, yet supported those who wished to isolate themselves. No one looked at the welfare of many churches whose members still met every week without epidemic illness.

Thankfully, that was the experience of this author. After the initial eight weeks of just streaming services as "ordered," our pastor spoke directly with our state governor and city mayor. He graciously explained that our church chose to abide by the dictates of our US Constitution which guaranteed our right to meet for worship. We respected some cautionary guidelines and our church never closed its doors again throughout the pandemic. Occasionally someone would be ill for a few days, but simply stayed home until recovered as we always had. No one suggested it should be otherwise. We worshiped, we sang, and we fellowshipped a bit farther apart, but face to face, and most of us chose to forget the masks.

There was NO serious illness in the body for almost an entire year. Each member of our body was beyond grateful for our church and each other and there is simply no doubt this weekly connection kept all of us so much happier, more hopeful, and saner. We knew of other churches/pastors who bought into the propaganda and their people lamented their loss, truly saddened by it. There was also frustration when this integral part of their lives was removed indefinitely. Strange as it may seem to some, this author believes that our faith in our Lord Jesus Christ and his promises was honored by our Father God, and He protected our congregation.

"Now faith is the assurance of things hoped for, the conviction of things not seen. For by it (faith) the people of old received their commendation. And without faith it is impossible to please Him, for whoever would draw near to God must believe that He exists and that He rewards those who seek Him." Hebrews 11:1-2,6 ESV

Ultimately, only a handful of our members, including my husband and me were ever hospitalized seriously, but our Lord graciously returned us home alive. Our experience as individuals and as a body of Christ became a great testimony to our community and more than that, it brought much glory to our Father.

So unfortunately for most people, especially those in bigger urban centers, there weren't adequate places to worship and still mind the guidelines. Many churches closed indefinitely, rather than jump the hoops and figure out how to do it. Worse, there were few plans or expectations of re-opening and no alternative plans were posited. Many felt they were fainting spiritually, if not physically. In the case of Ms. Wolf, even attempts at outdoor alternatives with distance were caboshed by the rabbis with no explanation given. She spoke up with good sense, and the rabbis let her know she was no longer a "fit" for their congregation. They essentially "broke up" with her and returned her membership fee! Single people, especially the older and widowed spent massive amounts of time alone and truly closed off from humanity. Obviously, the work of the globalist wolves who have no time for faith or religion and hate the strength and health it gives us wanted to be rid of it, and in most cases it worked.[55]

In the event of another pandemic or similar crisis, it has become terribly important to retain our ability to think and reason well. That includes our making our own good, personal choices for our health and well-being. We continue to build and maintain a healthy immune system. From the view of terrain health and good common sense, we must be outside as much as possible and in well-ventilated spaces, 'grounding' our connection to nature's resources of sun, water, soil, rain, and clean air. All of our normally good health choices remain good health choices and they give hope. One need NOT sit in helplessness and fear. Action is healthy—it freezes fear!

The restrictions didn't lessen and for many they became ever more insane. The CDC kept 're-citing' its own material! With each supposedly new study cited, there were more wrinkles, and more glaring flaws. The information was not peer-reviewed and 'researchers' did not perform the necessary scientific experiments to prove any of the conclusions. By making correlations, many erroneous assumptions were also made. "Correlation is NOT the same as causation." Decisions were made on correlation alone, and no real foundation existed, making them wrong decisions.

Ultimately, most were not made by scientists at all, but by the New York Times, or other media sources. For example: The New York Times continued claiming that bars and restaurants were a major source of the COVID illnesses. More and more, the information being cited was simply NOT reliable because none of the possible contributing factors to the narrative were even mentioned—factors such as whether dining was indoor or outdoor, was it well-ventilated, and did it adhere to the distancing and occupancy requirements. It simply blamed them all with zero rationale.

"Restaurant owners were driven to desperation. Their situations were already beyond difficult and so many owners had been forced to close their doors, never to be reopened. Owners began questioning the so-called "science" of the CDC, because it didn't even resemble science. Supposed science was being used to justify their keeping the entire restaurant industry closed or more restricted. Finally "the

National Restaurant Association, representing over a million restaurants and food outlets criticized the supposed CDC study, calling it an ill-informed attack on the industry hardest hit by the pandemic.

A letter was sent to their governors and groups representing the state regulators that there was no scientific evidence linking eating places to the surge in new coronavirus infections. They urged these groups to accommodate restaurants' ability to serve customers safely and not strangle the industry further with 'blunt-force' closings and other operational restrictions.

There was an unfounded impression that restaurants were part of the problem, and we were suffering as a result of inconsistent, restrictive mandates. Tens of thousands of additional restaurant bankruptcies—and millions of lost jobs—are now more likely, while the science remains inconclusive on whether any health benefits will accrue. We are too commonly labeled as 'super-spreaders' and have become a convenient scapegoat for reflexive shutdowns. Several pieces of research have been identified as deeply flawed. To date, we have found no systemic outbreaks of COVID-19 from the hundreds of thousands of restaurants around the country that operate within the Association's guidance and follow local public health and safety regulations."[56]

In truth, these restaurant owners proved to be 100% correct about the CDC and its faulty methods in every way, including factually, logically, morally, and ethically. Once again, after the dust settled, and thousands of restaurants had closed their doors permanently, a subsequent study showed that restaurants had only accounted for 1.4% of all infections. Unfortunately for these small business owners, they received no help or recompense for their losses. All the facts could not help them—it was far too late to save their livelihoods and this travesty was set in stone. Of course we must remember that killing small, non-globalist businesses was always one of the globalists' goals which they did beyond successfully.

Ms. Wolf tells the extent of lockdown in Northern England,

January, 2021. She had phoned a colleague at a University there. She found this man was only allowed one hour per day for outside exercise. Right in the middle of their conversation, the poor man began to weep. He was completely stressed out with harsh and totally unnecessary restrictions.

"An even worse account of the lock-down's effects is almost too horrendous to believe. Ms. Wolf helped many people globally, and one such way was to facilitate networking. She hired a technologist from the Philippines through a specific platform connecting other women 'techies' in the developing world to companies needing their expertise. The woman was a Word Press webmaster, a bright young professional, well-dressed, organized, and highly productive when the pandemic started. One year later, January, 2021, her once outstanding work was suffering. Over Zoom, she explained she was only allowed outside on alternate days and only then for groceries or medicine. The children weren't allowed outside at all. She had a boyfriend she'd been dating for years, but now if they walked in public, a public health officer placed a stick between the two young people, making sure they stayed six feet apart! They were not allowed to touch or hold hands. By the next month, her punctuation and grammar were erratic. She was unable to care if she made mistakes. On calls, this formerly ultra-professional and attractive young lady was pale and disheveled with dull, sad eyes. She seemed unable even to brush her once beautiful black hair. She was so depressed she was nearly immobile. With much sorrow, the company finally had to let her go. How many times and in how many places had there been similar scenarios?"[57]

As previously mentioned, the growing group of 'dissident' doctors were speaking up more and more on social media about the many health-related travesties being visited on people everywhere by the totalitarian ideas of the globalist wolves. "Dr. Patrick Philips of Ontario, Canada was one who began speaking out, doing interviews, and addressing COVID pathos. He told one reporter he often went back to the moment he knew, "something was wrong." He also attested to the fact that the Canadian government was 'cracking down harder than ever' on 'dissidents' like himself." But one of Canada's most important freedoms is their freedom of speech, as is ours in the US. Dr. Philips reported that he saw many elderly people arriving to his Emergency Room dying of starvation, not COVID. They were also dying of sheer depression. Many were dying because they had missed important diagnostic procedures and many other things had not been attended to, but rarely were they dying of COVID! Dr Philips spoke out more and more about the evils of what he saw every day. The Ontario government came down on him and took his medical license. He has not chosen to go through the process of restoring it, because his conscience will not let him ignore the travesties he still sees. He's living peaceably, but Ontario is already extremely short on doctors, in a socialist system and his loss has been felt by many. You can only be beaten back so long![58]

During the pandemic, a brilliant young PhD in Biotechnology working for a University in the Netherlands began writing and asking questions about all the unexplainable and inconsistent pieces of the COVID debacle that just didn't and still doesn't add up. "Dr. Simon Goddek first wrote about the need for immune building with Vitamin D. When it was published on Twitter, there was a firestorm, it was taken down, and he was fired from his job. It took an entire year to be restored to Twitter, but since it's no longer Twitter, his freedom to speak has been somewhat restored. Several vindictive occurrences happened to him after the first, when his truth-telling was not accepted. Today, Goddek lives in Brazil and does practical science investigation in hydroponics and other water-related projects, owning an associated business. He was basically branded and chased from Europe over his warning that there was something very wrong with the COVID PCR tests. He reported this in the journal Euro-surveillance claiming the PCR test for COVID had passed the peer-reviewed process for the journal's study in just over one day and had to be 'rigged' since it should require an average timeline of dozens of months. Once again, he faced immediate backlash but remained adamant that the truth be told. His outrage at this fraud was certainly that of a true scientist.

Once again, increased censorship, and continued vindictive harassment occurred because he spoke the truth, and globalists hate truth."[59] Interestingly, what he said is the truth, and many other scientists have been outspoken on the subject, as previously discussed.

Other scientists were also studying genomics, PCR, COVID tests, mRNA vaccines, and other such hot topics. One such was biotechnologist Kevin McKernan, who was the research director on the Human Genome Project at MIT. About a decade later he became the founder and CSO of Medicinal Genomics. He is a renowned leader in the area of DNA sequencing technology. First, it is interesting to note that Kevin's company laboratory was fully open and operating during the pandemic. Ms. Wolf, who interviewed Kevin stated, "The scientists there acted normally, dressed nicely, and conversed with one another easily without the mandated baggage, doing business as usual. The lab ventilation was exceptional and refreshing. Lush green plants flourished in the broad windows. Not one person there had been ill."[60] Mr. McKernan explained, "The PCR tests in use for COVID testing frequently pick up evidence of weeks-old cold or flu viruses in nasal passages and are often misidentified as COVID. After all, many colds are also coronaviruses. Viruses or 'the evidence of viruses,' since no one has ever seen an actual virus, being so miniscule that even the evidence of their possible presence can only be seen when mega-magnified by an electron microscope. Even then, the slides are prepared with toxic substances to 'stabilize' a dead bit of tissue in a process that renders the specimen to be something a viewer can only surmise about. So clearly, if the news reported 70,000 people had died of coronavirus without any further so-called identification, it would only mean there were deaths, but no one could say for certain they were COVID deaths.

The manner in which PCR tests were run was very subjective and so was the number of cycles needed to get an accurate test, which could turn out as falsely positive or negative, hence there was no guaranteed reliability; that's a very bad thing when so many people's lives were apt to be adversely affected by decisions made on the basis of potentially false information. Every day the dashboards reported the results of those PCR tests as if they were absolutes and proof that COVID-19 infections were rampant, and it simply was NOT true. There were also glaring flaws in data collection methods, as well as in the data displays themselves."[61]

Meanwhile, three other medical doctors from the "dissident" group warned that children should NOT be kept out of school. They were NOT at serious risk for COVID which from the beginning had been said and proven. Once again, these doctors were portrayed as wild-eyed, non-scientists or conspiracy theorists. Dr. Bhattacharya declared that older and more vulnerable people should be sheltered protectively, but young adults and children should be about the business of living normally. So many of them spent nearly two years marking time and losing educational ground needlessly. Time changed nothing. More and more of the finest doctors and scientists continued to be hounded and pressured over their solid, truth-based messages.

Messages continued from proven journalists, interviews, distressing first-hand stories from restaurant owners, and many others who were very close to their wit's end, but it was an ever-changing illogical environment almost everywhere. It was a continuous struggle to keep restaurants and small businesses open so that hardworking breadwinners could keep their families afloat and fed. As the perfect example of weird announcements: "Governor Cuomo of New York, on March 15, 2021 declared it would now be OK to have weddings and catered events, but all guests must remain masked, dance apart, and could only remove masks while seated, eating or drinking! Venues were restricted to 50% of their capacity with a maximum of 150 guests per event. All guests must carry proof of recent negative COVID testing or vaccination prior to entering. Guests must sign-in with contact information in case contact tracing became necessary. Venues must give notice to local health departments of large events above the social gathering limit of six in advance. Here's the real zinger—ceremonial and social-distanced dancing would only be allowed in designated areas!"[62] Doesn't that sound like an event to remember? We wonder if anyone actually did that for their wedding event, and if so, was there anything fun about it? All that could be said in retrospect years down the line, "It was certainly memorable!" One wonders how many extra people in the maximum 150, were designated monitors, or worse, spies!

Finally, by the start of 2021, millions were getting vaxxed, primarily because, more than anything else, they were sick and tired of their mundane lives of constant control and restrictions. Many took the jab only in an attempt to resume normalcy in their lives, and regain their freedom, which was, of course, a planned way of increasing vax compliance. However, there was no end of jabs in sight, but an exponential increase in the stories of the ultra-toxic adverse events people were having, including death. Everyone knew someone for whom the jab had been a really bad idea. Young, formerly healthy women were hitting social media speaking of appalling menstrual dysfunctions after the vax and just as many post-menopausal women started having cycles again. One mother reported her 12-year-old daughter had her first menses that lasted 14 days after she was jabbed. There were agonizing cramps, heavy bleeding, and even hemorrhaging of large clots with tissue reported. None of these reports were normal, but still became quite consistently reported. Women know normal and they know abnormal. Naturally all of this was also affecting fertility. One journalist spoke of these known problems on Fox News and her Twitter account was suspended. The reason she was told; she gave 'medical misinformation.' "CNN promptly added the label of "conspiracy theorist" which came as no surprise since the Gates Foundation had funded CNN $3.6 million for their next 3 years of reporting."[63]

The Secret Crimes of ALL Media, both Social and Legacy Media

By April 2021, increasing numbers of people were being

vaccinated with the mRNA 'vaccines' which aren't real vaccines. Many were even "double-vaxxed" and bragged about it. Throughout social media platforms people viewed the faces of smiling 'influencers' rolling up their sleeves to both be jabbed, and to proudly display the telling aftermath of band-aids! We can't even imagine how false and tainted was the propaganda, but we may be sure there were no ads of anyone being jabbed and fainting within minutes as the toxins hit their bloodstream! There were far too many of those to count!

The Blaze uncovered the money trail, traced straight back to the Legacy Media! We need to clarify the difference between social and legacy media groups in order to understand why this is such a telling statement. "Legacy media or 'Old Media' consists of the mass media institutions that dominated in the Information Age; particularly print media, film studios, music studios, advertising agencies, radio broadcasting and television. Demetrius Matthews is the CEO and founder of Legacy Media LLC. Legacy media conglomerates include Disney, Warner Media, Viacom CBS, Bertelsmann Publishers, and NewsCorp, owners of Fox News and Entertainment, and span from books to audio to visual media. The four largest social media owned by Meta, are Facebook (core platform), What's App, Facebook Messenger, and Instagram. Obviously, Legacy Media is much slower than social media and can take days for a piece of information to finally hit the airwaves compared to Facebook. Not as many people listen to radio, watch TV ads, or read the newspapers today, but we mustn't underestimate its usefulness and COVID proved that. A key strength of Legacy is its 'editorial control'. Its outlets have editors and fact-checkers who scrutinize content before it is published, 'ensuring the information disseminated is reliable and trustworthy'"[64] Don't you believe it, reader! Its editors and fact-checkers are just as heavily influenced by globalists and woke ideology as social media is. With that knowledge on media, once again "The Blaze, with its Freedom of Information Act at hand, emailed the Department of Health and Human Services (HHS) and found that it had bought advertising from major news platforms (Legacy) such as ABC, CBS, and NBC. Via the HHS, millions flowed to Fox News, CNN, NBC, the Washington Post, the New York Times, The Los Angeles Times, and Buzzfeed.com. The money came from the US Congress, which appropriated ONE BILLION Dollars in 2021 for HHS, who used the CDC as its distributor, to strengthen vaccine confidence in the US!."[65] Clearly the mission was the management of messaging we saw ramping up in 2001. The CDC and other agencies were allowed to award contracts to both private and public organizations to "carry out a national, evidence-based campaign to increase awareness and knowledge of the 'safety and effectiveness' of vaccines for the prevention and control of diseases, combat misinformation about vaccines, and disseminate 'scientific and evidence-based' vaccine-related information, with the goal of increasing the rates of vaccination across all ages…"[66]

This discovery revealed a whole new avenue of funding that in a few short months 'absolutely corrupted' American civil society… US taxpayer money was paying people and groups to promote, even drive the vaccines made by Big Pharma at the administration. It also carried a crossover business alignment with Big Tech, via the social media platforms that supported the entire propaganda machine. Therefore, it was a cleverly managed, circular current of influence from the same underlying sources on a massive scale, the likes of which had NEVER been seen before. Influencers were paid to report a variety of stories, from having vaxxed their teens, to deliberate lies about the vaccines. At that time it was NOT easy to find any reliable information about the vaccines, their ingredients, or their mode of operation within the body, but for a great many of us, red flags stood everywhere. Moderna claimed its vaccine was truly "the software of life." As with software that requires frequent updating, so would this "miraculous vaccine" function similarly.

Based on the Big Pharma pitch to investors, any person of medical knowledge could predict the need for vaccine boosters before the subject ever came under discussion. Investors in pharmaceutical products would obviously want to know that returns on their investments would not come to a stop anytime soon, guaranteeing greater profits. One could put good money on the bet that both manufacturers and investors planned on a big payday. Even more alarming than boosters was Big Pharma's glee about its lipid nanoparticles. We will see much more on this in a later chapter, but this discovery opened the door to a whole new exploding field of biotechnology that would revolutionize the transport and delivery of a wide-range of therapeutic agents. It gave massive potential for the integration of biotechnology and human bodily processes, as well as for drug delivery. "This technology presented a real 'gold-rush' mentality in the big venture capitalists who had 'dollar signs in their eyeballs,' and began running fully amok, just as the '49ers' did in 1849 as they ran for California gold. It is well-known that the world of Big Tech, and Big 'everything else' see nature and the human body as one of the last frontiers. To prove the point, by 2022, venture capital continued to exhibit immunity to the COVID-19 pandemic. Most people surely felt the economic dearth of two years in pandemic, but it had the opposite effect for venture capitalists."[67] There are some mind-boggling discoveries that could eventually be of value, but to get there will ultimately cost humanity an enormous debt we should not be willing to pay. Those of us who can still think and reason rationally already knew we wanted no part in this frontier of "playing God!" As the old adage goes, "If you think a thing is just too good to be true, in all likelihood, it is!"

There were so many red flags flying over this whole vaccination mess, it could easily make one nauseated and dizzy! A paper was written by a highly reputable group of physicians and epidemiologists, including renowned Dr. Sucharit Bhakdi and was sent to the European Medicines Agency. They warned that the mRNA vaccines were damaging the walls of blood vessels, even the tiniest ones, making people more vulnerable to strokes and blood clots, simply on the basis of 'How' the vaccine mechanism was created. They wrote: "It must be expected that endothelial damage with subsequent triggering of blood coagulation via platelet activation, will ensue at countless sites throughout the body. We request evidence of this probability which was excluded in pre-clinical animal models with all three vaccines prior to their approval for use in humans by the EMA...If such evidence is not available, it must be expected that this will lead to drops in platelet counts, appearance of D-dimers (protein fragments) in the blood, (indicators of blood clot demise), as well as myriad ischemic lesions (areas with diminished blood flow) throughout the body, including the brain, spinal cord and heart. Bleeding disorders may occur in the wake of this novel type of DIC (disseminated intra-vascular coagulation) syndrome—including profuse bleedings and hemorrhagic strokes. We request evidence that all these possibilities which were excluded in preclinical animal models with all three vaccines prior to their approval for use in humans by the EMA be sent and disseminated"[68] EVERYTHING about which they warned is exactly what happened in spades!

Multiple future warnings to friends and relatives continued to fall on deaf ears; it happened to this writer regularly. There was also a mammoth collective narrative promoting the mRNA vax as, "our only way out of this." In addition to that, the un-vaxxed were labeled merely as, "stubborn disease factories" to be shunned and ostracized wherever they were found. Vaccine promoters as much as said, "Don't bother us with your facts and warnings any more-they mean nothing!" Meanwhile the media continually cast all un-vaxxed as "Trump-obsessed, infectious racists" bringing both politics and race into the speak. They relentlessly depicted the vaccine as the only way to be a decent human being, willing to save the community. Massive delusion was perpetrated day and night.

Once again, Ms. Wolf and her husband decided to take a summer trip cross-country in 2021. After New York, what they found true was actually dramatically different than mainstream-media reports. The differences ran mostly along party lines and were therefore politically predictable. In red states, people were respectful of others' personal space and used hand sanitizer; otherwise, they just went about their business as usual. In South

Dakota, governor Kristi Noem had refused to lock down her state. There were lots of videos posted on CNN and NBC trying to show everyone just how bad things were in South Dakota without all the restrictions, but the pictures were neither current nor pertinent. South Dakota was actually thriving, but the mainstream-media couldn't show that! The large annual bike rally had still been held as usual in Sturgis Falls, but it too had been misrepresented by the media. The reality showed no unusual level of any disease had occurred. Media very intentionally reported on Sturgis Falls, implying that hundreds of people had been infected there. It bashed the happy people, their politics, their governor, and lied about everything. All of the numbers they used for cases and deaths were completely fabricated. They made bold, false statements that had absolutely no evidence links. There was the usual seasonal surge of COVID cases as had been true before, but that surge was happening in many states at the same time whether locked down or not. However, truth mattered little to those who bought into the lies. They continued calling the people of South Dakota, the governor, and the biker guests every ugly and spiteful name in the book while glorifying their house arrest and restrictions. The people of the pretty little town of Sturgis Falls greatly resented the horrid things said about them, but still looked forward to further rallies to come. Bottom line—it was/is relative and personal, just as we've always believed it should be.[69]

Consequently, we can easily conclude that "the science" being constantly touted as OUR guide to be followed, has never been followed accurately but it still became the mantra of the mainstream media. It was blasted across the country in feeds and news outlets, but it miserably failed to guide Americans with any solid or factual data nor any accurate assessment of true risk. It also flagrantly inflated all the numbers, especially of cases and deaths, and misrepresented cause and effect as well as the levels of risk to a predominantly healthy population. It's easy to see how so many citizens were disillusioned, even harmed by mental and emotional trauma as well as chronic sadness and depression from this cruel and reckless media propaganda. Ironically, at the same time, it also produced a certain sense of self-righteousness in some because they did what they perceived as the most compassionate and honorable things, even though it did not free them from it. Clearly, as we noted earlier, though the media called all anti-vax supporters "cultists," they refused to conform to the prevailing "vax" mentality, when in fact the constant promotion of vaccines was the real evidence of cult-like mentality which was easily exploited.[70]

As with most issues, there were at least two very divergent paths to take or ways to live in that time. Both camps saw sickness and hospitalization, and some died, though most deaths happened in the elderly, and in those with other chronic health issues. Surprisingly, the numbers of each camp were not significantly different. These two opposite belief systems did determine behaviors and lifestyles, but did not affect the ultimate outcomes. Many of the locked down and shut in folks grew increasingly vulnerable and some even severely mentally ill. Many succumbed to COVID-19 anyway, including some fully-vaxxed, and tragically died anyway, believing the lies of the 'wolves in sheep's clothing'. Some even believed and adhered to the lies to the end, also believing themselves to be justified, pure as the driven snow, and fully redeemed!

Globalist Big Tech Lies and the Real Agenda

Global masking enabled Big Tech and the CCP leadership to "train" the population in obedience and surrender of their human capital assets. It is abundantly clear that the Marxist mindset was utilized brilliantly by Big Tech. It demanded that all governments fight their "restrictions" war against the whole of humanity. The ultimate victory brought them both enormous profits, and the desired collateral damage. Big Tech's promotion of masks completely annulled the power, appeal, complexity, and communicability of the God-given human face. Big Tech also deliberately substituted the false "emotions" machines generated, for the real emotions of human beings. Developing children, mandated to wear masks, were sorely limited in their opportunities for normal play, to see faces, and interact socially. Withholding normal schooling from children taught them to avoid normal touch and correct social development.

During those 2-3 COVID-19 years, the mean IQ score for children born during the pandemic was diminished by more than 20 points from the averages of prior generations according to researchers at Brown University and Rhode Island Hospital. "We found that children born during the pandemic have significantly reduced verbal, motor, and overall cognitive performance compared to children born prepandemic...moreover, we found that males and all children born into lower socioeconomic families have been most affected. These results highlight that even in the absence of direct SARS-CoV-2 infection and COVID illness, the environmental changes associated with the COVID-19 pandemic are significantly negatively affecting infant and child development."[71]

Once again, Ms. Wolf related information of her experience of ten years spent in Big Tech space, seven of them as CEO of a tech company. She stated that human society is the competitor against which Big Tech MUST strategize. The majority of digital platforms intended to persuade people to stop living and operating in real time and work on the digital platform instead. That is their business model and it targets all private and community-based human time and space. Before the pandemic, most humans still did most things together in community. The goal of every digital company was to 'disrupt' any area of human society from which it was NOT profiting. The more 'Big Tech' can shut down human community and restrict humanity's freedoms, the wealthier Big Tech corporations become. Their invisible market of data purchasing and data warehousing is far beyond anyone's imagination. But all Big Tech business models acquired gargantuan advantages from the COVID-era suppression of normal human community and free assembly. Pandemic restrictions had absolutely no science behind them, but per agenda, they served the globalist wolves, and especially Big Tech extremely well for forcing people to rely nearly 100% on digital technology.[72] "Driving human interaction onto

Zoom and other non-secure platforms to do business was made to order for data-harvesting an enormous amount of personal information. It also ensured the old face-to-face human connections would eventually just shrivel up and die. Because of its basic simplicity, Zoom online quickly became a 'new normal.' Today it is rapidly approaching the setup for the 'Great Reset.'"[73]

Culture of a society MUST have human contact to be fruitful and grow. When the masses of people are isolated, they will fail to effectively teach, acclimate, and socialize their children. The culture of that society then dies, or lies in tragic disrepair, only to be replaced by something else, usually the Marxist doctrine of totalitarianism which is conveniently waiting in the wings ready to reset that society's original culture. This world has seen the likes of this despotic philosophy many different times, and though it may vary a little in use, its doctrines don't. Prohibiting the assembly of people kept us from attempting to gather and unite or form dissenting groups who might work hard to lead the masses away from these evil entities. It remains extremely important to remember the global forces of massive evil, led by the Prince of Evil himself, had been plotting, planning, promoting, and practicing for this upheaval for decades. Globalist allies are everywhere and involved in all areas of life. They already have vast wealth, power, and the will to control the world and make it over into their ideals. Every single tactic they used on all of us was meant to herald the complete disruption and overthrow of the current form of government while teaching them the need for transforming it to a far better system. "In the United States, this has been happening on university and college campuses for decades. A multitude of young adults have been brainwashed into seeing these Marxist ideas as a great improvement to the status quo! Other war tactics such as "divide and conquer" have been used liberally as well. Globalists understand that human contact is the greatest force underlying human freedom."[74] Clearly, martyred Charlie Kirk also understood exactly what was at stake in America, and worked tirelessly to give human contact and consistent truth all over American college campuses to turn the Marxist tide around. We desperately need an entire generation of Charlie Kirks!

Can you even imagine all of the rich and even necessary human education and sensory opportunities we were robbed of for at least two years? While it may be humdrum for some to go to the grocery store regularly and make personal choices of the merchandise, and perhaps a quick pickup of already selected foods is doable, but no one convinced most of us it was preferable. The cooking and preparation of our family's meals is no longer something we feel like dodging because its representative of the freedom we have to do so. If you've decided it works for you, it's OK, but you might want to ponder that and other things we completely missed the privilege of being able to do during COVID. Most of us are not unfamiliar with the benefits of Amazon, but knowing that in the first year of COVID alone, its revenues grew from $280.52 billion, to $386 billion as quoted in its annual report, becomes mind-boggling for several reasons. Building globalist corporations of extreme wealth and power is a major goal for the wolves. The colossal redistribution of wealth and investment accomplished during COVID, left the five largest companies in the world with more than $1 Trillion dollars. It is absolutely NO wonder that all the globalist schemes and goals were so lucrative and successful for these companies, since most people could only do most of their business through Big Tech's platforms. Globalists attained exactly what they planned for, and knew they would amass ever greater fortunes. At this point, the greatest wonder of all is that our nation has been able even to start recovering from the largest global debacle the world has ever seen, no thanks to the globalists and progressives among us.[74] Being thoughtful about such a statement, we might readily thank our Heavenly Father for His protection over our nation, and His unwillingness to give up on us.

Further, "the economic toll of the COVID-19 pandemic in the US reached US$14 trillion by the end of 2023. Putting a price tag on all the pain, suffering, and upheaval Americans and other people around the world have experienced because of COVID-19 is, of course, hard to do."[75] More than 1.1 million people died as a result of COVID-19 in the US, and many more were hospitalized or lost loved ones. Based on these findings, most economic losses were not due to health-care expenditures. The COVID-19 pandemic's economic consequences are unprecedented for the US by ANY measure.

The toll that it took on the nation's GDP was twice the size of that of the Great Recession of 2007-2009. Another perspective—it was 20 times greater than the economic costs of the 9/11 terrorist attacks and 40 times greater than the toll of any other disaster to befall the US in the 21st century to date. Other non-specific costs, like physical and mental health costs of the US population were even tougher to estimate and not included in these totals."[76]

By July of 2021, many people were gathering once again. This was the biggest pushback on restrictions yet seen. "State Senator Kim Thatcher and State Senator Dennis Linthicum, both from Oregon (Rs) called for an investigation into the CDC and FDA for their handling of pandemic data. They wanted to hold the CDC accountable for changing the way death certificates were recorded, and other concerns."[77] Big Tech continued censoring and suspending accounts of people who kept trying to inform the masses of the true reality. Twitter, CNN, and Linked In had all censored truth with their globalist "fact-checkers," one of the biggest travesties of the era. Big Tech also continued prohibiting anyone from raising any questions about the mRNA vaccines, especially from "known conservatives."

For conservative journalists, bloggers, and conscientious citizens the many forms of censorship were also constant. Sometimes, Big Tech would even rewrite their own versions of stories or blogs, present them completely out of context, twist words around, and make them say what was never intended at all. Some of these tactics would even set other writers against one another because of what was deceitfully said, and never had been written at all. There could be NO doubt it was an extensive, digitally-enhanced smear campaign. "Real journalism wasn't allowed, nor could it be trusted to be real, since anything deemed "misinformation" was automatically removed; in other words the real facts were not seen. It was impossible to demand corrections or retractions of Big Tech errors. Good editors were essentially intimidated to the point of helplessness. The vast majority of good and honorable writers were bashed with global headlines that declared, "they were shut-down for spreading 'medical misinformation' or 'vaccine myths.' In an incredibly short space of time good writers were often stripped of their income, their reputation, their friend groups, and their status. Many later had to start over or stop writing. It was impossible to speak to a governmental official, since Big Tech had frequently donated big money to electoral campaigns. This, incidentally was exactly what happened to Dr. Naomi Wolf!"[78]

The Vaccine Passport Controversy—End of Human Liberty

By the end of 2021, vaccine passports had been introduced in many states and nations. These passports were mandated along with the vaccination mandates and would allow Big Tech companies authority over the people. It actually amounted to a system of coercive bribery. It was like making an illegal deal with the people who were sick of lockdowns to get free from it, only to sell their souls to get it. It went like this: "If you want to do all the things you've always done including worship, visit family, keep a job to feed your family, go to a movie, or ride a long-distance train or plane—this is how to do it. You will need a vaccine passport. However, passports are central in the big transition into a world where all humans are at the mercy of Big Tech and global oligarchs. According to the World Economic Forum (WEF), "There is growing hope that in time the world's populations could become COVID-19 immune and there are promising signs that the vaccines are 'highly effective!'"(Massive Lies) The expectation is that with the vaccine, some aspects of life will return to normal—especially when it comes to travel—which has been particularly hard-hit. This is where a 'vaccine passport' or 'e-vaccination certification of compliance for border crossing regulations, might become a required travel document, to enable seamless border-crossing and the harmonization of varying national laws."[79] Such requirements requiring personal assault, were then and continue to be completely illegal.

"There are many truthful journalists, conservative politicians, and strategists who are clear that for our country's sake, knowing the above information promoted by the WEF, cannot benefit us! These people have warned us publicly about the heinous implications of vax passports. In addition, passports have also been heavily pushed by global health officials and that can't be good. It was also clearly understood to be a way to incentivize greater vaccine compliance. The vaccine passport was hailed as THE KEY to ending the pandemic and 'returning to normal life.'"[80] What it really is—blackmail, which is still illegal!

However, proof of vaccine has always been confirmed on a piece of paper! Consequently, passports were NOT needed. First, they signified far more than just proof of vaccine—the end of human liberty. Remember, it was also illegal in almost all instances to demand that proof—it's a violation of HIPPA and other laws to even ask that question. Employers aren't allowed to ask any personal medical questions of their employees. As many critics offered, if this war on passports were lost, no further resistance would be allowed. Everyone would simply have one all the time. Further, when the passport contained your entire vaccination history, any other desired medical history, financial information, etc. could be added very easily. Anyone who refused to participate, could easily be tracked anyway, and eventually the lack of that control piece could easily determine if you could shop for food, meet friends at a restaurant, or travel anywhere. "It would be the first step to a global, social credit system already being pushed by the WEF and others. A similar system in the People's Republic of China literally enslaves a billion Chinese people. The CCP can find ANYONE in five minutes flat because of its 360-degree surveillance system. "Good" citizens can get a boost in their personal score. "Bad" citizens have potential opportunities "closed" to them such as schools, jobs, and homes."[81]

The warnings continued—once the passports were rolled out—any other function the government decides to include could easily be included on the passports in a matter of minutes. Your bank account access could be switched on or off like a faucet, depending on what you might have said on a social media platform. The officials who have jurisdiction over and ability to manage it could very literally 'rule the world.' There is NO question about the massive push of the globalists toward digital currency— it's an integral part of the Global Reset agenda. Once the digital currency is initiated there will be no going back or fixing it. We MUST absolutely reject any attempt to get vaccine passports, because it's tantamount to opening a garbage dumpster full of snakes and it will be the immediate vehicle for digital currency and central banking. There will be no further capitalism as we know it, no free assembly, no privacy, no choices, and of course, no escape.

"In April, 2021, President Biden, "ruled out introducing mandatory federal COVID19 vaccination passports, saying citizen's privacy and rights should be protected. (Even now, that is hard to believe he said such a thing!) Schemes to introduce such passports had been touted around the world as a way to enable safe circulation of people while fighting the pandemic. Critics said such documents would be discriminatory. The US said it did not and would not support a 'system that requires Americans to carry a credential.' Addressing reporters, the White House press secretary…said there would be no 'federal vaccinations database' or a 'federal mandate requiring everyone to obtain a single vaccination credential'. Our interest is simple—Americans' privacy and rights should be protected; so these systems cannot be used against people unfairly."[82] Wow, for all the measures Biden 'rubber-stamped' to cooperate with the Globalists' plans for RESET, thankfully, that one didn't make the cut! Currently, the US is still in an exploratory phase with the Biden administration announcing an executive order in 2022 that led to further research into digital currencies. "Today, (mid 2024) 134 countries and currency unions, representing 98% of global

GDP, are exploring a Central Banking Digital Currency (CBDC). 68 countries are in the advanced phase of exploration— development, pilot, or launch. 19 of the G20 group countries are now in the advanced stages of CBDC development. The digital dollar has the potential to become the backbone of the United States economy, that would drastically change the face of global commerce. But there are still numerous conservative lawmakers in particular, voicing their concerns, because the electronic currency would give the U.S. government and the eventual New World Order unprecedented control over all our business transactions and private lives. While the US does not yet have a CBDC, President Biden and his administration have been systematically replacing our paper money with the digital dollar, so the work is in progress."[83]

The data show that all of the G20 countries, which have some of the largest economies in the world, are IN some phase of developing a CBDC. These include Argentina, Australia, Brazil, Canada, China, European Union (EU), France, Germany, India, Indonesia, Italy, Japan, Mexico, Russia, Saudi Arabia, South Africa, South Korea, Turkey, and the United Kingdom. In the United States, the 'digital dollar' is the proposed form of electronic currency that could be used to buy or sell almost any goods and services in the US just like the paper greenbacks are used today. However, a CBDC does NOT exist in paper form but would be solely transacted and represented in an electronic format.[84]

"The money would be directly issued by the Federal Reserve and live on a digital ledger, such as blockchain, which is a shared, immutable ledger facilitating the process of recording transactions and tracking assets in a business network. There is no need for traditional banks to handle certain types of transactions or record-keeping. A digital currency would require a fully integrated digital infrastructure and could take years of research and development to launch. However, CBDCs gained popularity in the late 2010s when global technology companies announced their own digital currencies, most notably Facebook's now-defunct LIBRA. Dozens of central banks and governments have since launched digital currencies or pilot programs, according to the data from the Washington D.C.-based non-partisan think tank, 'The Atlantic Council.'"[85]

China had high expectations for the performance of its central bank digital currency (CBDC), the e-CNY. Usage of online payments systems like WeChat Pay and Alipay are nearly universal and certainly widespread among the population, so the Chinese government expected its digital currency to take off quickly. In 2019, China began piloting its CBDC system. After a slow start, uptake accelerated rapidly, with 26 cities serving as test beds and 5.6 million merchants registered to use the currency nationwide as of 2023. Its implementation went into overdrive in 2024. China's embrace of digital currency is NOT going away and e-CNY is already involved in experiments with other central banks, aiming to trade directly with each other's currencies instead of going through the US dollar. That, in turn, could reduce the potential reach of US sanction and blunt Washington's financial power. The Bahamas, Jamaica, and Nigeria have CBDCs and Central Bankers in Brazil, China, EU, India, and the UK are at the forefront of the technology. The Central Bank of Iran launched on June 18, 2024.

As of July 2025, the US Federal Reserve has still not decided to transition to a CBDC or supplement its existing monetary system with one. It is researching the effects a CBDC would have on the dollar, the US, and the global economy. The Federal Reserve is committed to ensuring the continued safety and availability of cash and is considering a CBDC as a means to expand safe payment options, not to reduce or replace them. However, more than half of the world's banks are exploring or developing digital currencies. In December, 2023, Russia and China expressed their intent to abandon the US dollar in their bilateral transactions. Russia has already been using the Euro as their preferred settlement currency within BRICS. If the BRICS system continues to grow, it could become a challenge to the US dollar. The US will definitely proceed with the CBDC project slowly, using ten major banking firms, including: BNY Mellon, Citi, HSBC, Mastercard, PNC Bank, Swift, TD Bank, Truist,

US Bank, and Wells Fargo. With the global furor of a single currency for all, and the numbers of CBDC steadily growing, the US will not be able to fight the tide ultimately, but it is not in a hurry to transition at this time.[68] Centralizing a digital currency is not without its drawbacks, however. Digital currencies are particularly vulnerable to 'cybercrime' and efficiently regulating this new technology can require a massive administrative, financial and legal effort. By some critics, CBDCs are also seen as prestige projects with little to no impact. Adoption rates also seem uncertain due to concerns about data privacy and security. In the Bahamas, the first official implementation of a CBDC only led to an adoption rate of eight percent and a circulation of roughly 300,000 Sand Dollars."[86]

Contrary to the real facts, there has been much speculation about China's use of CBDC to the global economy. When discussing the vaccine passports and the possibilities of how China would use them as the basis of establishing a sophisticated system of individual buying and selling based on merit in following the rules. However, the reality is different. Over the past several years China has been steadily making progress towards digital 'renminbi' and now seems poised to become the first major economy to launch an official CBDC, but it's far more complicated than that, as China's digital currency project faces a variety of challenges at home and abroad. Though the Chinese government is further ahead in digital currency research than any other major economy, these economic and political challenges mean that after nearly a decade of development and several years of localized testing there is still no clear date for a full-scale launch of China's digital 'renminbi'(also known as e-CNY).

While a timeline for the final launch of the digital renminbi is uncertain, China's goals in creating one are much clearer. In addition to exploring the possibilities of using CBDC for cross-border transactions…"at home, the CCP has long been clear on its intention to limit the power and market share of both commercial banks and digital payment corporations that operate independently of the state, especially Alipay (owned by Alibaba) and WeChat Pay (owned by Tencent). Some observers have pointed out that a centralized digital currency would allow Beijing to more closely watch both individual transactions and the powerful Chinese private financial technology sector. Public perception is that the e-CNY offers no reason to change from the more developed and more convenient alternatives already existing. Some analysts speculate the e-CNY will not be able to overtake private-sector alternatives at all without substantial government interference to the point of mandatory use."[87] From the perspective of this author, the prospects of a soon-to-be, global currency, though an enormous amount has been done, is still not as close to fruition as we might have imagined. Will it happen? Yes, definitely! When will it happen? We don't see it fully implemented in the near future. Interestingly, this author believes that in God's New World Order where everything will be controlled by the Anti-Christ, including the money, he could set up a one-world currency very quickly, having nothing at all to do with current plans and technologies!

Chapter 12

Big Tech and Government Power Overreach

The Vaccine Passport Controversy—End of Human Liberty?

As we begin this chapter, we want to see how the concept of a vaccine passport would play out in God's coming New World Order as He has planned it. First, that New World Order will not look much like the plans of the World Economic Forum and its proponents. However, there are some details that even many believers in Jesus Christ may have missed. The books of Isaiah, Daniel, Zechariah, and Revelation within Scripture, in particular, give us a great many details about what that time will be like for people remaining on earth. This author believes in the grammatical, historical, and literal interpretation of God's Holy Word. It speaks of a seven-year period of judgment known as the Tribulation. In more recent times, many Bible students have tended to view this time in a very different light, but any student of Scriptural Eschatology (study of End Times) should carefully compare All such Bible passages. We believe that all those folks who previously accepted Jesus Christ as their Lord and Savior will be taken to heaven by Jesus Himself who will "rapture" them out of this earth BEFORE this horrible time of Tribulation is visited upon Earth. One of the most crucial parts of the Biblical New World Order is that it will NOT be run by this large group of Globalist Wolves we've learned so much about, though they obviously believe they will run it. No, the whole system will be administered by one man with a couple of assistants. Kingdoms and nations will all bow to that man's leadership. Scripture calls him The Antichrist, but he has some other names as well. One of those is 'the Beast.' There will be one ruler, one government, one religion, one monetary and economic system, one military, and one way to live. In the "New World Order" or Tribulation, every person will be "one of us" or life will be worth nothing. Everyone will be under the authority of the Beast, but later will be required to actually worship him to survive. All use and distribution of money will depend solely on one's loyalty to the Antichrist's authority. This will be ensured by requiring "the mark of the Beast to have the ability to buy or sell, that is to do the business of living. Scripture says:

"And he causes all, the small and the great, and the rich and the poor, the freemen and the slaves, to be given a mark on their right hand or on their forehead and he provides that no one will be able to buy or to sell, except the one who has the mark, either the name of the beast or the number of his name. Here is wisdom. Let him who has understanding calculate the number of the beast, is the number of a man; and his number is six hundred and sixty-six [666]." Revelation 13:16-18 (NASB)

The Bible clearly shows the universal mark of the Beast system with the coming cashless society. All the big plans of all the current nations will be worthless when the Antichrist comes into his Satan-controlled power. Vaccination passports of any kind will not be necessary—the entire globe will be under this system and record-keeping no problem at all. Anyone who fails to comply with the system, will be in constant danger of being eliminated. Here is the biggest caveat of all—anyone who takes that mark, no matter if he/she is starving, will have no other opportunity of an eternal home in heaven with Jesus Christ. To live and follow the Antichrist is the ultimate rejection and betrayal of God's Son. Famine, war, pestilence, and death will all be present in the Tribulation, but will be exponentially more life-threatening than anything ever experienced on earth before, due to God's judgments.

Revelation 6 speaks of the notorious Four Horsemen of the Apocalypse who deliver the first of these judgments:

> "...behold, a white horse! Its rider had a bow...and he came out conquering, and to conquer (war)...out came another horse, bright red, its rider was permitted to take peace from the earth, so that people should slay one another, and he was given a great sword (death)...behold, a black horse! Its rider had a pair of scales in his hand...a voice saying, 'A quart of wheat for a denarius (a day's wage), and three quarts of barley for a denarius, and do not harm the oil and wine! (famine)...behold, a pale horse! Its rider's name was Death, and Hades followed him. They were given authority over a fourth of the earth, to kill with sword and with famine and with pestilence and by wild beasts of the earth." Revelation 6:1-8 ESV

> "...You yourselves are fully aware that the Day of the Lord will come like a thief in the night. While people are saying, 'There is peace and security,' then sudden destruction will come upon them as labor pains come upon a pregnant woman, and THEY WILL NOT ESCAPE." I Thessalonians 5:1-3 ESV

From the perspective of this author, the prospects of a soon-to-be, global currency, while an enormous amount has been done, is still not as close to fruition as we might have imagined. Will it happen? Yes, definitely! When will it happen? We really don't see it fully functioning in the near future. It may well be that this piece of the plan will continue to defy international unity until our Lord's return for His saints. There is no doubt that the Antichrist will be able to get the job done in short-order!

Implications of Internet Data Harvesting

Many of us use an enormous amount of technology on our computers and smart phones as well as other devices fairly well, and we feel reasonably comfortable doing so. However, there is so much information regarding our regular use which we often don't have a clue about, even when it's a part of your job! There are several terms we need to understand at least enough to protect ourselves better. Not long ago there was a serious case of Google's piracy, obviously uninvited and trespassing on private information. We usually have no idea someone is hacking our platform accounts and applications, so we tend to forget about it and hope that no real damage is being done. Our Personal Identifying Details (PID) such as name, location, phone number, search history, etc. are really VERY easy to obtain from most accounts. Our Internet Protocol or IP address is not as easily located on our equipment, but it is part of the security protection of personal privacy and hides our online activity from stroke-by-stroke surveillance. Another protection we have is the so-called "Terms of Service." Most of us scroll right on by this Impossible-to-understand lawyer speak, but it is a legal document between the user and the media platform; spelling out the boundaries on those platforms' use of the user's personal data. These two forms of protection have stood squarely in the path of Big Tech's ability to do what they want to do, especially as it pertains to data harvesting. Big Tech wants to take full control and have the ability to take and use all data it finds however it wants to use it.[1]

"We can all have access to these platforms through "paywalls" meaning we must keep regularly paying for that access for whatever we want access to. But paying for that access naturally doesn't work in both directions. Platforms expect us to pay well for access, but they want to harvest as much data as possible for nothing and continue to use it any way they can. From the tech world's point of view (POV), the true genius of COVID restrictions was that Big Tech became the paywall!"[2] The intent was for each of us to get vaccine "credit cards" to swipe for access to goods and services, and keep those 'cards' current with continued "vaccine payments." The whole world would be the platform. Thankfully, to this day, that is still not the case, especially in the US and Europe, but it is still a part of the eventual plan. Today, there is a tight alliance between the US government and Big Tech, and the intent is for that alliance to stay tight, forming the desired global plan of corporate/governmental capitalism. (the brain child of the WEF) The ultimate intent is totalitarianism which is beyond dangerous. Now, the entire world has become a fully digitized platform, owned by five giant tech corporations, that can be switched on and off at will. Knowing this, it is not at all difficult to understand how the New World System of the Antichrist will know anything and everything about everyone!

There is still much to be understood about Big Tech because its given entities slip in and out of ranking position as their stock values fluctuate. "Tech stocks have been among the top-performing investments over the past two decades, but the tech rally hit a wall in 2022. For many years, Meta Platforms (META), Amazon (AMZN), Apple (AAPL), Netflix (NFLX), and Alphabet (GOOG, GOOGL), were consistently among the highest-growth stocks in the market—collectively known as FAANG. Unfortunately, some FAANG stocks lost their edge, and several of them have even changed their names. Market commentators and tech investors have coined a new acronym for the top five mega-cap tech stocks in 2023: MAMAA. Netflix has been hit particularly hard, and the company dropped behind its peers in growth and prominence. Google and Facebook rebranded themselves as Alphabet and Meta Platforms, while Microsoft (MSFT) grew to a more than $1 trillion valuation. Now the new Big (5) Tech acronym is MAMAA—for Meta, Amazon, Microsoft, Apple, and Alphabet. Each now has a market cap of more than $1 trillion."[3] It is NOT difficult to understand the enormity of this kind of power. It is still important to know these are the top five according to Forbes, however there are many other large corporations in the mix worth only a little less. Each of these top corporations has a monopoly in one or more products. Clearly, these fly in the face of our nation's anti-trust laws, but they seem meaningless when it comes to Big Tech!

As for the Global Predators who are currently betraying their own countries of origin; they believe they will always have controlling seats at the table along with these controlling Tech elites, but they are sorely mistaken. In the same way dissidents and others can be switched off and on, so too can the Globalist wolves be switched on and off, if Big Tech isn't liking the direction they want to go. Granted, Big Tech is mostly controlled by Globalist wolves, however, economic coups have happened with conflict-of-interest issues for decades and can certainly happen again. With upwards of $6-8 trillion dollars-worth of power, ANYONE can be turned off or on, including commentators, journalists, physicians, and even dissident technologists! All information grids could be gone. Worse still, supply chains could be annihilated to create global havoc the likes of which no one has ever seen. Personalities can be switched off—even whole populations can be shut off. If it can and is done now, it will certainly be no problem for Antichrist.

Note the following example: After rioters stormed the U.S. Capitol on January 6, 2020, some of the United States' most powerful institutions sprang into action to punish the leaders of the failed insurrection. However these institutions weren't necessarily the ones you might expect. "Facebook and Twitter suspended the accounts of President Donald Trump for posts supposedly praising the rioters, though that was Twitter's take. Amazon, Apple, and Google effectively banished Parler, an alternative to Twitter that Trump's supporters had used to encourage and coordinate the attack, by blocking its access to Web-hosting services and app stores. Major financial service apps such as PayPal and Stripe, stopped processing payments for the Trump campaign and for accounts that had funded travel expenses to Washington, D.C. for Trump's supporters. The speed of these technology companies' reactions stands in stark contrast to the feeble response from the United States' governing institutions."[4]

In 2021-2022, freedom was lost via the vaccine passports that made it into use in Europe, Canada, Australia, Israel, and several states in the US without a single shot fired. To this day, information on vaccines and PCR tests goes into a designated tech 'system.' Only a handful knows the who, where, and what of it! The only information of higher priority is probably that of nuclear power secrets. But the worst information of all is that there are no regulatory laws, no avenue to check for errors, and no transparency in the Big Tech corporations that compiled this data base. Consequently there is zero accountability. Your ability to say 'yes' or 'no' about any of your personal information is no longer up to you. It is all whatever the developers say it is. In the future, should another vaccine mandate be initiated, whether or not the actual science supports its use, there are a plethora of highly troublesome questions that will no doubt be ignored. What about individual bodily autonomy? What about our human rights? What about our freedom of association? What about informed consent? What about our democratic way of life? All of these were already done away with or simply disregarded the last time the subject was raised and questioned.[5] At the same time everything people do in this world is digitized. As our lives were digitized, they needed to be tracked. The second it was tracked; it was controlled! While there are numerous services offering protection of our personal information, and aiding in retrieving it, none are infallible. "There is no such thing as true privacy in the digital age."[6]

"States have been the primary actors in global affairs for nearly 400 years. That is changing as a handful of large tech companies rival them for geopolitical influence. "The aftermath of the January 6 riot serves as the latest proof that Amazon, Apple, Facebook, Google, and Twitter (now X) are no longer merely large companies; they have taken control of aspects of society, the economy, and national security that were long the exclusive preserve of the state. The same goes for Chinese technology companies, such as Alibaba, Byte Dance, and Tencent. Non-state actors are increasingly shaping geopolitics, with Big Tech companies in the lead."[7] Although Europe wants to play, its companies do not have the size or geopolitical influence to compete with their American and Chinese counterparts.

"All of the Big Tech corporations may also utilize surveillance and AI to monitor employees, which will definitely impact privacy and fair employment practices. Through control of e-commerce platforms, app stores, and other gateways, corporations have the power to extort fees from sellers and dictate business terms. Allowing Big Tech to monopolize AI is very risky business—digital content comes next. It allows them to exploit their role as so-called gatekeepers of digital infrastructures to make large profits."[8] That impacts the economy as a whole, the way people do business, their rights as employees and consumers, and the choices they can make. As tech companies continue to dominate virtual space, they increasingly exert sovereignty. Unfortunately all of Big Tech's policies served the CCP as much as they served Big Tech. A 'West', 'locked-down', 'restricted', 'masked' and an 'accepting, society-discrimination based on 'vax status,' mimics the CCP ideals. It was 'West', (primarily the US), that forfeited its historically competitive advantage over the CCP, including its individualism, its human rights, its universal equality, and its freedom. Now that our human spaces can be closed on the mandate of any random board of health, we have allowed a world where a vast hurdle has already been leaped, and the contest won. Big Tech companies have no need to compete with any of our former, smaller entities since most of those have been nullified and / or ruined.

Hypothetically, if we look ahead ten years, what are the most harmful, even menacing changes likely to occur in digital technology and human usage of digital systems? Some 300 experts identified five main areas of potential impact:[9]

The concern that digital systems will continue to be driven by profit incentives in economics and power incentives in politics. This would likely lead to advanced surveillance and data collection aimed at controlling people rather than empowering them to act freely and share ideas. Experts worry that ethical design will be an afterthought and digital systems be released before thorough testing. The impact would likely be to increase inequality and compromise democratic systems.

Experts fear the best of knowledge will be lost or neglected in a sea of mis- and disinformation and that systems previously informing the public will be further decimated. That would make the facts harder to find amid a sea of entertaining distractions, bald-faced lies and targeted manipulation. People's cognitive skills will continue to decline. "Reality itself is under siege," as emerging digital tools convincingly create deceptive or alternate realities, (like AI).

These experts fear new threats to rights as privacy becomes harder, if not impossible to maintain. They list surveillance advances, sophisticated bots, (automated programs that can mimic a user and are easy to use wrongly) embedded in civic spaces, the spread of deepfakes, (video of a person where a face or body part is digitally altered to make them appear as someone else) and disinformation, advanced facial recognition systems, and widening social and digital divides as looming threats. They foresee crimes and harassment spreading, as well as new challenges to humans' agency and security. A topmost concern is the probability that more sophisticated AI will lead to job losses, with a rise in poverty and diminished human dignity.

Humanity's embrace of digital systems has already spurred higher levels of anxiety and depression and this -will undoubtedly not improve with more technology. It's been fairly clear that mental and physical problems do stem from tech-abetted loneliness and social isolation.

Finally, concerns have been raised that norms, standards and regulation around technology will not evolve quickly enough to improve the social and political interactions of individuals and organizations. Two overreaching concerns associated with this one—a trend toward autonomous weapons and cyberwarfare and the prospect of runaway digital systems. Things could worsen as the pace of tech-changes accelerates. People's distrust in each other may grow and their faith in institutions deteriorate. Those, in turn, could deepen already undesirable levels of polarization, cognitive dissonance, and public withdrawal from vital interaction. Digital systems might actually get too big and important to avoid, making all users captives.[9]

"Ian Brenner wrote an earlier article than the one previously cited in this chapter that gives a touch of reality to the difference between Big Tech and Big 'anything else'! He said he never felt the same way about Big Oil or about Big Banking, or any other physically large entities. The reason was because these all existed in real physical space. As a consequence, they were regulated in physical space or sometimes not effectively regulated—nonetheless, they were inside sovereign government entities, and within existing territories. But now, tech corporations actually have sovereignty over their digital spaces. They not only determine what the rules are going to be, but they actually create them from the ground up. They are the architects—they drive the algorithms—they own the data—they decide what to do with it—everything about that space is the mandate of the tech companies themselves. That is the kind of power in digital space that increasingly feels like a parallel world to physical space where governments are in charge. During COVID, Big Tech responded to issues almost instantly and made decisions. No one voted for their rules. They just decided what they would do or not do, exerting their own sovereignty. That thought remains and so does that sovereignty today. There are no boundaries, and no accountability. It's a little bit scary, no-WAIT! It is actually a whole lot scary![10]

Systematic Larceny of Lower and Middle Classes

By June, 2021, this author and her spouse were both critically ill with COVID-19, Delta variant. We were both hospitalized with very high oxygen consumption for two weeks and 4 weeks respectively, but thankfully we were given the usual drug regimen of steroids, regular meds, anticoagulants, and system-related meds—NO Remdesivir. We managed, with our Lord's direction and protection, to survive without intubation and ventilators. The illness was NOT without its trials and sequelae, but again, thankfully, we have been able to manage post-COVID scarring and other post-issues—all without taking the toxic vaccination. If we had it to do again, we would still make the same decisions. With that said, we may address a few other issues in a later chapter, but for now, we believe this late infection and time line was an important turning point for a number of significant pandemic factors, most of which occurred while we were ill.

First, the public health agencies had usurped a level of power unprecedented in US or world history, which was NOT hard to realize as their decisions were increasingly obnoxious at every level. There was no real need to continue the charade they had created in terms of ANY of the mandates, but continue them and exacerbate them they did. There were occasional normal and seasonal rises in numbers, but the numbers were proving in many ways greatly exaggerated and did NOT represent true risks. Nevertheless, the public health agencies such as the CDC and WHO seemingly had the power to reshape our society and intervene in our capitalist economies in ways we'd never known before. They had not yet reached the zenith of their expectations for the pandemic and they would keep it going as long as possible. With their aggressive and deplorable dictates, they simply ignored the laws of democratic lands, bypassing our Congresses, Parliaments, Cabinets and Commonwealths, described by Ms. Wolf as "nothing short of a slow-motion coup!"

At first, the masses didn't recognize what was happening and it was touted as 'good-for-all," which of course wasn't true. It was good for higher-classed elites and globalists, but few others. CDC moratoriums were perpetrated on owners in majority black communities. As could have been predicted, that led to the massive transfer of assets from middle-class working people, to the coffers of large institutional and corporate investors. More than 110,000 eating and drinking venues closed in 2020 because they were FORCED to stop doing business under the lockdowns. Without the business making the necessary revenues, owners often had to sell their buildings to live, which fed right into the pockets of the wealthy who COULD buy them, making more money.

By the end of March, 2021, those same corporate investors purchased over 15% of ALL homes for sale in the U.S. In many parts of the country, single-family homes to buy were not easy to find in many markets and American companies were NOT the only entities buying them; very often it was a foreign government, especially China and the CCP, or foreign globalists and investors—that is still true today in 2025. Boards of Health and their unnecessary restrictions killed the livelihoods of tens of thousands of people, leaving poverty and destitution behind them. In fact, as this process was well under way, the carnage of people's homes and businesses were a clearly large part of deliberate societal breakdown and a part of the global agenda. This brought another kind of epidemic where wealthy local buyers made regular calls, posted signage, and sent cards and letters through the mail, sometimes anonymously, announcing they would pay cash for any properties in the area, no matter their condition. This eliminated the ability of others who were looking for and able to buy a home, to find anything suitable. All possibilities had been snapped up to make more money, either on high-priced rentals or over-priced houses.[11]

The worst lockdowns and restrictions were in the very large cities and surrounds of San Francisco, Boston, New York, Los Angeles, and Chicago; all areas where real estate was most in demand in the beginning. However, as the communities began to look abandoned and then uncared for by commercial owners, residential owners wanting to get out to freer areas and states had to sell at big discounts because other would-be buyers didn't want a home in a now nearly-abandoned neighborhood with little value. Worst of all, it wasn't just businesses and homes that were ruined, but in many cases, whole communities were decimated. They looked nothing like their former pleasant and well cared-for residences or towns. But there is yet far more information on the ramifications of this housing/community travesty. "An excellent research project was conducted in 2020 through the UCLA Luskin School of Public Affairs till June of 2020. They looked at the question: How can LA's working-class communities of color disrupt the devastating impact of speculative capital that is raising housing costs, creating displacement, and destabilizing neighborhoods?"[12]

Project rationale was spot-on. "Globally, there has been a shift toward land and housing serving as an investment tool rather than satisfying the basic human need for shelter. Residential real estate now constitutes 42% of global wealth. In Los Angeles, there are major racial and ethnic wealth disparities, with Latino and Black households having about 1% of every dollar of Whites' wealth.

Renters who make up 63% of all Angeleno households—have not fared well as their homes have been commercialized, and they have almost no opportunity or leverage to intervene in the real estate market to protect their families' interests or to keep their communities whole. Low-income neighborhoods of color such as those in South and East Los Angeles are disproportionately vulnerable to regional economic changes in the city. Considering the current public health crisis and the economic crisis projected to follow, low-income neighborhoods of color will face a growing impact of speculation and displacement by financial actors with greater, more immediate access to capital."[13]

Three years later, in June, 2023, a new study found that racial disparities in homeownership within Los Angeles County continued to persist. The report based on pre-pandemic data... "reveals that despite anti-discrimination laws and regulations, households of color continue to face significant barriers to accessing low-cost mortgage credit, hindering their path to homeownership and exacerbating the racial wealth gap. The report highlighted the central role of homeownership in wealth creation in the U.S. and emphasized how limited access to this wealth-generating vehicle impacts households of color. Specifically, the analysis exposed the inequitable treatment of people of color in the mortgage market, particularly among Black and Latino applicants in L.A. County."[13] The bottom line is that non-equitable dealings on houses for minorities are still inequitable regardless of credit histories and creditworthiness, and COVID-19 did nothing to help their situation, which does NOT bother globalists or the execution of their agenda in the least.

Further disparities resulting from the Globalist larceny of COVID-19 within the racial and ethnic minorities in the U.S. have included higher rates of infection, more hospital stays, and more deaths caused by the virus than white, non-Hispanic people. Income, access to health insurance, occupation, and housing security were all issues of disparity. Minorities infected with COVID-19 also experienced greater negative aftereffects in health and work loss than did similarly infected white participants. Those negative impacts affected their poorer health status, activity levels, and ability to work. "Though we can't specifically pinpoint the cause, we know that, historically, these populations may have a harder time accessing health care, which in turn complicates their recovery, in spite of displaying very few symptomatic differences across clinical study groups. This leads researchers to believe that the differences may be associated with socioeconomic disparities."[14]

Going back to the larceny of the lower and middle classes, we look at our reality now. "In the post-war era, the average hourly compensation of American workers rose with our productivity gains. The economy grew and the middle class expanded with more purchasing power. However in the late 1970s, while productivity gains continued much like they had been, wages started to flatten. In the mid-80s the median household's income stopped growing completely when adjusted for inflation. Today, if you are an hourly-wage worker (the majority) you are earning no more than you earned in 1969, proportionately, and job security has also declined. So, despite an economy that's far larger and more productive than 40-50 years ago, the typical American worker has gone essentially nowhere. "The standard explanation calls this 'neutral market forces,' especially globalization and technological innovations that have made many working Americans less competitive. However this standard explanation doesn't account for much, (just a few years). It also doesn't explain why other advanced economies facing similar forces didn't succumb to them. Worse yet, it doesn't explain why so much of the nation's income and wealth have risen to the top like cream in fresh milk."[15]

America's middle class has shrunk because of its declining bargaining power—orchestrated and directed by America's oligarchy (globalists). The economic gains that should have gone to the middle class went instead to the hyperwealthy interests at the top. Post-war corporate governance by business owners and managers was considered a public trust, a stewardship, that was operated for the benefit of the people. However, by the late 70s and early 80's, a radically different corporate ownership emerged from "corporate raiders" who mounted hostile takeovers with high-yield junk bonds. Raiders used leveraged buyouts and undertook proxy wars against the 'industrial statesmen" who, in their view, were depriving stockholders of the wealth that properly belonged to them. Raiders assumed that stockholders were the only legitimate owners of the corporation and the only valid purpose of the corporation was to maximize shareholder returns. This did NOT happen by accident. It was a product of changes in laws governing corporations and of financial markets—changes that were promoted by the monied interests, America's oligarchs (globalists). Changed laws made it possible for corporate raiders to get the capital and the regulatory approvals they needed to force unfriendly takeovers. During the 70s, there were 13 hostile takeovers of companies valued at $1 billion or more. In the 80s, there were 150. CEOs began to see their primary role as driving up share prices. The easiest and most direct way to do this was cutting payrolls, a firm's largest single expense.'[16]

Ultimately, the corporate statesmen of the 1950s and 1960s were replaced by the corporate Butchers of the 1980s and 1990s, whose nearly exclusive focus was to "cut out the fat" and "cut to the bone!'" With these 'unethical corporate transformations,' the purpose of the American corporation was forever changed. Share prices soared as did the salaries of CEOs. Results have been touted as "efficient" because resources theoretically have been shifted to 'higher and better uses.' The human costs of this transformation have been astronomical. Millions of workers have lost jobs and wages. Many communities were abandoned. Any benefits were not widely shared. As corporations have steadily weakened workers' bargaining power, the link between productivity and workers' income has been broken. Almost all gains from growth have risen to the top—most workers are less economically secure, and very few can afford any shares of stock in their own companies. Now the richest 1% of Americans own 52% of all the shares of stock owned by Americans. The richest 10%, own 93%. The nation's economic gains, once distributed broadly to the working and middle class—sit squarely on top.[17]

In summary, "making the progression of the history of American oligarchs make sense, we can easily understand how these American corporate leaders became the greedy and powerful monsters who have robbed the American lower and working classes systematically for decades. Most of the wealthiest of these acquired their wealth and power in this manner."[18] Having now rubbed shoulders for several decades with the oligarchs of the world, they have all become the Globalist wolves of today. The COVID pandemic was just one more way to increase that power and wealth to these same elites, to continue doing what they intend to keep right on doing. The costs and damages done to all global citizens is not now nor has it been a cause of concern to them. They have no consciences, nor compassion for all the masses they've harmed. The New World Order will in their minds be the ultimate prize where they can sit atop their self-constructed thrones and rule without hindrance. Now, grand luxury buildings await the children of these Global wolves. In London, New York, Paris, San Francisco, and many other showcase cities, their towers and mansions just keep on rising and flourishing.

The Vaccine Mandate—Damage and Illegality

September 9, 2021 was a day many Americans think of as a disaster for several reasons, but mostly because of the horrible and tragic aftermath. President Biden gave his infamous, and angry speech to those folks who had NOT yet been vaccinated. The rudeness and crudeness of it was breath-taking in its presumption. Most American citizens had NEVER heard a sitting president speak to his constituents so aggressively as he did that day. The basic message was, "If you people can't get the necessary vaccinations, we will force you to get them in whatever manner we need to use." He repeated the lie that vaccines were "safe, effective, and free!"[19] This was a three-fold piece of misinformation and he knew it! Most of us didn't have all the information on the vaccines at that point, but we knew enough to be very cautious about them and we didn't believe they were safe, or effective and didn't care If they were free or not!! Biden then announced new vaccination mandates which were NOT legal because our laws are legislated by our Congress and it is supposed to represent "We, the people." Our country had been 'taken over' by unelected, self-appointed officials who were making their own rules. The mandates would force 100 million American workers to submit to taking the mRNA vaccine or lose their jobs.[20]

Before, we continue with the aftermath of this hideous speech, we need to "address the plethora of either implied or deliberate pieces of 'disinformation' perpetrated by the President of the United States. He admitted that "this same week, the weekly death toll was decreased by 70%. They claimed this was the result of the vaccines already given. Epidemiologically, this was not true, because the natural course of the disease had been waning already before vaccines were introduced. Going to the unreasonable and dangerous lengths they went to attain herd immunity simply was not necessary at that point. Another piece was the bold statement that vaccines provided strong protection for the vaccinated, but the efficacy of the vaccines was questioned from the beginning,"[21] People having had the disease, had natural immunity for an indefinite amount of time, but 'public health authorities' were not even considering it as adequate or having no need for further immunization. We also knew that having a second jab increased the risk of adverse effects more than it inferred additional immunity because of the "vaccine" mechanism. Without repeating the entire speech, it is completely safe to say that Biden made a lot of assumptions he said were based in the facts, but they weren't facts. They were specially selected lies, declared to make people believe he was right, when he could scarcely have been more wrong. Finally, Biden said, "This is Not about freedom or personal choice, it's about protecting yourself, those around you, and those you love." Many of us diametrically oppose that statement. That wasn't what it was about at all—it was about absolute control of the majority, and that's what it's still about.

Immediately, there was widespread unbelief, fear, anger, and a sense of helplessness, because the institutions and workplaces didn't care that the mandate was illegal. They too were threatened to comply at risk of losing money or being shut down. Colleges and Universities didn't want their federal money drying up. Most of us will NEVER know what incentives, nor how many were utilized to force the vaccines. Threats were of job losses, suspension of college educations, and loss of military commissions. They were workers, their spouses, college students and their parents, all medical personnel, and military men and women who were desperate to keep their jobs and careers, but never wanted to be vaccinated potentially jeopardizing their own health. The mandates completely removed personal autonomy and informed consent from everyone; also illegal. These folks were forced into a 'Catch 22 dilemma!' They faced grief and hardship if they refused to take the vaccine and lost their livelihood, or they would live with the real possibility of crippling adverse events, even death from being jabbed. That was in every way an impossible choice to have to make. Many succumbed to the vaccination under much duress because they simply couldn't afford to lose their jobs. A far greater number of those forced to take the vaccine, wound up with critical adverse events and no recourse, and many died. This author personally knows people who lost their lives from the toxic vaccines. Naturally, though the various health agencies were well aware of this outcome, they had no intention of ever admitting the truth of how extensive death by vaccine had been and continues to be until this very moment. After all, they had already made sure no one could be liable for those with health issues or death, because vaccines were issued under Emergency Use Authorization. (EUA) However, the plan was to vaccinate everyone, no matter the safety, because globalists' goal is depopulation, and a tiny matter like critical adverse events and deaths to them was of no consequence to achieve the goals.

It is still beyond belief that our nation would promote this whole, evil agenda without any compunction, compassion, or need of recompense. Whatever the decisions people ultimately made, there was suffering and horrific loss, and worst of all no hope of going back for a redo. This merciless, and criminal act was just one of the many heinous crimes the Biden administration perpetrated on the American people. At the very least, religious, health, and other exemptions should have been honored without argument across the board as vaccination exemptions have always been available, but proportionately, very few were given. Perhaps one of the most stunning facts in all of this charade, was how few people actually recognized that our nation, during that time, was under totalitarian measures; all were anti-Constitution and antiAmerican. In researching the question of legality, many contend that mandates are NOT illegal, because it is not illegal to demand something be done for the benefit of all citizens. Just as many disagree because when something is deemed personally damaging under any circumstance, and there was certainly plenty of reason to question the safety of an experimental vaccine allowed under EUA-only status with highly questionable red flags all over it, NO MAN has the right to force it on another for the benefit of all. A substance of potential danger, even death, should NEVER be forced on anyone. The Law of Man prevails.[22]

As also mentioned in the president's speech, children 12 years and over were NOT exempted from the vax. An experimental vaccine, barely tested, and then NOT scientifically proven safe should have never been forced on a single teen. And the "health officials" were working feverishly to make it available for children. Teens and children were considered very low risk for the disease, and only a rare case, usually with an underlying medical problem, had any problem if they got COVID. The obvious rationale for doing it became getting them all back in school; that being nothing but a ruse, because it did not reopen schools quickly as promised, and the reasons for our children 'going to school' were totally ignored in the politics of the teachers' unions. Our system of education was established as the single most powerful ideological training ground for what it means to be a Democratic American. It is meant to pass to upcoming generations the vital lessons of our heritage, based on fairness, justice, and freedom— that there is an inherent relationship between hard work and just reward.[23] As we have seen, these ideas are absolutely foreign and nonsensical to the Marxist or totalitarian mindset. American children engage in freedom of thought, and critical inquiry, expecting to have their individual rights and bodily autonomy honored; expecting an essentially free and fair future. Even when children are taught in somewhat less than the best environments, they still understand their right to have that.

In 2020-2022, the normal education of our children changed drastically. The globalist efforts to destroy all of this social contract was very clearly a conscious and systematic process. Our time-tested model was quickly replaced with schools, administrators, and teachers willing and being compelled to bully, torment, and even abuse our children. The former message of respect and support for parents and their children was everywhere replaced with the message to parents they now had no say in their children's education or bodily autonomy. With new protocols being dictated from education "officials" above who intentionally aimed to dissolve the entire practice of educational merit, they couldn't care less about fairness. In fact, suddenly, it looked just like the type of education forced on children raised in countries under Marxist dictators. It stressed the full enforcement of silence, compliance, suppression of any rebellious or independent thought. Next generation children would always be fearful of the consequences of "stepping out of line." They would remember the ever-present use of "restrictions." They would be so broken by the threat of isolation from their peers, they would readily submit to ongoing mistreatment and abject control. Indoctrination of our children with wrong ideas is abuse in its worst form. [24]

"James Lindsay has been exposing the Critical Race Theory and Wokeism for several years and has written a book entitled, *The Marxification of Education*, focusing on how Marxism and Critical Race Theory infiltrated American education in preschool,

K-12, and universities. He was motivated to write it because of the insane insistence of liberals and progressives that these things are NOT being 'taught in school.' "Even the United Nations Education, Scientific, and Cultural Organization (known as UNESCO) had already tipped their hand on that. The primary fountainhead of the ideas being smuggled into our educational system is Brazilian Marxist education theorist Paolo Freire, and the ideas go under the name of 'critical pedagogy'...which is being forced on children under false pretenses, (i.e., the perpetrators of this conspiracy are telling parents that critical pedagogy is one thing when it is in fact something else, namely brainwashing)."[25] It was replacing actual necessary education, when many of our students aren't even near proficiency in math, reading, and writing, as reflected by nationwide NAEP assessment scores. All of the teaching of Freire and one Henry Giroux, an evangelist of Freire's work is 'Woke Marxification' which began making its way into our education, starting in the 1970s. Lindsay says, "The theft of North American education by Freirean ideas is nothing short of a crime against humanity."[26] There is so much information on the extent of the indoctrination and what has been taught, we lack time to cover it well, but all parents of school children MUST be aware or become aware of what has been happening in their children's education. Increasingly, parents are turning to home-schooling networks for their children's education to protect them from this abuse.

Masked classrooms, as previously discussed, were a plus for reinforcing this teaching. Fearful children under the teaching of heavily indoctrinated leftist supporters, (the NEA, in particular, which heavily supports the hiring of such teachers) who bought into their ideas. They are joyless adults who promote the idea of children barely being seen and almost never heard. Individualism and original ideas are crushed. 'Gifted and talented' programs have been termed '*racist*'; cultural and aesthetic studies were halted. Sadly, when teens and young adults begin to understand the ideological changes, many just plain give up because there is no longer a reason to try. Most young people today cannot answer the simple question: “Where do you imagine you will be in five years?” It might be answered with silence and / or tears, because they realize their new world views offer no real expectations for their future. Classrooms have become increasingly silent these days, students stare aimlessly ahead, more immobile and sadder than they can ever remember being. Education reform became a top priority for the new Trump administration. We long to see positive changes in all our young children, and new incentives of help for those in higher education. That certainly includes the instruction of all young adults, no matter their area of interest.

In some parts of the country, particularly in large cities, politically blue, school edicts banned extracurricular activities when students refused the jab. Of course without it, the student could be separated from his team, the team could be decimated, and it might even mean a loss of scholarship. This ruling did NOT come from the state but was an unjust freelance act of deliberate cruelty by local school administrators who wanted to control. All lockers were removed from hallways, to keep students from congregating during COVID. Worse, still growing bodies were forced to carry their entire locker contents (most 75+ pounds) around in their backpacks all day long. The rule was: “no mask—no voice.” There was literally so much unwarranted abuse of both parents and their children in schools when it finally did convene that many parents simply brought their kids back home for schooling—an excellent choice! Treatment in school was just too intolerable and damaging. Not surprisingly, there is scant documentation of classroom and school abusive controls on students. No one wants to talk about this travesty that occurred far too often in that era.

Because of an unproven “virus” that was unleashed globally on all peoples and nations, unspeakably heinous things were perpetrated in the name of saving lives, when the reality was not even about an illness, it was about a small minority of greedy, power-hungry people who still intend to one day control our planet. A final example of abusive control was a dastardly picture:

children seated on their classroom floor, fully separated from one another, having scant conversation as they ate their lunches. They ate nothing but finger-foods with their hands, just like puppies in a kennel. Why? They blamed the bug, but the bug had nothing to do with it!

Vaccination Cruelty Results from a Cult Mentality

"By the end of 2021, study after study regularly appeared, all confirming each other. It became perfectly clear that ANY vaccine protection attained was rapidly dwindling over time and they had never prevented people from sickening with COVID-19. "Statistics soon proved more vaxxed people were being hospitalized with COVID infections than were the un-vaxxed, and by April 2022, the U.S. CDC data showed about 60% of adults dying of COVID-19 were vaxxed or boosted, and that remained true through 2022. What explains the rising share of COVID-19 deaths among vaccinated people? The CDC basically brushed it off as inconsequential since the majority of the people had now been vaccinated. More of those tended to be older with more underlying health conditions, which was clearly why there would be more deaths in the vaccinated."[27] This reasoning was false, because if the vaccines were doing what they were supposed to do, there still should be far fewer deaths in the vaccinated, proportionately. This is another example of double talk from "health officials." With these stats showing more vaccinated people dying, there was clearly no reason to keep pumping toxic vaccines into people![28]

"CDC and other researchers have shown that protection from COVID-19 vaccines can diminish, or wane, over time and booster doses were needed to maintain a robust immune response."[28] Remember, this author and her spouse each succumbed to COVID without having been vaccinated, however, four years later, the natural immunity we received has been far superior to that of the waning vaccinated. Neither of us has had COVID-19 again in the last four years. Given the choice, we'd still take our chances with the illness over the known toxicity of the vaccines!

As of January 2022, the harmful adverse effects of the vaccines continued mounting rapidly, and three years later, we can easily see much of the longer-term known sequelae. Many more people are finding heart diseases, cancers, immune deficiencies, and systems illness of chronicity never seen before COVID vaccines. Had it been a different vaccine, at a different time, the previously diligent Health and Human Services department, CDC, and FDA would have yanked the COVID-19 vaccine from the market almost immediately as reports came in exponentially! There have been significant concerns about the safety of many vaccines for as long as they have been available in the US. From 1955 on, there have been no fewer than ten different vaccines reported for adverse effects. In each case, including polio, simian virus 40, swine flu, hepatitis B, rotavirus, meningococcal, Hib, H1N1, porcine circovirus, (PCV) and HPV were all pulled for specific known effects to do further testing, but NEVER the COVID-19 vaccines, though there were exponentially more concerns than ever before.[29] However, to the sheer amazement of any thinking person, the FDA simply rolled out the needed boosters to compensate for the incomplete job earlier vaccines had not accomplished! We all know good marketers can make the very worst of products look desirable. The insanity of people who had bought into the utter travesty of the vaccinations, was soon proven when we heard them boasting of being "double-vaxxed and boosted!"

Meanwhile, the horrendous adverse effects of the vaccinations became impossible even for the CDC to ignore. Those of us caring about this travesty were doing our best to keep these facts noted on social platforms, but millions of others, who were vaccination brain-washed, seemed totally oblivious to them. By now, there was a "true cult following of vaxxers." Along with the cult members, a clear, two-tier society was forming of the "haves' (vaccines) and the "have-nots."(antivaxxers) starting in the countries and states that had practiced vax-discrimination and used 'vaccine passports.' In addition to the two-tiered society, another culture of cruelty was launched. The 'forced' vaccinations were ramped-up almost hysterically. Divisions were becoming crystal clear. "Since 2021, public and political disclosure had normalized stigma against people who remained un-vaccinated, often woven into the tone and framing of media articles. Political leaders singled out the un-vaccinated, blaming them for the continuation of the pandemic; stress on hospital capacity; the emergence of new variants; driving transmission to vaccinated individuals; and the necessity of ongoing lockdowns, masks, school closures and other restrictive measures. Political rhetoric descended into moralizing, scapegoating, and blaming with pejorative terms and actively promoting stigma and discrimination as tools to increase vaccination. This became socially acceptable among pro-vaccine groups, the media and the public at large, who viewed full vaccination as a moral obligation and part of the social contract. The effect, however, has been to further polarize society—physically and psychologically—with limited discussion of specific strategies to increase uptake especially in communities where there would be disproportionately larger individual and societal benefits. There is rarely a discussion of who and why people remain unvaccinated. Vaccine policy appears to have driven social attitudes towards an us/them dynamic rather than adaptive strategies for different communities and risk groups."[30]

Many nurses quit their jobs because they could no longer stand by watching people get vaccinated and then incur a full-blown anaphylactic reaction or code scene within a few minutes of the vaccine hitting their bloodstream. Many other nurses, and health personnel quit or were fired for refusing to take the jab—and many others, some now dead, should have quit sooner. Firefighters and paramedics went on strike. Doctors were fired from hospital staffs. Hospitals faced a major healthcare crisis due to lost staff. Denying the unvaccinated appropriate medical care was actually discussed and suggested. How bizarre and surreal to watch all of this happening when, by this time, in reality, tens of millions of people had already survived COVID-19 and had their superior natural immunity, however, reality simply didn't matter. There were nearly constant verbal attacks from every direction on the unvaccinated.

The cult became increasingly insane over their wrong perceptions of the characters of the unvaccinated, attributing heinous things to them, while they continued saying and doing heinous things even to their friends and loved ones who had chosen not to be vaccinated. You, the reader, will recall "our friend, Ms. Naomi Wolf, who herself was not vaccinated either, as a writer and journalist experienced some of the most hideous discriminatory acts imaginable. She told of a lifelong friend she had cherished coming to her home for a visit, and refusing to enter her home. He told her he didn't sit inside with un-vaxxed people! She was even more stunned when their pre-arranged meeting couldn't happen outside due to rain. He repeated his original statement high-handedly and canceled their meeting completely. Ms. Wolf also told of receiving important invitations on several occasions stating, "Fully Vaccinated Only!"—even when the events were to be held outside. She found that nearly all the things she had normally done, she could no longer do—without the vaccination, they had all become off limits. Even potential travel was off limits without being fully vaxxed and she found entire countries were only open to the "fully vaxxed."[31]

"The longer the insanity lasted, the more cloistered her world became. Per mandate, the un-vaccinated were being charged $100/week for the testing required to be able to keep doing their jobs. An immune-suppressed individual would want to think long and hard about vaccination that could make them extremely ill. But Ms.Wolf knew of an immune-suppressed woman who was denied a vital kidney transplant because she was not vaccinated! Meanwhile, the masking mandate was as unbending and unnecessary as ever. In a local library there was NO accommodation for the ADA law (adults with disabilities) which clearly states such an individual cannot be discriminated against for not doing something that could be personally harmful. A provision MUST be made—but it was NOT made. The librarian simply referred her to a city attorney. Single study rooms were provided to "Friends of the Library"—those who were vaccinated! All common spaces were closed. The porch would have been fine, but it was being enclosed! The nice librarian was 'so sorry—but there is nothing I can do.' Today, most everyone is fully aware of the ADA law. With any disability, there is always some accommodation that can be made and so many ways a problem could be quickly and easily solved, but none had been tried. They could have just designated a separate space for disabled people—the law for all public spaces. But this particular city had made its own law and also made medical decisions for everyone. In many cases it made using the public library virtually impossible. The library itself had been converted into a scolding, mean, and intrusive overseer at its best—we can't talk about its worst!"[31]

"By year's end, 2022, the utter cruelty and complete segregation had approached the point of raging sadism. Believe it or not, Australia was in chains if the un-vaccinated were not in full quarantine. Austria locked down the un-vaccinated. Often, the un-vaccinated were denied access to very special and emotionally important events such as graduations, recitals, weddings, funerals, and one-time happenings that would be missed forever. It became difficult to even recognize some of the people (family and friends) that could say and do such cruel things. It had definitely become a two-tier society, where the vaccinated were enabled to sit on top to exclude, shun, and mistreat the second (lesser) tier of the un-vaccinated and feel quite superior and righteous in doing so. Indeed, the cruelty on display nearly everywhere had become far more contagious than any virus ever could be."[32]

> "And when He (Jesus) comes, He will convict the world concerning sin and righteousness and judgment." John 16:8 ESV

Consider this: There will be a final reckoning someday, maybe soon. Jesus will be the ultimate judge of all. When He returns to judge the world, who do you suppose will be judged more harshly—the individual conscientiously attempting to make the best decision regarding the body God gave him/her, or the one who follows the greedy, and powerful crowd's rules and treats all other people as if they are dirt under foot because they didn't do what that self-righteous person thought they should? Just a thought! This author is NOT the judge, but in Scripture, Jesus had a good deal to say to the self-righteous Pharisees who supposedly followed the laws to the letter, but had no time or compassion for the common folks they had been called to lead. When all is said and done, we are told Jesus will do the judging based on what is in the heart of a person.

Daily, new reports were surreptitiously surfacing about the abusive treatment of the un-vaccinated in hospitals and of normal therapeutic treatments being withheld. Once again, this is very interesting when you understand that most any medical facility has NEVER been allowed to turn away people in need of medical care. What changed? Granted, there are a few reasonable things for which a hospital might not treat a patient, but discrimination of ANY kind is NOT one of those. Individuals who do not carry health insurance are still entitled to hospital emergency care, including obstetrical care, regardless of their ability to pay. "The Federal Emergency Medical Treatment and Active Labor Act, as well as COBRA mandate minimum standards and a patient must receive treatment to the extent that any Emergency condition is medically stabilized."[33] Discovery of the highly-effective use of monoclonal antibodies as a treatment for COVID was withdrawn by the corrupted FDA. Yes, we can say corrupted, "because its top two regulators had resigned from it due to their disagreement over the advisability of boosters!" The booster decision was the bailiwick of the FDA only, but President Biden had stuck his nose into that business announcing a booster rollout by his own deadline without regard to the fact it wasn't his business to do so![34] We may always be sure that insanity feeds insanity. One observation many of the remaining thinkers made was that some friends and colleagues who were born skeptics their entire lives would be predictably cautious about the vaccines. They tested the validity of everything, taking no potential health risks of foods, beverages, or excesses, and isolated themselves from any possible danger, yet were the first ones in line with their specially-protected progeny to get their little bodies injected with mRNA poison, still listed as experimental until 2024! They even bragged about doing it on social media! They had simply been 'bewitched' by the vaccine spirit and their minds took complete leave of every bit of wisdom they'd ever known. Ever wonder WHO was responsible for that 'Spirit feeding the vaccine insanity? Don't wonder too long!! It couldn't be more obvious.

> "Now the Spirit (Holy) expressly says that in latter times some will depart from the faith, giving heed to deceiving spirits and doctrines of demons, speaking lies in hypocrisy; having their own conscience seared with a hot iron; forbidding to marry, and commanding to abstain from foods which God created to be received with thanksgiving by those who believe and know the truth." I Timothy 4:1-3 NKJV.

> "Satan, who is the god of this world, has blinded the minds of those who don't believe. They are unable to see the glorious light of the Good News. They don't understand this message about the glory of Christ, who is the exact likeness of God." 2 Corinthians 4:4 NLT

In light of this Scripture, we can better understand how the entire knowledge base and belief systems people had known all their lives were suddenly abandoned and forgotten almost overnight. Seemingly intelligent, informed people started seeing things that simply weren't there to see and were unable to see the things that remained right in front of their eyes. Many of us who hadn't lost our footing tried in so many ways to remind them of truth, and speak out about women's health and women's bodies and what the vaccines were capable of doing to them both immediately and in the future, not to mention the health of their infants. They would have an effect on their young daughters' future lives in so many possible ways. However, this evil delusion was alive and well, as the Destroyer would have it. Compassionate, well-meaning writers and speakers were trying to spare people a large potential measure of grief, but these same were only labeled, smeared, threatened, and silenced by Big Tech, and the warnings fell on deaf ears. "People like Senator Ron Johnson (R-WI) regularly called for caution and investigation of vaccines to ascertain safety, but Big Tech 'fact-checkers', the biggest bunch of regularly biased and ill-informed speakers out there, regularly discredited and belittled him and his concerns.[35]

An extremely interesting turn of events happened, when the "two feminist Supreme Court justices, Sonia Sotomayor and Elena Kagan were heard discussing vaccine mandates. It was just like they'd never heard of any of the legal claims of Roe v. Wade, such as the 'right to privacy'. Justice Kagan's career-long view has been that all citizens have the 'right to physical privacy in medical decision-making— 'my body, my choice'! and 'it's between a woman and her doctor,'—all vanished into thin air! All of her ultra-expensive education and her superior knowledge of the Constitution also flew right out the window! Part of Justice Sotomayor's reasoning mind must surely have blown a fuse at the word, "vaccines." She has been a life-long activist for justice, inclusion, human rights, the Constitution, and the rule of law. Many other 'progressive' professionals always argue against inclusion in any form. But, almost every last one of them went dumb, as a comprehensive, systematic, cruel, top-down, discrimination 'cult' was established in a matter of months in New York City. States like California adopted systems that looked shockingly like apartheid with its physical characteristics. It's almost funny—now these former fighters for human rights and equal justice under law have enthusiastically signed on to this massive structure of pure discrimination. It happened so quickly, they didn't even see it coming, but now they embody what they've spent their lives hating in just one year!"[36]

Here is the greatest irony of all! "As the anti-vaccine contingent has notched several successes in their arguments, the abortion rights movement has taken hit-after-hit, culminating in the June 24 Supreme Court decision that ended the federal constitutional right to abortion! The ruling leaves it up to states to decide, and up to 26 states are expected to ban or severely limit abortion in the coming months. Now that anti-vaccination groups have laid claim to 'My Body, My Choice,' abortion rights groups are distancing themselves from it—marking a stunning annexation of political messaging... It strengthens the meaning of choice in the anti-vaccine space and detracts from the meaning of the word in the reproductive rights space."[36]

But, looking back, what has been accomplished gives us no pleasure. Now, we Americans, a formerly proud and independent people, have experienced a travesty we never wanted or saw coming. Those who submitted to the COVID-19 vaccination debacle, received a personally intimate, permanent, and probably damaging intrusion that most didn't choose. Americans as a whole have been a kind, compassionate people, but a great many have been transformed, accepting a culture of cruelty. Historically, America has been known for its equality of treatment for all and a kind of light for the world to emulate. That character has been replicated in other parts of the world. Now, however, it has become a society of horrible discrimination, pretty much emulating that of ignorant, and non-enlightened peoples. We can't realistically hold our heads as loftily as we once did. The virus and the vaccines were merely tools, utilized effectively by the globalist wolves to accomplish the planned, systematic, and tyrannical breakdown of America.

Is COVID-19 Still a Pandemic?

When the pandemic started as declared by the World Health Organization (WHO), after testing positive for COVID-19, we all had to isolate for a full 14 days. As time passed, isolation was 10 days, then 7 days, then 5 days, and now the CDC has cut it to just 24 hours after a person is fever-free and symptoms are improving. "All of these changes, plus the widespread relaxation of mask policies in public places, begs the question: Are we still in a pandemic? Or has COVID-19 reached the endemic stage, meaning it's here to stay, but not spreading out of control? Terminology can be confusing—for example, the WHO still calls COVID-19 a pandemic, even after declaring an end to the public health emergency last spring, 2023. An endemic is the constant presence of a disease or infectious agent within a given geographic area or population group...Endemicity does not mean that a condition is benign or without consequences...approximately 2,000 people were still dying every week from COVID in the US and we continued to learn more about long-COVID and its consequences, so there were still reasons to remain vigilant. SARS-CoV-2 appears to be here to stay; and that makes it endemic."[37]

In a regular sense, our lives and times are linear, meaning they flow from past to present to future. However, events in our lives can simply unfold in non-linear and unpredictable ways, making it difficult to pinpoint an absolute past, present, and future. The non-linear theory of time suggests that ALL moments, past, present, and future, may actually coexist. Many things do not progress smoothly from one stage to the next in a logical or expected way. This is what happened to all of us, when our normal moved into "pandemic time." For example: obesity rates skyrocketed—a problem that COVID caused but also made COVID more dangerous. Then COVID mandates shuttered gym activities, dance, and Weight Watchers' classes, the very healthy measures needed, had become health hazards with COVID. As previously discussed, the WHO was the only organization that could start or stop a pandemic. The globalist Gates Foundation had funded $780 million to the WHO and it did not want WHO to stop its ongoing gold mine any time soon. Some people vowed to never stop wearing masks, and some never have! Yes, the real pandemic was officially over, but would forever be endemic. Similarly, from 9/11, the war on terror was declared, but it has never really been declared over. It was effectively redefined as an everywhere battlefield—your airports, your schools, your home, your mall, your... It generated an era of wartime rules invoked yet again during COVID by all the "non-elected officials like the TSA. By every objective measure, COVID remained a disaster, and the 'rules' still don't work, but many of them are still in place, such as the mandated vaccination schedules for all children. It also generated untold billions in profits for the very same globalist wolves.[38]

In the same way, the pandemic has been a horrible misfortune for all of humanity, but the very same minority of globalist wolves did not consider it a misfortune at all. The very same small minority of privilege is still at the center of power and still fully capable of ensuring that it will keep us forever on at least a semi-war footing, and those pesky rules of a free, peaceful Western nation safely in abeyance. Now, much of what America has been is seriously ill, perhaps needing life support. The eradication of Western cultural wealth is largely complete. It is now generally accepted that people could and would willingly police other people's behaviors. The end of the sovereign individual with free will who decides for his or herself will never be universally seen again. The reasons for all the closures of public venues and erasures of important American history are reminders, promoted by Big Tech and the CCP. The elimination of that evidence ultimately promotes the wicked agenda of the World Economic Forum with its clear hostility to any form of nationalism or national identities. However, there are efforts being made to stem the tide of CCP and Big Tech interference.

Former National Security Advisor Robert C. O'Brien said, "National Security officials all agree on one thing: TikTok poses a clear and present threat to America. We cannot allow the Chinese Communist Party, our chief adversary and an organization notoriously devoted to propaganda and censorship, to control the platform that America's youth overwhelmingly rely on for news. To do so would be akin to allowing Soviet control of several major American newspapers and TV channels during the Cold War. Congress must pass this bill and finish the job the Trump Administration started in 2020: forcing a sale of TikTok to remove it from CCP control, or prohibit its operation in the US."[39]

Heritage Foundation Tech Policy Director Kara Frederick; "With each passing day that TikTok remains operational in the US, the CCP can gain further access to sensitive data on American citizens and continue to refine its ability to manipulate and exploit our population—particularly the next generation. TikTok poses a grave threat to our national security. TikTok's unchecked growth and infiltration into the fabric of our society will only make it more difficult to extricate ourselves and our children from its grip. We must confront this crisis head-on and immediately prohibit TikTok from operating in the US. The Protecting Americans from Foreign Adversary Controlled Applications Act is a crucial step forward in this fight and will be a powerful tool in our arsenal to put an end to this noxious, CCP-beholden surveillance platform once and for all."[40] This House committee contained no fewer than 29 major spokespersons speaking to the urgency of this legislation. There were at least 20 known instances of CCP manipulation and exploitation investigated on at least 12 highly concerning issues. This current committee is dedicated to working on a bipartisan basis to build consensus on the threat posed by the CCP and develop a plan of action to defend the American people, our economy and our values.

Another interesting perspective is the BIG, Big Tech picture now. Beginning in the 90s and accelerating after China joined the World Trade Organization in 2001, China became the tech industry's foundry. That relationship brought benefits to both sides. "But more recently, it began to unravel, as US distrust of China's government mounted, American awareness of China's human rights abuses grew, and China began to flex its muscles on the world stage. Now all that, plus the pandemic, has left the US in a 'bring production home from overseas' mood. At the same time, the Ukraine war is causing many countries, particularly those with authoritarian leaders, to think twice about welcoming US tech giants. Putin's war is also driving Russia deeper into an alliance with China, and any effort by China to supply Russia with arms will further deepen the gulf between Washington and Beijing. The result is the start of a vast withdrawal from a single tech market. More broadly, the changes cast a long shadow over the tech industry's internationalist vision, suggesting that the past three decades of upward growth may have peaked."[41]

So, the question remains: Is the COVID-19 pandemic over? We

believe the actual pandemic, by definition is over, but it has most definitely become endemic. We will not see the end of COVID-19 no matter how many people get vaccinated. "A disease is said to be endemic in a specific population or populated place when that infection is constantly present, or maintained at a baseline level, without extra infections being brought into the group as a result of travel or similar means…an endemic disease always has a steady, predictable number of people getting sick, but that number can be high or low, and the disease can be severe or mild. Also a disease that is endemic can become epidemic. A short, incomplete list of some endemic infections includes the common cold, malaria, polio, rotavirus, hepatitis C, measles, RSV, and influenza."[42] Therefore, we do expect to see continuing cases of COVID-19 indefinitely, from now on. However, as seen above, all of the global changes that took place during the pandemic by design, will continue as planned, and in fact will get closer and closer to world domination if all goes as planned. In addition, as this book is being written, the push is to develop a global reliance on other vaccines for new and existing infections. Currently, that infection is the "bird flu," and the push has already started for that vaccine. If it can be managed, the beginning of a new pandemic may be on its way!

Evil Humanity Meets Its Spiritual Father

Many people have come to believe that the era of COVID-19 and all of the multifaceted parts of it was the result of a long-range pre-planned event by a relatively small number of very wealthy and powerful people who decided they wanted to own and control the entire world system, turning it into the New World Order they envision it ideally to be. The pandemic set that agenda onto a rapidly-moving timeline toward that global goal, with very little pushback. Is it possible that a small powerful group of people could do so much damage in a relatively short period of time all by themselves? Was it just human vanity with a large helping of moral irresponsibility? There is no doubt the infection was not just physical, but soul-deep. There was a deliberate abandonment of the most cherished of post-war values we'd held for nearly 75 years. Almost overnight, these globalists most of us were barely even noticing much, brought their money and power to bear on a mostly unsuspecting world with a demonic vengeance, in less than two years. Most of this driving force consisted of heads of state, of medical boards, of school boards and teachers, of heads of unions, of heads of all levels of government, and a cabal of global wolves.

"This edifice of evil is too massive, too quickly erected, too complex and really, too elegant, to assign to just human depravity and human inventiveness. It suggested a spiritual dimension of evil—an evil like a gigantic cultural spacecraft that landed on Earth, with unfolding technology and immediately setting loose upon the egalitarian, post-Enlightenment West, a global dystopia run on cruelty and cognitive dissonance. Now we are actually engaged in spiritual combat and stand in need of help from a higher 'Being', better armed to fight true darkness than ourselves alone."[43] How could such 'normally' nice, sane people have been enabled to do so much pure evil? How could they have allowed an unqualified system to place masks on babies and little children and suppress their normal breathing? How could they have required friends and colleagues to eat in the streets like a whole caste of untouchables? How could New York City police arrest a woman and her terrified, nine-year-old child for visiting the Museum of Natural History without the proper "papers" (a vaccine passport). US citizens actually held those "exposed" to a contagious disease in forced quarantine who weren't even ill, without a charge or trial! Others were banned from their jobs by the thousands, stigmatizing them as criminal threats to health and decency.[43]

Every one of these things happened in the USA and so much more every day while our government had been hijacked by the globalist mandates. Our America, with its principles of equity and equality that had always governed its human relations by law; where our laws against the abuse of corporeal punishment of children in public schools are on the books in every state. Under abusive management, our laws were ignored or abandoned altogether. Many commentators and journalists compared 2020-2022 to the early years of Nazi leadership. "In Germany, the psychological preparation for totalitarianism had already been laid for the heinous abuse and vice that would soon come to pass. Scores of new ideas and policies were already established and policing them had already begun. Casual, but steadily increasing cruelty was already an enormous part of Nazi culture. They had created the two-tiered society, where the top tier was the chosen "Aryan race" with its privilege and leadership, and upper-class citizenry, and the lower tier were the hated Jews and their sympathizers, and other lower and middle-class worker bees, for which there was increasing degradation, abuse, and death to the undesirables, all by varying degrees. It had been a modern, civil society, but it quickly degenerated into an authoritarian despotism capable of committing the most unimaginable evil ever loosed on its society and the world at large. Its heinous evil was seen, heard, smelled, and endorsed by doctors, medical associations, journalists, famous composers and filmmakers, universities, teachers, shopkeepers, and neighbors who participated in the evil to save their own lives. Other peoples and countries were aware of most of this, including Americans, who literally looked the other way as long as they weren't involved in it. When America entered the war, it fought the battles against that enemy, but it was already way too late for the millions of maimed and murdered. We must NEVER forget the atrocities committed then or even more recently. It could easily happen again."[44]

It was a very short, downward glide from the creation of the two-tiered society to the actual embracing of the horrors of eugenics. Men taking it upon themselves to play God, decided which people were simply unworthy to keep living! They used some of the same key words recently used in the pandemic, such as "hygiene" and "public safety" and 'for the good of all" in their constant propaganda, which led to establishing the first Nazi "euthanasia" programs. "The code name Aktion T4 or T4 Operation, was the term meaning 'mercy killings', which the Nazis used to euphemistically refer to their systematic extermination of certain groups including the mentally ill, aged, disabled, and others. It was part of the Nazi's attempt to preserve the purity of their master race—in order to create a superior group of 'Aryans', the Nazis needed to destroy all those with racial defects...by the end of the war approximately 62,000 Germans had been killed as part of this program alone."[45] One of the most heinous aspects of the Euthanasia Program was the fact that its staff members were trained medical doctors, sworn to help care for their patients. At its inception, the program was illegal, yet its practitioners seemingly had no moral, religious, or legal doubts about what they were doing. Supposedly harmless language, unauthorized "medical authority," and the excessive multiplication and concentration of power in each, created a top-down multiple authorization process, that would eliminate the possibility of any one office making final decisions. In that manner, much harm could be done by many and no one got blamed for the heinous decisions made. It would be analogous to a large firing squad that's only partly and anonymously armed so that no one can actually be blamed for killing the "offenders." This leadership pattern could hide the true nature of what was a visibly-hellish, abominable, every-day evil.[46]

> "Then the Lord saw that the wickedness of man was great in the earth, and that every intent of the thoughts of his heart was only evil continually. And the Lord was sorry that He had made man on the earth, and He was grieved in His heart...The earth also was corrupt before God, and the earth was filled with violence. So God looked upon the earth, and indeed it was corrupt; for all flesh had corrupted their way on the earth." Genesis 6: 5-6, 11 NKJV

The above passage of Scripture reminds us of just how wicked were the people on earth as far back as Noah's time. God was actually sorry He had created them and had to judge them with the flood before there remained no one righteous to propagate humanity. As it was, there were only eight humans left to start humanity over after the flood. Since the wickedness of men today, is very little better than it was then, we might easily expect, based on the promises of Scripture, that God is considering what He will have to do to bring repentance on earth today! However, there is another bit of Scripture that Father God would remind us of—humanity has an ultimate enemy. He was created as a very special and lofty angel, long before humanity existed. At that time his name was Lucifer. But, because he began to think he was more important than his Creator, God cast him from heaven with a third of all the other created angels, who became demons on earth. Because of their estate, they became God's enemies, and because we are His creation, also our enemies. We need to know our Enemy and his forces will do whatever they can to destroy us. Jesus, Himself, called Satan "the enemy." Who is he?

> "Be alert and of sober mind. Your enemy, the devil, prowls around like a roaring lion looking for someone to devour." I Peter 5:8 ESV

> "Put on the full armor of God, so that you can take your stand against the devil's schemes. For our struggle is not against flesh and blood, but against the rulers, against the authorities, against the powers of this dark world and against the spiritual forces of evil in the heavenly realms." Ephesians 6: 11-12 ESV

This last verse was used by a well-known medical freedom activist when asked how he was able to stay strong in his mission, when his name was constantly smeared and he faced career attacks and social ostracism. We who would live according to God's ways must keep this in mind. We aren't fighting flesh and blood, but neither are we fighting alone when we know our Father, and His Son, Jesus Christ.

As we look back at this whole pandemic agenda and all of the ways and means of evil visited upon us from every direction, by using our own ability with critical thinking, we can clearly determine that everything was well-planned and elaborately executed. It was also not just a human effort. Proof is in the malevolent cruelty, the darkness of its spiritual source, its giddy flamboyance resembling a magician with some new tricks, its elaborately detailed imagination, and its very creation by the father of innate indifference to his monumental desire to cause pain and suffering. It is impossible to believe this whole conspiracy was conceived by mere humans. Many of those humans, without naming obvious names, work mostly at a bumbling brain level only slightly above the highest animal species. They have difficulty making governmental entities work at all because they can't agree on whose ideas will likely fly best in the political arena. We are probably grossly understating the forces of darkness we faced then and will continue to face in the decades ahead of us. Yes, Satan, the god of this world has never ever backed away from a battle. The fact is, as our Father God allows it, he still wins a good many. However, Scripture teaches us his time is running shorter and shorter and he knows it. He won't give up, but his days are numbered, and we know he ultimately will not win the war. Believers in Jesus Christ and His Word have shown us the true end of the story.

Globalist Authoritarians vs. the Individual

Suddenly, in 2022, the tide began to turn. In January massive anti-mandate protests started in several nations. By February, many other nations and several states in the US had also begun pulling back from the worst of the tyranny. It was almost like everything had been turned on with a switch, and then suddenly turned off with the same switch. Pfizer had planned to conceal their internal documents regarding the COVID vaccines for 75 years and desperately sought to do so. However, a US court had made the decision that it could NOT do this—the documents would be disclosed immediately, 1000s at a time, which may have helped to flip the switch.

Soon, several countries were reporting higher rates of COVID infection among the already vaccinated! The former cheerleaders of the many mandates started covering paper trails and talking desperately to their lawyers. Many of the vaccinated had become very nervous, quiet, and somber. More and more people were being harmed by the jabs and many had died very soon after being vaccinated. Many more were ill and not getting better. This very sad, and tragic outcome was a long way from getting better also. In January 2022, the US Supreme Court ruled against President Biden's vaccine mandate for everyone except military and healthcare workers, and it should have been for everyone. Military databases and the massive numbers of injured and dead healthcare workers have proven that mandates were completely irresponsible from the very beginning, a fact that we will see in far greater detail in the next chapters.

"In Canada, Prime Minister Justin Trudeau killed a truckers' convoy protest. The Canadian Trucking Alliance stated most protestors had no connection to trucking. Near a blockade in Coutts, Alberta, multiple weapons were seized. The protests and blockades were against vaccine mandates and restrictions, and were called the Freedom Convoy by organizers. Starting on January 22, hundreds of vehicles formed convoys from several points and traversed Canadian provinces before converging on Ottawa five days later, rallying at Parliament Hill. The convoys were joined by thousands of pedestrian protesters. Canada and the US had previously accommodated unvaccinated cross-border truckers by exempting them from COVID mandates to prevent additional problems to supply chains, but those exemptions ended with about 85% vaxxed. However, up to some 16,000 Canadian truckers were still affected by the restriction."[47]

Protesters occupied the downtown core of Ottawa and stated they would not leave until all COVID restrictions and mandates were repealed. Both Biden and Trudeau discussed ending blockades at the border, but on February 14, Trudeau invoked the Emergencies Act and a large joint-operation police presence in Ottawa arrested organizers and protesters, removed parked vehicles, and dismantled blockades from streets. In a week, most of the protesters had been cleared from Ottawa.

The convoy was condemned by the trucking industry and

various labor groups. Ultimately, four men were charged with conspiracy to commit murder of Royal Canadian Mounted Police officers. Some sources called the protests an occupation or siege. "Politically, Trudeau condemned the convoy, while many conservative Parliamentarians and Republican politicians in the US, as well as many other conservative politicians and media figures endorsed the convoy. Many said it wasn't an anti-vax movement so much as a freedom movement. Sources said the Freedom Convoy blockades cost the Canadian economy as much as $3.9 billion in loss of trade activities and cost downtown Ottawa millions per day in sales and wages for almost one month. Arrest, charges, and detention were used on several organizers and protesters. There has been much disagreement over Trudeau's actions, but most seem to believe his handling of the trucker crisis was not stellar, and actually harmed public confidence in his leadership both at home and abroad.[48] He "stepped down in late 2024!"

Many supposed the West with all its troublesome freedoms and democracy was probably over. However, hope springs eternal. As defeated as the Canadian truckers were after the above experience, they definitely inspired many similar grassroots actions around the globe. Flags and banners went skyward with words like, "Freedom"; "Liberate," and "La Libertá." "Perhaps the truckers did actually win—that rally may have been the most successful protest in human history!"[49] The truckers haven't always gleaned the credit, but it is highly significant that all the Canadian provinces dropped their COVID-19 vaccine passport systems. In spite of the globalist predators' overwhelming power and the certainty that they will continue their vicious agenda, those truckers reaffirmed what is most vital—the power of the individual to refuse to submit!

In March, 2022, a former investments portfolio manager began warning the world about Pfizer's data fraud. At first, he was primarily trying to caution all his peers in the investment community that betting on the 'Pfizers of the world' was a bet against our freedoms forever. "Edward Dowd reported that CDC charts showed 'boomers' had died, after being vaccinated, on the same scale of deaths from the 'Viet Nam War.' He fully expected that fraud investigations would sink Pfizer stock and drive Moderna into bankruptcy. Then he wrote a book entitled: *Cause Unknown: The Epidemic of Sudden Deaths in 2021 and 2022*. Mr. Dowd included a favorite quote of Carl Sagan, "'If we are not able to ask skeptical questions...to be skeptical of those in authority, then we are up for grabs for the next charlatan—political or religious—who comes ambling along.' 'It wasn't enough,' Jefferson said, 'to enshrine some rights in a constitution or a bill of rights. The people had to be educated, and they had to practice their skepticism...otherwise, we don't run the government, the government runs us.'[50] In other words, if we blindly accept everything authorities tell us, we are not educated, and if we are not educated, we are slaves of government. 'Without disagreement, science not only stagnates, it degenerates into an intolerant cult.' We are seeing that today, and we should also see that it is never in the best interests of power-hungry governments to have an educated population."[51]

Edward Dowd is well-educated and has an impressive track record as a BlackRock fund manager who grew a fund from $2 billion to $14 billion. He knows how to crunch the numbers and understands what they mean. He looked at multiple sources of data on all-cause mortality over several years and noticed a very disturbing 'signal' in the data. Many others have also noticed it, but have not pulled the data together and analyzed them in nearly as much detail as Edward has. "When insurance giant OneAmerica announced a 40% increase in all-cause mortality in the 18 to 64 age group, there was barely a ripple of media reaction. For context, a 10% increase would represent a rare, once-in-two-hundred-year event. We haven't seen a spike like this since animals paired up by twos for an extended cruise on Noah's shiny new boat. But this is a catastrophe of Biblical proportions. As Dowd puts it, the 60,000 excess deaths among millennials—over just one year—were roughly the equivalent of another Vietnam war. Other sources of data, including the Society of Actuaries Research Institute and the CDC itself, were confirming the same alarming signal."[52]

"What is more concerning—the people who are dying should

not be dying in such large numbers. Dowd filled several pages with data and pictures of young athletes who died under very unusual circumstances. Health authorities have tried desperately to normalize this by fabricating the label "SADS" (Sudden Adult Death Syndrome). SADS offers absolutely no explanation, but it makes it sound like you know what is going on! Later the 'A" word was changed (Sudden Arrhythmic Death Syndrome), as they speculated further on a possible cause. With an airtight case showing the skyrocketing death rates, we should ask why this is happening. There are plenty of clues."[53] One very clear sign that something is really fishy is when authorities start changing definitions—such as the definition of a vaccine. Another sign would be when you ask the FDA for their data on the so-called "vaccines," and they tell you they will get back to you in 55 years, and then amend it to 75 years! We must know these are data morally and legally owed to the taxpayers who paid for these studies. Then the CDC sets up a new system called a v-safe to monitor vaccine safety but doesn't care to share those data with the public—do you think there is a problem?

There is more. Joe Biden got fully vaxxed and had COVID several times. Jill Biden got fully vaxxed twice and got COVID twice. So did the prime minister of Canada, Anthony Fauci, and Pfizer's CEO. Is there a problem?!!! The VAERS system shows more deaths after COVID vaccination than deaths for all other vaccines combined for the last thirty years. Is that a problem?!!! Then there was a sudden shift in excess deaths from older people to younger people following COVID vaccine mandates in 2021…hmmmm! Apparently, Denmark thought it was a problem because it stopped all COVID shots for people under the age of 50! Then Dowd looked at disability stats from the Bureau of Labor Statistics, where he found a large increase among working-age people in 2021 and 2022. He did not elaborate on the details of those disabilities, but stated that the things you would see there can often be worse than death! A slight increase in the death rate in 2020 was among older people with serious co-morbidities, so why was there such a panic over

COVID! The main reason was the computer model generated by the infamous British epidemiologist named Neil Ferguson. From 2001 to 2020, this quack had made grossly erroneous predictions many times—he was never even close. No one knows why anyone was still listening to him in 2020, but they did, and here we are.

The original outbreak of COVID was not dramatic, yet in 2020, mandates and lockdowns swept the world in just a few months. This heinous holocaust was not an accident and was not due to mass incompetence. Yet, the response to the far more dramatic morbidity and mortality in 2021 and 2022 was almost nil. Governments and media puppets were almost completely silent. Clearly, they all knew what was really going on and why, and saw nothing concerning. "Nothing to see here, move along now and please die quietly!" Ms. Wolf's book contains many photos putting faces on this horrendous disaster—faces of beautiful young, talented people, who were set to make their marks on this world, but were denied their very lives by murdering power grabbers.

"The most cited study on the topic of sudden death in young athletes was done in 2006, where experts in Switzerland looked at sudden cardiac death in athletes under 35 years of age, between 1966 and 2004; there were 1101 deaths over 38 years, an average of 29 per year. Now since June 2021, there hasn't been a single month with fewer than 29 such deaths."[54] Even though these oft repeated figures are damming, fact-checkers continue to make the claim that SADS is caused by an undetected genetic heart condition often occurring in young adulthood. The obvious question is "Why did these deaths from supposed genetic heart conditions NOT show up exponentially until the onset of COVID-19 jabs?!!"There were 90 reported in December 2021 alone, and about the same the following month. For at least another year and a half, it became crystal clear that this crisis was never about "the virus," but about a global bid to kill off our free world and suppress all of our freedoms. Today, many people would now agree and refuse any further jabs, but various reasons remain for why they still feel they can't refuse them. These still want you to tell them that it's OK, but it's NEVER going to be OK! It's just a way to guiltlessly offload any personal responsibility. There is simply no way left to equivocate or ride the fence on vaccines, especially those that ARE NOT vaccines! Many brave souls have battled this travesty from the beginning and even lost a lot, but at least retained their personal self-respect. But where in the world is everyone else who now knows what really happened? Aren't we all called to rise up against evil? The heroes and heroines are those who are still just doing their jobs as conscientious human beings with responsibility to fellow human beings. Many in jeopardy of losing their jobs realized that if they didn't speak out, they would no longer have a career worth saving!!

Not all the time, but frequently, peaceful refusal to follow restrictions could be threatened, but seldom accomplished. This is important information to know about and understand. There should have been far more peaceful protesting of COVID restrictions but far too many people simply 'rolled over and played dead' in submission to them. Had there been greater pushbacks on the loss of personal rights, we might well have managed to keep them. Governmental officials and law enforcement all knew the mandates were NOT lawful. There were a few who displayed their bully-demeanor and spoke roughly and gruffly to offenders, but most of them knew if anyone wanted to exercise their rights, there was little they could do, though it might take a few frightening moments to prove it. There are many testimonials of people who stood strong in the face of confrontation and experienced little pushback. It could and should have been done far more than it was. This also proved for the most part that the mandates were technically meaningless. Far more should have been done by citizens to express their displeasure over the restrictions—that was their guaranteed right as a citizen.

The ACLU, for example, has stressed that citizens KNOW their rights, including free speech. The typically peaceful way to protest is called Civil Disobedience.[55] It is both a political tactic and the basis of movements advocating social change. It is a non-violent action engaged in by an individual or group of individuals who refuse to obey a law for moral or philosophical reasons. It is marked by the deliberate "violation of the law" for social purposes. It is NOT merely conscious law breaking, but rather it is law breaking with the express goal of correcting a perceived injustice. "It is non-compliance intended to convey a message of discontent to the government, media, and public. The acts of defiance are overt, public acts aimed at marshaling collective opposition to unjust or unconstitutional laws and policies. Civil disobedience can emanate from different motivations and assume a number of forms. It may be active or passive, direct or indirect. An individual can either actively commit a prohibited act or passively refuse to conform to a prescribed action."[56] Examples of non-violent resistance are bus boycotts, Freedom rides, marches, and mass demonstrations, as were used in the Civil Rights Movement. Over 10,000 of these—nearly 95%—involve peaceful protesters. The questions of our freedoms remain questionable following COVID-19! When it comes down to the alternative of everlasting servitude to totalitarianism, our future decisions on whether or not to speak up will definitely determine what we wind up with. The certainty is that tyrannical leadership only falls when everyone is involved in resistance. Millenia of history is exceedingly clear on this point. If we confront the dangers of tyranny head-on, it enables each of us to use our God-given opportunities wisely to serve all of our fellow citizens. When we conscientiously stand up for ourselves and our freedoms, we can all hold our heads up high, having become so much more than we've ever been before. If we leave the responsibility to others, we all will lose our opportunity, perhaps forever. If they could, a large percentage of the one billion Chinese would warn free people passionately of what we MUST stand against. Before we finish this chapter, we need to recognize the heroes among us who did stand up, and for many of them, at significant personal cost.

Heroes and Heroines of the COVID-19 Debacle

From near the beginning of COVID-19, there have been real live American heroes and others globally who stood for truth and integrity amid constant persecution, maligning of their character, abuse and frequent attacks. This author would count it an honor to be in the same room with any of them. These "dissident" doctors, nurses, scientists and other professionals put their careers, jobs, licenses, reputations, and so much more on the line to stand for all they believed and knew was right. Dr. Wolf actually interviewed many of them first hand to ascertain their views on everything pertaining to the pandemic. We will hear from some of these in this chapter.[57]

Dr. Harvey Risch, PhD at Yale University's School of Public Health and Yale School of Medicine, is Professor Emeritus of Epidemiology, and has a stellar history of work in multiple disciplines. He is the author of more than 400 original peer-reviewed research publications in medical literature, and cited by other scientific publications more than 53,750 times. Dr. Risch was asked, "What is the biggest myth about this pandemic? and what actually happened to him as a result of his stance?" He replied, "The biggest myth…the people are freaking out about the numbers of cases occurring: people have the idea that every case of COVID is bad, and we have to be rid of every one of them before we will be completely safe…one of the things we've learned is that cases themselves don't really matter. What matters is what happens to those cases. Yes, having a respiratory illness can be both unpleasant and difficult, but as long as it is manageable, we get through it…it's just part of life, and we try to manage it the best way we can. All of the freaking out about cases and more cases, different cases, new cases, new strains, etc. is an anxiety-generating panic mechanism to cause people to lose their senses of judgment and reason because they are panicking about the uncertainty and perceived risk. What matters is hospitalizations and mortalities."[58]

Over the course of that interview, Dr. Risch made comments about many things related to the pandemic including:

- Over time, COVID-19 acted precisely as expected for respiratory illnesses.
- Mutations became steadily more transmissible, and more

infectious, but steadily less harmful.

- More people contracted it, but fewer died—death rates flattened.
- Given a predictable course, it was better for more people to get the illness and receive good natural immunity, than to vax everyone.
- Anthony Fauci was THE primary pusher of misinformation.
- Every person who contracts the illness produces millions of variants whether vaxxed or not.
- Reality was—most people had already had COVID, whether they had any symptoms or not. That means there was absolutely NO NEED for vaxxing anyone.
- When the disease peaks, and begins to wane, herd immunity has been reached, by definition.
- Many states had already reached herd immunity by Nov and Dec of 2020, well before immunizations had even been introduced.
- He strongly defended the original ivermectin and hydrochloroquine because they had been highly effective in real time treatment.

Dr. Wolf also interviewed Dr. Howard Tenenbaum, DDS, Perio., PhD and Professor of Mt. Sinai Hospital—University of Toronto, Canada (the PhD is in Bone Cell biology). He is also a Professor in the Dept. of Laboratory Medicine and Pathophysiology and credentials go on and on. His research peer-reviewed studies have been largely focused on mechanisms that might link periodontal diseases (gums) with other conditions including cardiovascular disease and diabetes. His diverse and indepth studies have led him to many concerns regarding COVID-19 including the following:

- COVID was very treatable with the early intervention, in fact quite easy to treat. But...
- There is a vaccine with questionable efficacy and comes with very significant risks, esp. in the younger population, young men in particular.
- Having studied inflammation in cardiovascular illness, the young men are at much higher-than-normal risk of developing myocarditis. When someone who is clearly pro-vax speaks of this danger, he calls it a "mild condition" but that is completely untrue. It kills frequently!
- There's no such thing as mild myocarditis and in fact, it's a very dangerous condition. Even if the person with myocarditis doesn't die from it right away, he is still at a much higher risk of developing early and longterm cardiac diseases, including cardiomyopathy.
- Dr. Tenenbaum believes it is still critically important to get the message disseminated—COVID vaccines do not appear to be the panacea most people hoped for and in fact have far too much high risk. What the CDC has told us is exactly the opposite of what we know is true. It's also completely the opposite of what you would logically conclude.
- This is so important to know because Big Pharma and the health agencies are determined to vaccinate children and he believes that is CRIMINAL! Children statistically have zero risk of dying from COVID, and do not transmit it to others.
- Governments want to start vaccinating our children with these dangerous vaccines at Two Months of Age for no sound reason whatever! There is no medical or logical reason for it and the potential life-long dangers from adverse events can't be fully known as yet.
- Adding to that, we do already know many of the potential

adverse effects that will sentence our children to permanent disabilities.

- Consequently, giving this KNOWN toxin to ANY CHILD is CRIMINAL[58]

Dr. Paul Alexander, formerly of McMaster University and also formerly of the US Dept of HHS was also interviewed by Dr. Wolf. He spoke about the biggest problem to date being the vaccination. "Due to the fraudulent manner in which the vaccine trials were conducted and the information we know has been withheld from the global community, we don't know...the long-term implications. When clinical trials are conducted properly, it is followed and safety checks are conducted for as many years as possible. When the product is proven to have safety concerns, it is pulled back, not produced in mass quantities and used anyway. This process NEVER happened with the COVID vaccines, beside the fact that the clinical trials themselves were completely faulty and inappropriately done."[59]

The simple and reasonable opinion of Dr. Alexander was just to allow the well, the healthy, and the young in our society to just get out and live their lives as normally as possible, in the way we've always done before. They should NOT stop doing what they want to do out of fear. In all likelihood, they had the illness already and have their own natural immunity to it. Getting a case of COVID would be very little different for them than having a cold or influenza.

Then Dr. Wolf asked Dr. Alexander what he would say to a young expectant woman (perhaps at only 2 or 3-months' gestation), who also works for a federal agency and has been told she must take the vaccine or lose her job. Clearly, the good doctor could do nothing to change her situation, sad as it certainly was. "Every one of us would love to have presented her to President Biden and said, "Do you see what your stupid mandatory vaccines are doing? You have become the Hitler of the USA!" But, of course, we all know that he and all his minions have no conscience with which to reason anyway! Prior to COVID, we never gave pregnant women anything that wasn't absolutely necessary for the safety of both mom and baby. We certainly did NOT force things of unknown or questionable safety. Once again, giving this known toxin to any pregnant woman was not only irresponsible, but CRIMINAL! In reality, from the beginning, the FDA and vaccine developers all KNEW that pregnant women and women of child-bearing age were to be excluded, because of the potential harm. So if you looked at the vax protocols from the initial incomplete studies, and administered the vaccine to pregnant women anyway, there is absolutely no doubt, YOU CROSSED THE CRIMINAL LINE!"[60]

Further, Dr. Alexander cited some additional information. It was known that the spike proteins produced by the vaccines, continue producing them for at least six months and are found throughout the bloodstream. In some instances, they may also have been transferred to infants through mother's milk. One of the problems with the spike proteins is clot formation, a condition called thrombocytopenia. Some infants have died of the same clotting problem associated with the vaccinated mother. It's a condition producing low blood platelets which causes bleeding, and the infant is far more at risk then its mother because of small blood volume. Clearly the spike proteins are being made all over the body, in many places where it's risky. So, they are inducing almost immediate and significantly diverse damage.[60]

Another Canadian physician tested patients who had been vaccinated, for the genetic marker of blood clot formation. With no doubt, he found that at least 60% of the people who had just been vaccinated had elevations in this marker. This means these people were already developing micro-clots which often show up in the lungs and patients start having difficulty breathing and shortness of breath. The most minute of clots can get caught anywhere in the body and keep growing, and can easily lodge in the heart or brain, causing heart attacks and strokes which we all know can be fatal. If severe damage is developing, the person can be a walking time-bomb. Lower platelet counts are also associated with Immune Thrombocytopenic Purpura (ITP) which may also cause hemorrhage. "Vaccinations are a common environmental trigger of

ITP induced by vaccine adjuvants. It has also been an adverse event with other vaccines, including MMR, HBV, HPV, Varicella Zoster, DTaP, Polio, Influenza, and Pneumococcus. A French study that evaluated drug-induced ITP found that approximately 45% of the cases were post-vaccinal."[61] Despite reams of information about serious adverse events, studies continue to iterate there are extremely few instances where these risks outweigh the advisability of the vaccinations. The literature continues to push the vaccine narratives regardless of what is considered very low risk for the diseases. ITP can cause large purple bruises and can also cause reddish purple dots on the skin resembling a rash. Children often improve without treatment, while adult illness often lasts months or years.

Finally, Dr. Alexander was asked, "What happens to the spike protein? How does the body get rid of it?" Dr. Alexander spoke of a well-known pathologist in Canada who had done a lot of autopsies since the beginning of the COVID pandemic. In deceased women, he found the endometrium of the uterus had the highest expression of the ACE-2 receptor—another protein that allows the virus or the vaccine to affect human cells. This receptor provides the 'entry point' for the virus or the spike protein from the vaccine to be received and further affect a wide range of human cells. The spike protein was also highly expressed in placentas, and testes in males. Dr. Risch added, "when the spike protein 'sits' on the surface of a cell and protrudes into the blood flow, platelets brush up against the spikes and start clumping, then clotting. This much is still something of a theory, but it makes complete sense, when you understand the whole clotting mechanism."[62]

Dr. Wolf subsequently interviewed Dr. Peter McCullough, of whom we already spoke in an earlier chapter. The reader will remember his massive extent of knowledge, ability, and high-level experience in the fields of medicine and science. He has been embedded in the fight for truth since the very beginning of COVID. "As an example of the efforts of Big Tech to squelch the truth, when Dr. Wolf posted these interviews on You Tube, her account was temporarily FROZEN for "medical misinformation! The information cited was 100% truth, and provable."[63] The next time she posted on You Tube, they FROZE her account completely.

Many nurses who knew and witnessed the truth firsthand were often told they would be fired for dispensing such "medical misinformation." One year later, every bit of the information given in warning was abundantly and tragically confirmed. Another entire year passed with all the forced vaccinations on innocent people who never wanted to take them, only to find out it was one of the worst decisions of their lives, with no means of rectifying the probable damage. After considerable evidence and continued pressure, the CDC finally admitted the truth that post-vaccination, young men were definitely suffering from myocarditis at high rates, which if not immediately severe would increase the probability of other serious heart problems later in their lives. Almost daily, young athletes, some even in their teens and more often male, were collapsing on the athletic fields globally, and most died. Daily, a large number of concerned citizens pointed out the improbability of the young, healthy, and fit collapsing and dying for any other reason but the COVID vaccines. Social media sites didn't even try to deny it! Others were hospitalized with critical blood clots in vital organs. Young people were never at high risk for the COVID-19, but now many of them were dying either almost immediately or within just a few days of receiving vaccines. More warnings were proffered from very concerned citizens and parents than at any other time in the history of vaccines. Most would happily avoid the vaccines if they could afford it, but far too many were coerced into taking them to preserve their jobs.

The next year, VAERS reported thousands of cases of adverse events or reactions to the vaccines. Reports included blood clots in varying degrees of severity, myocarditis and other heart concerns, severe disruptions of women's menstrual cycles, and miscarriages. However, as previously mentioned, VAERS reporting is not easy, but lengthy and time-consuming, and medical staff are hard-pressed to get the job done. Individuals can do their own reporting, but most don't have the personal understanding and patience needed when they are suffering the issues. It is estimated that those reports received amount to only about one-tenth of what should be the total in real adverse events, in real time. With the added exponential numbers associated with the COVID vaccines, only a small fraction of actual events was reported. Any restitution for the harm caused on average was slim to nil, and it's highly unlikely to get any better.

By January 5, 2022, a study funded by the National Institutes of Health (NIH), confirmed COVID vaccines, "caused a small increase in menstrual cycle length. Despite the evidence, the Mayo Clinic declared menstrual cycles return to normal a few months after being vaccinated and there were no reported long-term impacts. Menstrual irregularities and heavier bleeding were even more common. With one or two extra days per cycle, for a woman it could mean an extra 12-24 days of discomfort per year. It may sound like nothing to the gentlemen in the crowd, but very few low-risk women would have opted for that choice if this information had been reported to them! The question became "With the average of a 20% distortion of cycles, what had happened to women's fertility, especially if it had been problematic before the jab?" A University of California @ Davis study claims, "there is NO evidence the COVID-19 vaccines affect anyone's fertility or cause infertility."[64] Far worse than the misinformation produced by Big Tech is the knowledge that millions of women could have had early warning from whistleblowers on media about their risks, BEFORE risking their reproductive health. Even more maddening today is the fact that institutional and public health officials are still 'doctoring' stats and rabidly denying that any of the concerns have merit. It remains nearly impossible to get past the "allopathic system" of Western medicine to find unadulterated truth about today's vaccines and drugs and the real risks involved, while Big Tech and globalists still carefully filter what is allowed online. If you dear reader want truth in medicine, you will have to do some careful digging for it.

With regard to a final thought on women's reproduction and

vaccinations, you need to read this # 1 recommendation for pregnant women about vaccinations, quoted directly from the "Key Recommendations" of the American College of Obstetricians and Gynecologists (ACOG) for use in pregnant, recently pregnant, lactating, and nonpregnant women aged 12 years and older: "The American College of Obstetricians and Gynecologists recommends that ALL eligible persons aged 6 months and older, including pregnant and lactating individuals, receive a COVID-19 vaccine or vaccine series...Vaccination may occur in any trimester, and emphasis should be on vaccine receipt as soon as possible to maximize maternal and fetal health. A single dose of the 2023-2024 updated COVID-19 vaccine is recommended for ALL adults, including pregnant and lactating adults, at least two months after their last vaccine dose."[65] In case someone hasn't caught on yet, the expectation for COVID-19 immunization is that everyone will continue to get a regular annual vaccination, and there are no exceptions...AND just so you know, COVID-19 vaccines may be "updated," but the changes are minimal. The best news we have now—"as of August 27, 2025, the EUA status for COVID vaccines has been rescinded, by order of DHHS Secretary Robert F. Kennedy, Jr.! COVID-19 is no longer considered a public health emergency. COVID vaccines are still available, but no longer mandatory. In addition, the FDA is now requiring COVID SHOT(not vaccine) manufacturers to provide randomized, controlled, clinical trial data in order to ensure that the COVID shot approval is evidence based."[66]

We have chosen just a few of the heroes and heroines of the COVID era in this chapter and named many more in a previous chapter. There are hundreds, maybe thousands of courageous souls in the US and globally who are still doing their utmost to keep providing truth. It is extremely difficult with the weight of the globalist agenda behind everything they do, still propagandizing as hard and as fast as they can. They will NOT give up—there is too much money and power-mongering at stake. So God bless those who love the TRUTH. Scripture tells us:

"You will know the truth; and the truth will set you free...
so if the Son sets you free, you will be free indeed."

John 8: 32,36—ESV

Here, then, is the greatest of questions—"Who were the good guys in this whole scenario? Even more to the point—-who were the real villains?"

Part IV

Vaccinations—All Ramifications

Chapter 13

What and Why Are Vaccines Really?

The Definition and History of Vaccines

There is so much information on vaccines, it's nearly impossible to weed out the truth from the massive amounts of disinformation that have been compiled by Big Pharma, the FDA, the NIH, the WHO, and the CDC among others. They were present and being effectively used to maintain the vaccine farce long before COVID-19 ever surfaced. Vaccines have absolutely nothing to do with good health. As with most things, the main reason is the LOVE of MONEY:

> "People who long to be rich fall into temptation and are trapped by many foolish and harmful desires that plunge them into ruin and destruction. For the love of money is the root of all kinds of evil. And some people, craving money, have wandered from the true faith and pierced themselves with many sorrows." I Timothy 6: 9-10 NLT

With the clear influence of the globalist wolves' agenda, and the full cooperation of the globalists' Big Tech machinery, the disinformation and propaganda continue full speed ahead to their most extreme extent. Those professionals with a conscience, and integrity, also continue to tell the truth about vaccines, but it's much harder to hear them amidst the globalist din. The good news is that since the Trump administration resumed, the appointment of Robert F. Kennedy, Jr. to the office of HHS Secretary, a good many travesties and potential health issues have been addressed with panache, and our nation is definitely in a better health era for now. Therefore, it behooves us, the truth bearers, to study, learn, and know the truth thoroughly and be adept at disseminating that information far and wide, in order to minimize vaccine damage, and known mortality.

To do that, we need a good working definition of exactly what a vaccine is. According to the Cambridge Dictionary, a "vaccine is a created substance that is put into the body of a person or animal to protect them from a disease, often containing a weakened or dead form of the disease-causing organism, causing the recipient to produce antibodies (proteins that fight diseases)."[1] Hippocrates described the infectious diseases of mumps, diphtheria, epidemic jaundice, and other conditions in 400 BC but there were no proposals on treatment. However, by the 1100s, a technique called 'variolation' was developed, that involved the inoculation of children and adults with dried scab material recovered from smallpox patients. Variations of variolation have been noted in China, Turkey, Africa, and Europe at this time. It was not until 1721 that variolation was introduced in Great Britain.

The first disease that critically bothered mankind enough to seek a way of stopping the infection was smallpox. According to researchers, inoculation with material from smallpox lesions to trigger immunity against smallpox, dates back to antiquity in China, and the first written account of the procedure was described in 1549. There are versions of an earlier time of practicing inoculation in China before it was written down from oral histories. According to Arthur Boyleston, "the oral tradition in China was invented by a Taoist or Buddhist monk, or possibly a nun, about 1000 AD and practiced by Taoists as a mixture of medicine, technique, magic, and spells which were transmitted orally and covered by a taboo so that they were never written down. There is no firmer evidence for this...than the fact it was a widely accepted tradition. An editorial commentator wonders whether it is realistic to believe that something with the importance of inoculation would have remained completely secret for over 500 years. Secret or not, the practice of inoculation traveled west toward the Ottoman Empire in the 1500s, reaching Constantinople (modern day Istanbul, Turkey) in the mid-1600s. From there, it traveled to Europe and Northern Africa. Then it traveled to the Massachusetts Colony via an enslaved man named Onesimus. He told the Reverend Cotton Mather—of Salem Witchcraft Trials fame—about being inoculated by enslavers to resist smallpox and get better pay for his enslavement. Cotton Mather, together with a local doctor in Boston, adopted and promoted inoculation as a deadly smallpox epidemic arrived in Boston in 1721."[2] Is it not interesting that the first instances of vaccination included the use of witchcraft with magic and spells, hidden by a tribal taboo! About the same time, Lady Mary Wortley Montague, wife of a diplomat in Constantinople, decided to have a local physician inoculate her son, and later her daughter in Scotland. By 1723, it seemed clear, based on evidence, that inoculation by a physician in a controlled environment must be better than waiting to catch smallpox 'the natural way'. Later Benjamin Franklin became a champion of inoculation when his son died of smallpox in 1736. In a document he wrote in 1759, he included some numbers on death rates of those who had been inoculated which gave additional proof that the risk of death was lower in those who were variolated, making common the practice in Europe and North America. Then General George Washington ordered his American troops to be inoculated as part of their joining the Continental Army during the Revolutionary War.[3]

Consequently, by the late 1700s, Dr. Edward Jenner realized that milkmaids and others previously infected with cowpox were immune to smallpox. Cowpox caused pustules similar to smallpox, but cowpox was far fewer, the disease was much milder, and not lethal. Jenner devised regulated experiments where people who had never been ill with either disease, were inoculated first with cowpox, and later with smallpox. This approach worked; people showed a mild reaction to the cowpox, and no reaction, nor disease to the smallpox inoculation—the first vaccine was born! The cowpox inoculation remained the only vaccine in use for smallpox around the world for almost 80 years. Science and technology were not yet ready to create other vaccines, until "Louis Pasteur, a French biochemist, who began working on a treatment for the rabies virus using rabbits. The most well-known human guinea pig was Joseph Meister, who had been bitten by a rabid animal. To save his life, physicians allowed Pasteur to practice his experimental vaccine procedure on Joseph. Without it, Joseph would most likely die a painful death from rabies, so there was nothing to lose. After the 21 days of incubation, Joseph did NOT show any signs or symptoms of rabies. Using the infectious agent in a less virulent or "attenuated" way, other vaccines were created, based on the same principle of weakening the pathogen before giving it as an inoculation."[4]

Later in the 1800s, scientists were studying the immune response of humans and other animals and discovered "antibodies." These proteins were created some time after infection; they would bind to the pathogen and inactivate it. Without antibodies, a person could develop the disease and die, so scientists worked on safe ways to create those antibodies in large numbers and give them to people as a sort of immune "patch," to enable people to develop their own antibodies. This was the beginning of the concept of "anti-toxins." This discovery and usage resulted in problems with allergic reactions and injuries from the animals used to make them which led to the creation of toxoid vaccines. In 1902, contamination of one anti-toxin with actual tetanus toxin led to several injuries. The US federal government responded by creating the agency now known as the Food and Drug Administration.[5]

Scientists have subsequently continued working on vaccines against all types of virus groups to prevent more diseases. By 1954, Jonas Salk and his team developed the first "killed virus" vaccine against polio. It went against the vaccine norms of the time. It was believed that a vaccine MUST contain live/attenuated virus, and that a dead virus would NOT cause an immune response. Dr. Isabel Morgan and other women led the way to the vaccine which saved thousands of children's lives. The 1960's brought the oral polio vaccine developed by Albert Sabin as a replacement to Salk's vaccine. However, there was a very big fly in the polio ointment in April of 1955, known as the "Cutter Incident." Right in the middle of the vast public acclaim for the Salk polio vaccine, "Dozens of people who had recently received shots came down with what appeared to be vaccine-induced cases of the disease. The CDC's recently-formed Epidemic Intelligence Service swung into action and traced the cases to vaccine lots from Cutter Laboratories, whose manufacturing procedures had been insufficient to inactivate the virus. A lawsuit against Cutter subsequently found that the company had not been negligent but was nevertheless liable for damages. The case established the legal doctrine of liability without fault, according to which pharmaceutical companies could be held responsible for harm caused by their products even if they had acted in keeping with the best-available methods and standards."[6] That doctrine should have been kept and enhanced long before they tried anything as dangerous as a 'vaccine that wasn't a 'vaccine!'

Critics have seen the successful litigation against Cutter and the "legal doctrine of liability without fault" as the root of many of the difficulties plaguing today's vaccine system. A series of suits followed, especially when two important rulings against Wyeth Laboratories, established that vaccine manufacturers had a legal duty to warn recipients of the tiny risk of paralytic polio that was an inherent property of the live attenuated virus. These cases held ramifications for vaccine liability. The Cutter Incident eroded the public's trust in vaccines, even though polio was essentially eliminated from the America's, Europe, and most of Asia by the early 2000s. "The greatest cause of vaccine reluctance in today's issues is the ways and means that the most current COVID-19 'vaccines' were produced. As we have discussed previously, there were MANY things done in the process that have rightfully caused people to take their chances with COVID rather than take the jab, including the following: the rapidly produced, under-tested 'vaccines' that had multiple problems but were released anyway under the EUA law; the now known toxicity of the 'vaccines' that has never been admitted by the manufacturers; the mandates which forced compliance on so many people who were not allowed individual autonomy in the decision; some losing jobs over it; some losing health and life over it; ongoing adverse events and ill health causing great frustration and pain in their lives; the inability to get retribution for damages; the multiple lies told and the misinformation rather than facts about the 'vaccines', and so much more."[7] Any literature you can find throughout Big Tech sources still contains propaganda and misinformation everywhere you look. All questions asked are answered ambiguously, real facts and figures are hidden, and no real information on risks, numbers, and real incidences of adverse events are ever given. There is NOTHING on the world-wide-web that is fully trustworthy.

Here is the thing that characterizes the push for full vaccination compliance for every person on the planet. The use of vaccinations started out with a genuine desire to help obliterate infectious diseases and their spread. For multiple millennia, humanity had various diseases but they also had a God-given innate immune system He created in every way, to protect and heal itself perfectly. For the most part, when men lived relatively healthy lives with natural foods, few toxins and natural untainted resources, they did quite well in the war on disease. Early in man's civilization, humanity was able to live as much as nine times longer than we do today, relying on God's provision instead of trying to improve on it. It took humanity a long time to systematically break down what had been provided. Today, too many people are convinced that God's provision is not enough and His resources are going to run out, when real science informs us there are just as many untapped resources today, as we had when we started. This author believes it's imperative to question the global narrative on everything, including immunizations, because humanity has so badly skewed what God, in His infinite wisdom so perfectly provided. There are plenty of great answers to perceived problems today, which don't now, nor will they ever come from the globalist agenda. It is 100% anti-God, and destined to utter failure. It is imperative we humans, created in the image of God, question all of this propaganda and seek the Source of all truth today! The sole reason for promoting universal vaccination has NOTHING to do with better health and those promoting this agenda have only one motivation—more wealth. Of course they do love the control that came with it as well.

> "I praise You because I am fearfully and wonderfully made; Marvelous are Your works, and that my soul knows very well." Psalm 139:14 NKJV

> "Jesus turned and saw her: 'Take heart, daughter,' He said, 'your faith has made you well.' And instantly the woman was made well." Matthew 9:22 ESV

> "The joy of the LORD is your strength," Nehemiah 8:10b

Before we discuss pros and cons of vaccines in more depth, we should try to understand how vaccines actually work. Pathogens or disease-carrying organisms are all around us, both in our environments and in our bodies. If a person is susceptible and encounters a harmful organism, it could lead to disease and even death. However, as we previously said, our bodies have many ways of defending themselves against these pathogens. Skin, mucus, and cilia (microscopic hairs that move debris away from the lungs) all work as physical barriers that prevent the pathogens from even entering our bodies in the first place. When a pathogen does infect the body, our body's defenses, called the immune system, are triggered, the pathogen is attacked and either destroyed or overcome.

A pathogen is a bacterium, virus, parasite, or fungus that can cause disease within us. Each pathogen is made up of several subparts, usually unique to that particular pathogen and the disease it causes. The subpart of a pathogen that causes the formation of antibodies is called an antigen. The antibodies produced in response to the antigen are a very important part of our immune system. They are like the soldiers that do the fighting. Each antibody, or soldier, is trained to recognize one specific antigen. We each have thousands of antibodies in our bodies. When the human body is exposed to an antigen for the very first time, it takes some time for the immune system to respond and produce antibodies specific to that antigen. In the meantime, the body may become ill. Once the antigen-specific antibodies are produced, they work with the rest of the immune system to destroy the pathogen and stop the disease. The antibodies to one pathogen generally don't protect against a different pathogen unless the two are very similar to each other, like cousins. However, once the body produces antibodies in its primary response to an antigen, it also creates antibody-producing memory cells, which remain alive even after the pathogen has been destroyed. If the body is exposed to the same pathogen more than once, the antibody response is much faster and more efficient than the first time because the memory cells are at the ready to pump out antibodies against that pathogen.[8] Therefore, if a person is exposed to the dangerous pathogen in the future, his immune system will be able to respond immediately, and protect him from the disease. This process is described as "attaining natural immunity"—just as our Abba intended.

In the past, science has been able to both understand and help our bodies form antibodies for various diseases by the use of vaccines. "The process of making a vaccine uses weakened, non-dangerous, or inactive parts of a particular organism (antigen), introduced into the body to trigger an immune response within the body. It is enough to help our body's immune system learn to build the specific antibody needed to help it fight that disease. Then, when the body encounters the real antigen later on, it already knows how to fight it."[9] The current process of making vaccines such as for COVID-19 does NOT contain the antigen itself. Instead it uses a genetic "blueprint" for producing antigens rather than the antigen itself. For many of us, this newer process is very problematic, because the "blueprint" contains genetic material from many sources, even animal sources instead of human ones, and there is no way for any of us to determine whose DNA and mRNA strands have been used in the vaccine to be placed into our bodies. Health officials, Big Pharma, the CDC, the WHO, and the FDA have all approved this form of vaccination, and continue to insist it is safe, effective, and reliable. However, it's impossible to find out ***exactly*** what has been utilized in these vaccines unless you have medical and scientific bio-research ability to do so, and there are no voluntary disclosures on the part of Big Pharma. Somehow, they don't believe it is necessary to disclose the sources of ingredients in their vaccines, but still insist we allow it to be put into our bodies, on their say-so alone. This is NOT acceptable, no matter how much they may have refined them since the experimental first vaccines rolled out. The blueprint manufacture is the same. All of the above so-called "scientific" entities have mass-produced their propaganda and continue to push these vaccines 100%. Every bit of "official" literature on the web insists these vaccines are both safe and effective and we MUST accept them even for our 6month-old infants. Anyone with the audacity to disagree with the narrative, is immediately dubbed as a misinformation spreader. However, it is important for you, the reader, to look and listen to the information they refute, for yourself. There are hundreds of doctors and scientists who do not adhere to the narrative for many reasons we will be discussing. It is imperative that you do your homework, though admittedly, it is not easy. Good and true information does exist along with the proof needed to help you make informed decisions. Just be aware that the internet is NOT necessarily your friend when truth is needed.

In the case of COVID-19 "vaccines" which are NOT vaccines in the truest sense of the word, there is an entire body of truthful information, procured by many of the finest physicians and scientists in our nation and across the globe. We have mentioned many of their names already. Most specifically, what needs to be said here is the fact that the narratives we have ready access to, all tout the marvelous benefits and reasons for these vaccines, but they rarely mention side effects or adverse events in tens of thousands of people who have taken them. They might tell you some of the possibilities, but will immediately inform you that such events are very rare. They will give numbers and graphs that are meant to portray what they want them to say. There are some overt lies but much of the time they come through simple omission of truth. If we pay attention to their own Big Tech news media, and follow the daily numbers of young people who either died after COVID-19 jabs or were left with lifelong disabilities, there is plenty of evidence clearly reported, but "official" public health authorities continue to deny most of these facts, saying they can't "prove" the casualties were vaccine induced. Also, we regularly hear of other ways people have been affected by these jabs, and the list has grown exponentially. As we mentioned previously, fewer than 10% of adverse events and deaths from the jabs have even been reported, and those that have been are just the tip of the iceberg, as we will also learn. Consequently, you may call this paragraph your WARNING!

There is a "Vaccine Information Fact Sheet for Recipients and Caregivers" giving some information. First, it tells you that the recipient will be given one of three possible vaccines and until August 2025 said it was authorized under the Emergency Use Authorization (EUA) by the FDA as of August 31, 2022 for each vaccine. "The term 'MONOVALENT' used with the vaccine name refers to any authorized or approved COVID-19 vaccine that contains or encodes the spike protein of only the Original SARS-CoV-2. The fact sheet specifically states you should NOT get any of these vaccines if: you had a severe allergic reaction after a previous dose of a COVID vaccine or if you had a severe allergic reaction to any ingredient in these vaccines."[10] Dear reader, do you know how many people under the mandatory vaccine rule were still coerced into taking a second dose of the vaccine or boosters when they had incurred severe reactions to the first dose, and either died or were severely injured by the second because they couldn't afford to lose their jobs?!!! We know it happened over and over and most were NOT documented by anyone. Without proof, legally, nothing happened!! But this author, and almost everyone she knows, is completely aware of a relative, friend, or acquaintance to whom it clearly happened. Further, almost anyone to whom you, the reader, has spoken, can also affirm such reports. That number alone, if they could somehow be counted, is exponential.

Following are the "stated ingredients in the three main COVID-19 'vaccines:' messenger ribonucleic acid (mRNA—source unknown), lipids (SM-1029, fat molecules), polyethylene glycol [PEG] 2000, dimyristoyl glycerol [DMG], cholesterol, and 1,2distearoyl-sn-slycero-3-phosphocholine [DSPC], tromethamine, tromethamine hydrochloride, acetic acid, sodium acetate trihydrate, and sucrose. The FDA added a warning label on the mRNA vaccines regarding 'serious (but rare) cases of inflammation of the heart muscle (myocarditis) and of the outer lining of the heart (pericarditis) in adolescents and young adults, more often occurring after the second dose of an mRNA vaccine- on April 24, 2022"[11] Note that as is usually the case, the first ingredient listed is the main and most prominent one in that product, and we have no idea as non-scientists what has been used to make that genetic main ingredient. More will be said in the next chapter about the actual ingredients and the reasons they are present.

Ever since the very beginning of the COVID-19 pandemic, the statistics have always indicated that children and infants have a very low risk of sickening with SARSCo-V-2, and should they actually succumb, an even lower risk of it being significant, and certainly NOT life-threatening. Today, in the "Early Childhood Vaccine Schedule, from birth to six years, there are already approximately 30 doses of various vaccines required by the state in order to start school. There's also a minimum of six others, not including influenza and COVID-19 annually in the adolescent years following. In most states, since August 30, 2021, non-medical exemptions are no longer issued."[12] This is a critical indictment of governmental overreach in all our lives and particularly our children, who have no personal control at all. We are shooting foreign substances into our children FROM BIRTH, before their immature immune systems have had opportunity to naturally do what they would do if left alone, with absolutely no moral or ethical compunctions, and literally scant possibility of avoiding it, because our governmental bodies say we have to do it. Does this NOT bother parents anymore? It should bother every freedom-loving citizen of this United States, that our government has the implicit ability to hijack our children for what they deem is in their best interest, and more importantly in the best interest of all citizens. Parents have been completely robbed of their ability to decide what is or is NOT best for their children!

We also want to look at benefits vs risks for infants and small children re: COVID-19 immunization. Going back to the FACT SHEET for all recipients, we see that the ONLY benefit for this age group is whatever measure of protection against COVID19 is attained. Based on their known risk for the disease which is next to nil, the benefit is truly negligible! On the other hand there are significant risks in getting the COVID19 vaccination. The fact sheet claims there is "a remote risk" the vaccine can cause a severe allergic reaction, though the stats do not show it to be "remote." Signs of such a severe reaction include:

- Difficulty breathing
- Swelling of the face and throat
- An accelerated heartbeat
- A bad rash all over the body
- Dizziness and weakness

Myocarditis (inflammation of the heart muscle) and pericarditis (inflammation of the lining outside the heart) have occurred in some people, most commonly in young adult males. Reactions usually occur within a few minutes to one hour after the jab. Many with such reactions were nowhere near emergency help when it was needed.

How would you as a parent of an infant or small child receiving this unnecessary vaccine feel if you witnessed this life-threatening (anaphylaxis) reaction in your helpless child just 10 minutes after leaving the clinic, and you couldn't get help fast enough to save him? HELPLESS! So your child might be one in a hundred or a thousand that has a reaction—how much comfort would that be if it is your child? All of this is done to protect your child from an illness similar to the common cold to him. Can we all see how little sense this makes? During the two weeks after a jab, your child could experience:

- Chest pain, headaches, fever/chills
- Shortness of breath or difficulty breathing
- Feelings of having a fast-beating, fluttering, or pounding heart
- Excess sleepiness, fainting
- Unusual and persistent irritability, crying
- Unusual and persistent poor feeding
- Unusual and persistent fatigue or lack of energy
- Persistent vomiting
- Persistent pain in the abdomen, muscle or joint pain
- Unusual and persistent cool, pale skin
- Serious, unexpected side effects, still being studied

If any or many of these symptoms occur, call 9-1-1, or go to the hospital immediately.[13]

Following treatment, it is imperative that the adverse event from the vaccine be reported to the FDA/CDC Vaccine Adverse Event Reporting System (VAERS). The VAERS toll-free number is 1-800-822-7967 or report online to https://vaers.hhs.gov/reportevent.html Thousands of people have received no help or restitution of any kind after adverse events, and statistics remain skewed as to their incidence because the necessary reports were not filed. If necessary, see a lawyer qualified in such cases to help you. There is also a Countermeasures Injury Compensation Program

(CICP). The federal government may help pay costs of medical care and other specific expenses of certain people who have been seriously injured by some specific medications or vaccines, including COVID-19. A claim must be submitted to the CICP within one year from the date of receiving the vaccine. To learn more, see www.hrsa.gov/cicp/ or call 1-855-266-2427. If any restitution is given, it is considered a rare event.

Traditional Arguments For/Against Mass, Compulsory Vaccinations

While vaccines have aided many global public health successes, such as the eradication of smallpox, they have long continued to be the subject of multiple ethical controversies. The key ethical debates related to vaccine regulation, development, and use most often revolve around: 1) mandates, 2) research and testing, 3) informed consent, and 4) access disparities. In the US, state policies mandate certain immunizations, including school entry requirements, which cover vast numbers of children. Ethical debates and objections to school and other mandates arise frequently, as they should, because individuals and even whole communities disagree with the mandates, and/or have religious or philosophical beliefs conflicting with the ways and means of doing them.

For example, public health vaccine regulators who want, supposedly, to protect the greatest number of people, have badly infringed upon individual autonomy and liberty. However, when this public health monopoly has become a system of compulsory control over everyone, and the numbers of vaccination requirements have increased exponentially over a few decades, there is plenty of room to question real motivation. That is especially true when a small minority of extremely wealthy suppliers continuously grow wealthier by the day from this mandatory process! Since the advent of COVID-19, this has become increasingly clear; the mandatory process became even more suspect for a large number of reasons we've already discussed. Excessive infringement on individual rights and loss of personal freedoms certainly did nothing to decrease the distrust and obvious questions on motivation. Since that time, tensions have run high, and distrust even higher as individuals hated the massive control, and now more than ever wanted to exercise their rights to protect themselves and their children by refusing to comply with compulsory vaccinations. That is especially true if they don't accept the existing and ever-present "EVIDENCE" of so-called medical or safety information, or if their ideological beliefs do NOT support mass vaccination.[14]

The standard argument for restrictions on individual rights is that they are justified for two reasons—for the benefit of the individual and/or the benefit of the community. However, in the excellent company of a great number of other individuals, this author vehemently objects to this statement. It implies that the "powers-that-be" have the right to make that determination, supposedly because we other individuals are unable or incapable of making our own decisions as to what will or will not ***benefit*** us. That does NOT justify their restrictions, particularly when the FACTS being presented are NOT absolutely true, and are partially a matter of the opinion of someone with letters behind their name. Big deal, many of us have equally impressive letters behind our names! There have been instances where, for example, the health of a child was considered at risk by authorities, who sought to override parental autonomy. However, even the American Academy of Pediatrics recently concluded, "Continued vaccine refusal after adequate discussion should be respected unless the child is put at significant risk of serious harm. Only then should state agencies be involved to override parental discretion on the basis of medical neglect."[15] AMEN!!

Another standard argument for compulsory vaccination is that individual autonomy law may be curtailed to protect the community from infectious disease because unvaccinated individuals pose a risk to the entire community—including other unvaccinated individuals. However, vaccines are NOT 100% effective, some children are too young to be vaccinated, and there are some persons who have medical vaccine contraindications.

There is often either real or perceived disagreement between individual and community benefits and it may be based on current scientific evidence which supposedly overrides individual autonomy. The problem with that as we saw so clearly during COVID, was that even "official" public health people couldn't agree with each other, nor could any one official make up his mind as to the scientific evidence which frequently did 180-degree shifts, followed by subsequent policy changes that left most of us shaking our heads. We were to 'Follow the Science,' but those of us who know science reasonably well, couldn't find the science in the morass of lies.

When the state does curtail individual freedoms for the collective good, it should also address several issues including the magnitude of the individual and community risk, the strength of the individual's conviction, wider and long-term consequences of restricting individual autonomy, effective risk communication, best available scientific evidence, and transparency in the decision-making process. It is beyond fair now, for the purpose of this book, to point out that none of these things were legitimately cared for prior to mandates for COVID-19. They simply didn't exist anywhere. However, one of the most influential and enduring philosophies in history, developed by Immanuel Kant, and known as "***categorical imperative***," states, "Act only according to that maxim by which you can at the same time will it to become a universal law which preserves individual autonomy and emphasizes ideas such as informed consent."[16] That idea clearly wasn't considered either.

In continued discussion of this controversy, we have an exceedingly arguable issue brought up frequently concerning who decides if a particular vaccine is really safe or not. The truth is that safety studies are NEVER done by the CDC or the FDA, but by Big Pharma and its billion-dollar manufacturers. This by any legal standard is known as a direct "conflict of interest." Naturally, the manufacturer of a vaccine stands to make an incomprehensible amount of money if it states its own product is both safe and effective. That simply is NOT good enough. Such a statement by a company with regard to its own product wouldn't fly in any other business but medicine/drugs. A competitive company wouldn't stand for it in the market. The reality of the entire testing process for a new drug or vaccine is normally arduous and necessarily lengthy. Drug safety testing is a very complicated process involving many different steps to ensure the highest level of safety, including preclinical research and preclinical safety assessment testing. Then clinical trials include phase I, II, III, and IV trials, the last being post-marketing surveillance. The first three trials are to attain FDA approval. It is all complex and extremely time-consuming, averaging 14 years to complete phases I-III.[17] However, the caveat is that knowing you have new drugs/vaccines you want to have approved for use almost immediately, there is no time for this lengthy process and you must CREATE an emergency like a pandemic enabling you to utilize the Emergency Use Authorization process so that the normal lengthy process is NOT necessary and all the majority of the safety testing process is omitted. That is exactly what happened with the COVID-19 vaccines and the drug Remdesivir. They were all experimental drugs with known toxicity and the strong potential of adverse events, but the FDA approved them under the EUA very quickly. No other regulating body was necessary for its approval.

To further understand the ramifications of the above method of approval by the FDA under the Emergency Use Authorization, we need to look at the vast number of COVID-19 vaccines that went through it and were later removed from authorization:

- The Johnson & Johnson Covid vaccine- early in the vax process, 100 suspected cases of Guillain-Barré syndrome. Thrombosis and thrombocytopenia (TTS), blood clotting disorders, caused pauses in its use, and was later revoked entirely.
- Janssen Covid vaccine, FDA revoked EUA 6/1/23
- Oxford-AstraZeneca Covid vaccine withdrawn—blood clots still a problem

- Moderna Bivalent is no longer authorized
- Pfizer-BioNTech is no longer authorized

All original COVID-19 vaccines were replaced by updated versions, however these, too, were still under EUA.[18] Many other vaccines produced in the past for other infections were also found flawed and were discontinued. It's an extensive list that came largely because of court cases regarding vaccine injuries. We will give a few examples that were especially tragic, to give the reader an idea of the extent of the real problem.

Worst Case Adverse Events and Deaths BEFORE COVID-19

The first example is taken from the film, "Vaccines Revealed," by Director, Patrick Gentempo, DC, CEO of Revealed Films Library, which contained decades of documented facts about real-life people. The good doctor's goal was and has always been to disseminate truth.[19] The first story is of an infant, Porter Bridges, whose mother, Sarah shared her child's story. Baby Porter was vaccinated with a live-virus Pertussis vaccine, to which he severely reacted and was later diagnosed with Pertussis-induced Brain Injury. As usual, at his very young age, giving this highly unsafe vaccine was NOT about healing or even protecting anyone, it was all about control.[20]

Sarah Bridges was awakened the same night of Porter's vaccination by his eerie, high-pitched screams and a temperature of 105 degrees, but was unable to wake him. They arrived at the hospital emergency room just in time for a grand mal seizure that lasted for two full hours. He was intubated, ventilated and sedated, and finally woke to mental retardation and autism. At age 20, he is still fully brain-injured with borderline irreversible encephalopathy, which is usually caused by infections or long-tern exposure to toxins such as drugs and chemicals. Sarah was able to find a vaccine 'court', a very long and drawn-out process—taking almost seven years to finally resolve his case. That pertussis (live-virus) was still on the market for a full six months after Porter's brain injury, but had been on the market for decades before it was removed. Most of his medical bills were still paid for by his parents, but because of the court case, they were able to get some decent resources for Porter. Without it, this type of lifelong travesty would devastate, even sink most people in similar situations.

In the decades-long process of compulsory immunizations, most people are NOT fully informed of real risks they are taking, nor anything of the consequences they will face in the occurrence of adverse events. Having worked in doctors' offices and pediatric clinics, this author can attest to the ways that children's shots are given. Parents are mostly resigned to their seeming inevitability ,and are shown and given fact sheets for each vaccine, listing some of the risks, but not all of them. There is usually no time to read through the sheets before their child is vaccinated, and very often, any questions go unanswered. With a bit of good fortune they might at least get a few verbal precautions to watch for before leaving. Worse yet, as a parent, you can't even imagine the reality of an actual adverse event, or what the eventual ramifications might be unless you've done your homework and/or heard some horror stories. For the Bridges family, this debacle resulted in a broken marriage, governmental representatives' denials of the realities and needs Porter incurred, as the doctors, therapists, and others had all said. Pertussis vaccine encephalopathy was first reported 56 years ago, and the compensation system was extremely poor. There was no humanity exhibited, and in fact the parents felt very blamed and shamed most of the time, as authorities even today continue denying the clear and proven 'correlation between vaccines and autism.' Hundreds of kids/families have been compensated in some measure for damage done. However, the entire system from the Journal of Pediatric Medicine on down swears there is NO link at all, and using the word "autism" negates any further cooperation; you will certainly not be heard.

Here is a brief excerpt of what the Journal says, "Analysis of the recent literature does NOT support the existence of such a syndrome and suggests that neurologic events after immunization are chance temporal associations of neurologic conditions that occur in the target age group, even in the absence of immunization. (meaning it just suddenly happens in a perfectly normal infant for no explainable reason, and just happened to occur on the day of the vaccination). Population-based studies do not prove a causal relationship with acute encephalopathy, (they don't prove it doesn't either). There are no consistent neuropathologic findings suggesting a specific pathophysiologic process, and hypotheses concerning possible mechanisms of damage are not supported by reproducible studies in children...There clearly is an increased risk of a convulsion after DPT immunizations but no evidence that this produces brain injury or is a forerunner of epilepsy. Studies have also not linked immunization with either sudden infant death syndrome (SIDS) or infantile spasms."[20] Increased numbers of children with autism have become exponential. Government is fully aware of it, but still denies it. In a very real sense, this quote from the journal as good as admits the potential correlation when it states the potential of convulsions after DPTs. Convulsions ARE seizures and seizures are the most common anaphylactic responses in children. Even in the area of the NICU in this nurse's experience, seizures VERY often cause acute brain injury, no matter the cause, and the effects of them are usually not known till later in the child's development, sometimes much later. Does the reader begin to understand why there is often a clear element of distrust of what medical literature has to say? It is often not trustworthy by virtue of what it doesn't say. Any hint that there may be fault in treatment protocols promptly gets danced-around or covered up. Beyond this problem, good factual and provable information is available, but 95% of the time it will be labeled as "misinformation" by Big Tech, and too many medical and scientific professionals choose to play the globalist game, because they will not risk being shut down, banned, or any of the things that do happen to the professionals who refuse to play the globalist game.[21]

The reader will note that when a child has a severe adverse event or dies, the parents are often bashed, bullied, treated as pariahs, and not supported while they try to do the best they can for their child. What often happens to such a family who fights the battle for their child is much like what happened to Sarah Bridges in the story we've already shared. Under the worst stress anyone can imagine, once happy marriages fail; the health of one or both parents, as well as of siblings crashes, causing further stress and expense; decent sleep is often rare; there is intense and unrelenting grief in the constant fight; the dreams once held for the injured or lost child die, like a death, without an actual death; the normalcy of life as they knew it is gone forever, and it's all just too much for the family to handle day to day. There are NOT just a few stories that happen only rarely; there are thousands just like this one.[22] Adding to all of the above, there are tons of issues with the court systems. Only a handful of lawyers can personally afford to keep trying these cases, because it takes so long for the government to pay them. Most chemicals (vaccines) will cause both an environmental and a genetic event. Porter was given no further DPT vaccine, but he was given other vaccines later. He wound up in the intensive care unit again, crashed and regressed. Their doctor finally agreed there would be no further vaccines for Porter, and ordered extreme caution with his siblings. Why did it take so much trauma, for a professional to finally agree that vaccines were NOT wise for Porter? The reality is that they very often aren't wise about many other children either. All chemicals and drugs have potential side effects, and half the world swearing it isn't true of vaccines is not fixing a very serious and ever-worsening problem. There are many alternate ways of using vaccines more judiciously, such as waiting until children are older and their immune systems more mature, rescheduling them, or staggering the various vaccines given instead of hitting the child with several at one time. Some of these ideas are used in other countries, like Sweden, with far less adverse events exhibited.[23]

Who should be handling your child's health care, vaccinations, and decision-making? Exemptions for the hyper-scheduling of compulsory vaccinations are gone or going in most states, however it's a huge issue among professionals and one being addressed by HHS. But parents should be making these decisions, NOT the government-sponsored public health agencies. This problem has been compounded by an enormous overreach of government power, analogous to totalitarian health care, which of course is part of the globalist agenda. Current systems failed its citizens in a massive way during COVID. Isolation from the world at large is really impossible, but vaccine safety, with all its failures, MUST be better discussed and investigated.

Victimized parents and children have been treated abominably, as pariahs, for advocating for their injured family members—a travesty that knows no bounds today. Now it is necessary more than ever before, for parents to BE EDUCATED!! Understand what this governmental overreach has done to our medical system and the damage that has been done to so many of our children. The incidence of autism alone in this country knows no bounds, and continues to rise exponentially. There is no conceivable chance that Big Pharma will ever back away from its billions in drug/vaccine profits. There is no motivation to do so, and there is no accountability or liability. It will take an act of Congress to redeem this system and that can only happen when parents and concerned citizens rise up and demand it. What tragedies have happened in children's and family's lives are seldom even heard, and even in a court win, the ultimate results in those families are seldom ever heard, or mourned.

Another, very well-known supporter of vaccination reform is Robert F. Kennedy, Jr. Despite what you may have heard from all Big Tech globalist supporters, he has definitely been able to raise awareness as to what Big Pharma, public health honchos, and globalist politicians want the world to believe about vaccinations. He is the chairman and founder of the Children's Health Defense. He is constantly accused of being the leading proponent of anti-vax advocacy and COVID-19 vaccine "misinformation." As such, he is constantly bashed, bullied, fact-checked by the same globalist media base, and accused of being a conspiracy theorist. While all of that is beyond annoying to hear constantly, this author views that accusation as a "badge of courage" since it occurred throughout the COVID-19 era, and the majority of conspiracy theories have since been proven factual.[24]

RFK, Jr. has in fact been a huge advocate for vaccine-damaged children and their parents. With his political advantage, and connectedness, he's had a lot to potentially lose battling his foes, but "he is passionate about all he has seen and learned about vax-related problems and injuries. He has also been especially critical of the mercury and other environmental pollutants found in monumental levels in our water, soil, fish, etc. The mercury contamination in our fresh fish supply is still high. Mercury in the vaccine supply became very problematic because few people read the science. The federal government tried to sweep the whole issue under a big rug. Many studies existed about mercury poisoning and there were many links to autism. The general public had a total disconnect to the issue because it had been journalistically buried for so long and lied about,"[24] Up to 70% of advertising money came directly from Big Pharma. While it might be true that media peons actually believe they are helping families and kids by promoting vaccines, it's highly unlikely. The worst behaviors in public health have been incentivized by MEDIA which works hand-in-hand with the CDC and Big Pharma. They MUST sell vaccines!! Huge financial incentives push more and more vaccines, so that the compulsory immunization schedule of vaccines for kids has grown exponentially. It's very hard to have faith in this massive increase in vaccines; more than anywhere else in the world, when there is clear conflict of interest. Allowing the decisions for more and more flies in the face of necessity, when its clear there is a massive profit margin for all of Big Pharma and its many globalist supporters.

"These are all issues frequently voiced by Kennedy, to the chagrin of Big Pharma and its entire system. No wonder the accusations fly. To make the entire vaccination scene even worse, in 1986, Congress was complicit with Big Pharma when it passed the Vaccine Act. That ACT effectively exempted the industries of vaccines and drugs, so that no matter what they decided to do or say, true or false, they can do pretty much as they please. There is NO liability, giving complete freedom to bring to market whatever they want, some without any real testing or clinical trials at all. Pure pay dirt! This ACT launched a literal "gold rush" in the vaccine business. The profit margin was enormous with comparatively scant cost involved. There was a massive increase in vaccines and a huge increase in mercury from 70 mcgs to 230 mcgs; the numbers of vax-affected kids increased exponentially."[25] Disorders scarcely ever known in children for 2500 years, showed up in one of every 68 kids. While the "unbiased" science heroically tried to attribute the huge increase in autism to various and sundry environmental potential causes, an excellent article was written about the clear correlation of mercury and autism. This review focused specifically on mercury exposure with an exhaustive 91 studies examining this correlation.

"Examination of the relationship between mercury and autism spectrum disorders (ASD) from 1999 to February of 2016, the vast majority (74%) suggested that mercury is a risk factor for ASD, revealing both direct and indirect effects. The preponderance of the evidence indicates that mercury exposure is causal and/or contributory in ASD"[26] This was despite the "experts" claiming that the whole idea had been debunked, and Kennedy was accused once again of conspiratorial theories. It simply comes down to who you want to believe. This author has a very large tendency to believe the persons who have no "skin in the fight!!" Those wanting to make many more billions in vaccine profits do not qualify! At the same time, there were multiple other increases in mercury exposures in areas beyond vaccines. Clearly, it was also an oft-used environmental toxin as well. Based on the timing of the 1989 Vaccine Act above, from that marker there was also an exponential increase in many neurological health problems. In addition, any person exposed to mercury poisoning as a precursor, might also find other health problems occurring due to mitochondrial cellular damage throughout the body. Yet these multi-billion-dollar industries are virtually unchecked, and there is NO liability for the damages they directly caused. Mercury is used to produce chlorine gas and caustic soda, and is in thermometers, barometers, batteries, and electrical products. Workers in facilities where electrical equipment is manufactured are at risk of exposure. The inhalation of mercury vapor produces harmful effects on the nervous, digestive, immune, pulmonary, and urinary systems. The mercury salts are corrosive to the skin, eyes, and digestive system. Meanwhile, "efforts have been made in industry to cut mercury contamination."

Expectant mothers in particular are warned not to eat mercury-affected fish to protect their infants in the womb, yet thimerosal, a mercury-based preservative is still used in some vaccines. In 1999, Public Health Service agencies, the American Academy of Pediatrics, and vaccine manufacturers agreed that thimerosal should be reduced or eliminated in vaccines as a precautionary measure, though they all swear there is no evidence of harm caused by these low doses of thimerosal in vaccines, except for minor reactions like redness and swelling at injection sites. However, in 2001, thimerosal was removed from all vaccines except influenza."[27] The various health agencies in 1999, perpetrated the idea that the mercury in thimerosal was not in a dangerous form and was excreted from the body in days. "What they didn't tell the public, is that the mercury was actually metabolized to an organic form that was 2-3 times more toxic, and in fact was NOT excreted, but crossed the blood/ brain and placental barriers and sat IN the brain. People in the production of mercury-laced vaccines KNEW they were toxic, especially to infants under 6 months of age."[28] However, to change them all would largely reduce the profits from the pocketbooks. The CDC had a secret meeting, not well-known but well-documented with a large email trail in the Vaccine Safety Data Base, established for this very reason. 75 vaccine makers met with health officials on what to do! At first, the problem was hidden, the vaccines continued unaltered, but were NOT given to their own families. On official vaccination websites where vaccine ingredients are listed, there is a large, colored caveat stating that "some websites may claim that ingredients are harmful; make sure you seek information from credible sources." Another caveat in a second, colored box stated, "CDC and FDA take great care to make sure that a vaccine is safe both before it is licensed and after the public begins using it. Making sure that all vaccines are safe is a top priority for CDC."[29] After the era of COVID-19, we all can readily trust that!! NOT!!!!

So, after all the information was presented, an in-house epidemiologist reviewed it all. Mercury was deemed a potent neurotoxin. It was decided and verified that an infant under 6 months of age had from 760% to 1100% greater risk of autism, speech delays, ADD, ADHD, and many other neurological risks. The epidemiologist instructed the CDC to do a wide range of studies on all the data, and they have NEVER done that to this day, though many other independent groups have done so. However, in other countries where the exposure to mercury was far less, autism was exploding, especially in Sweden. They changed their vax schedules, removed the thimerosal, and their figures improved dramatically. So the American CDC clearly deceived and defrauded the American public in all the mercury-related vaccination issues. The proof of this exists, but it is NOT allowed in court and the folks who have all the facts in hand have NOT been allowed to testify. It also proves, at any given time, decisions may seem rational and good for the public, which fully justifies what they did at that time. However, this kind of decision is far from rare.[29]

A well-known case in point was the wisdom of a Hungarian physician, obstetrician, and scientist of German descent who in 1850 was an early pioneer of aseptic procedures. He was even described as 'the Savior of Mothers.' Postpartum infections, also known as puerperal fever, were rampant after childbirth and often fatal. "Ignaz Semmelweis discovered that the incidence of these infections could be drastically reduced by requiring all healthcare workers in obstetrical clinics to disinfect their hands. When done, the mortality rate of these mothers dropped from 18% to less than 2%, and he published a book. Despite his research, his observations conflicted with the established scientific and medical opinions of the time and his ideas were rejected by the medical community.

Many doctors were offended at the suggestion they might be at fault with contaminated hands."[30] Fifteen years later, the increasingly outspoken doctor allegedly suffered a 'nervous breakdown', was committed to an asylum by his colleagues, beaten by the guards, and died two weeks later of a gangrenous wound on his right hand." He was just a few years before Pasteur's and Lister's work! Many times, especially in the presence of other egotistical colleagues, it just doesn't pay to be right!

Here's the crux of the problem—the Centers for Disease Control cannot withstand a Public Debate! It may have started out with right motives in its glory days, but today the CDC is a mere 'tower of deceit.' The mainstream media is completely compromised and backs the deceit of the CDC almost all the time. The US government also backs and protects it. Before, during, and since COVID, medical doctors can lose their licenses by disagreeing with the CDC. Once highly-respected professional Journals of Medicine, that gave provable facts have been compromised by the weaponized CDC. Now their bottom-line abstracts may be edited to make them say what public health officials, some doctors, and scientists want them to say. To reverse the damage and subsequent inability to trust any of them, the powerful light of the sun itself needs to be shown on it from many sources. However, no one is allowed to talk about it, under threat of great personal damage. There should be forced debate in the Public Square. This system is akin to their religion—it's cruel, it's vicious, and it vilifies victims. Never before have very normal children been damned to only partial lives for the rest of their lives simply because they became overt victims of public health dictates. Thousands of parents, especially moms, face constant demeaning from this false religion, because they have the audacity to question it. Ruthless, damaging agendas assaulted and killed our children long before COVID came on the scene. Now, an estimated 100 million kids are exposed to the toxic COVID vaccines annually, while the Big Tech gurus will NOT allow the proven facts to be exposed. Despite all evidence of the toxicology of the COVID vaccines, an entire generation plus of our children have been poisoned. We must keep writing, talking, and printing information to governmental leaders, media representatives, social media platforms, and every American grassroots citizen who can and will disseminate truth wherever and whenever possible. Health freedom is worth fighting for, and saving our children from systematic poisoning is one of the most important battles in the war. After continuous research on public media, it is clear that the truth will NOT be found there, because truth advocates are not allowed there to declare it. But there are still plenty of conscientious doctors and scientists telling the truth and proving it; you, dear citizen, must ferret it out and stand firmly on it. This author has found Epoch News, Newsmax, and Substacks are all especially good for accuracy despite their being bashed by Big Tech regularly.

There was a time in America when iconic institutions like the CDC, FDA, WHO, NIH, and more, and the professionals who ran them were honorable. We citizens were rightfully trained to trust their knowledge and experience. Today, especially post-COVID, these professionals, like Anthony Fauci still want and demand that similar trust continue unchecked, but that is no longer possible—they are NOT trustworthy!! Their track records for the last several decades actually prove just how untrustworthy they have become and much of it is a matter of public record. Every one of the entities listed have taken the word of Big Pharma far more often than the word of lifelong scientists. Big Pharma is first and foremost an enormous monopolized business conglomerate of power second to none in today's world. It has the money, it writes the safety info, it makes the rules, and it's accountable to no one. Reading their product information often reveals how little real knowledge is actually imparted. Even the doctors prescribing their noxious drugs haven't the time or inclination to wade through it all. Parents and people with health challenges are doing the reading. For example, "when the really big kerfuffle surfaced about asbestos in baby powder, it was parents who first understood how misplaced their trust had been! Big Pharma insisted it was a 'tempest in a teapot', but the parents stood up and said, "NO—that's a lie!" The drug company Johnson & Johnson had known for decades that asbestos lurked in its Baby Powder. While facing thousands of lawsuits alleging that its talc caused cancer, J & J insisted on the safety and purity of its iconic product. But internal documents examined by Reuters show that the company's powder was sometimes tainted with carcinogenic asbestos and that J & J kept that information from regulators and the public. J & J didn't tell the FDA that at least three tests by three different labs from 1972-1975 had found asbestos in its talc— in one case at levels reported as 'rather high'."[31]

Why are we still trusting the very people already convicted of fraudulent dealings? J & J has already been ordered to pay out millions of dollars several times in court actions. The most recent trial ended in a $270 million settlement June 4, 2024. It was also determined on June 12, 2024 that the company will pay another $700 million in a nationwide settlement over allegations that it misled customers about the safety of its talcum-based powder products. That's called fraud!! J&J now needs the support of 75% of the remaining plaintiffs to get approval for a bankruptcy settlement that would finally end the litigation, shut off future cases and prevent people from opting out of the deal. However, the courts rejected two previous efforts by the company to resolve the talc cases in bankruptcy. What is more ironic than this story is that Big Pharma often uses the high cost of litigation to justify its massive drug costs to consumers. The irony is that if they were working their end correctly, taking care of known problems before harm is done, giving appropriate information to cut risk rather than conceal it, they wouldn't need additional money for litigation!

After all the deception and monstrous lies associated with the whole COVID-19 debacle which continued ad nauseum, many people started to understand they had been lied to, tricked, cheated, mandated, manipulated, jabbed, and locked down for essentially nothing, the information dam started crumbling. Many more scientists and physicians started speaking out more, and being heard more. They spoke about how dangerous mass vaccinations were. More people started listening to them as media couldn't hide

ALL the damage they were doing. The mortality rates for COVID-19 vaccinations were / are higher than for all other vaccines combined. President Biden and his handlers were 'hell-bent' on vaccinating everyone as we previously discussed. However, the mania and chaos that resulted caused multitudes of people to start speaking up and asking the questions no official wanted to answer. At that point, only about 42% of Americans were fully vaxxed. Lies about how effective the vax program was, began to be challenged. The more pressure for everyone to be vaccinated coming from the hierarchy, the more pushback from the people was happening. This was finally a good and positive sign that citizens were starting to think for themselves once again. The constant threat of death from disease had now become possible damage or death from the vaccine. Now hospitals and clinics were reporting weird and aggressive cancers, exponential increases in many other diseases, and strange phenomena that could not be explained except by the surge in COVID vaccinations. Young, healthy, and fit athletes who had been coerced into the jabs were dropping like flies on sports turfs around the globe. It was feeling very scary, unhealthy, and tragic!

VAERS reports of Adverse Events were coming in rapidly to the CDC, capturing less than 1% of suspected vaccine injuries, when normally they only captured a dismal 10%. All the while, the CDC tried to maintain damage control and alleviate panic from the masses reading the social media platforms and legacy news sources. The normal rate of vaccine mortalities in a year is 40,000, but with COVID, vaccine mortalities were off the charts and getting far more difficult to hide. VAERS reporting is so time-consuming that reporters couldn't keep up, but professionals are mandated to report. One woman tried to do this job responsibly and was shut down and threatened by the hospital she worked for. With all of this, there is absolutely no question that actual mortality numbers had gone exponentially and ponderously to such levels, no one would EVER know the truth if it could be buried well enough. We will get to more issues and stats with professionals soon, but for now, the reader must remember that we aren't even talking about real vaccines. The COVID-19 intervention is NOT a vaccine as we know them or as they are defined. It is nothing more or less than Gene Therapy! Any work surrounding this questionable technology is new, very costly, still highly experimental, has toxic elements, unproven benefits, and though the powers that be will push them until the sky falls, they have not been tested for the necessary numbers of years. Reformulating the original preparations has not changed the main ingredient which is mRNA/gene therapy. All caution was thrown to the wind when the plan for a pandemic was formed. We may all bet big money that this snowball already made it down the mountain and there's no stopping it now.

In addition to all of the above issues, prior to rolling out the 'vaccines', one step in the trials is testing on animals before it is ever tried on humans. "These mRNA formulations had NEVER been tried on animals. The safety baseline was established on humans against saline placebos. Almost IMMEDIATELY, the studies were shut down, and the world was given the mRNA 'vaccines' that turned into an experimental clinical trial with no previous clinical trial, and was NEVER documented."[32] Here is the most distressing thing about this documented information. Without the help of medical and legal professionals who have produced video and book information from the antivaccination perspective, there would be no viable perspective at all. When anyone makes an attempt to find web-based information on this material, everything printed is from the totally skewed perspective of vaccination necessity because it's the only narrative allowed by Big Tech. One might find acknowledgment of those professionals in an article, but their credentials, degrees, professional opinions, and right to speak of them are all considered misinformation, and are vehemently denied because they can influence people to look at ALL the facts; not just those that the global narrative wants to promote. It is a total wasteland loaded with nothing but pro-vaccine propaganda. Subjects such as: lies they tell, their focus on civil liberties, that their experts(real ones) aren't real experts, though they have the same legal certifications, that science won't save us, that the science they use is skewed, and that all the official governmental, globalists, public health agencies, and Big Pharma do not have citizen's best interests at heart, and should not be trusted. Ironically, the things they accuse anti-vaxxers of propagandizing are along the same lines of their own propaganda, which they claim is truth.

Following is an abstract statement from one of the multitude of articles full of misinformation that narrative groups such as CDC, NIH, WHO, FDA, and Big Pharma publish constantly, and are loaded with outright lies, lies by omission, innuendos, exaggerations, name-calling, etc. Dear reader, you can see for yourself, how difficult it is to discern who is really presenting true ideas, and you must also remember to ascertain their motivation. Anti-vaxxers do not stand to make themselves a ton of money, and they have a far better motive of true protection of people, especially children than does any party in the "official" narrative. Here is a direct quote from the National Institutes of Health re: Anti-vaccine advocates: "The article draws on a broadcast popular among the anti-vaccine community and maps out six 'themes' used by the broadcast to ***mislead viewers about COVID-19.*** The themes are the claim that government and pharma are lying to you, claims that COVID-19 is an excuse to remove civil liberties, viewing people as experts that aren't really experts, claiming that science cannot save us, claiming they are skewing the science, and that 'they' are out to harm the viewers. The article points out that similar themes are used to mislead followers with anti-vaccine information. It highlights the concern that such themes will not only mislead people who are already anti-vaccine about the pandemic, but may also draw in people seeking information about COVID-19, and suggests options for dealing with the misinformation…antivaccine organizations are built around a deep belief that vaccines are harmful and operate within an alternate reality. The anti-vaccine world is characterized by deep mistrust of government, and a set of ***'alternative facts'—incorrect views about reality***—held by people in the movement. This alternative reality lends itself easily to negative claims about COVID-19."[33] Can you, dear reader, see that this whole derogatory statement is exactly like "the cauldron calling the teakettle black?"

The bottom line on understanding the rollout of the COVID-19, according to Dr. James Chestnut, DC and Dr. Toni Bark, MD; it has NEVER been about the merit of vaccination, but the fact that it's globally unthinkable that the COVID vaccine was OUT and disseminated BEFORE it could be verified for safety and effectiveness. There was simply NOT enough data, or if there really was enough data, it was NOT uncovered even to the professionals involved. Real scientists can't tolerate the lack of data, especially with such an enormous potential of toxicity. As it turned out, there was very good reason for distrust. Entirely too many people will believe and trust the people they have been led to believe they CAN trust. Policies, however, have been bought! Few doctors are in a position to assist in policy making, so they get little chance to question the policies made by those who do. Government makes policies and its rules are based in the power and money of Big Pharma, no matter how much denial you hear and read.

If we want a perfect example of the policy, we could minimally expect with the COVID vaccines, by looking at the policy designated for influenza vaccines. In the beginning it was considered 'mandatory' that seniors 65 years and older MUST have one annually. In ten short years, that policy included everyone. As always, the data was manipulated, numbers of cases were totally exaggerated, and even doctors didn't trust the proposed necessity, but the POLICY was now in place and there was no published data to support the policy. In the case of the flu, there is no antibody issue, and it isn't even the same every year. However, by skewing the data figures, it could look however they wanted it to look. Doctors and nurses as frontlines for patients are expected to believe in and trust the policy makers. After over five decades in the medical field, this author has never trusted allopathic medicine (Big Pharma-based) less! The path of policy implementation starts with the producers—Big Pharma—not the science! Doctors must obtain real data from independent researchers who 'have no dog in the fight'. But that is all very time-consuming and doctors have been sold a bill of goods from Pharma reps through incentives. They should put their own questions and faith to the real scientific test instead of putting blind faith in the CDC and other agencies. Medical doctors need to be pro-evidence from medical school on in order to be decent patient advocates. In addition to all of that, no one wants to be the next whistleblower, but the conclusions in drug studies are seldom supported scientifically—absurd beyond belief.[34]

Hundreds of Red Flags Waving Everywhere You Looked, But Too Many Paying No Attention!

To see the reality of how this actually works, we need to look again at the story of Dr. Peter McCullough. This man is a highly-respected North Texas cardiologist with absolutely impeccable academic credentials. He is a full professor of medicine at Texas A&M College of Medicine in Dallas. "Dr. McCullough is an internist, cardiologist, epidemiologist, and holds a Master of Public Health degree. He is known as one of the top five most-published medical researchers in the US and is the editor of two medical journals."[35] From the very beginning of the COVID-19 debacle, Dr. McCullough, as a researcher and practicing physician at Victory Medical Center, along with colleagues, developed a protocol for the early treatment of COVID-19. He recommended that all of their patients keep a ready supply of OTC items to help build their immune systems and fight off the effects of the SARS-CoV-2 virus. Those were as follows:

- Povidone Iodine—a topical antiseptic wash (Betadine)
- Zinc 50 mg/day
- Vitamin D—5000 IU/day—increased to 20,000 IU/day during active treatment
- Vitamin C.—3000 mg/day for active treatment
- Quercetin, 500 mg/day for prevention—500 mg/day for active treatment

- Famotidine or Pepcid at a high dose, 80 mg/day active treatment
- R_X of antivirals per physician protocol as needed [35]

The reader will recall that in addition to the above treatment protocols, through research and practice, they also utilized two very reliable drug treatments to treat COVID-19 very successfully. Those drugs were ivermectin and hydroxychloroquine. These drugs were/are safe, cheap, and very effective treatment and kept a large number of COVID patients from needing hospitalization. He wrote journal articles that clearly supported his studies and practice and prepared to present his work before the US Senate. However, his work and plans threatened to stand in the way of globalist and Big Pharma plans for their drug and vaccine choices, to be pushed through the FDA approval process on the Emergency Use Authorization (EUA) plan. This could only happen if there were no other effective treatment options available. So they briefly ran bogus testing on the ivermectin and hydroxychloroquine to disqualify them as treatment options so their new choices could be approved. Dr. McCullough used $3500 of his own money to publish his findings ahead of the Big Pharma plan. However, the National Library of Medicine pulled his paper. He went to the Senate anyway, but his published protocols had been censored and the drugs were now rare and scarce. Suddenly, there was no other research, no other papers, and nothing offered from major medical centers, and he was left as the lone ranger with his protocols. He tried to reach out to other doctors treating COVID-19 to hear what they were doing, but the pushback was like a tidal wave. He flew back to D.C. as a witness for a majority of doctors trying to support him and was accused of having insufficient evidence—because most of it had been "killed" over that year. Hydroxychloroquine was disqualified as ineffective and its EUA revoked. Ivermectin alone was considered lacking in the globalist camp as "no serious illness could be effectively treated with just one thing!" The academically-superior doctors like Dr. McCullough were called "SNAKE-OIL Doctors" by a bought and paid-for bunch of lowly, junior physicians with little to no real experience. From this time forward, all of the aforementioned, studied and proven treatment information was and has been forever dubbed 'misinformation' in all narrative-published materials since.[36]

"The upshot for Dr. Peter McCullough is that his life, because of his courage to keep fighting the tidal waves of globalist money and deceit, has changed quite radically. Big Tech determines what may or may not be seen and heard on media. The whole purpose of Senate hearings was to disseminate real information to Americans. Halting and defying that was far beyond unprofessional, but the COVID agenda wanted America to believe COVID couldn't be treated effectively without vaccine mandates. It was too late to start treating COVID in the hospital, and only the vaccines could assure that patients wouldn't get sick enough to need a hospital if they were vaxxed. Efforts of the good doctors to save lives were, however, thwarted at every turn. The monoclonal antibodies were great and effective, but too hard to come by for everyone. As with most infections, early treatment was always most effective, but it had been shut down in lieu of ineffective Remdesivir and ventilation in the hospital, which killed more people than it ever saved. However, vaccination never kept up with relative risk, and it was later discovered that people were actually more vulnerable to infection after only one dose, than they had been without it. Yet those awaiting a second dose were given no additional precautions about the danger of exposure. Today, despite the total vilification, censorship, threats, and losses of jobs, titles, salaries, and professional respect Dr. McCullough suffered, "he has had years of dedicated academic and clinical practice in combating the SARS-CoV-2 virus and in doing so, has reviewed thousands of reports, participated in scientific congresses, group discussions, press releases, and has been considered among the world's experts on COVID-19"[36]

As of a WCRDC annual meeting in November, 2020, Dr. McCullough registered his McCullough Protocol for the treatment of acute COVID-19 because of its large range of clinical severity from asymptomatic to fatal. "In the absence of clinical trials and guidelines, and with hospitalizations and mortality mounting, we must deploy treatment for COVID-19 based on pathophysiological principles. As a result, he developed a renowned protocol based on age and co-morbidities that allows for many people to be monitored and treated at home during self-isolation—reducing the risks of hospitalization and death."[37] Just as important today is his own clinical practice, The Well Integrative Medicine. There he and his team now use the McCullough Protocol for Base Spike Detoxification (BSD), used in post COVID-19 and vaccine injury syndromes. We may discuss this further in a later segment. Meanwhile, Big Tech maintains a constant stream of villainous propaganda against this beyond-exceptional doctor, still accusing him of misinformation when the proof of his accuracy is right in front of our faces. If it bothers him, it doesn't show as he goes courageously forward saving lives and helping heal COVID vaccine damage one patient at a time.

Since the time of all the vaccine whistleblowing, there are many medical and scientific experts operating along with legal advocates to rectify as much of the damage done by the globalist agenda as possible. They do NOT push the vaccine because of its proven toxicity. They have to fight the effects of the vaccines and toxic spike proteins every day. The VAERS reports are completely off the charts, and never has there been a time when the CDC and the FDA cared less about the damage they continue to push. Safety and ethics boards for vaccines are a thing of the past. There are no ongoing reviews of the vaccines, because if there were, the vaccines would have been discontinued years ago. Consequently, nothing happened to alter or halt the whole vaccination program. There were no safety guardrails and no road signs, as they continued pushing the vaccines for every age group except 6 months and under, which they aim to get before they quit. It's still fair game for pregnant women, despite the professionals who decry them. Online and paper-driven information continues to push absolute need for everyone, and continually makes the bold statements that the vaccines are now considered perfectly safe for everyone, with nothing but insignificant side effects except in rare cases, which is the most heinous lie of the century. Beware folks, lying is now perfectly acceptable if you want what you want, and the bigger the lies, the less apt people are to sit up and pay attention. The rule of thumb is: tell a monstrous lie long enough, and consistently enough and it will eventually be accepted as fact. That's exactly what the internet has done to the exclusion of almost every bit of truth it can block. It is very nearly to the point now, where if you want truth, the internet is NOT the place to find it.[38]

The bio-physiology of the COVID-19 vaccines is now very well known. Good doctors and scientists around the globe have done due diligence in studying both the SARS-CoV-2 and the chemistry of the COVID vaccines at length. The truth of their toxicity, ingredients, all potential adverse events and more are now known far more specifically than ever before, but you will not get the truth from those pushing the globalist and vaccine agendas. For the truth you must hear and see all the information that has been written and filmed on individual protected websites and seminars that Big Tech has not been able to shut down. T.V journalists like Jonathan Otto and professional doctors who interview these experts will allow us all to learn the real facts when we seek them. "Jonathan is an entrepreneur, filmmaker, and warrior for health freedom. He has traveled widely and has a huge global network of connections. He is a wonderful source of true, documented information, especially on alternative approaches on healthcare, shown effective in many other parts of the world. His humanitarian documentaries are second to none in professionalism. He and his wife Lori are committed believers in Jesus Christ and reflect His love for humanity in all they do. They are involved in their local church in San Diego, CA."[39] Many of these work under private non-profit funding and many also freely share what they have personally learned at little cost, because they have seen first-hand the results and the people tragically affected by post COVID and COVID vaccine syndromes.

As we earlier said, it is not really appropriate to call the "Jabs" vaccines. They are and should be recognized as "gene-transfer" technology. The preparations they call vaccines are formulated with DNA and mRNA materials from a variety of sources, not even all human. These genes carry genetic information into human cells and they make spike proteins which are toxic to our body cells. It is a method being used to force the body to make antibodies against these foreign proteins. "The mRNA spikes of the molecules are not only toxic, but can be carried to any part of the body." In the beginning, the COVID bio-genetics researchers insisted that the spike proteins given in the jab were only a temporary problem, would not leave the area of the injection site, and any reaction would be local. We now know that this was mere wishful thinking. The spike proteins multiply rapidly. Dr. Peter McCullough has written more than 45 scientific papers on the mechanism of mRNA and the production of spike proteins, along with other highly respected professionals. The physical and psychological damage that has been done in the bodies of the 'vaccinated' due to the toxic spike proteins is enormous in scope and severity and mortalities are off the charts. Autopsies and histories are now known and spike proteins have been found in every type of tissue throughout the body, even mingled in the notorious blood clots. The CDC, FDA, and Big Pharma continue to deny this vehemently, but the proof of the spike proteins' presence is an irrefutable cause of death. Dr. McCullough spoke of breast tissue so distorted from vast changes that mammograms either couldn't be done or were badly delayed. Measurable spike protein was found systemically for a full two weeks after vaccination. Ovaries, testicles, and other reproductive organs were affected. None of the process of spike production took place just locally, but throughout the body, and was often found in dangerous areas with potential systemic organ damage from permanently high spikes and chronic organ issues. These problems and more continue to arise long after vaccines were given, and now COVID 'Jabs' are commended for annual usage.[40]

In addition to all the toxicity issues, the bogus vaccines are in every way an inferior product. There is no satisfactory efficacy or duration, and what there is relies heavily on a constant and regular booster to keep it working, which of course increases the constant potential of additional toxicity. A very real problem arising from the vaccines is that they created most of the viral variants or mutant strains. Any antibodies of any value within the body are not effective in the presence of heavy mutations, part of the reason for the appearance of the deadly Delta variant. In the US, in June of 2021, all health care workers had been fully vaccinated, creating a 1000-fold increase in the environmental viral load. By August, it was estimated that most hospitalized patients who died had been vaccinated or had contracted the Delta variant. The CDC touted that over 90% of hospitalized patients had NOT been vaxxed, but it simply was not true. Barring the Delta variant, the vast majority of hospitalized were fully vaxxed early in the process and immunity was already seriously waning. The truth was that most of the people incurring COVID were vaccinated because they admitted it— while if not vaccinated, few admitted it for fear of active discrimination.

Next, we look at the "contributions of Dr. Andrew Kaufman. He has a background in molecular biology and chemistry from MIT, specializes in mental and emotional health in psychiatry, and lately has been heavily involved in the area of natural health. In his main area of practice, when COVID arrived, he studied all of the health issues affected by it. In practicing psychiatry, he quickly became frustrated with the high degree of dependence on drugs, particularly antidepressants, but people weren't getting better. He began taking his patients off all the drugs and they got better. The same was increasingly true in treatment of cancer and other problems when using drugs. He got to the point where he increasingly distrusted allopathic medicine. Many natural treatments frequently worked better. So he spent over three years studying the world of natural healing and different paradigms, and basically changed his life's whole direction at the risk of losing his professional reputation. The results have been amazing across the board, to his own surprise. He now just wants the truth of health going out to regular people who are searching for it, and help them understand reality."[41]

In the case of COVID, Dr. Andy, as he likes to be called, began to note an extraordinary amount of damage in patients from COVID itself, and from COVID policies. Later in the hospital, he began seeing severe illness related to employment issues, and criminal and forensic issues relating to mental health, but these were most unusual for a psychiatrist to see. He began to comb through reams of documents looking for the smallest of clues, and trying to disprove the prevailing thought processes due to COVID. He knew a whole lot of crazy was being seen in medicine, from cancer patients, death and dying issues, and end of life notions which had a big mental influence on people and were exacerbated by COVID. With COVID, he observed huge spikes in psychiatric cases and questioned why. He studied virus papers, trying to find basic common elements and uncovered a huge psychological mess. "Virus data had been horribly misinterpreted and basic policies were set on complete fallacy. In the lab, for example, various sources of RNA were never separated in fluids, even as to their being animal or human. They were utilizing extremely tiny segments of RNA which were certainly NOT identifiable when they couldn't even be seen to isolate them. There were NO control experiments, yet they passed peer reviews. Once they uncovered seriously flawed information, they stopped trying to isolate the virus, seeing the whole thing was manufactured on pure theory, no proof ever seen. That genetic 'material' used to make the diagnostic testing was a *complete molecular 'house of cards!'* It was represented to the general populace that the virus was identified, but it NEVER was. Isolation by its real separation NEVER happened, therefore it couldn't possibly be purified. There was NEVER microscopic proof, because it could NOT be verified by the process with electron microscopes. Therefore, there was NEVER, essentially a real SARS-CoV-2 or COVID-19. By any scientific terms, it was pure simulation—just smoke and mirrors. You simply cannot test and identify what you cannot find!"[42]

Further, a number of issues were NOT seen that would have been typical of an actual pandemic. These known issues are critical to understand to gain proper perspective on reality. We discuss them briefly as follows:

- Death Reporting—"all-cause mortality"—Far more people would truly have been dying exponentially than what looked like near-normal figures as usual. Numbers of deaths were constantly tweaked. Comparing the numbers to previous years, they were almost identical and seasonal. Week to week, including seasonal increases, causes of deaths were all considered due to COVID-19.

- The Constant Campaign of Fear was abnormal—there were two million deaths in the US, but that was far LESS than the expected number of deaths which normally averages about 30% of the total population. After the lockdowns, spikes in rates occurred because of the changes in policy on DNRs, nursing home care, fear at home, etc. (suicides were definitely a part of that too). Collateral damage increased—COVID-19 didn't.

- All reported deaths were NOT from COVID, based on COVID testing, because there was no good, consistently reliable test available.

- If there was even a hint that COVID-19 was involved in ANY way, doctors were instructed by Medicare to call the cause of death—COVID-19, because the reimbursements of cost were much higher if the death was due to COVID. There was so much mislabeling according to a later study from funeral homes, directors simply didn't buy it—autopsies had been nearly eliminated because they didn't want real proof of death listed. Consequently, COVID must have "CURED" a lot of heart disease, cancer, pneumonia, strokes, etc., and even the number of accidental injuries diminished nearly miraculously.

- Why? There were a lot of cultural changes, impacted mostly by deliberate changes in governmental policies.
- Many others like Dr. Kaufman believed what they suspected was happening, but were unwilling to admit that modern American allopathic medicine as we/they knew it simply ceased to exist. But Andy refused to wear a mask that was contraindicated by the science and then was fired from his medical job. Opportunities in the healthcare industry changed vastly. Further, as Artificial Intelligence took over more roles; real doctors who understand medicine, as no AI ever could, were far less necessary and usually AI was far more focused on optimizing revenue, per its programming.
- People can and generally do recover from most illnesses most of the time, if their innate immune systems are left alone to do the work they were CREATED to do. Dr. Andy wanted to write new and improved medical curriculums, much as Dr McCullough did with his protocols, but far too many doctors, trained in the drug-oriented allopathic system wouldn't or couldn't take the risk of bucking a really bad "official" system.[43]

A few last things require some additional consideration. Repeated COVID testing was just as worthless as relying on the tests for true results—the results of two tests could even be different, done 15 minutes apart! As we said before, the nature of the PCR, which was never intended to be an assay, cannot be efficient because the steps in the test itself are so variable, thus regularly producing possible false positives and false negatives. Anything a person does day-to-day in normal life can skew results. In addition, the PCR test was never validated for any ONE specific virus. It only indicated that a virus was more or less present. It was NOT done for SARS-CoV-2 specifically, so there was NO GOLD STANDARD of reliability. At best it was very much like Russian roulette!

Without an accumulation of real, thoroughly tested data, there was only a false foundation on which to build. So, increasingly, as additional data was added to the whole, the entire thing was built on a false foundation; so any new data was not reliable either. As is the case of influenza, designated as 'seasonal', there may be varied symptoms year by year. For example, with COVID, one of the perceived defining symptoms became the loss of taste and smell, making the assumption it must be COVID and not the flu. But ENT doctors say 20% of the population experienced those symptoms before COVID ever made its appearance. That would be one in every five people having loss of taste and smell from ANY virus! But this false information has continually been reinforced, including by the CDC, that the loss of taste and smell IS a hallmark of COVID-19. It is simply NOT so.

Now if we take another look at the whole vaccine campaign, in truth, we should say NO to getting this poison, if we value our own health. It's NEVER been about an ongoing illness that should be prevented, because clearly the vaccine doesn't prevent COVID! Since there is no true increase in mortality, why the hyped-up urgency? It normally takes at least ten years to get a vaccine to market, and COVID took about 3 months, not counting all the secret development of a potential SARS-CoV2 vaccine, that would be needed shortly after the 'virus' was introduced!! Despite all the glorified explanations of its years of potential planning for the need of such a vaccine, and the claim they didn't know what would turn up, and then being able to adjust what was developed to the "novel" virus safely in 3 months, it was nothing but a scam, and/or else the whole thing is a heinous lie. You can't have it both ways. We also know from current claims that "risks of adverse events are still VERY HIGH, and despite supposed reformulated vaccines, they are still very high per all the doctors who are having to treat post-vaccine patients needing to regain some semblance of normal function, if possible. The jabs do not prevent transmission, and do not guarantee immunity which continually wanes. The attempts to make vaccines with gene technology for some types of viruses have been in the works for years and have NEVER been successful, but all of a sudden, when needed, they hit it right!! It supposedly works through RNA altering genes, completely different than any other 'vaccine' previously created. Its mRNA is transferred to each person's RNA who receives it. The exact sequence is NOT known, but it uses our own cells' protein to make the new spike protein that is toxic, and has never been shown to work effectively in the lab before. Any kind of gene may be transferred, including animal-based genes."[44] Artificial Intelligence software was used to project the potential side effects. It found a HIGH volume of possible adverse events, including death. There were more than TWENTY severe illnesses projected to be seen. Despite swearing to the contrary, both before rolling out the first vaccines, and those that have been slightly reformulated, there was very little safety testing, all for NO conceivable benefit, except the accumulation of magnanimous wealth. Unfortunately, there will NEVER be any 'Going- Back to square one.' The die is cast, and the deeds are done. The facts remain extreme and chilling, and it's just the beginning of anything else Big Pharma decides to foist upon us all in the probable near future. Whatever else you do now or in the future, do NOT take a jab if you haven't, and never ever take another one. Your life is IN YOUR HANDS!

A final question might be, "Why do so many seemingly intelligent people succumb to being jabbed?" We now know that taking them will NOT keep vax mandates away from our doors. These dangerous and worthless vaccines are still being pushed with every sign and internet entry. Eventually, they will be used to limit all normal access to products, services, and freedoms. Had they been ready to facilitate vaccine passports and digital credits, it would already be limiting us. But we MUST say "NO" now. As of January, 2025, the everlasting push for continuing all vaccines, including COVID-19 is unchanged from the rollout. COVID-19 vaccines are NOT going away, and we may be just as certain that other such 'vaccines' for additionally contrived gain-of-function 'viruses' are planned and will be introduced to the masses just as soon as they can create another EMERGENCY!! The long-term expectations of this global reset will not be going away, but will get worse and worse. The psychology behind vaccines and the global reset is to control all people everywhere, and those who desire it have the power and money to make it happen. It's time for all concerned citizens to spread real facts, and stay educated for yourself, your family, your communities, and our nation.

What this agenda has already done to us globally is just like a game to the globalist wolves and their cronies. Each time they choose to play this game; they can work out some glitches they missed the last time. The game can be played relentlessly. All they have to do is pick another "bug" with their fraudulent science. Having done that, they can easily replicate the former results and a whole lot more. Remember, we live in a day when our lives can be destroyed by the next scammer or hacker quite easily and most of them are NOT professionals. With AI now available, figures, pictures, people, and more can easily be altered at will. It can present almost anything to the public and make the majority believe it is what they tell you it is. Perhaps, a quick look at what Jesus said can give us the very best of advice, "Behold, I am sending you out as sheep in the midst of wolves. Therefore be wise as serpents and innocent as doves." Matthew 10:16, ESV

> "For such men are false (leaders), deceitful workmen, masquerading as leaders of good. And no wonder, for Satan himself masquerades as an angel of light. It is not surprising, then, if his servants masquerade as servants of righteousness." 2 Corinthians 11:13-15 NLT

> "They claim to know God, but by their actions they deny Him. They are detestable, disobedient, and unfit for doing anything good." Titus 1:16 NLT

> "Do not conform to the pattern of this world, but be transformed by the renewing of your mind." Romans 12:2 NLT

> "In everything set them an example by doing what is good. In your teaching show integrity, seriousness and soundness

of speech that cannot be condemned." Titus 2 7-8 NLT

Long-term, But Scant Consideration of Problems in All Vaccines

Gynecologist/Obstetrician Dr. Gary Goldman has a stellar history of education and is board-certified by the American Board of Obstetrics and Gynecology. He trains medical students and residents in Ob/Gyn at Cornell Medical College. He also completed his certification in Functional Medicine in 2018 and remains a member of the teaching faculty since 2020. He has published multiple articles in peer-reviewed journals and books. During the 2009-2010 H1N1 influenza pandemic, he clearly "documented a four-times increase in the flu vaccination of pregnant women with an increase of 4000 times the effects on pregnant women and a massive spike in fetal deaths over 19 annual influenza seasons, but without thimerosal, the vaccines were deemed safe. In addition, he noted an increased risk of non-influenza respiratory viral infections. There were four times more infections in those taking the vaccines. In his own long-term study, "Dr Goldman noted that internationally, the nations with the lowest infant mortality rates, vaccinated the least. He also noted that in 20 years of VAERS reports, the higher the number of influenza doses given, the incidence of other illnesses were also higher and continued to increase with each vaccination given."[45] Yet, there is never a decrease in the numbers of vaccinations on the childhood immunization schedules! Dr. Goldman once worked at the CDC and also noted that varicella vaccine goes to over four million children. Researchers knew that given the basic mechanism of varicella vaccine, and giving the heavy increase in varicella vaccines, there would be a certain correlation between those and the vastly increased need for shingles vaccinations in adults![45]

Next, we have the extensive story of a courageous British doctor, whose experience treating vaccine-injured children with gut and neurologically correlated issues, "came down to a major confrontation with pro-vax perpetrators—a compromise in medicine, corruption of the science, and a real and present threat to children in the interests of policy and profit. It is a story of how 'the system' deals with dissent among its doctors and scientists. In the pursuit of possible links between childhood vaccines, intestinal inflammation, and neurologic injury in children, "Dr. Andrew Wakefield lost his job in London's Royal Free Hospital, his country of birth, his career, and his medical license. He has been maligned by the medical establishment and the mainstream media, and so set the record straight in his book: *Callous Disregard: Autism and Vaccines: The Truth Behind a Tragedy.* In it, he clearly explained what really happened, and he called out the organizations and individuals that are acting not for the sake of the children affected by autism, but in their own self-interests."[46]

Dr. Andy was trained in old-fashioned medicine that says, "the patient always comes first." He believes that the patient's history dictates the kinds of testing needed, which he did, as parents presented their affected children to him. However, modern medicine is frequently NOT done that way anymore. Then, he became very interested in a child presenting with autism and heinous gastrointestinal symptoms. He previously didn't know a lot about autism, but began studying it at length, and found a clear, documented interaction between bowel and brain functions which has currently taught us a lot. Oddly, there was an increasing flood of children with the same story. However, Dr. John Walker Smith, a world-renowned pediatrician and specialist in gastrointestinal issues was also a firm believer in vaccines, their safety, the money to be made, and the science behind their 'safety.' He mounted a major pushback against Dr. Andy's studies and observations. Authorities were being informed about the suspicions of MMR vaccine causing autism as early as 1991.Wakefield began studying it in 1989 and did his homework. Dr Smith got wind of it in 1998, nine years of research later, and was among the first to deny the possibility. After all, children do sometimes regress developmentally—it's not uncommon, and nothing was done about it. However mothers KNOW their children and witnessed what happened to them. Education is always the ONLY real answer. Dr. Andy would tell them to trust their maternal instincts. Much of today's medicine uses direct, one-way, programmed, and automated information designed to be fully authoritative, if NOT always accurate, and requires us, especially parents to trust it, and buy into it no matter what your gut tells you. Please, Parents!— DON'T DO IT!! Use your own brain and your own gut instincts. If you get pushbacks from authority figures, push back and keep asking questions. The more dodging of questions you encounter, the less you trust what they say!

The risk of autism from vaccines has increased continuously and exponentially, despite all the adamant and authoritative narrative which is almost the only thing available in mainstream media and internet. It is actually of epidemic proportions. When you look at the top ten presenters of information on any given topic, you will not see a balance of good / bad, pros / cons, rights / wrongs, etc. and they will all be unequivocally written by globalist-directed agencies, professionals, and institutions. No controversial information is included unless it has been fully and efficiently debunked. But now we CAN identify the causes quite easily knowing the complex equation. Having given almost every child a continuous cocktail of vaccines, all of which contain either toxins, or ingredients proven to cause sensitivity and allergic reactions in many children, the correlation of vaccines and autism is clearer than ever. Pro-vaccine adherents will declare adamantly on a stack of Bibles that each vaccine is perfectly safe, but they have no clue about the safety of any given cocktail of them. Adverse events are very well known to Big Pharma, and all of its cohorts, but if a vaccine causes only one problem in a thousand, or even a million children, it is not deemed a problem!! All of the collection of toxins, viruses, and array of foreign materials that make up the vaccines can so shock an infant's or child's immune system, that they can never recover their God-given immune system again. The powers that be simply DO NOT CARE that this happens as long as they make their money, and control this evil system operating in the falsehood of health. It is true that some of the perpetrators genuinely believe they are helping children to grow up healthier—but it simply is NOT true. It most assuredly should be stopped, but it will NEVER be stopped because there is too much money in it, and it ultimately controls our entire healthcare perspective.

Destroying literally tens of thousands of lives of children and their families simply cannot be justified under any circumstances. The Pharmaceutical industry has previously and will continue to rake in the largest profits from vaccine development because of its universality. Manufacturers of vaccines have NO liability or loss by law. Safety studies remain inadequate because they are NOT done correctly or ethically— there are no real scientific proofs of safety. So, the question remains—does the MMR vaccine cause autism NOW? The answer is YES! In vaccine courts, facts of true experience are testified to regularly, but a hundred other potential excuses beside the vaccine are offered, refuting parental knowledge and experience with exact timing, emergency room records, steady digression of behavior post-vaccine, etc. There is extraordinary injustice and discrimination against these families to keep companies from paying restitutions. This can very literally destroy a family as well as their child's life physically, mentally, emotionally, socially, financially, educationally, and more. The PLAGUE of neuro-developmental disorders is well and fully present in our society. Further, when parents are gone someday, who will care enough to take care of their child, many of whom are far from able to take care of themselves. These dilemmas have led to murder/ suicides that society condemns, but the parent knows—there will be no one to care for their remaining debilitated child.[47]

How can we even start to fix this? First, we must listen to parents, especially the 24/7 mother!! Exactly what happened? Listen to the whole story. What was its origin— what started it? We MUST assume there is an organic origin FIRST, until proven otherwise. DON'T start throwing more drugs at the problem. When you find the sometimes-subtle inflammation, and treat gut symptoms appropriately, the child starts to improve, and you may hear, "My child is coming back!" The neuro-regression stops. Autism may be far more treatable than it was ever thought possible when symptoms are early and the root of the prevailing problems is treated correctly. The child is NOT irreparably broken after all!

"Dr. Wakefield was told that his work was NOT going to be good for his career. But all our lives are about choices. His choice was stark, as we've seen earlier. He lost an awfully lot personally, but he didn't lose his self-respect and good conscience, and he didn't let these innocent children and their families suffer the irreparable losses they most certainly would have suffered without his intervention. To him, it was still his only viable choice to be the patient advocate. Many of the industry came after him, filed complaints, told whopping lies, manipulated questions, and skewed his answers, and defined the difference as fraud. Then they sued him for defamation in a court of law and said they would let the people decide who they would believe. Despite all this, they can no longer DENY the correlation between MMR and autism. Even with the reams of adamant and determined denials in every globalist narrative, the onus of proof is still more than ever on the manufacturers."[48] However, the money and power have used artificial means to increase efficacy of the vaccine on the short term (rabbit blood), fraud, cheating, changing numbers, etc., but a whistleblower told the FDA about mumps vaccine claims. The case went to federal court and Merck stood to lose billions. The hope was that all the fines would put them out of business. Merck's attempts to have the case thrown out were dismissed. This author was unable to find the result of the case, because surprise-surprise, all evidences and decisions were removed from the public domain. How convenient, that without that information, the claims of no correlation between MMR and autism can still stand uncontested!!

Anti-vax proponents are still very active in trying to prevent the vaccine injuries in our children. As most of us know, one of the leading proponents is Senator Robert F. Kennedy, Jr. Anyone associated with the globalist, 'progressive' narrative will promptly accuse him of promoting misinformation and conspiracy theories.

However, RFK, Jr. has done his homework and has been there for the vax-injured children and their families, and knows their stories intimately. What is somewhat refreshing is the fact that it's much harder to avoid or omit the influence of an American scion running for the highest elected office in the land!! Breaking News!! Kennedy dropped from his race for the White House, but in our new Trump Administration, he has been selected for the pivotal role of the new Secretary of Health and Human Services. Hopefully, this will be instrumental in righting some big wrongs which he is doing regularly now. He is also "targeting institutions such as pharmaceutical and tech companies; a very good thing. He does still believe autism is tied to vaccines, and definitely opposed state and federal COVID-19 restrictions which of course set him up for loud accusations of spreading misinformation. Largely, he believes that every American who wants a vaccine for themselves or their children should have access, but he will continue to increase scrutiny of the efficacy and potential consequences of vaccines."[49]

"The "Vaccines Revealed" video stated that 87% of parents today do NOT believe all of the vaccine rhetoric they are constantly exposed to. This author hopes and prays this is so. More than 50% of parents believe there are problems with the efficacy and safety of vaccines. There is growing mistrust of them and of government over bad decisions, fraud, lies, vaccine failures, vaccine dangers, adverse events that are too often either ignored or excused, and deaths of children. If the government, FDA, and Big Pharma want to continue to swear all vaccines are truly safe and effective, it is high time that such studies be done openly and all results published accurately BEFORE they are ever licensed. Those who cannot prove the same for existing vaccines should be required to do the same. This has never happened, and the average citizen is never privy to the kind of information proof they want before subjecting their children to these foreign substances. Also vaxxed vs un-vaxxed studies MUST be done! Even if the safety and effectiveness is proven, are they really better than allowing children to develop their own immune systems as the Creator intended!"[50] This medical professional and author, has big, serious doubts of it. She still believes our PERFECT Creator did a perfect job with our bodies, and they are far more resilient without man's faulty products and continuous interference.

Real People—Stories of Real Families, True Professionals and Their Traumas

The Story of Dawn Loughborough

This is the story of how Dawn began to investigate the real deal on vaccines. Her first child was born in 1997. In 1998, at 13 months of age her child was given the first MMR and reacted almost immediately. By the evening, the crying was screaming and the child was inconsolable. Over a number of weeks there was a kind of cascading effect and an integrative doctor noted inflammation in the form of allergies, and placed her vaccines on an elongated schedule. The baby was seen by a cardiologist and a chief of pediatrics, Dr. Paul Offit, who confronted Dawn. She spoke of her daughter's needs and the man turned vicious, and she was 'set-up' because of her concerns. He actually called her a baby-killer for delaying her child's vaccines and shouted at her. He was beyond intimidating, but thankfully lost his license later. Her daughter, 16 years old at the time of the 'Vaccines Revealed' video had developed autoimmune illness, and missed a lot of school because of it. In her senior year she physically "crashed" with multi-symptom regression. When Dawn's son came along, they were very cautious and gave him a modified cellular pertussis vaccination. That night he awoke with high-pitched screaming, was also inconsolable, had a golf ball-sized hydrocele in his left groin, a fever, and was rushed to the emergency room. He was given an IV, and fever medications, but started seizing and his whole left side was swollen and edematous. Dawn told them about the vaccine given that day, but they were not well-informed about this potential. He had full left-sided affect with clumsy, uncoordinated movements (similar to a stroke) for about six months. She initiated physical therapy to help him and his case was reported to VAERS, which again only happens about 10% of the time. The emergency room staff had no idea how to treat such adverse events—even ice bags would have helped, but were not used. His pediatrician had trouble navigating the VAERS report system. Dawn said that if this had happened to most parents, they would be stuck in a paradigm with these hidden issues; unless they had prior experience as she did. She was able to make the connections, but few parents at that time would have figured it out.

Today, her son is autistic, but he is doing well. He had severely regressed, but continues to gradually come out of it. She left a thriving career to stay home and care for him. She managed most of his care which became her main priority. They moved back to the family farm, growing herbs and vegetables, grass-fed animals and living holistically and sustainably. Dawn stated she loved her experiences and spoke of her children connecting with nature and beginning to heal. They benefited tremendously. She also came into contact with Dr. Andy Wakefield over her son's gastrointestinal problems who recommended Maalox to contain severe inflammation. Prayer was an essential part of the healing process. There were lots of other doctors and tests. He had gluten and/or casein migraine-like headaches, vomiting, and poor sleep if he was exposed to them. When his symptoms were effectively treated, his speech started returning. Dr. Wakefield had established protocols that worked, but other doctors were afraid to back them and bad-mouthed his ideas. Dawn had to deal with these other doctors' bullying, fear-mongering, and vindictiveness toward Dr. Wakefield. There were more reactions to vaccines and many problems for many years, especially with MMR, rotavirus, oral polio, and influenza vaccines.[51]

Ms. Barbara Loe Fisher came along and established the Vaccine Information Center to work in conjunction with VAERS reporting. Dawn actually worked with her on research in 2009 during the H1N1 pandemic (not an actual pandemic), tracking it worldwide, and hoping for breakthroughs in vaccine safety. The beginnings of the ideological war between so-called anti-science vs empirical science were ramping up even then. The appropriate management of all this could have been so great because there was no corporate accountability of vaccination laws as yet (1986). After that, there has simply been no incentive for manufacturing to work any harder on efficacy and safety. "Dr. Brian Hooker found a Price study where pregnant moms who got mercury in the flu shots connected with the regression of autism in their children later on. Once again, there were no studies to compare vaccinated children with unvaccinated kids. Authorities claimed it would be unethical to do such studies because some children would not have received the benefit of needed vaccines to do them. It was not a truly viable argument, because they could very easily have found parental volunteers who would happily agree to at least delay vaccinations in their children to do such needed studies. Though all the pro-vax authorities will NOT admit it, it still has become quite clear that children have far less ADHD, Autism, Asthma, and so many other health chronicities when they have NOT been vaccinated. Further, vaccinated children in the US are 54% sicker than are non-vaccinated children in many of the undeveloped countries of the world."[52]

Why is there so much resistance among mainstream doctors to use good nutrition and alternative but proven treatments? One sound reason is that most medical doctors of allopathic (Western) medicine are pathetically lacking in the knowledge of good nutrition because they don't learn it in medical school. Our views tend to be shaped by our experiences, such as the influence and use of the food pyramid. Big Pharma, however, has massive influence in medical schools. Students are NOT taught to go deeper into the "art of medicine." Most doctors who have some decent knowledge of functional medicine, worked extraordinarily hard on their own research and practice to acquire a more integrative approach. It is NOT necessarily evil or cynical of all allopathic physicians to be lacking in the same way that Big Pharma is. Parents who do special diets, elimination of toxins, elimination of psychotropic drugs, and other good ideas are up against a massive system of its own misunderstanding. Much healing happens. But there are simply no evidence-based scientific studies because Big Pharma has no incentive to see that such studies are done. In that same thought process then, parents have been falsely accused of negligence and even had children removed from their home, because they refuse to comply with the standard operating procedures and do alternative treatment instead. These are the real crimes against parents who simply want and need to help their child get healthier. Consequently, advanced learning in other good forms of medicine, such as mitochondrial work are NOT readily available to mere parents. In the same way that standard allopathic medicine is scared to death alternative treatments will somehow 'put them out of business,' the propaganda goes on everywhere. Their fear-based industry has so influenced available information, that parents, too, become fearful of really good alternative treatment for the same reasons. Medical logic has claimed a plethora of victims without good reason. One example would be that of giving vaccines to pregnant moms who have no documented need of them, just to play it safe. Failing programs are still being forced on people militarily. The US gives the most vaccinations of ANY other nation, yet our children are sicker—the numbers are proven, but seldom shown to the public. Once again, the internet allows absolutely nothing antivax reported, gets fact-checkers to debunk almost every statement Kennedy has ever made, makes lists of all his so-called 'conspiracy theories' and decries the medical opinions of any professional that refuses to agree with their pro-vax stance.

The CDC has freely admitted that one major reason to give the first Hepatitis B shot to newborn infants on day one is that it helps program parents into the continued habit of scheduled vaccinations from then on. "Infants who received Hep B vaccine during their birth hospitalization had higher odds of receiving ALL recommended vaccines by 19 months."[53] This is the "official public health officials" psychologically betting on the early (BIRTH) establishment of habitual indoctrination to their lifelong programs! Don't you just love being systematically brainwashed and manipulated? Vaccines are still essentially artificial immunity. Children have innate immunity from their creator and continued immunity from their nursing mothers. Why not utilize efforts to do immune boosting naturally with nutrition and other good health habits to build a child's natural propensity to immunity. It works in underdeveloped countries by necessity all the time—it would surely work in the US! The answer is because Big Pharma has 100 industrial lobbyists to every one other person like this woman who advocated for her child. Their highly-paid roles are to do nothing but influence political policy toward DRUGS!! It is a hugely false marketing influence that is almost impossible to compete with. The market used predominantly to influence adult immunization is NOT their personal doctor—it's Hollywood that does almost all the actual influencing. If you don't believe it, watch your television alone for about two hours and determine what percentage of the advertising is dedicated to Big Pharma!! If you haven't already discovered this truth, this author monitored family programming only for a couple weeks, and the advertising for Big Pharma was minimally above 50% of the total! There are other studies where families are NOT helped despite the hype. Many have been channeled into immunization programs of experimentation which are hidden, removed from all records, and cannot be found again later by protection of the law.

The Story of Barbara Loe Fisher

Going back to the families of vax-injured children, we need to give a bit more attention to Barbara Loe Fisher, co-founder and president of the National Vaccine Information Center (NVIC). She, too, is a parent of a vaccine-affected child from the older version of DPT vaccine. She co-founded the center with other parents of children affected or who had died of the effects of a vaccine. Barbara was a highly educated woman at the time, but she did not recognize a serious vaccination reaction. Her child had just received his fourth DPT vaccine and went unconscious. He could not be wakened, and she had not been instructed on how to recognize such a reaction.

He finally wakened, but continued to regress afterwards. Her son had been exceptionally smart very early but could no longer do any of the really advanced things he had previously done. He developed constant infections, exhibited failure to thrive, gastrointestinal issues, and constant diarrhea. All of the medical tests were supposedly unremarkable. "In 1982, a woman named Lea Thompson wrote a book and did a video entitled, *DPT: Vaccine Roulette*, and in 1985, Barbara Loe Fisher co-authored the book entitled, *DPT: A Shot in the Dark*, both of which had a profound influence on parents who also had injured children from what they believed to be the DPT. Lea Thompson had shown that vaccines could cause brain damage to children. Many doctors were NOT well-educated either, so these productions did considerably slow the use of the DPT shots. Naturally this history didn't thrill vax advocates, and they still have nothing good to say for these ladies who tried very hard to prevent further DPT vax injuries."[54] Barbara's son had become very learning disabled, due to his injuries, but at the time of the film "Vaccines Revealed," the young man was into his mid-thirties, had become both a videographer and a competitive weight lifter. Shortly after the "Shot in the Dark," there was a big spike in the numbers of SIDS deaths occurring after vaccinations. Big Pharma believed this could potentially happen in groups of infants if there were nearby contaminated vaccine lots. The government began widely dispersing various vaccination lots, but it never admitted to doing so. Because there were so many cases of vaccine-injured children going through vaccination courts and costing Big Pharma a lot of money, the "government and industry were pushing for the National Childhood Vaccine Injury Act of 1986, created the National Vaccine Injury Compensation Program (VCIP), a no-fault alternative to the traditional tort system. It provides compensation to people found to be injured by certain vaccines. Whether a vaccine manufacturer or administrator is afforded the liability protections of the (1986 Act), depends upon whether the vaccine is covered under the (VICP). Under the Act, persons with petitions of vaccine-related injuries or deaths resulting from covered vaccines must first exhaust their remedies under the VICP before they can pursue legal actions against vaccine manufacturers or administrators."[55] Just another way of punishing people for being victimized, while the perpetrators go free or nearly free and continue their same money-making endeavors.

The entire system is still crippled by lack of compliance with the designated rules. There are no sanctions in the law for non-compliance—it all needs to be codified by law so it can work right. There is still very low compliance from all factions in reporting processes. The majority of doctors' reports generally get to Big Pharma instead of to the CDC, the FDA, or other agencies. The American Academy of Pediatricians and the CDC have NOT done a decent job of education on adverse events or in reporting them. Further, doctors don't want to acknowledge that what they think they are doing to 'help' children, really hurts and injures them. Nurses who are often also mothers are better at listening to moms, but even nurses have learned there are tons of mixed messages of cause, and many more conditioned responses. They should never ever immunize sick children, but even parents are not excited about making another trip to the doctor's office for a later shot, if her child only has mild possible symptoms. A child used to receive 23 vaccine doses, today it is approximately 69, depending on annual requirements or options. 49 of those doses are before the age of six. There ARE massive increases in adverse events. One in six children are learning-disabled. All numbers are exponentially higher than they used to be and so are those either chronically ill or disabled. It is only in the United States where the numbers are so appalling. Most countries do NOT mandate childhood vaccinations as we do. There are very few contraindications listed today, so doctors just keep on pushing them. Doctors don't write many medical exemptions either. Choices by parents should NEVER be sanctioned as parental choice in their views. Doctors are also greatly discouraged from signing medical exemptions. A child had to have had a documented adverse event in order for a medical exemption to be valid. There is no such thing as protection or prevention in siblings of a vax-injured child. There are now gaps in the science of vaccine knowledge. Family biological and genetic issues are NOT considered. These policies are morally and ethically unconscionable! The argument is always but— isn't there also a moral obligation to protect everyone else and prevent disease outbreaks?!! The parental duty is to keep their children safe FIRST! Vaccines are given to healthy children and adults, BUT there are two health risks inherent in that—vaccine failure or adverse reactions.

Today, the general directive in the United States works on the basis of herd immunity. In many cases, like in pertussis for a time, it was NOT given because it wasn't working efficiently. The reality is if vaccines are efficient, it shouldn't matter if a small number aren't vaccinated. According to epidemiology, it is NOT unvaccinated children that spread disease! However, as is common, the markers keep moving and changing. Varicella started out as a voluntary vaccine, but within a very few years it too became mandatory. Now, as we said before, the adult population has major issues with shingles which were NOT problematic before, and recently we had to have a second shingles vaccination to get higher efficacy so that all levels of immunity remain high throughout adulthood. But vaccine immunity is ARTIFICIAL IMMUNITY! Because of all the fake immunity, our own natural immunity is challenged as never before. The problem of chronic inflammation becomes worse with every new inflammatory exposure. If a person must deal with chronic inflammation, why in the world would we deliberately INCREASE it?!!! This whole set of issues begs another set of questions that every single citizen should be thinking on long and hard.

We haven't even addressed the 'WHY so much mandating?' There is clearly a WAR on our personal health freedoms—one size MUST fit all, but one size doesn't ever fit all. There are still tens of thousands of people who are marginalized by various extenuating problems. After 9-11, legislation gave police and military authority to enforce health guidelines mandated in emergencies. The Federal government has a full-on cooperative business relationship with the FDA and Big Pharma that can fast-track medications and vaccines to bypass the standard, delayed safety and effectiveness routes to licensure. All control is in their hands. But FAST is NOT SAFE! Safety and effectiveness are conflicting goals. When the standards are lowered, there is NO assurance of safety or efficacy. The extra money necessary is 60% funded by Big Pharma, so there is NO problem financing or fast-tracking it.

A much more crucial question is: How many people are we willing to sacrifice to this ideological KILL?!! Big Tech has avidly discouraged and usually banned any media sources from even addressing policy issues in the vaccination realm. There is no respect or even civility toward those who refuse to play the Big Pharma game—if it ever existed, it certainly doesn't exist today. The last seven years have been even worse, even for those taking the neutral ground on advocacy. The almost complete lack of informed consent reveals the fear of all the entities who refuse to relinquish their full control. They are scared-to-death of the possible paradigm shift. What they refuse to acknowledge are the questions: NOT about WHO is right or wrong, or somewhere in between—it's about the health of our nation and our world!

Dr. Kelly Brogan is a medically holistic psychiatrist and best-selling author and self-proclaimed "Reclamation Queen." "She specializes in a root-cause resolution approach to psychiatric syndromes and symptoms. It is evidence-based proof that we can change our personal stories about health, beginning with awareness of what's possible, doing radical self-care, and expanding into our own sovereign wellbeing."[56] As an advocate for women, Dr. Brogan began to look at the idea of informed consent, especially for pregnant women, most of whom worried about all the toxic exposures they encountered and how these might affect their unborn babies. She questioned if the flu shots were really safe. Bottom line was—they had NEVER been approved for pregnant women and very few were told of informed consent. There were no real, sound data bases available regarding the safety and efficacy of the flu shots in pregnant women—yet they were/are constantly pushed as necessary for them. Most people don't connect the dots or ask enough questions. Toxicities FILL our environment beyond any other time in human history, but people do not know how to defend their own bodies; there is even apathy about harm done to our bodies.

A massive example of such harm is the incidence of autoimmune, thyroid conditions that often appear in women after pregnancies. Preventive medicine is still difficult to teach people because traditionally, the vaccine programs are almost the only treatment modalities that are considered preventive. But the one-size-fits-all mentality brings certain collateral damage to individuals, and ultimately to society. The science of epigenetics is key to treating individuals genetically different from others. The little that people know of drugs or vaccines has come largely from skewed media commercials. In Dr. Brogan's practice, psychotropic drugs are NOT the basis of treatment for functional psychiatry. She began weaning pregnant women off of these drugs because they cause body imbalances and issues of their own. She often witnessed a physiological withdrawal too uncomfortable for the woman NOT to go back to. But the symptoms they experienced were not depression-induced, but medication-induced. Women needed to be instructed about the potential symptoms of taking the drug and offered true informed consent up front, about all that science has to say so they can CHOOSE what they want to believe. Dr. Kelly then described her entire protocol for physical and spiritual awakening and transformation. Thousands of women have achieved complete, drug-free healing with her methods.[57]

The studies of Dr. Robert Whitaker and *The Anatomy of an Epidemic* support the ideas and practice of Dr. Kelly Brogan, but trying to change or even explode the current medical paradigm is anything but easy. Many people will display horrible defensiveness, and a feeling of persecution, even from the maverick doctors who question the old paradigm. They want to protect their status quo. Anyone sick and tired of the old must be willing and aware that there is a possibility that their prior knowledge and assumptions may well be wrong. This is KEY! Dr. Whitaker asked the question in 2010: "Why did the number of Americans who receive government disability for mental illness almost double since 1987, and a 5-fold increase since 1955? He spoke to several reasons; Thorazine, the world's first 'wonder' drug was introduced in 1855, and Prozac rolled out in 1987. There are now nearly 6 million Americans disabled by mental illness and the number increases by 400 people every day. It IS this drug-based paradigm of care that is fueling the epidemic. Drugs increase the probability that a person will become chronically ill, and induce new and more severe psychiatric symptoms in a significant percentage of patients."[58] Psychiatric treatment with drugs is often so aggressive as to be highly questionable, and may also suggest that those doing the treating are needing to hide something.

Another consideration posited and addressed, by Dr. Peter McCullough, when he stated that the COVID vaccines didn't work well enough in ALL people to warrant the idea of "one-size fits all." He advocated for "a program that limited vaccination to the high-risk people within the population, namely the elderly and those who had co-morbidities—they had far more to potentially gain and less to lose if they were vaccinated. A more-narrow focus would have prevented over 13,000 deaths when vaxxing first ensued; half of those within the first 48 hours! VAERS reports at this point showed 545,000 total injuries, and 10,000 of those were deemed permanent injuries. Malfeasance was denied by the CDC and the FDA twice and also vehemently claimed the vaccine had caused no deaths. Any attempts to give clear, true data were crushed by the media, and the goal continued to be 100% vaccination for everyone. They continued to declare Pfizer's complete approval (of course they did—no conflict of interest here!) However, Pfizer had NOT given unqualified approval even of its own vaccine. Pure propaganda (lies) was constantly repeated by both the CDC and the FDA, while the evidence of harm mounted exponentially."[59]

As the SARS-CoV-2 virus began mutating and producing new variants, the efficacy of the COVID-19 vaccine diminished even more. Efficacy was only about 50% and would NOT last a full year. Naturally, the drug companies maintained that vaxxed immunity was still better than natural immunity gleaned from actually having the disease. Epidemiologically, that is essentially impossible, nevertheless, without checking immune levels on every person, vaccinated and unvaccinated, that would be impossible to prove. Many of us know a fair number of vaccinated people who have had serious COVID-19 several times! From a personal perspective, this author and her spouse had COVID seriously (Delta variant) in June, 2021 and had NOT been vaccinated, nor sick for a full 18 months prior. After recovering, we were both pressed regularly by almost every medical person we encountered to get the highly ineffective vaccine, which would likely have destroyed our newfound natural immunity. We are so thankful we never succumbed to the almost constant browbeating. Our Father God did protect us before, during, and after our illnesses. Four years later, we have never had it again. There has been a minimum of 15+ case studies done that totally refutes/denies the above claim of better immunity procured with vaccines. ALL pushing of authorities to vaccinate already naturally immunized persons is absolutely wrong and irresponsible from the perspective of true epidemiology. There is NO evidence that this is helpful and a large body of evidence that it could be very harmful epidemiologically. The CDC and WHO constantly tell us to "stick to the science" but they don't. Pregnant women and small children are least at risk for infection and do NOT warrant a vaccination risk, but all authorities concerned are still profusely pushing both. Where's the previously practiced science of avoidance of foreign substances in pregnancy and infancy? This is still criminal and unconscionable to even consider. There is NO compelling clinical benefit for COVID vaccination in children. In spite of swearing it isn't so, VAERS has over 5000 cases of myocarditis IN children with the spike protein, but the CDC will not admit actual numbers officially! However, the VAERS system reported "from December 2020 to August 2021 alone, there were 1,626 cases of myocarditis."[60] That represents only 8 months of vaxxing, with averages of only 10% of cases being reported, as discussed, and those vax rates have increased exponentially in the 3.5 years since! Reports increase daily in children being diagnosed with blood clots, seizures, Guillain Barré syndrome and other neurological issues. The CDC does NOT list these possibilities when giving the COVID vaccine and there is NO informed consent with mandates. Nothing now happening is RARE, and it may well be that the current numbers of adverse events are just the tip of the iceberg in vaccination injury and death.

COVID-19 vaccination has NEVER been anything less than continued and regular gene therapy, which under any scientific definition is still just experimental, because of all the ramifications of gene therapy. The regular manipulation of the building blocks of life itself will always be experimental and the results are far from being regularly predictable. We also know that succeeding jabs and boosters DO NOT PREVENT further infections, but they do increase the numbers of spike protein-based entities in the human immune system. Men may call it biotechnology, but the essence is still deliberately, yes, even defiantly, messing with and trying to manipulate God's own creative domain. The God of this universe has intervened in man's deeds in past history, when he aimed to prevail against God's laws; He can certainly do it again if necessary! However you the reader may view the "science," we still have to call it the way our Father God calls it! However, too often the evil shenanigans of men go unchecked by our Father, because men were often being judged, throughout Scripture, for the disasters they made for themselves, while ignoring God's laws. This genetic engineering, with all it's potential for disaster, is another one of those follies.

When it came to the multiple issues surrounding COVID-19, doctors and nurses regularly found themselves in some bad spots, between a rock and a hard place. They know the ethical and moral aspects of having knowledge and ability to help people. We believe most of them don't want to harm their patients or other people in that process. As for Dr. Peter McCullough, persecution has been severe for trying to tell people the truth. He has family members who took the jab. Real medical freedom has been taken from him. He had personal and professional licenses canceled and has been sued. We now have a health system that will prosecute doctors because truth is NOT what they are promoting. Dr. Peter was constantly threatened at every level of his life. Opinions are not subject to fact-checking but they were 'agenda-checked.' The system wanted to "save lives by hurting the people with mandatory vaccines, while suppressing early treatment that would save far more lives without potential vaccine harm." That is what the pandemic was about—a deliberate, fully intentional effort to push a harmful agenda on the global population by abjectly controlling it and making tons of money doing it. Had SARS-CoV-2 been treated the same as SARS-CoV-1 was, it would all have gone away in a few months, but that was NOT the planned agenda. As public health officials (criminals) continue pushing mandatory vaccinations against the will of the people, there will continue to be an exponential increase in adverse events, because it's the essence of this 'vaccine' that shouldn't even be called a 'vaccine'. About halfway through the pandemic process, two prominent CDC employees resigned positions where they "had it made"—a very telling decision for prominent staff. It would be very hard for folks who still have a conscience to keep playing such hurtful games!

It would be negligent in a chapter speaking so thoroughly about gross damages of all kinds, not to at least see some of what Dr. Robert Malone saw through the COVID pandemic through his unique role. Interestingly, "he is regarded as an inventor of mRNA and DNA vaccines and a world-wide expert in RNA technologies." He received his medical training at Northwestern University (MD) and Harvard University (Clinical Research Post Grad). He was scientifically trained at UC Davis, UC San Diego, and at the Salk Institute of Molecular Biology and Virology laboratories. He is internationally recognized in virology, immunology, and molecular biology. His own discoveries in mRNA non-viral delivery systems are considered the key to the current COVID-19 vaccine strategies."[61]

"When Dr. Malone first 'invented' the original mRNA vaccine technology as a medical and grad student in the late 1980s, he could not have imagined he would become a leader in a movement to expose the dangers of mRNA vaccines that billions of people have received—too often without being informed of the risks. For voicing opposition to the mainstream narrative, he was censored by Big Tech and vilified by the media. But he continues to speak out and alert the world to the web of lies we have all experienced. From vaccine safety and effectiveness to early treatments like ivermectin, to lockdowns, masks, and more. He is THE signature, dissident voice telling the other side of the COVID story, the role of corporate media, censorship, propaganda, and the brave new world of transhumanism promoted by the World Economic Forum (WEF) and its acolytes."[62]

The long-term chronic effects of vaccines such as Guillain Barré Syndrome, cardiomyopathy/cardiotoxicity, seizure disorders, neurologic disorders, gastrointestinal problems, etc. have long been known possibilities, but all of these and many more have been seen from the use of COVID vaccines as we have seen previously. The CDC and the FDA are clearly aware of these adverse events, but continue to see them as rare possibilities, despite the clear volume of VAERS reports. They maintain the lies that the vaccines are very safe and effective when they clearly are not. An interesting fact is that in the beginning of the COVID vaccines, Israel had a written contract with Pfizer that adverse events could NOT even be reported. Doctors were NOT allowed to talk about it and patients were denied the freedom to speak of it on social media like Facebook. Anthony Fauci ***SWORE*** the vaccines were safe and effective. People who experienced adverse events and tried to share it on social media were immediately shut down, designated crazy, and the censorship was complete. "Nobody spoke of the concept of, absolute risk reduction which would have given some measure of accountability. Instead, the CDC elected to use a fully outdated system of reporting to minimize the appearance of risk. But the method was NOT sensitive, it's inaccurate, and obsolete, also giving the appearance of hiding information and minimizing it was their intended goal. The effectiveness of a vaccine or drug is relative. The belief that a vaccine is 60-75% effective, is enough to use it. According to the CDC, even now, age is the strongest risk factor for severe COVID-19 outcomes. Patients with one or multiple certain underlying medical conditions are also at higher risk. Additionally, being unvaccinated or not up to date on COVID-19 vaccinations also increases the risk of severe COVID-19 outcomes (however, that statement has been proven false many times over, the CDC continues to tout it)."[64] The Delta variant was nearly as infectious as Varicella, which is 3-fold more infectious than all other vaccinated illnesses, so it didn't even approach the 60% standard of effectiveness by the CDC's own graphs, but this fact remained confidential and was plugged anyway. It had already stated that the spread of COVID-19 wouldn't be stopped if its effectiveness was 100%, so that continued masking could be justified. However, information leaked that new infections were occurring primarily in previously vaccinated people. So there was deliberate lying and deceit across the board on the effectiveness of the vaccines, and there still is today! Worse, if there was ANY good news it was attributed automatically to the use of the vaccines. If any not-so-great news, that was attributed to the failure of those people who refused to vax. However, the public at large bought the lies and the constant repetition of the narrative—they were safe and their communities were also safer.

"But what effect did the COVID policies really have on lives, livelihoods, and our democracies? How was it possible that the lies spread by governments (and health agencies) would persist, and that our institutions would fail to correct them?" Dr. Malone's book we've mentioned took a hard look at these questions and illustrated how data, information, and psychology were/are distorted during and since the pandemic. "Governments intentionally weaponized fear to mold behavior. The media smeared anyone who objected to the narrative. Big Pharma—aligned with larger globalist interests exemplified by the likes of Bill Gates and the WEF—had captured the agencies that are supposed to regulate it long before the pandemic began. Dr. Malone explored these perverse connections between Pharma, government, and media, and told us what can be done about it. Since Dr. Malone is never satisfied with a simple answer or easy solution, he proposed multiple action plans for a better future."[65] The MOST important thing is for each of us to find our own ways of resisting the control of fascist, corporatist, and totalitarian overlords. If we desire to step out of this past darkness toward a nation and a world that defends the principles of the Constitution, upholds individual rights, and honors free speech—we must ALL be involved in that transition back.

Today, we KNOW people are just as much at risk of contracting COVID-19 whether they were vaccinated or not. The vaccines have NOT protected and given us any better immunity than the natural immunity we received by having the disease. In fact, there is still poor durability of the vaccinated immunity, requiring those vaccinated to boost at least annually to maintain some of it, which of course doesn't bother Big Pharma at all. It simply means an enormous and continued flow of the money almost indefinitely. There are many studies, both previously and currently that prove natural immunity is better. Just be aware, that you will not find this proof on social media platforms or through Big Tech, because truth is whatever CDC, FDA, WHO, NIH, etc., via Big Tech, says it is at any given time, even if they changed their minds! The risk/benefit ratio for vaccinating infants to 18 years is "upside down"! The benefits of the vaccine MUST outweigh its risks of use for each intended indication. "In basic terms, any benefit/risk ratio greater than 1 is favorable. With COVID vaccine, the benefit/risk ratio as reported by pathologists is far better in unvaccinated children, so it makes absolutely no sense to vaccinate infants and most children for COVID, scientifically."[66]

The National Vaccine Injury Act of 1904 is the supposed gold standard. The ONLY thing that really matters is 100% mass vaccination. The ACT was an attempt to encourage and ensure vaccine production by creating a no-fault compensation program as a required first resort for those who believed that they or their children had been injured by certain vaccines. If a parent wants to refuse vaccinations for their children, there are actually some states that have ruled that refusal to vaccinate constitutes child neglect. Dear reader, can you see how much power as a parent has long since been removed from you? If doctors, in their sincere medical judgment believe a child's health would be jeopardized by vaccinations, a medical exemption will be granted. Even a religious exemption is VERY difficult to acquire today. The safety of the vaccines is adamantly declared, and your doubt of it does not mean a thing. The law also states that any opposing idea to Big Pharma MUST be shut down. With the current administration, and the work of Robert F Kennedy, Jr. in particular, we may hope that at least some of this nonsense and yes, abuse, will be mitigated in these next four years. This type of fear-mongering has driven many a concerned parent to go ahead with their child's vaccinations, only to lose the perfectly normal child they had to life-long adverse effects and even death. This law is NOT equitable or Constitutional and it's existed for 120 years to the detriment of thousands of children and their families ,just so Big Pharma could suffer no loss! If vaccines were really VERY safe, this law would not be needed, and even the very common side effects possible could NOT be a potential risk for some children. This author is among a vast number of professionals and parents in every health related field who believe the truth presented here.[67]

Dr. Anthony Fauci is one of the most powerful lobbyists in the nation because of his high-volume philanthropic efforts in most congressional districts. He has been able to ramrod policies through Congress that almost every other doctor in the country could never have gotten away with. What most Americans don't know is that the money is procured from Congress for his various projects, and that same money isn't his, it's taxpayer money! So "when he allotted vast amounts of money to various virology labs to keep the highly-questionable value of gain-of-function experiments going, he did it with our money, not his. His efforts were largely responsible for driving Big Pharma's unlicensed products such as COVID vaccines, and drugs like Remdesivir under medical experimentation through the FDA licensing process at warp-speed, through the Emergency Use Authorization act. Normally "informed consent" is required by federal law. It requires FULL disclosure of risks, understanding of the disclosure, and acceptance of free-will consent of recipients. NONE of that happened with COVID vaccines—it was 100% against bioethics laws—failure to comply. There were no rules, no consequences and the end fully justified the means."[68] On top of all this, universal vaccination sets the population up for the selection of a super-escape mutant of the disease that would be untouchable by prior vaccines. The idea is considered a very bad one by most scientists and epidemiologists, causing a loss of any potential vaccine that could work when it might truly be needed most, especially another pandemic. But this concept, too, has been totally ignored. In fact, dissenters of the COVID vaccines were actually accused of murder for refusing to protect society with vaccination! The real murderers were those who made and promoted the toxic vaccines, those who pushed mandatory vaccines for whole segments of our society, and virtually killed tens of thousands of them in that process.

Last, but far from least is the mention of huge damage done to purveyors of real COVID truth, is Dr. Joseph Mercola. Governments created a list of a dozen men and women (called the Dirty Dozen). Dr. Mercola has the rather dubious distinction of being number ONE on that list as the man who spread the most disinformation according to the White House. Discrediting campaigns against this "dirty dozen" generally backfired. In general, physicians are vaccine advocates because in the allopathic system of modern medicine it has been trained into them and they can't question what they are doing without a sort of identity crisis. Despite learning and knowing basic scientific principles of traditional medicine of centuries, they must avoid most of it in lieu of drug-based treatments. Consequently, any information that does NOT follow what they learned and are expected to practice, can quite easily fit into a misinformation paradigm because it doesn't fit their paradigm of medicine. Globalists and their agenda have the money to defend this drug-based paradigm and will use any means to do so. They have created a delusional mass psychosis that includes fear-mongering, censorship, and isolation of people from people—much like the Salem Witch trials—totally irrational and untrue. Naturally, it can't be rational because a rational thought process was totally abandoned. This is the system that has sought to control any thought process that contradicts their own and shut it down along with anyone who dares to think for themselves. Such was the case for Dr. Joe.

Dr. Joseph Mercola is a highly qualified and educated osteopathic M.D. who had already written dozens of books and peer-reviewed articles before anyone ever heard of COVID-19. As an osteopathic physician, he has great respect and belief in natural and traditional medicine and therapies. What's more, given the patience and time, alternative natural protocols generally do a really good job of helping our bodies heal as they were meant to heal—naturally. "Silencing Dr. Mercola's Voice, of course, was the Medical Cabal's early priority (with COVID). For decades, he has been among the most effective and influential advocates against the pharmaceutical paradigm. He is an eloquent, charismatic, and knowledgeable critic of a corrupt system that has made Americans the world's top consumer of pharmaceutical drugs. Americans pay the highest prices for drugs, and have the worst outcomes among the top 75 nations. Putting opiates—which kill 50,000 Americans annually—aside, pharmaceuticals are now the third biggest killer of Americans, after heart attacks and cancer. Like a prophet in the wilderness, Dr. Mercola had argued for years that good health does NOT come in a syringe or a pill but from building strong immune systems. He preached that nutrition and exercise are the MOST effective medicines, public health officials ought to be pushing policies that discourage reliance on pharmaceutical products and that safeguard our food supplies from Big Food, Big Chemical and Big Ag. These predatory industries naturally considered Dr. Mercola to be Public Enemy #1."[69]

Big Pharma banned Dr. Mercola from the airwaves and newsprint long ago and at the same time turned Wikipedia—which acts as Big Pharma's newsletter and propaganda vehicle—into a massive source of lies and defamation against Dr. Mercola and every other integrative and functional health physician. At the beginning of COVID, all the social media platforms joined the campaign to silence them. "It is a damning omen for all of democracy when citizens can no longer conduct civil, informed debates about critical policies that impact the vitality of our economy, public health, personal freedoms, and constitutional rights. Censorship is violence, and this systematic muzzling of debate—which proponents justify as a measure to curtail dangerous polarization—is actually fueling the polarization and extremism that the autocrats use to clamp down with ever more draconian controls."[70]

A very well-known communicator and journalist and previous CBS newsman named Edward R. Murrow, in the era of McCarthyism, once said, "The right of dissent, or if you prefer, the right to be wrong, is surely fundamental to the existence of a democratic society. That's the right that always went first in every nation that stumbled down the trail toward totalitarianism."[71] Personal threats were leveled at Dr. Mercola and on his company. His First Amendment rights were horribly threatened like hundreds of others. He was called a bio-terrorist, when in fact the entire operation was done by bio-terrorists. Censorship NEVER allows a public debate of ideas. Its, "Agree with us or die," is the agenda. It was impossible to get informed consent. Dozens of well-documented studies disputed what public health officials perpetrated. Their intention was always to suppress offending ideas, no matter what it took. Fellow citizen!! It is imperative we all understand that this mess was NEVER a vaccination issue. It was and still is a FREEDOM issue. Our freedom of speech was very nearly wiped out! Almost everything the mainstream media tells or prints IS NOT TRUE! False information was blasted out everywhere. We were all told what WE must do to protect the health of our loved ones and friends by vaxxing. The truth was and is that it didn't protect anyone.

Today's propaganda is more sophisticated than at any other time in history, and now the social media platforms were ready-made to support it completely, as planned at least two decades ago. Naturally, it was/is proven irrefutably that almost every bit of information gleaned by those who were censored and vilified for it, was true and provable.

The real criminals, deceivers, and liars like Anthony Fauci, who had been given such enormous power by the US government via the NIH, appropriated over a TRILLION dollars to pay for the gain-of-function experimentation in both CCP and American labs; determined to increase viral transmissibility, viral replication, virulence, and much more of the SARS-CoV-2. Fauci's part in all of this fraudulent science makes him one of the most vicious criminals of all time. He is directly responsible for the deaths of millions of people globally, both from COVID-19 and from his heinous manipulation of the AIDS epidemic decades ago. He almost makes Hitler look like the candy man!

Dr. Joseph Mercola, like Dr. Peter McCullough, and so many others knew the best ways to build natural immunity to the virus. He, too, had outlined very specific directives for staying well and for treating the COVID-19 if a person succumbed to it. They were highly effective and hundreds recovered well with early treatment. Dr. Joe has a simple email address that could be accessed by anyone interested in real help— Mercola.com. As Dr. Mercola began his book, *The Truth About COVID-19...*, he spoke of just how the pandemic has shone a harsh spotlight on the fundamental 'dis-ease' and ill-health of the nations. It exposed our vulnerabilities to a whole plethora of life-threatening co-morbidities, medical errors, and the corruption of the entire pharmaceutical industry. In addition to its effects on our health and on the health care industry, it also empowered the global elite more than ever before to manufacture lies and half-truths. Besides Big Tech and Big Pharma, "the WHO and Bill Gates bought politicians and scientists from across the political spectrum to do their bidding. There is a shadowy network of military contractors and bioweapons specialists hiding behind the facade of biomedical and vaccine research while Big Tech silences their critics."[72]

As Robert F. Kennedy, Jr of the Children's Health Defense pointed out, "Machiavellian manipulation of this pandemic amounts to nothing less than an attempted coup d'état by big data, by big telecom, by big tech, by the big oil and chemical companies and by the global public health cartel led by Bill Gates and the WHO. It wants to magnify and amplify its wealth and its power over our lives, over our liberties, and it wants to subvert our democracies and destroy our sovereignty and our control over our lives and our children's health."[73] However, there is mounting evidence and increasing certainty that a growing number of independent scientists, investigators, and lawyers have begun to deconstruct and critique the "official story" on the origins, nature, dangers, prevention, and treatment of the COVID-19 pandemic. "The 'official story' dogmatically upheld by the CCP and military, Big Pharma, Bill Gates, the CDC, the NIH, the mass media, and Big Tech, is that the SARS-CoV-2 virus emerged 'naturally' from nature and then inexplicably jumped the species barrier from bats to humans, precipitating the most serious and deadly epidemic since the Spanish flu one hundred years ago, which infected one-third of the world's population at the time and killed up to 50 million people. "Here's the kicker—according to establishment virologists and gene engineers (who get their money from military bio-defense programs, government funding, and Big Pharma), a relatively innocuous and heretofore noncontagious coronavirus quickly mutated into a deadly killer, leaving behind no biological or epidemiological traces whatsoever of its rapid evolution."[74]As the saying goes, "If you believe that, we've got some swamp land for sale in Florida!" PREPOSTOROUS!!

Chapter 14

All About the 'Vaccines' That Aren't Vaccines

Introduction to COVID-19 'Vaccines' in Depth

There is so much information about vaccines that people should be aware of it is difficult to determine where to begin. A great effort has been made by Investigative Health Journalist, Jonathan Otto, and his team to not only find the real facts, but to disseminate them in independent video series that were / are NOT subject to the censorship of Big Tech entities. He accessed, interviewed, introduced, and disseminated reams of information these doctors, scientists, journalists, lawyers, and other professionals gave him. They spoke the truth and clearly do NOT agree with nor support the established globalist agenda. There is more proof of the real facts than of the false narrative—it just takes courage, creativity, sensitivity, ability, and hard work to document all of the information through the back door approach, but it has been an enormous success and people have been well-informed of the truth. To that end, this author intends to bring as much information to this book as there is time and ability of the reader to utilize it.

The docuseries we'll discuss first was entitled "New Hope" and covers background information on the COVID vaccines. Back in the 1980s and early 1990s, Dr. Robert Malone of whom we've already spoken, understood through his gene research with DNA and RNA ,that a lipid nanoparticle technology would encapsulate the DNA and RNA molecules. They were to be used to target cancer cells via various toxins, including ricin toxin, king cobra venom, diphtheria toxin, etc., utilizing toxins as therapeutic agents. The actual patent for the mRNA gene therapy of the Covid vaccine is not owned by

Dr. Robert Malone, but by Katalin Kariko and Drew Weisman at the University of PA. Starting in 2009, the research was primarily shifted to the leadership of the NIH for funding and documentation of gene therapy technology. In the research, they disclosed the use of RNAs and snake venom phosphodiesterase in every single one of their gene therapy mRNA vaccine research development papers! The fact that so many toxic effects of the COVID vaccines were attributed to snake venom derivatives with patents on them, and replicated in the vaccines, easily explains the toxicities and causes of many really heinous effects. "One man in particular is very concerning, Paul F. Reid, a scientist who has the patent from the US government as of 1993-1996 per his personal biography, was paid to take snake venom neurotoxins and manufacture them synthetically in bacterial and yeast systems, purify the venom, then apply it in the large-scale production of vaccines," as described by Dr. Brian Ardis.[1] The question was: Did Reid accomplish this task for which he was paid? The answer is a resounding "YES!" In "2010, Reid was awarded a US patent for a detoxified king cobra, common cold and influenza vaccine! Within that patent, Reid specifically stated, in fact, the advantage of using venoms for anti-viral vaccines is that they don't need to be virus specific; because all venoms target the exact same receptors that all viruses target. It could be used to stop global pandemics in mass production!! This was just ten years before COVID."[2]

All viruses actually target nicotinic acetylcholine receptors as do the venoms. So giving the venom-based vaccine, blocks the viruses in the body from entering the receptors. How convenient, right? Wrong! The major problem with using snake venom is it's deadly, and toxic which the patent says again and again.

When using them, the venom must be detoxified, in one of four designated ways: hydrogen peroxide, ozone, formalin (a form of formaldehyde), or heat (destroyed at 131 degrees F) which our bodies couldn't tolerate. Many different venoms have also been patented for use in vaccines—the "V" in vaccines stands for venoms. All of Big Pharma was moving to full-on venom-based vaccines. "In

January of 2020, the known toxins of king cobra venom were listed in a patent and over 300 were identified; only 19 were venom-specific, and capable of organ-targeting (killing organs). Perhaps COVID-19 has nothing to do with the year 2019 and the name is no accident! Many of the antidotes being used to treat vaccine-damaged people have been identified by knowing the details revealed in those patents, which by necessity must reveal all the mechanisms of action. As the reader can probably surmise, it is clear that this information provides the reason why the COVID-19 'vaccines' could be rolled-out so quickly, because the technology and wherewithal for making them was present for nearly three decades before needed!"[3]

So, why was it necessary to turn our bodies into a toxic spike protein factory using mRNA? It was easier to get to the end product of antibody production without using another harmful technology to go along with it. Dr. Shankara Chetty stated, ... "in the first seven days of the illness, COVID-19 is a virus, but after that, it is very literally a cytokine storm," defined as a pathological reaction of our innate immune systems causing an excessive release of pro-inflammatory, signaling molecules called cytokines. They are a normal part of our body's immune response to infection, but their sudden release in large quantities can cause multi-system organ failure and death (a true 'STORM'). COVID-19 disease and other respiratory diseases in particular are capable of causing this response due to a hypersensitivity trigger. Dr. Chetty realized very quickly it was a lab-made virus and "they were using the most pathogenic part of the virus to make a very ill-conceived 'vaccine.' If the leak had been a mistake, they would have done their best to cordone that area off and do everything possible to contain it, but if it was intentional and they wanted it to affect the entire planet, the first thing they would do was develop a fake test for it (PCR) to hype the numbers and blow it all out of proportion. If that happened (which it did), I would immediately know it was all part of a very big plan."[3] I'd seen the spike protein, engineered on the virus which is the primary pathogen.

The CIA man told me, "You know, Dr. Chetty, they have taken an ordinary coronavirus, and weaponized it. They had been looking for this piece on the virus— they have put a military trade package on this virus and we've been searching for this package and were shocked to hear this spike protein was it."

Dr. Chetty then asked, "If you know now that the spike protein is the primary pathogen, what is it doing in the 'vaccine?'"

He said, "The mass vaccination program is actually part of the military strategy. It has nothing to do with health. Dr. Chetty, you watch now—they will soon insist that every person on the planet must take this 'vaccine' whether they like it or not. They will challenge your freedoms, take away your job opportunities, curtail your movements, all in their effort to force this 'vaccine' on all humanity, including women and children; everyone is fair game."

"Certainly we were dealing with a global military campaign![4] (Dr. Chelli)

"Now, given that the spike protein is a toxin, obviously, so is the 'vaccine.' The projected outcome of that is very clear and the following is what it looks like. If someone has poison sitting around it cannot kill anybody unless it is used. If someone voluntarily drinks that poison, it was certainly a bad choice to make. But the day I start to force someone to drink it, it takes on a whole new meaning, and it's called poisoning, with intent to kill. That is a criminal act. So we understand if anyone started down the road forcing people to take the toxic 'vaccine', we could be certain it was a global poisoning taking place. So when the first mandate occurred, we knew that yes, it truly was a global military campaign, despite all protests to the contrary. It was meant to poison people."[4]

A peer said to Dr. Chetty, "You know there are just two things that cause the type of responses we're seeing—an allergen or a venom."

"However, there was a clear pattern of the transmission of the pathogen which ruled out allergens, leaving venom etiology, There have been literally thousands of studies with cultures from all parts of the body, especially in conjunction with long COVID. It has been discovered without any real surprise that the gut health is affected, and affected even longer than respiratory health. The various venomous toxins can remain in the gut for many months without proper treatment. It's important to understand how toxic the 'vaccines' are, despite the constant misinformation propagandized that it isn't so. If a person suspects he may have long COVID, particularly if he was vaccinated, it is imperative to get medical attention from a doctor who recognizes it for what it is, and is in the camp of doctors that understand its cause and know how to treat it."[4] The best place to seek medical help is from members of the American Association of Physicians and Surgeons, as previously discussed because they will listen and respond correctly.

Now that we know a bit about the patented spike protein being the actual manufactured primary pathogen, we need to understand how it was designed to infiltrate human DNA. "The most concerning aspect of the COVID 'vaccines' is the type of novel technology that is being used to create them. Today, not a single expert has been able to pinpoint every single ingredient in the shot, but the ones they have identified are all extremely harmful to the body with absolutely NO known benefit to our health. Now we know that not only did the patents for these bioweapons exist long before the planned pandemic, but that the mRNA technology has been shown by various experts to infiltrate the DNA, making a spike protein production factory that wreaks havoc on multiple organ systems and is responsible for the enormous amount of damage being done constantly."[5]

The very best description of the spike protein and how it works, that this author has seen, was done by Dr. Peter McCullough, one of the most prestigious and prolific authorities on COVID-19. He started by letting us know that the Emergency Use Authorization (EUA) mechanism was used in conjunction with the US Military via the Defense Advanced Research Projects Agency (DARPA). Historically, the EUA IS a military mechanism to be used whenever a National Emergency is activated. It was a National Security Authorization to streamline the production process of needed items. You, the reader, should know that those within the military are accustomed to this process, but this was the very first time it was ever used on the public. You should also know that a coronavirus is normally not a dangerous pathogen; but similar to a simple cold virus. However, it was COMMISSIONED by our US military via DARPA years ago to be potentially used as a bioweapon. Once again, the Big Tech media denies this fact, but it's a matter of public record which the web will not publish. Dr. Peter Daszak, President of EcoHealth Alliance, and recipient of massive amounts of funding for research from the NIH, was the subject of a major hearing by a House Oversight Select Subcommittee on the Coronavirus Pandemic in April, 2024. This hearing served to hold Dr. Daszak publicly accountable for discrepancies between his closed-door transcribed interview and the available evidence. "During the hearing, Dr. Daszak was pressed to explain EcoHealth's relationship with the Wuhan Institute of Virology (WIV), and scrutinized on his abuse of taxpayer dollars to fund dangerous, potentially pandemic-causing research. Forthcoming testimony to Congress described evidence showing EcoHealth 'absolutely' facilitated 'gain-of-function' research at the WIV on the American taxpayer's dime. Chairman Wenstrup said, 'It is important to understand that you intentionally downplayed the role of China. Between your actions to DARPA and those with NIH, you have failed to be a good steward of taxpayer dollars. So our recommendation is that you receive no further funding."[6] In addition, the committee planned to take further steps to address Dr. Daszak's complete contempt for the American people. But the quote proves that EcoHealth was supposed to be accountable both to the funder, NIH, and to DARPA (American Department of Defense).

Moving onward to the information about the spike proteins which were deliberately manufactured in the lab in 2012, via mRNA, under the authority of BARDA (Biomedical Advanced Research and Development Authority). Part of HHS's role is to develop medical countermeasures addressing the public health and medical consequences of chemical, biological, radiological, and nuclear (CBRN) accidents, incidents, and attacks, pandemic influenza, and emerging infectious diseases. It comes directly under the authority of the NIH, which engineered the spike protein to make it more lethal and invasive in the human body. Two different research papers describe how SARS-CoV-2 would be introduced to human populations, and how they could make the spike protein "lock to a human ACE2 receptor in a humanized respiratory epithelial tissue receptor, then get the spike (pathogen) to jump from bat to human. All of this was done by American ingenuity, funded by the NIH, then subcontracted to the Wuhan Institute of Virology, the Biosecurity Annex—level 4 (top security level) under the authority of the CCP military complex. Subsequently, a French contractor working in this area took his science to Moderna (Big Pharma) for development. Now, we are describing a Bio-Pharmaceutical Complex or organized consortium, working actively together on two things 1) SARS-CoV-2 as a biologic threat, and 2) A Defensive strategy for it, such as monoclonal antibodies and vaccines."[7]

"The Messenger RNA (mRNA) is genetic material loaded onto lipid (fat) nanoparticles. It is standardized with a synthetic nucleotide (5 prime-3 prime analog capsules). A nucleotide is a molecule that is the basic building block of DNA and RNA, the nucleic acids that carry genetic information in cells. These capsules are NOT digestible so they keep the mRNA stable. Because the nanoparticles are lipids they can travel everywhere in the body, and can also cross the blood-brain barrier into the brain. They go readily to the heart, muscle, adrenal glands, reproductive organs, etc., so we know that loading the genetic material onto lipid nanoparticles is a widespread delivery mechanism. Once the mRNA itself is taken up into the respective organs, the spike protein is produced by the mRNA material in the cytosol or fluid volume in the body's cells by human ribosomes (protein synthesis) that read the mRNA and produce copious amounts of the spike protein. The really tragic result of this is that spike proteins are produced for an uncontrolled duration, in an uncontrolled quantity. This is the FIRST time we've ever given a 'vaccine' or any other product where there is NO control and NO safety boundaries on how much could be produced. Shockingly, we now know that the mRNA is present throughout the circulation for a minimum of 15 days, and maybe a month or more. Once the spike protein is represented on the cells' surfaces, the body attacks its own cells in an autoimmune response that causes widespread inflammation. 'Spike protein is taken up by antigen-presenting cells (markers inside or outside the body that help the immune system determine if something in the body is harmful to it), which ultimately present to B cells that mature into plasma cells and produce 'antibodies'."[8]

Consequently, the reader can get the idea of what we now must deal with. It is still being touted that there are no actual changes to one's own DNA in the cell nucleus, but thoughtful scientists, journalists, medical professionals and many of the masses are concerned that with so many bodily changes being affected, it certainly has the potential of changing human DNA and the genome. Indeed, it's highly unlikely that all this genetic engineering will NOT affect the DNA and cell structures based on what we are certain it does. The 'vaccines' DO appear to alter human DNA permanently although Big Pharma and the 'official' public health agencies vehemently deny this. We now have the genetic code for a lethal, foreign protein in our bodies permanently if we are among all those who have taken the vaccine. The ongoing and casual dismissal of all these possibilities is even more worrisome because it gives no heed to ethical/moral medicine, science, or previous public health policies. Hence, justifiable concerns abound. We are reminded of a plethora of effects to both vaccines and drugs that were once deemed perfectly safe, even harmless, and were later determined they weren't harmless at all. Indeed, most had shown concerns when they were originally approved for use.

The CDC, NIH, WHO, etc., regularly touted the supposed fact that 'vaccines' do NOT change the human genome. Clearly, this bold-faced lie was a huge piece of the mass deception perpetrated around the globe. Indeed, it does change the genome, and the CDC and others have a responsibility to come clean on this information in the interest of warning people of the health issues pursuant of this knowledge. Further, we have been told by the perpetrators themselves, that gene therapy is the only technology Big Pharma, and the globalists backing it, intend to pursue in the future. That is, the globalist agenda requires the production of more and more 'vaccines' to prevent the multitudes of new diseases expected to present in the near future. We have seen this intent escalating with each "new" viral manifestation that has already surfaced. Every new 'vaccine' developed will have the same potential of toxic adverse events and death because the technology is NOT going to change. None of them will be truly beneficial or a development for better health. The standard is to simply make more and more money with each rollout. However, just like so much other propaganda subsequently proven wrong, the global powers running this narrative will never back down and do the right thing by global citizens, as they have now clearly proven. Therefore, those who have taken the vaccines must understand that their own genomes are permanently altered and therefore may change health outcomes for any of them.

To continue the explanation of spike proteins, the research has been done since 1904, but it really ramped up during the 1940s. Paul F. Reid has the patent for the spike protein, paid for by the US government in 2010 as we saw previously. Today, the spike protein can now be synthetically produced and is nothing more or less than the toxic production of snake venom. and other venoms. The primary responses to the toxic spike proteins in the human body are blood clotting, neurological issues of all kinds, and cytotoxicity, which is the death of any kind of cells. According to Dr. Brian Ardis, "All venom proteins are glycoproteins and all are neurotoxins."[9]They will destroy all vital cells in the body. The spike proteins of COVID-19 vaccines are chemically identical to snake venom proteins. As the spike proteins circulating in the blood stream and binding to cells continue producing toxin, the amount of toxin in the body increases little by little every day. Eventually any and every disease process known to man will occur—hence the dire predictions for shortened life spans of survivors and early deaths are highly likely, though the vaccine narrative NEVER goes near the vaccine prognosis, continually claiming that vaccines are "safe and effective!" One of the earliest signs of toxicity is paralysis and it was also the first side effect published in the Pfizer documents, in the form of Guillain Barré syndrome.There were 1300 known diseases listed in these documents as possible side effects. No wonder it took so long to be able to acquire the Pfizer documents—they were NOT happy or anxious for findings to be aired when trying to sell 'vaccine!'

There is a super-twisted concept that is prevalent in Pharmacia today similar to the concept of treating unhealthy cancer patients with chemotherapy. The idea is that hopefully the chemo will kill more cancer cells than healthy ones. Similarly, Big Pharma has developed anti-viral drug therapies. They are convinced that venoms will actually bind to the same receptors on your cells that viruses bind to—therefore if you give vaccine or drugs that are venom-based and they fill those receptors which they can, there will be no room for the various viruses to fit into those receptors. Considering that up until COVID-19, most of the viruses were NOT very innocuous, and venom is poison, it should be an obviously bad idea, but Big Pharma is convinced it will work. However, This clearly hasn't worked with COVID 'vaccine' and instead has harmed the receptors that venoms target. This explains every immune-deficiency reaction that's been seen with COVID-19 'vaccine' injuries. In Italy in June 2020, there was a study where scientists took the blood, mucus, urine, stool, etc., of COVID-positive patients as well as control studies of negative patients. The COVID-positive patients had 36 kinds of animal toxins, including 14 conotoxins from all of them with nothing in the negative patients. Another study was done of mammalian brain cells in the glial center of the brain. By placing spike proteins in the alpha-7 nicotinic glial receptors, new neurons were replicated rapidly, and it was possible to create a new glioblastoma brain tumor there in just 3 days. That should give anyone pause![9] Incidentally, glioblastomas were once extremely rare, which was good because they are very fast growing and almost always lethal. Now, however, they are being found quite regularly. The author personally knows several people diagnosed with glioblastomas since the pandemic officially ended. Many other "super cancers" have also shown up exponentially in sizes and numbers never seen before. Yet, though Big Pharma's patent papers show these are strongly possible in vaxxed people, they deny the 'vaccines' caused them and remain adamant it can't be absolutely proven.

Another very crucial aspect of the glycoproteins relates exactly to the whole global agenda. When young adults in particular were given the COVID 'vaccine,' both males and females were effectively sterilized—a far greater percentage of the next generation will be unable to reproduce. All the other succeeding generations will be sicker and die younger with all manner of exacerbated diseases including supercancers. All of this damage has been shown whenever tested but globalists see this news with glee. After all, this whole result has completely augmented the globalist agenda of depopulation. Immune systems are fighting themselves. The worst problem of all according to Dr. Henry Ealy, is known as glycosylation. "In it the red blood cells are coated with a sticky substance (due to the attachment of carbohydrates to the backbone of a protein through a wrong enzymatic reaction), which forms the glycoprotein. This causes the red blood cells to stick together decreasing their surface area's ability to carry oxygen and take away the carbon dioxide. The gas exchange gets worse and worse until it gets very hard to breathe. The clotting grows; some clots may run the length of an arm or leg. The clotting prevents blood plasma from breaking the clot down; (this is no accident knowing the agenda). This only occurs as a result of venom protein due to its substance, Ecar, that causes the clots, but removes the textillinin which is needed to break down the clots. Therefore, by its very mechanism of action, known by everyone involved in the 'vaccine manufacture', the 'vaccine is very literally a bioweapon.' It is certainly not 'safe or effective' as propagandized and it is still required for infants and children intentionally. It is a 'wrecking ball' to the body because every cell is energy-dependent, needing the energy for its mitochondria to survive. In addition, it inhibits the production and use of nitric oxide, which is necessary for the lining of blood vessels and helps nerve cells communicate, among many other functions. Because the body's DNA literally becomes mutagenic and incompatible with life, we know it is a bioweapon. To destroy the human genome is not an accident—it is the goal."[10] Dr. Ealy's explanation of this process was the best this author could find; and while it isn't super easy to understand, perhaps the reader can get an idea of the deliberate use of this well-known process to take out as many people with the toxic 'vaccines' possible. This phenomenon has been extensively proven by coroners doing autopsies. They describe these enormously thick and long snake-like ropes of blood clots they remove from major blood vessels. At first, before the cause was fully known, these forensic doctors were absolutely 'blown away' by the repetitive presence of them in the blood vessels of people with known history of vaccination, These were completely unlike anything they had ever seen. If the person died of COVID-19, the strands could also be present in a far lesser presentation.

Proving the intentionality of the mRNA technology is not difficult. Katalin Kariko had been working with mRNA and lipid nanoparticle hydrogel wrapped around the mRNA, since 1978, along with Drew Weissman. They are both scientists at the University of Pennsylvania and are literally "the creators of the COVID vaccine."

They are the ones who received a $3 million dollar royalty check for all the COVID19 shots produced. Their research studies go all the way back to 2009, and they were funded by Anthony Fauci and the NIAID of the NIH to do ONE thing—mRNA gene therapy! The global world prefers to ignore all of this information because it doesn't want people to know what's causing all the harm in the 'vaccines.' They created the mRNA injections—mRNA instructions to your body to make from your own genes supposedly—spike glycoproteins which also happen to be cobra venom factor. They disclose in their studies that in order to cut RNA and DNA they use two substances— snake venom phosphodiesterase, the RNase which is also a component of snake venom. In April of 2020, Katalin Kariko was interviewed by her undergrad university in Europe. She was asked where she started using mRNA. She said, "In 1978 right here at this university! It was literally the lipid nanoparticle hydrogel with mRNase that created the immune response. These two components cause every bit of neurological damage seen from the 'vaccines'."[11]

Dr. Christina Parks, PhD, scientist, expert in cellular and molecular biology has studied the action of this technology and the physiological damage that it does in the body for many years, and can give a fairly concise explanation that allows us some understanding of why the damage happens where it does. She was shocked that drug manufacturers were planning on using this experimental gene therapy to do "vaccines. "In the past, the lipid nanoparticles have been extremely inflammatory and continued to be so when it came time to make the 'vaccines.' Also, because the lipids are FAT, the molecules will naturally seek out areas of the body that are more heavily fatty. Initially we were all told the 'vaccine' would stay in the area of the deltoid muscle (injection site). but that wasn't possible, nor was it consistent to its composition; hence it wasn't true! The design of gene therapy is to get as much of the product diffused throughout the body as it possibly can—proof of the lie. They want it to get to the T-cells, a type of white blood cell that helps protect the body from infection and attack from cancer cells. They aimed to make the mechanism of the 'vaccines' work as long as possible. So, what we can expect is that it makes as much spike protein as possible for as long as possible to as many cells as possible. The spike protein will stay in the cells, anchor to the outside of cells, or go into blood circulation. Bottom line is all the things you suffered with contracting COVID will likely return if vaccinated because you have the spike proteins in your body to keep on making the same. Since our immune systems are supposed to attack the foreign protein which the body is now producing exponentially, and increasing the massive inflammation, the body must now try to neutralize or destroy the offenders. This will cause extreme immune infiltration to areas of mass spike protein, causing an even greater inflammatory response and a lot of tissue damage. Remember, the fatty areas of our bodies will concentrate more of the spike protein action than others, so you should know the ovaries are encased in fat as are the adrenal glands. The heart is a muscle encased in fat. Lymph nodes figure largely and because the mRNA is not broken down, this will cause chronic long-standing inflammation in lymph nodes because it will keep making the spike protein. Over time, the inflammation causes all systems to tire of trying to keep up and start suppressing the immune system that was supposed to be strengthened. Being worn out, unable to keep up, it stands down and starts attacking itself, causing autoimmune responses. Now the body is even more susceptible to infections, and as we've seen, cancerous propensities stand up strong because the T-cells scanning for cancer are also suppressed. Indeed, we have seen this played out in the reappearance of cancer and turbo-cancers. Any other infections or illnesses present in our bodies at that time, get a green light to go ahead as well."[12]

Every day, the numbers and types of adverse events to the 'vaccines' grow and expand. Another area very affected is the eyes, and even young people who have been vaccinated have had small strokes in the eyes which can easily lead to blindness in a teen or child. Dr. Seema Nanda, OD is another professional with very real concerns for patients who were vaxxed. Dr. Nanda compares its action to an atomic blast instead of a drone strike. It (mRNA), used in these fake 'vaccines', is being used so randomly and irresponsibly it's like a loose cannon. It should be an entity with known actions, programmed to strike in a localized, precise mode. Instead, when it is released into the body randomly, and with an unregulated and highly diffuse action impossible to track, it's not doing what it is supposed to do. Is it an accident? Whatever the reason, the entire charade needs to be stopped just like other problematic vaccines and drugs of the past were stopped until a lot more investigation could be done and done effectively and scientifically. What is happening is completely unacceptable for a myriad of reasons. This 'vaccine' was supposed to stop the virus from spreading and from replicating and it's done neither. It requires constant boosters to no avail and little if any protection. We've established that vaxxed people are far more susceptible to repeat infections than those not vaxxed, though everyone in the global camp vehemently denies all of this known information. The body that God created heals itself well and Dr. Nanda completely supports natural medicine.[13]

Multiple and diverse issues are occurring in the eye, including retinal hemorrhages, small strokes, optic neuritis, cancers in the iris, and on the cornea, corneal transplant rejections; the body rejects a tissue that has never been a rejection problem before COVID. But, as Dr. Nanda wisely pointed out, "What if we treat a teenager with optic neuritis who is going blind, and ultimately his eye finally heals? Who can say how many times the same problem could recur, or a different eye problem surfaces, or a different problem occurs somewhere else in the body."[13] The mRNA is so random and so unique in its action with every single person, that any predictions are pointless. NO ONE KNOWS! WHY do we NOT know about all the possibilities we may face in our lives if we were vaxxed? Why was there no information given to all those who succumbed to the vax? Completely beyond the facts of forced vaccinations for a large segment of our society, there was NO informed consent. Now, with the children's vaccine schedule requiring COVID-19 vaccination for ALL children, 6 months of age and older, it's virtually impossible to protect our own children from the ravages of this 'vaccine' travesty. The powers that have been controlling America's public health are working with the global wolves in their agenda of control and depopulation. They will stop at nothing to further that agenda. Parents!! Please educate yourselves about these 'vaccines' and do whatever it takes to protect your precious children from this evil travesty. If they have been vaccinated already, and they are showing signs and symptoms that their bodies are NOT right or NOT what they used to be, stop all vaccines and do your homework. See a doctor who will pay attention to your concerns, and ask if your doctor has any experience in treating vaccine injuries. DO NOT believe the information plastered all over the web and social media. It has been completely hijacked by the globalist agenda and there is very little truth to be found there.

Myriads of Irregularities in Various Vaccine Studies

Early in the process of studying the experimental 'vaccines' by suspicious doctors and scientists, a vast number of anomalies were found in simple microscopic amplifications. There was no need for extremely high-powered electron microscopes—the process for studying so-called viruses made very little sense anyway. By the time they managed to prep a slide in a multi-layered, death-producing, chemically contaminating process, anything seen on the "doctored" slide was of the purest speculation and probable imagination. A vast number of researchers deny the presence of viruses, since no one has any visible proof they exist outside the realm of the laboratory. In the same way we do NOT know exactly what is in the 'vaccines' with absolute certainty. There has NEVER been any open and honest ingredient list accessible to public scrutiny. Only those having access to Big Pharma documents or to their patents, which by law must list every item and its intended use, can understand the highly concerning and scary reality.

There are some people who do have this access and when its known, it's far beyond concerning to actually see the proof of the depopulation agenda before your eyes. Worse, the ingredients of any one vial of 'vaccine' are variable, depending on factors such as gas-lighting, use of placebos, and all the differing lot numbers of vials, showing non-uniformity.

Since the rollout of the first 'vaccines,' hundreds of doctors and scientists have studied the contents of the vaccines all over the globe, and almost every one of them have seen the 'vaccine' under various types of microscopes at various powers. One such committee of experts known as the International Crimes Investigative Committee (ICIC) includes the following people and the committee gleans more experts all the time: Dr. Reiner Fuellmich,

(JD and host); Dr. Michael Yeadon, (the former Pfizer Chief Science Officer and Vice President, who left Pfizer as he began to witness the crimes in front of him); Dr David Nixon (of Brisbane, Australia who began viewing the vaccines under dark-field microscopy) along with Dr. Ana Mihalcea, (of Romania, Germany, and the US who has collaborated with Dr Nixon, and studies shedding phenomenon as well); Dr. Shimon Yanowitz (of Israel, doing his own set of vaccine microscopy study); and Karen Kingston, (also a former Pfizer employee, whistleblower, biotech analyst of mRNA technologies, etc). Nixon, Mihalcea, and Yanowitz all describe extremely abnormal structures they've found present in the COVID vaccines within minutes of thawing the frozen vaccine vials. The obvious claim of the vaccine companies is that the 'vaccines' are frozen and kept frozen until ready to be given to keep them stabilized! At least that much we know is true, because the molecular structures change drastically with scant time in room temperature. Nothing remotely like these structures, regardless of what they may turn out to be, is normal, nor should they be in the 'vaccines'. "The structures have strange and complex crystalline growths that self-assemble with any energy source such as EMF radiation waves, light, air currents, temperature changes, etc. Structures are highly mobile and grow/change rapidly. There are beads, ribbons, tubes, needle-like connectors, liposomes clearly seen. All complex structures have the distinct appearance of electronic circuitry, as confirmed by Matthew Taylor,(an electrical engineer collaborating with Nixon). He confirmed that structures have an amazing advanced technology present. The electronic circuitry self-0assembles right before your eyes! There are known lipid nanoparticles, toxic heavy metals, and ribosomes in the 'vaccines' as well. NONE of these ingredients should have been in any so-called 'vaccines' ever! They should all have been recalled from the beginning of these discoveries; at the very least, the affected vaccine lots should have been recalled and gone through strenuous testing. None of these ever happened."[14]

Kingston analyzed mountains of legal documents including

patents for vaccines and drugs, and stated that 80% of the injectable's ingredients have been redacted as compared to the patent designates, which cannot be altered. Redaction means to hide or remove the confidential parts of a text before publication or distribution or to examine a text for this purpose. There are no fewer than 60 different manufacturers globally producing lipid nanoparticles, primarily for use in 'vaccines', and we've proven over the last several decades that vaccines don't work, the example of influenza vaccines alone when looking at real numbers proves this, despite what Big Pharma and all the various public health agencies claim. We can't even imagine this much buy-in on products that aren't even needed and are toxic, ever going away or even slowing down, and neither can the billionaire magnates that make the products! Remember, the FDA approved all of this criminal activity over two years ago under the Emergency Use Authorization Act which gives carte blanche to Big Pharma with no accountability and no liability for making these poisonous and deadly products, knowing 100% what they were and what they were capable of doing! It is extreme regulatory fraud against no fewer than 5.3 billion vaccinated people globally. It goes without saying—the previously planned for and executed use of the EUA for this reason is a monumental problem. This law was secretly planned by globalists to work exactly the way it did decades before they used it. No other groups on the planet can operate without impunity, with no accountability and no liability for the travesty they deliberately perpetrated. Worse, any and every crime they've brazenly committed is legal under the EUA and they are completely confident the system will remain totally broken. As Yanowitz commented, "the investigative committee and any other groups of honest researchers who want to stop the crimes against humanity legally, must go in through the back door and work outside of this legalized criminal system."[15]

According to Yanowitz who has a vast amount of microscopic proof of what has been found, the injectables (he refuses to call them 'vaccines') aren't just electronics-oriented, but are heinously toxic. Now, many scientists have been able to replicate them. In addition, "we now know that people who have been inoculated do emit some type of essence when interfaced with EMF radiation, and people with bluetooth capabilities on their mobile phones can pick up a plethora of addresses in the same room, emitting from those previously vaxxed."[15] We know through our VAER system and the systems of other nations that millions of people have died globally, and tens of millions have been adversely affected. Because of these discoveries, it is hoped this is the avenue by which this committee and many other entities will be able to stop at least a good amount of 'vaccine fraud.' With these proofs of ingredients in the injectables which are NOT organic and lack biologic content these vaccinees have been injected with known "medical devices" which are NOT protected under vaccine law, but are specifically included in their patents. These and other components do NOT immunize a person. This is the kind of proof and information that will hold up in a court of law and could finally change everything legally. The blue tooth technology is easy to detect and shows serious ramifications. The proof has been noted even in graveyards with the blue tooth, where recent deaths of vaccinated people still emit the waves—in one instance they were received from 96 of 112 corpses tested! This is easily replicable—anyone can do it! The evidence can also be irrefutable with autopsies of known vaxxed people. The EMF radiation continues to react in two ways—one is continued communication as we have seen; the other is when it can still function in the self-assembly of the molecular components of the injectable."[15]

Yanowitz continued with additional information from his microscopic studies in the dark field with very low magnification. He clearly demonstrated very large structures. "The process within the cells in still nanotechnology, but grows out so quickly that it approaches simple microscopy for size. He showed that in just one week of development, sophisticated ribbons, tubes, strands of beads, and detailed electronic-like structures. They appear as carbon and oxygen-based artificial organisms and possibly some metals. It has been posited they may be graphene oxide (carbon & oxygen), being bound by a hydrogel cloud. Besides being seen in the injectable molecules, it can also clearly be seen in the blood drawn for lab procedures of both vaxxed and non-vaxxed patients. Thus it would not represent the shedding of some imaginary virus, but of the growing components which continue to discharge their own contents. While they are clearly seen IN people's blood, they are NOT biological and cannot occur naturally. The program for all of this is IN the vial, but it must grow outside the vial after thawing, into the self-assembly."[15] "There are also enormous numbers of liposomes defined as various-sized round sacs of phospholipid molecules enclosing a water droplet, formed artificially to transport drugs or other substances into the surrounding tissues. Naturally, these should NOT be present either. Some of the liposomes burst, spilling contents. When dry, the needles and hydrogel are still visible but the liposome is gone. Some never burst. The self-assembly starts in just five minutes at room temperature. Chains assemble with fine filaments. Some are multi-compartmented ribosomes made of RNA and protein, the site of protein synthesis, and can spill from all compartments. These were all found in the injectables, freshly thawed from frozen and sealed vials. The Pfizer product self-assembled even faster than Moderna. This is akin to embryonic development technology as large as 50 microns. Different kinds and sizes could contain almost ANYTHING. There is certainly enough proof globally from enough experts that ALL injectables should be instantly banned and never seen again!"[16] Clearly, this is once again proof of probable bioweapons; the reality is this whole agenda is World War III. It was NEVER about health in any way, but it is a matter of life and death. At least 1.6 million Americans have died of the COVID injectables and counting. We will examine some of the practical work of a vast number of health practitioners who are working diligently to neutralize and nullify the adverse effects of those still affected.

In the meantime, the reader should investigate and examine all the excellent data and encouragement available through the 5-year-old, Truth for Health Foundation. It contains pertinent and factual information from a faith-based perspective in regular and professional, weekly articles. It will help you report vaccine injuries, offer guides for treatment and correction, give medical and legal advice, educational material, whistleblower reports, and faith over fear. Its vision is: "We envision a world where people choose their path to live fully as human beings according to the physical and spiritual laws of life as God designed us." Its mission is: "To provide truthful, balanced, medically sound, research-based information and cutting-edge updates on prevention and treatment of common medical conditions, including COVID-19 and other infectious diseases, that affect health, quality of life and longevity. To present faith-based integrative approaches to medical treatment, health and healing services that encompass all dimensions making us human: physical, psychological/emotional, spiritual, social and environmental. To advocate and provide legal defense of basic human and civil rights related to preservation of life, the right to bodily integrity, health, and quality of life, medical freedom, and securing the autonomy of the doctor-patient relationship and the ability to engage in unconstrained professional medical decision-making tailored to the needs of the individual person."[17] "Foundation Officers, Directors, and Staff are grounded in Judeo-Christian principles of honesty, integrity, respect, kindness, compassion, humility, and commitment to preserving God's gift of Life as we serve our patients and communities. We strive to honor God and Jesus Christ in all we do as we conduct business, and to follow Biblical principles exemplified in Jesus' Healing Ministry throughout the New Testament as we implement health programs for the people we serve."[18] The President and CEO is Dr. Elizabeth Lee Vliet, one of the influential people we discussed earlier in this book. Many of the other doctors of the American Association of Physicians and Surgeons (AAPS), which do NOT adhere to any of the globalist narrative are also leaders, members, and supporters of the foundation. Its web site offers a myriad of excellent, well-resourced materials to help us all learn more and be able to stand firmly in the truth. It is also imperative to know that as Christian Conservatives, we have been marked and tracked as a threat to the entire globalist agenda—we are public enemy #1 to Washington D.C.'s 'federal democracy.' President Trump is also a key threat and has been ever since he entered the political maelstrom. Globalist elites and their hordes will NEVER give up trying to remove him in ANY way they can. That is the reason he has suffered so much persecution—he won't give up either. He certainly needs the protective prayers of God's people every day. Currently, with several months into the new Trump Admin, we feel more hopeful that preserving our nation is once more possible; and we pray, many of the wrongs we've discussed in this book will be righted with a God-led President and other leadership chosen to help mend our nation. It's time that every believing and freedom-loving citizen do everything our Father God would have us do to support our new leaders under God.

> "If my people who are called by my name will humble themselves, and pray and seek my face and turn from their wicked ways, then I will hear from heaven and will forgive their sin and heal their land." II Chronicles 7:14 ESV

Going back to the ICIC committee, Dr. Nixon first examined his own blood under the dark field microscope (live blood analysis) and using a 3D microscopic camera verified his views. Dr. Mihalcea corroborated the studies with her own equipment and the shared findings over Zoom. At a 100x magnification, they both saw the odd structures floating—nothing normal for live blood. Other experts could not identify them either. The examinations continued to the actual 'vaccine' where similar structures were seen, but no such structures were disclosed in vaccine information. Critics said the structures were mere artifacts of the experiment, but there was absolutely no external manipulation on the one drop of vaccine on a slide. Unlike electron microscopy, it was a very small amount of magnification. Twenty-six plus independent teams globally have identified exactly the same things:

- The RNA was sequenced from various vials, but never

conformed to the label on any given vial.

- DNA and protein impurities were detected in massive quantities.
- A large number of heavy and rare metals of unknown origin or purpose including: cesium (nuclear), barium, cobalt, iron, chromium, titanium, cerium, gadolinium, aluminum, silicon, sulphur, thallium, and antimony.
- Large structures seen: blobs, particles, crystals, flat square shapes, fibers, ribbons, and assembly and movement were visible immediately from the frozen state
- Different forms of graphene are possible (containing carbon and oxygen)
- There were leftover magnetic beads (it was seen and known that simple refrigerator magnets would stick to people after injection).
- The RNA was not always present, but DNA and impurities were always present in massive quantities.

A researcher several years ago examined 44 different vaccines and found many of the same structures even then, but apparently no one has been able to identify them consistently, though they functi*on the same way. The same struc*tures are seen in vaccinated blood that are seen in the 'vaccines'. The structures become larger as the serum dries out and they do NOT degrade. In 2 months, 4 months, and even 6 months, they are even more prominent and have evolved quite weirdly. Today, there is a huge consistency of the crystals and fiber seen in blood samples. No one has chemically analyzed it because continuous advanced research is very expensive unless you have a direct line to NIH funding and the favor of self-appointed donors!! Big Pharma has literally billions of dollars invested in producing 'vaccines', and various producers and serum lots are NOT consistent with each other. We now also know that these same structures are not limited to blood samples anymore—they may be found in other body fluids and tissues of vaxxed people. Some of the structures actually look like computer chips, and have given rise to various conspiracy theories and a plethora of questions. More mature samples show clear patterns of structures with connecting fibers. Hydrogel, the molecules of various polymers, has been shown to be programmable and able to grow. It can create biosensors because it is able to merge with human cells. It is now the world of artificial intelligence merging with biology. As previously discussed, it has the uncanny appearance of electrical circuitry, and there are nodal points attached that appear to be firing. Now the structures are also appearing in increasing amounts on PCR swabs, meat, rain water, and garden vegetables. There is NO doubt nanotechnology is affecting everyone, and it can NEVER be normal. This is serious stuff folks!

The "concept of "shedding" has become recognizably important. It is happening largely because of the proliferation of EMF radiation. Many non-vaxxed people have been found with the same kind of structures in their blood and tissues as those who were vaxxed."[19] We know that some people are far more sensitive to EMF than other people, and some people get far more exposure to it in their daily lives than others. Additionally, we are seeing far more non-vaxxed people with the same known effects of vaxxed people, including turbo cancers and myocarditis. Integrative, functional, and naturopathic physicians are strongly recommending regular, active detoxing be added to their lifestyles. Obviously, two of the greatest sources of EMF radiation are our cell phones and computers, and they will NOT be going away anytime soon! There are sensible protocols available for limiting the amounts of EMF exposure that bear some careful consideration. The billion-dollar questions become: "What else are they hiding in the 'vaccines' that Big Pharma clearly knows is not only potentially harmful to humans but often lethal.? Why is there such an all-out obsessive/compulsive agenda for pushing toxins on all peoples, at every age, when they clearly don't work, and have helped no one? Obviously, there is the greed factor of money, money, and more money, However, given all the points of the globalist agenda, there is *SO MUCH MORE AT STAKE!*

If you listen to any of the representatives speaking for the globalist views and agenda, you will very quickly discover the ways they perceive our world is not just changing daily, but has already changed drastically. For example, Dr. Yuval Noah Harari, advisor to the World Economic Forum (WEF), wrote a book entitled, Sapiens, and another book entitled, *21 Lessons for the 21st Century.* He says, "politicians could soon have the technology to create heaven or hell." An even more striking quote that has been widely repeated is, "Humans are now hackable animals. The whole idea that humans have this soul and spirit, free will…that's over. Today we have the technology to hack human beings on a massive scale. Everything is being digitalized; everything is being monitored."[19] While Harari goes on to explain his point of view as a historian, the fact that intellectual leaders are thinking this is what humanity has come to, is indicative of the globalist mindset, and what it intends to do with it.

In light of all the structures that have been noted in both blood and injectable serums, and given that we have no apparent positive answers as to what this all means, we must look beyond the realm of the ideas of genetic engineering and see what may be hidden in plain sight to explain what we see. There is plenty of evidence to explain— other possibilities to explore. The giant questions now are: Are the touted mRNA serums really based in genetically-based technology or is it predominantly a huge series of smoke and mirrors, hiding technology that is actually far more sinister? If they are not mRNA, what are they? Dr. Lee Merritt is one of America's Frontline Doctors (AFLDS), who has studied deeply and thoroughly about the whole COVID-19 debacle and believes, as do so many, that it was a highly-planned and contrived set of global propaganda, full of smoke and mirrors—she is NOT alone! Most of her conclusions have obviously been dubbed as misinformation, while in fact, this author has seen no claims that she doesn't agree with wholeheartedly, along with an ever-growing group of believers. Much of the labeled misinformation has already been debunked for truth, except of course from the whole globalist narrative. You, the reader, may judge for yourself, when you've viewed more details.

Based on a series of very practical insights, Dr. Merritt has discussed four main reasons why she believes the COVID injectables do NOT even contain the dreaded mRNA. Those reasons include the cost, the production capacity, the known degradation, and the philosophy behind them. There is a philosophy behind any WAR scenario, and the COVID conflict is no different. It is often described as the 'dark occult' which generally means that which is secret or hidden. Usually, one of the darkest of occult practices is association with blood sacrifice, a prerequisite of war. In all wars, there are languages unique to the event, e.g. the Navajo Code Talkers of WWII. This whole scenario is associated with and surrounded by a so-called "virus." The Latin meaning of the word "virus" is "poison." Poisoning has often been the weapon of choice for millennia of conflicts historically. Hence, we have a simplified philosophy for COVID.

Like NASA programs, there is an exponential COST involved in this war. Over the entire decade plus, prior to the COVID onset, roughly 60 billion dollars was spent on research, which yielded relatively little in terms of usable information, and even that was not provable. One program managed to find an ophthalmology treatment in 2018 for about one million dollars of the 60 billion, or about 0.002% of the whole! However, we are supposed to believe that just 2 years later in 2020, they were suddenly able to mass produce 'vaccines' for around $30 per shot for the world. Highly unlikely!! As to the actual production of 'vaccines.' In October of 2022, Pfizer claimed it produced 638,734,000 doses at eleven of its facilities. That would be enough from just one company to immunize every person in about 10% of the globe. At the EUA rapid response rate, they would have needed to produce 18.7 doses/second without pause.

That makes NO sense—even if they had started way earlier—mRNAs are very short-lived. They would last about 3.5 minutes if super-chilled, longer if frozen. "Scientists are currently looking at research advances on nanoparticle-based mRNA delivery for liver cancers and liver-associated infectious diseases. Due to the poor thermal stability of mRNA, a cold chain is required in order to ensure that mRNA formulation is at optimal stability, prior to clinical use, which is very costly, especially when considering that infectious diseases are most prevalent in developing nations of the tropics, amplifying the need for mRNA products that do NOT need ultra-low temperature storage."[20] So we can see that the road blocks are many when the global infrastructure has no means of ultra-cold protection, even in transit globally. Since we knew all this in 2023, how were they able to keep this massive number of vaccine doses ultra-cold globally in every injection locale in 2020? It just wasn't possible.[21]

Once again, smoke and mirrors—a total sham! "Despite attention to and investment in quantifying global burdens of disease, the diagnosis in the majority of COVID-19 related deaths remained unclear over one year into it—over 360 cases per prominent pathologists."[22] This is NOT scientific stuff at all. For most of this time, autopsies were seldom done at all because they feared it might spread the disease. Laboratories reported that blood tests revealed hydrogel, metal fragments, and graphene oxide, but they did not find any mRNA. Most have reported the same things and say they don't see any mRNA. But what do the known ingredients have in common? They are all parts of 'current transfer'(electrical) and nanotechnology. So, if they are NOT mRNA, then what are they? The answer to this question is "Hybridized Opsins" in the field of optogenetics. This means that scientists can change the function of the output of genetics which is DNA with mere wave lengths, thus changing the function of the cell. All humans have opsins that don't respond very quickly, but bacteria, for example, has a lot of opsins which can be hit with a current, making them like an off/on switch. When bacterial opsins are mixed with human opsins or hybridized, then beamed with wave lengths, they can either cause or halt heart arrhythmias. It is perfect, silent, and direct energy. They respond both to wave lengths and to light pulsation. "The field of optogenetics integrates optics and genetic engineering to measure and manipulate cells (frequently neurons) and their governing bio-molecular processes. The tools and technologies developed for optogenetics research utilize light to detect, measure, and control molecular signals and cells in order to understand their functions. Optogenetics tools can be broadly classified based on their functions into two groups: Actuators are genetically-encoded tools for light-activated control of proteins, and Sensors are genetically-encoded reporters of molecular signals. Opsins are light-gated ion channels or pumps that absorb light at specific wavelengths. Upon activation by light, these channels and pumps respond by opening or closing, which conducts the flow of ions into or out of the cell."[23] This is NOT new technology, and was being used in diagnostics early in the twenty-first century.

Another, somewhat related field of research being used increasingly is known as Biophotonics. It involves the interaction between electromagnetic radiation (EMF) and biological materials including tissues, cells, sub-cellular structures, and molecules in living organisms. It is being used to examine, to track, and to control biological processes at these various levels of biology (photonics is the simple science of light). Cell cultures may be split in two, allowing whatever is happening in one side, to be electromagnetically passed to the other side, which speaks to the close association of "shedding" as discovered from the coronaviruses. It can also be used to facilitate the early detection of diseases. A point of concern is that this process works equally well, whether the subject is human or just bioengineered materials. Currently, the process is another form of imaging to be used, but it has an enormous potential for so much more. Dr. Carmel Mothersill of McMasters University is a highly acclaimed radiobiologist and researcher who has co-written a plethora of research papers on this technology, using low-dose non-DNA targeted radiation as a treatment modality. "There is strong laboratory, as well as human evidence for 'bystander information transmission' from irradiated cells to non-irradiated cells/tissues/animals. Whether in a petri dish or in real life, this speaks to the close association we know as 'shedding.' The cell creates a field around itself of tangible action that enlarges and grows as directed by our DNA. People like to trivialize the natural way our bodies work. Our DNA contains 3.1 billion base-pairs of chromosomes. We can't do a quick swab for DNA and make an accurate diagnosis! After all, an entire 50% of our DNA is common to a banana!! The whole idea of the DNA as a 3-dimensional special configuration may actually NOT be so. The reason is we were electromagnets long before we were DNA-based!"[24] This author strongly disagrees with that statement. There is plenty of proof that DNA is the foundation of every living creature. It's a magnificent and complex unit whose physical shape is even replicated throughout all nature, God's own design. We may be electromagnets, but that doesn't have the miraculous character of our DNA 'blueprint.' Of course, the reader is free to explore the idea and determine what he finds most possible.

Nikola Tesla famously said, "Alpha waves in the human brain are between 6 and 8 hertz. The wave frequency of the human cavity resonates between 6 and 8 hertz. All biological systems operate in the same frequency range. The human brain's alpha waves function in this range and the electrical resonance of the earth is between 6 and 8 hertz. Thus, our entire biological system—the brain and the earth itself—work on the same frequencies. If we can control that resonate system electronically, we can directly control the entire mental system of humankind."[25] However, since Tesla's time, there has been vast discovery of frequency resonances, of which there are many. Other frequencies have been used very effectively with multiple body systems to do a kind of reset—as alternative medical treatment. This is information we had in the 1940s! Clearly, Tesla knew that humans could control other humans mentally! Now we know a high-frequency current intensifies the action of the brain. It is a mental stimulant like alcohol, but instead of being hurtful to the brain cells, it is beneficial. Tesla had no doubt of the beneficial effects that would follow the installation of electrical wires, carefully insulated, in classroom walls, and saturation of the atmosphere in the rooms with millions of electrical waves! It was tested in Stockholm, Sweden on the same children for 6 months. The results were startling. The students in the electrified classroom grew more in stature, weight, and physical development and mental acuity increased dramatically.[26]

Defense Advanced Research Projects Agency (DARPA), division of the US Military that is doing neurotech research resonates with Tesla's acoustic mind control. Their research into brain-computer interfaces (BCIs) using sound waves uses Tesla's idea that the entire mental system of humankind could be controlled electronically. Interestingly, we mostly hear about Tesla as 'the good guy', but he certainly understood the potential of some very dark technology—aka artificial intelligence. "DARPA is pursuing a range of minimally-invasive approaches that use optics, acoustics, and electro-magnetics to record neural activity and/or send signals to the brain at high-speed resolution. DARPA's Next-Generation Nonsurgical Neurotechnology (N3) program that launched last year, was just awarded funding from six different organizations on May 20,2024. DARPA wants 'telepathic' soldiers! Here are just some of the technologies DARPA's N3 program is pursuing:

- A device that uses an acousto-optical approach to record from the brain and interfering electrical fields to write to specific neurons using ultrasound waves to guide light into and out of the brain to detect neural activity.
- An acousto-magnetic device for writing to the brain that pairs ultrasound waves with magnetic fields to generate localized electric currents for neuromodulation.
- A magneto-genetic approach to make neurons sensitive to magnetic fields.
- An integrated device that uses focused ultrasound for writing to neurons.

According to DARPA, these 'interfaces could ultimately enable diverse national security applications such as control of active cyber defense systems and swarms of unmanned aerial vehicles, or teaming with computer systems to multitask during complex missions.' The individual devise can also be combined to provide the ability to interface to multiple points in the brain at once. DARPA wants soldiers to use BCIs to augment their own abilities—essentially communicating telepathically with machines through various frequencies, including sound waves which convert into electrical signals. The question everyone wants to know: 'Can frequency-based technology also be used to control people's minds, soldiers or otherwise?' Tesla would say, 'yes!' DARPA tells the public this technology is more like a mere continuation of centuries of military innovation,"[27] however, we may be sure that, like every other useful technology, there is a lot of potential for misuse and harm as well. This is the stuff of what used to be science fiction, realized.

During a lecture in 1995, nearly three decades ago, Dr. Pierre Gilbert, PhD, a Canadian theology professor warned that it would NOT be long before the world would see "magnetic vaccines" that would make it possible to control people. They would have the ability to harm All of humanity. "The 'vaccines' will have liquid crystals in living systems that will be hosted in the brain cells, which will become micro-receivers of electromagnetic fields where waves of very low frequency will be sent. The liquid crystalline scale is singularly well-fitted to provide complex forms with organizational ability, can be uniquely combined with living cells and are highly permeable. Through these low frequency waves people will be unable to think, you'll be turned into a zombie. When the 'vaccines' are made from the creation of intentional infections and mandated by law, everyone will be thus prepared. Whatever we've been looking for in the current COVID vaccines in terms of genetic material, is really NOT necessary—this technology is far more universally viable. They can precisely target specific areas of the brain and change all behaviors centered in the brain. Don't think of this as a hypothesis. This has already been done. Think of Rwanda!"[28] He was suggesting this technology was behind the 1994 Rwandan genocide in which radio was a weapon of choice and constant propaganda the ammunition to the point of brainwashing.

The current 'vaccines' are truly toxic on so many levels. Though the global narrative will always deny it vehemently, it's very possible that all who received 'vaccines' have actually "killed" themselves literally in a variety of potential ways. No one wants to accept this as fact; even a vast number of physicians cannot and will not accept the facts because that would infer a good deal of responsibility for what happened and will continue to happen. They used the idea of infectious disease protocols to cover what they were really doing. So, for example, why do you want the population at large to develop the eating of insects to augment our protein intake? It has nothing to do with protein intake, and potential limited food supplies. You see, insects contain chemicals called chitin and chitosan which are 'biomimetic and photonic' materials. A biomimetic chemical is synthetic but can mimic actual biochemical processes and photonic means the transmission of photons as in fiber optics. However, they are both very toxic in several ways. They are crystalline and also indigestible. Can you even imagine how these two highly toxic chemicals could wreak havoc in the processes of which we spoke earlier?

Now for the really scary news! "A team led by US science and technology development firm Battelle has won a contract from DARPA for its next-generation non-surgical neurotechnology (N3), aimed at developing bi-directional brain control technology interfaces for able-bodied service members, five years ago! Currently, the BCI research is being used to help people with disabilities. An example is a quadriplegic man being able to move his hand again using brain control technology. It is called BrainSTORMS (Brain System to Transmit Or Receive Magnetoelectric Signals). Battelle's N3 concept involves the development of a nano-transducer that could be introduced into the body via injection and directed to a specific area of the brain to help complete a task through communication with a helmet-based transceiver."[29] The nano-transducer would use magnetoelectric nanoparticles to establish a communication channel with the brain. The magnetic core of the nano-transducers would convert the neural electrical signals into magnetic signals that would be sent through the skull to the helmet-based transceiver worn by the user…Battelle will also use neural decoding, artificial intelligence, hardware engineering, in vitro electrophysiology, and systems integration to combine the various aspects of the project.

Numbers of other such global headlines are available. One is: 'China Unveils Brain-Computer Interface Chip.' "China has achieved a breakthrough in Brain-Computer Interface (BCI) chip research, with its first BCI chip "Brain Talker" making its debut…at the ongoing World Intelligence Congress held in northern China's Tianjin Municipality. BCI is a system allowing a person to control a computer or other electronic device using his or her brainwaves, without requiring any movement or verbal instruction. The chip can identify minor neuron information sent by the brain wave from the cerebral cortex, efficiently decode the information and greatly quicken the communication speed between the brain and machine."[30]

Another very concerning headline is: *Weaponizing the Brain: Neuroscience Advancements Spark Debate.* "The rapid advancement of neuroscience and its corresponding technologies has prompted renewed and growing interest in both its development and the ethical concerns about the use of such techniques and tools in military and security contexts. Advancements in neuroscience could be used to create 'super soldiers', link brains to weapon systems for command and control, or even manipulate groups or leaders into taking actions that they normally wouldn't do. New developments in brain science are improving neurological and psychiatric care, However, there is also considerable potential for dual-use applications of neuroscientific methods and tools that extend beyond the hospital beds to the battlefields. There are big concerns for the negative effects that the field might have on 'neuro-modified' individual's health. There is trepidation about using such approaches to turn warfighters into amoral, combative automatons and questions about what responsibilities and burdens might be incurred for—and borne by—the military, and perhaps society at large, when dealing with such effects. Certainly, the internationalization of brain science, taken together with the speed of its progress, fosters additional concerns about the development and use of neuroweapons."[31]

As we contemplate all of the ways that men have discovered, studied, and developed for the potential welfare and benefit of society, we can and do see good things that have come from these. However, in the same way that gain-of-function research utilized deliberately to enhance the virility and transmission of deadly viruses that have NOT in any way benefited the well-being of man, except to pad the pockets of globalist predators and others, we see the development of all the technologies we've mentioned in much the same way. Any of these technologies also have the tremendous potential of creating harmful, even deadly monsters that once unleashed will be extremely difficult to halt. Man always wants more, and wants to exceed the boundaries of ethics and morality given by our Father God in his Word, that can keep our world from destroying itself. Too many evil men and women have too much information and wherewithal to be the next destroyers. There is NOT a lot that most of us can do to stop this runaway train from the ultimate collision course it is on, but each one of us can take specific steps to protect ourselves and our families. Doctors have a motto: "First, do no harm!" It's simple but brilliant. In this age of toxicity where almost everything we interface with is potentially harmful, we must be educated and devoted to God's wisdom in our lives. At this point, an extremely wise idea would be simply to not allow ourselves to be injected with ANYTHING, if we can prevent it. This is especially true of any product that identifies as a 'vaccine,' when it isn't, because every one of them contains things unnecessary to optimal health, and many are toxic. Despite the claims of Big Pharma and all public health officials, with the support of the mainstream media which are largely false, it is nearly impossible to know all we need to know about everything we come into contact with. It's fair to say, don't trust the media, and don't trust anyone with the bottom line of making more money. They should be avoided until proven trustworthy. All pharmaceuticals are mostly synthesized chemicals with the potential of dozens of serious side effects. Do your homework. Don't take something that is potentially more harmful than the problem you already have. Look for good alternatives, especially NATURAL ones, and there are many. Remember, there are excellent doctors still practicing real medicine that do NOT rely solely on these chemicals. We can all be healthier than we've been, intentionally.

'Vaccines' to Transhumanism in the New World Order

As noted, "DARPA N3's next-generation nonsurgical neurotechnology program has developed the high-performance, bi-directional brain-machine interfaces for able-bodied service members. Such interfaces enable technology for diverse national security applications such as control of unmanned aerial vehicles and active cyber-defense systems or teaming with computer systems to successfully multitask during complex military missions. Noninvasive neuro-technologies such as the electroencephalogram and transcranial direct current stimulation have already been used for years, but the new integrated service device does NOT require surgical implantation. It has the precision to read from and write to 16 independent channels within a 16mm^3 volume of neural tissue within 50 milliseconds. Each channel is capable of specifically interacting with sub-millimeter regions of the brain with a special and temporal specificity that rivals existing invasive approaches. Individual devices can be combined to provide the ability to interface to multiple points in the brain at the same time."[32]

Today, we have an entire system of scary technology in light of what the military and other scientists have already developed, the context of which becomes more sophisticated every day. "There are two interfacing parts of it; the Internet of Bodies (IoB) and the Internet of Things (IoT). The IoT is a network of physical devices, machines, and other objects that use sensors and software to collect data and exchange it over the internet, enabling remote monitoring and control. An IoT device has a sensor that transmits its data automatically without human or manual interruption to an IoT platform that processes the data and triggers automatic actions. The IoB is an ecosystem of internet-connected devices that monitor the human body and collect personal biometric data. IoB connects a person's body or actions to the internet; IoT connects the internet to objects. The IoB is a subset of IoT devices that interact far more intimately with the human body. They connect the body to an online network through technology that you wear, ingest, implant, or otherwise link to a human body. There has been a distinct shift from a world in which we 'use' technology, to one where we 'become' the technology. Naturally, all of this is being touted as a huge potential medical breakthrough, but it also poses a plethora of potential moral, ethical, legal, and even liability issues that could wind up looking very much like a hornet's nest."[33]

The natural progression of all the above ideas and technology is the upsurge of transhumanism, one of the goals of the globalist agenda. By definition, "transhumanism is the belief or theory that the human race can evolve beyond its current physical and mental limitations, especially by means of science and technology." In 1951, Julian Huxley popularized the term for his view that humans should better themselves through science and technology, possibly including eugenics and the improvement of the social environment. Both Julian and his writer brother, Aldous Huxley, were extreme leftists in philosophy and supporters of Darwin, evolution, and natural selection. He was director of UNESCO and president of the British Eugenics Society and first president of the British Humanist Association, and as an atheist, a signer of the Humanist Manifesto. With that in mind, the Humanist Manifesto is one of the most ungodly documents ever written, seeking to put humans above and beyond anything Jehovah God intended. It's no surprise that Huxley stood for almost every one of the ideas of the globalists today, at a time that it was far less popular, including unscientific ideas on genetics in agriculture, all aspects of evolution, cell biology, eugenics, planned parenthood, restraining population growth, climate change, etc. However, he struggled as an academic brainiac, sought various sexual and marital infidelities, had a couple debilitating nervous breakdowns, and, no doubt suffered from bipolar depression. Strange, ungodly ideas, extremes in his thoughts and desires, often a societal outcast, a kind of academic dropout, Huxley was a blueprint for the globalist mindset of today, and the 'father of transhumanism.'[34] He was a textbook model for today's evil globalists. Scripture, written in the first century by the Apostle Paul as the Father inspired him, describes them perfectly:

> "For the wrath of God is revealed from heaven against all ungodliness and unrighteousness of men, who by their unrighteousness suppress the truth. For what can be known about God is plain to them, because God has shown it to them. For His invisible attributes, namely His eternal power and divine nature, have been clearly perceived, ever since the creation of the world, in the things that have been made. So they are without excuse. For although they knew God, they did not honor Him as God, or give thanks to Him, but they became futile in their thinking, and their foolish hearts were darkened. Claiming to be wise, they became fools, and exchanged the glory of the immortal God for images resembling mortal man and birds and animals and creeping things. Therefore, God gave them up in the lusts of their hearts to impurity, to the dishonoring of their bodies among themselves, because they exchanged the truth of God for a lie and worshiped and served the creature rather than the Creator…and since they did not see fit to acknowledge God, God gave them up to a debased mind to do what ought not to be done. They are filled with all manner of unrighteousness. They are gossips, slanderers, haters of God, insolent, haughty, boastful, inventors of evil, disobedient to parents, foolish, faithless, heartless, ruthless. Though they know God's righteous decree that those who practice such things deserve to die, they not only do them, but give approval to those who practice them." ROMANS 1:18-32 ESV

The irony of the transhumanism goal of the globalists is that they have a culture of death, and have done all in their power to depopulate the earth, yet "It is their belief that we can and should eradicate ageing as a cause of death; that we can and should use technology to augment our bodies and our minds; that we can and should merge with machines, remaking ourselves, finally, in the image of our own higher ideals…ultimately by merging man and machine, science will produce humans who have vastly increased intelligence, strength, and lifespans; a near embodiment of gods."[35] This quote was from an article already more than six years old, as an excerpt from a book entitled, *To Be a Machine* by Mark O'Connell. It made some strong arguments about the very real problems inherent in men becoming like gods. Humanity has a long history of desire to be like gods or become gods! In Scripture, the chief perpetrator of this philosophy was none other than the Prince of Tyre whose 'father' was Satan himself. Almighty God said this about him:

> "Because your heart is proud, and you have said, 'I am a god, I sit in the seat of the gods, in the heart of the seas,' yet you are but a man(or angel, both of which were created beings), and no god, though you make your heart like the heart of a god…Because you make your heart like the heart of a god, I will bring foreigners upon you, the most ruthless of the nations; will you still say, 'I am a god,' in the presence of those who kill you, though you are but a man, and no god, in the hands of those who slay you? You shall die the death of the (heathen) by the hand of foreigners; for I have spoken, declares the Lord God." Ezekiel 28: 1-2, 6-7, 9-10 ESV

(Satan himself held the heart and soul of the King of Tyre;) Isaiah 14:11-15 speaks of Lucifer's(the angel's name became Satan) demise as well.

The next idea that fits in with the race to transhumanism is the subject of nanobots (microscopic robots). "Scientists propose putting nanobots in our bodies to create 'global super-brains.' Nanobots would create the 'internet of thoughts' where instant knowledge could be downloaded just by thinking it. An international team of scientists led by members of UC Berkeley and the US

Institute for Molecular Manufacturing predicts that exponential progress in all nanotechnology modes will bring the development of a human 'brain-cloud interface' (B-CI). That B-CI would connect neurons and synapses in the brain to vast cloud computing networks in real time."[36] "The concept has been presented by writers of science fiction such as Ray Kurzweil, for decades. He said, "By 2030, nanobots will flow throughout our bodies—this fleet of tiny robots would keep you healthy and connected to the cloud. He is Google's director of engineering and a well-known futurist who is quite successful with his predictions—this one was in 2017. Cell-sized robots can sense their environments and store data."[37] There is a myriad of other potential technologies that we only have time to speak of briefly here.

"Brain-chip-interfaces are hybrid entities where chips and nerve cells establish a close physical interaction allowing the transfer of information in one or both directions. There is a huge uptick in the usage of implantable microchips as neuronal probes for investigating brain circuits, using chip-based microelectromechanical systems (***MEMS***) to establish communication pathways through close physical interaction with brain cells."[38] "Until recently, local inflammation and scar tissue from the so-called 'foreign-body response' has prevented the development of in-body sensors capable of continuous, long-term monitoring of body chemistry. Today, scientists are presenting results showing tiny biosensors that become one with the body have overcome this barrier, and stream data to a mobile phone and to the cloud for personal and medical use. The one company is developing a whole family of tiny biosensors composed of a tissue-like hydrogel similar to a contact lens, that is painlessly placed under the skin with a single injection. These biosensors work within the body's tissue— without any metal device or electronics, thereby overcoming the body's attempts to reject it. Some have functioned for as long as four years. The biosensors can continuously monitor any number of specific body molecules, including glucose, lactate, oxygen and carbon dioxide, with others constantly being developed as need occurs."[39]

Naturally, Artificial Intelligence (AI) is involved in almost every aspect of the nanotechnological advances. AI is the science of making machines that can think like humans. It can do things that are considered 'smart.' AI technology can process large amounts of data in ways, unlike humans. The goal for AI is to be able to do things such as recognize patterns, make decisions, and judge like humans. It works by simulating human intelligence through the use of algorithms, data, and computational power; the ultimate goal being learning, reasoning, problem-solving, perception, and language-understanding as well or better than humans. Currently, one of the most used and popular AI applications is Google Maps. Siri is Apple's virtual assistant using voice recognition and is powered by AI. However, the very term itself induces an uneasiness in many people and rightly so. "Elon Musk has warned that AI is 'one of the biggest threats' to humanity. This is because humans face the threat of being outsmarted by machines for the first time!" When you share personal or sensitive information with an AI chatbot, you lose control over where that data goes or how it may be used—and chatbots store data on servers that are vulnerable to hacking attempts and breaches. Many AI systems have already 'learned' how to deceive and manipulate humans! One very scary fact—it appears that humans are not only capable of forming deep emotional connections with AI but can even experience romantic love toward it!! Also, the overwhelming majority of smartphones today have silicon that drives some integrated AI capabilities. Futurist Ray Kurzweil has predicted that by the 2030s, AI will have achieved human levels of intelligence, AND it will be possible to have AI that goes inside the human brain to boost memory, and turn users into human-machine hybrids. For believers in Jesus Christ, AI should be used very cautiously. While it can provide answers to factual questions and solve some problems, it cannot offer any sense of personal purpose or fulfillment. A dependency on AI could easily usurp the place of God in our lives as a god, and we already have an overabundance of those around us! One really good thing to know is you can turn off AI on your mobile phone if you prefer not to have it in current phone models. "Go to Settings >Advanced Features >Advanced Intelligence and then select each item (phone, keyboard, interpreter, notes, voice recorder, etc.) and ensure it is toggled off."[40] On Apple IPhones, go to Settings>Apple Intelligence and proceed similarly.

One of the most current, cutting-edge technologies is Synthetic Biology, better known to us as Genetic Engineering. Every technology we've discussed is crucial to the overall field of biotechnology, but no other area carries as much potential for playing God than this one. Its principles have been used for decades in multiple areas of agriculture, manufacturing, botany, etc.; we would know such products as genetically modified organisms or GMOs. In so many ways this technology has already jeopardized the integrity and quality of these products, such as our food sources, mostly in the effort to yield more product and make more money. Some things genetically modified are best left in their packages for lack of value! By definition, "genetic engineering is the alteration of an organism's genotype (chemical composition of DNA that determines the observable traits of an organism), using recombinant or recombination DNA technology to modify an organism's DNA in the form of recombined DNA vectors *typically generated by molecular cloning*. By modifying the DNA of organisms using specialized tools, cells can 'learn' to behave differently. The justification of this technology is that it allows scientists to find solutions for 'global problems' such as climate change, cancer, or almost anything they think should be changed or improved on! In reality, they are ultimately making biologic slaves!"[41] This is touted as the technology utilized to make the COVID 'vaccines' that are NOT truly vaccines.

Finally, we come to the place of connecting all the dots in what we know we've observed in the bloodstream of vaccinated individuals and via shedding, the blood even of non-vaxxed persons. Electrostimulation is used to remotely program user-designed genetic elements within designer cells to generate desired outputs. The following article titles only will give the reader a good idea of the technologies being utilized:

1) "Electrogenetics: Bridging synthetic biology and electronics to remotely control the behavior of mammalian designer cells;"[42]

2) "Therapeutic cell engineering: designing programmable synthetic genetic circuits in mammalian cells,"

3) "Living Electronics: A catalogue of engineered living electronic components," (including wires, capacitors, transistors, diodes, optoelectronic components, spin filters, sensors, logic processors, bio-actuators, information storage media, and methods for assembling these components into living electronic circuits),"

4) "Exploiting synergies between microbial electrochemical technologies and synthetic biology," and 5) "Digital and analog gene circuits for biotechnology." For every one of these articles, there are scores of additional ones. Here is an article that appeared 8 years ago entitled, *Genetically Engineered 'Magneto' Protein Remotely Controls Brain and Behavior.* [43]

This new (8-year-old) method uses a magnetized protein to activate brain cells rapidly, reversibly, and non-invasively, by activating specific groups of nerve cells from a distance. Understanding how the brain generates behavior is one of the ultimate goals of neuroscience. "The most powerful of these is a method called *optogenetics*, which enables researchers to switch populations of related neurons on or off on a millisecond-by-millisecond timescale with pulses of laser light. Another currently developed method, called chemogenetics, uses engineered proteins that are activated by designer drugs and can be targeted to specific cell types. Both methods are powerful but have bad drawbacks. More recently, another method, totally noninvasive, can be genetically engineered so they can become sensitive to radio waves and magnetic fields, by attaching them to an iron-storing protein called ferratin, or to inorganic paramagnetic particles. This new protein, TRPV4, is sensitive to both temperature and stretching forces. These stimuli open its central pore, allowing electrical current to flow through the cell membrane, evoking nervous impulses that travel into the spinal cord and then up to the brain."[44] This latest development is a system so simple, and needing only a single carrier virus that can be injected anywhere in the brain. By all indications, this is so brilliant no one even addresses the fact that it only works this well when a virus is injected into the brain of the subject. Apparently, that fact is not disturbing to anyone!

Last, but far from least, is the use of the now prominently touted CRISPR electrogenetic technology system that can turn human cells into biocomputers to connect with and control biological information systems. "In 2013, MIT molecular biologist Feng Zhang transformed the field of biotechnology when he first adapted the CRISPR bacterial genome editing system to edit DNA in human cells. In eleven years, an impressive array of individuals across an equally impressive collection of labs, departments, and centers at MIT have produced a toolbox of CRISPR-based enzymes to measure, improve, and repair cellular functions. Biologists, neuroscientists, and molecular biologists have used the system in a multitude of applications and for a host of devastating diseases for rapid diagnoses. This system can now be turned on and off with light, provide unprecedented control over when and where it cuts DNA, and can even be reprogrammed by synthetic biologists and computer scientists into a new form of memory storage. The rate and diversity of CRISPR applications continue to accelerate rapidly and prolifically. However, there are still some serious risks when you speak of altering humanity's own building blocks. The primary risk is the potential for off-target genome editing effects. This system can induce site-specific DNA mutations in human DNA. There is also the potential risk of certain types of cancer, allergic reactions, and damage to organs or tissues if an injection is involved. Modifications made to sperm, eggs, and embryos can be passed to future generations, raising the stakes exponentially for any mistakes made along the way."[45]

We simply cannot finish the subject of' vaccines and technology without addressing the moral, ethical, and spiritual implications of what we know is happening today globally. Ethically, it is a founding principle in the field of human gene therapy that the human germ line (those that can become reproductive cells) in patients should NOT be disturbed genetically, but of course there are risks of spontaneous germ line alterations in embryos. Direct intentional editing of the germ line carries additional risk in the potential alteration of entire gene pools. Editing for the purpose of 'improving' the genome is fraught with even more ethical questions because we don't even know what that would look like. The greatest moral issue is that even with the best possible intentions like removing a diseased allele (a variant of a DNA sequence at a particular location on a chromosome), present technology cannot assure us that unintended modifications created through an editing procedure would not result in a devastating long-term outcome such as cancer or adverse developmental effects. Other potential risks too involved to get into here are also present.[46] The bottom line for many of us may come down to a purely spiritual aversion to doing something very potentially risky when it smacks of "playing God," by trying to manipulate His building blocks of life. Some would say that much of the medical manipulation done today is akin to this, and perhaps it is, but it doesn't make any of it morally and spiritually right. Our Father is the Great Physician, and as the Creator of our bodies, He should be the ONE maintaining them. He heals us when it's His will to heal us. Naturally, that is a faith-based mindset that many don't aspire to, but it's the only mindset that pleases Him, if a great relationship with Him is what you desire. Scripture has much to say about living a life of faith which in these days of evil and chaos is our only firm foundation:

> "Faith shows the reality of what we hope for; it is the evidence of things we cannot see...By faith we understand that the entire universe was formed at God's command, that

what we now see did not come from anything that can be seen...It was by faith that Enoch was TAKEN UP WITHOUT DYING; 'he disappeared, because GOD TOOK HIM.' For before he was taken up, he was known as a person who pleased God. And it is impossible to please God without faith. Anyone who wants to come to Him must believe that God exists and that He rewards those who sincerely seek Him." Hebrews 11:1, 3, 4, 5 NLT

Standard Composition of 'Vaccines'—Standard Responses

According to trustworthy scientists who have studied the composition of the COVID-19 injectables, there are just five basic components that have been identified on a very elementary level:

- mRNA (life), encoded form of optimized SARS-CoV-2 spike protein;
- Graphene Oxide (aqueous solution)
- Nanoparticles (lipids and various metals)
- Spike glycoproteins (SP) (altered SARS-CoV-2 pathogen)
- Polyethylene Glycol or PEG (glue)

Metal nanoparticles can be found almost everywhere including copper, silver, gold, aluminum, silicon, carbon, other metal oxides—present in foods, cosmetics, clothing, environment, vaccines, and drugs, for example. Graphene Oxide consists of Carbon and oxygen and can be found in a plethora of aqueous compounds such as intravenous medical solutions, cleaning solutions, cosmetic preparations, and physiological saline. It can be used for everything, everywhere. "The present invention (COVID-19 'vaccine') relates to an injection solution, a physiological saline solution, a glucose solution, and an IV, which are to be administered in a blood vessel and subcutaneous tissue of the human body for the purpose of curing a disease. This solution containing graphene is dispersed therein according to the present invention and a corona virus 'vaccine' using the same, is intended to be used for each known disease including dementia, Parkinson's disease, Lou Gehrig's disease, Huntington's disease and the like. They are also intended to be used as a therapeutic agent for viruses such as MERS, SARS, Corona viruses by dispersing graphene powder with a size of 0.2mm or less in an injection solution, an I.V., a physiological saline solution, and a glucose solution used in conventional hospitals. The solution with the graphene powder dispersed therein is injected into the human body where the virus has penetrated, and when the virus and graphene powder meet, the virus and the powder are attracted to each other by nanocohesion. When the graphene powder adheres to the body and the spike projections of the virus, the virus can no longer function properly, cannot proliferate, and eventually dies, supposedly resulting in a coronavirus 'vaccine'."[47]

Graphene is supposedly quite compatible with life, but if it goes toxic in process, it can cause a cytokine storm (severe immune reaction), bilateral pneumonia, blood clots, oxidative stress/cell damage, and effects to the neuro system. Pfizer's OWN Vaccine Safety Data sheet document shows the ingredients of the vaccine as previously mentioned and even as minimal as they are, they are clearly toxic in nature; but the company still makes the claim that the 'vaccine' in NOT hazardous! They could not even be safely given to animals, which was done at length before the need for the COVID vaccines was clear, and the trials never went beyond the animal stage because they couldn't. Pfizer also claimed at the rollout of the vaccines, that they would remain at or near the injection site, but that was intentionally NOT true. After just ten minutes, the vaccine was clearly dispersed all over the body. After eight hours the liver is full. (The liver is our body's first-line organ of detoxification.) The mRNA is not even of human origin—it is made with bacterial RNA. It had to interfere with all normal bodily functions, because it is toxic and fully distributed throughout the body. Everything about the 'vaccines' was too much, too fast, and presented too soon. Initially, scientists were unable to find the evidence of spike proteins on examination because the toxicity produced such a profound inflammatory response.

In the process of immune pathology, apoptosis is the normal process of programmed cell death. In adults, it is used to rid the body of cells that have been damaged beyond repair. It plays a role in preventing cancer. If apoptosis is for some reason prevented, it can lead to uncontrolled cell division and the subsequent development of a tumor. Apoptosis normally happens in cells that have been around in the body long enough that they're kind of worn out, and they need to make way for nice, new, young cells. If that doesn't happen, its cancer. However, too much apoptosis in an otherwise normal human being will result in a number of so-called neurodegenerative diseases where cells die when they aren't supposed to die. Apoptosis plays a crucial role in the maintenance and control of the immune system's normal balance (homeostasis), immune response, and immune tolerance. Immune cells that recognize self-antigens must be deleted or killed. Apoptosis is not the same as necrosis where cells die because they've been injured, but is an orderly process in which cell's contents are 'packaged' into small packets of membrane for 'garbage collection' by the immune cells (lymphocytes). Old cells die 'neatly' without damaging their neighbors. Four main things can trigger apoptosis: oxidative stress, alkylating agents, ionizing radiation, and chemotherapeutic agents internally. Normal apoptosis does NOT induce any inflammatory reaction, Deficient apoptosis is associated with cancer, autoimmunity and VIRAL INFECTIONS! Apoptosis IS one of our body's best defense mechanisms. Doesn't it stand to reason that injecting toxic substances must overstimulate this mechanism, creating much of the neurodegenerative responses? Doesn't it also make sense that the massive destruction of cells involved can also exhaust and deplete the necessary responses to so many dead cells and cause abnormalities in those cells still trying to survive the onslaught? Apoptosis in lymphocytes is regulated by 'GENE' products that either induce or block this process. If that process is NOT originating from our own 'GENES', what are the odds that direction from a fake 'vaccine' will mess up the natural process entirely? [48]

Much of this information is based on the Big Pharma lists of ingredients as well as the elements listed in patent documents (about the only thing they can't get by with lying about)! The disclosed ingredients of the vaccines have at least helped scientists and doctors find antidotes, particularly if the vaccine instructions tell you what NOT to do after taking the jab. Doctors have disagreed over the presence of spike proteins as the chief toxins or just various other added toxins added to the vaccines, as we previously discussed in regard to the presence of snake and animal venoms. Dr. Ryan Cole, a board-certified pathologist insists on the presence of the spike deposits, often persisting as long as 128 days post jabs. He insists the spikes cause abnormal blood clotting, and a whole plethora of bizarre things have been seen in vaxaffected people by the hundreds of thousands. As we noted above, the 'vaccine' will block the normal immune system function, and the suppression of it opens the whole body to other illnesses as well. Dr. Cole fought the legal system of Idaho over his presentations on COVID-19 and the 'vaccines'. "He impugned the mRNA 'vaccines' created to combat the coronavirus, claiming that they cause cancer, increase COVID-19 infections, cause blood clotting, hurt reproductive organs and alter DNA. The 'Commission' noted his claims were 'demonstrably false'(NOT) and that he could endanger the public by voicing them as a doctor. He told the crowd to whom he spoke to never take a genetic shot again, and said the 'vaccines' should be 'pulled immediately.' He said all of his claims were backed by data."[49] Dr. Cole says his speeches 'cost me my career,' and he would not be the first or only professional punished for telling the truth. This is a travesty!

- Dr. Richard Fleming, a highly qualified physician, cardiologist, and pathologist spoke at an American Association of Physicians and Surgeons seminar in Kansas City entitled, "The Tyranny of Evidence-Based Medicine," in the company of several other AAPS professionals. He spoke about the exponential incidence of inflamothrombotic response or ITR, from the basis of his cardiology findings. Dr. Fleming has studied the microscopic blood samples of hundreds of his patients, both vaxxed and non-vaxxed, with and without saline. "Normal, mature red blood cells (RBCs) are devoid of nucleic, ribosomes, mitochondria, and other organelles, which are important in other cell types. This enables the RBCs to accommodate the maximum number of molecules of its protein hemoglobin that is iron-rich and gives blood its red color. This is what enables red blood cells to transport oxygen and carbon dioxide. Having no nucleus allows them to change shape (flexibility) more easily as they move throughout the body."[50] We need this information to understand the significance of what has been seen in the blood slide samples. About 84% of the body's cells are the 2030 trillion red blood cells and these make up almost half (40-45%) of the blood's volume. Just so you know, dear reader, your body manufactures 17 million red blood cells per second!! Each cell's life cycle is between 90-120 days. With its normal plasma, red blood cells remain a vibrant red and they do NOT clot.

- Now having reviewed this above information, when viewing the blood slides under normal microscopic exams, adding normal saline did not change the character of the blood at all, as expected. However, "when a drop of COVID-19 'vaccine' was added to the slide, it remained red for less than one minute; the color disappeared. Clearly the oxygen was also gone, but it wasn't gone because none was available in the environment, it was gone because the cells were damaged. The cells changed shape and began clumping all in under one minute! Not only was oxygen gone, but the hemoglobin molecule damaged permanently and irreversibly. The mRNA and lipid nanoparticles will

> breakdown very quickly unless it's VERY cold from its frozen state, leaving debris, air bubbles, and crystals on the slide. Given the almost immediate desaturation of oxygen and clumping of red blood cells, it is NOT difficult to understand how a vaccinated individual might faint soon after a vaccination, and even move into the need for resuscitation quite quickly if there is a severe lack of oxygen. Anyone having received a vaccination 4-42 days prior to the onset of any concerning symptoms should be suspected of potential life-threatening ITR, regardless of the 'vaccine' manufacturers statements of its extreme rarity!!! Symptoms indicative of potential blood clots, are severe headache (brain), visual changes, abdominal pain, nausea and vomiting, back pain, shortness of breath (clot in lungs), leg pain, redness, or swelling, and petechiae, (tiny capillary bleeds) bruising or bleeding. There are two prominent blood tests that can quickly indicate clots when seen together—the platelet count is usually low and the 'D-dimer' (a protein the body makes to break down blood clots) test will be elevated, often four times the normal upper limit."[51]

Early in the COVID-19 pandemic it was known that blood clotting was a definite hazard of the illness and patients in the hospital in particular were treated for them prophylactically, as was this author, as well as for 40 days post-COVID! So think about what was clearly an automatic problem in a 'vaccine' using SARS-CoV-2 to make it!! Soon after the 'vaccines' rolled out, manufacturers knew the blood clots were a problem, but there were no warnings when the 'vaccines' had already failed to meet FDA standards pre-EUA. Even now, the United Kingdom, France, Czech Republic and Slovakia have a suit pending against the 'vaccine' producers in the International Criminal Court for product liability, which is NOT protected under the vaccine laws (SMART Nations). Liability simply means it's proven to be harmful. All of these studies by Dr. Fleming and multiple others have been repeated over and over.

Every one of the vaccine products should have been pulled from the market years ago, but they simply tweaked them a bit, and rolled them out again in August 2024. The toxic elements have not changed, and neither have the completely false claims of the manufacturers on the safety and efficacy of their poisons, let alone all the damage they still claim happens VERY rarely. Reality and numbers speak for themselves and most people, if they are paying attention, are fully aware of it. However, despite proofs everywhere, Big Tech continues to lie and deceive the public, the federal government has continued to mandate them even for our infants and pregnant women until just 3 months ago and Big Pharma marches on in the globalist cloud of lies. It should be noted that the President of the US takes an oath to uphold our Constitution which states that no citizen can be forced to take treatments of any kind. When President Biden mandated the vaccines, he removed informed consent, and did not uphold the Constitution—That is clearly TREASON!!! Legally, the Supreme Court could take care of this, if the case is ever presented; better yet, a US Military Tribunal could arrest, try, convict, and prosecute him for treason. No one, including Benedict Arnold ever gave them more grounds for doing so!

Meanwhile, there are some treatments, including Ivermectin, that are able to reverse some of the damage, but not in everyone damaged.[52] Research continues every day and constant progress is being made toward new and even more effective treatment options. Many nutritional, functional, integrative, chiropractic, and alternative medicine professionals have developed multiple effective treatments that also help greatly in reversing damages, which we will see a bit later.

Now that we've discussed all the toxicity of the 'vaccines', and we know there are elements in them which clearly do not belong in so-called 'vaccines', including electromagnetic components, we can clearly understand that there is a probable reason the globalist agenda promotes the whole vaccine narrative 100% and it's clear that the reason is NOT for our health's sake. As for Big Tech and vaccines, you cannot find much truthful information anywhere in their bailiwick about anything vaccine-related. They categorically deny that 'vaccines' alter human DNA when the mRNA in the 'vaccine' does NOT even use human RNA. They continue claiming the 'vaccines' deliver only the encoded messages, not genetic material. However, once the encoded mRNA is injected into human beings, it certainly doesn't leave the body voluntarily. In addition, "there are proven disadvantages to using DNA 'vaccines'. There is a risk of affecting genes that control cellular growth. Constant repeated dosing is required to maintain any acquired immunity, so there is no end to the amount of toxin acquired in one's life. The degree of immunogenicity is far lower than that of the inactivated vaccines of the past. It can only be done with a very limited number of protein antigens—COVID 'vaccine' only works, if it works on COVID-19. While the 'official' health-care 'pros' insist loudly and constantly that the 'vaccines' are extremely safe and very effective, the opposite is true. One statement the CDC has made on almost every occasion of questioning about heart risk is; "there is a *VERY* minor risk of myocarditis inflammation of the heart muscle and pericarditis or inflammation of the outer lining of the heart that is usually both mild and rare in adolescents and young adults after receiving the COVID-19 'vaccine.'"[53] (all provable lies). However, the CDC itself finally admitted that it's not really rare, and it's not possible to have MILD inflammation of the heart. Any inflammation of the heart, especially in a young person is a serious risk and it isn't mild!! It has been known on many occasions to drop a strong, and fit young athlete on the playing field, where he or she is gone on the spot. There are cases reported someplace nearly every day—that's hardly rare. Another narrative claim you can see everywhere is that "it's much safer to get the vaccine than the disease." Under the worst-case scenario there is relative truth to it, but for most people, it simply isn't true either. All infants, young children, adolescents, and young adults have a very low risk factor for getting a serious case of COVID-19, but the vaccine can certainly kill them or do a lifetime of damage from which they may never recover."[53]

If the CDC and FDA were functioning under previously normal

conditions, actual reports of over 4,000 deaths, much less the exponential number there really are, officials would have halted the use of these toxic agents—100%! However, the entire mindset under full-on globalist wolves has been revamped and turned on its head. Tragically, rather than the once firmly held motto of 'First, do no harm,' in the current climate has been altered and dictates, "Do any harm necessary" to meet the goals of the globalist wolves. Sell more and more vaccines and drugs and crush the American spirit. While the slaughter continues, until very recently the CDC refused to even examine this travesty. But, by 2023, there were so many provable stories of fit young people, especially athletes, dying of vaccine-induced myocarditis, the CDC was finally forced by the public to look at it much more seriously. By contrast, in 1976 when following swine flu vaccinations, it became clear the vaccine was causing a small increased risk of Guillain-Barré Syndrome (GBS), federal health officials decided it was necessary to stop immunizations until the issue could be studied more thoroughly; the risk was just one in 100,000 people. Formerly, vaccines were recalled even for a potential issue as a precaution. Now, all caution has evaporated. In 2012, eight years before these vaccines even existed, an important review was published warning that human experimentation "Should NOT Proceed," much less mass global immunization. Based on animal studies, the SARS-Co-V vaccines induced extreme hypersensitivity. It urged extreme caution in proceeding to application of such 'vaccine' in humans. Many animals got very ill, and died. The obvious conclusion is that these same 'vaccines' were rushed through the EUA process to AVOID any real examination of their known hazards. Normally in the past reality, existing documented animal results would have been enough reason to prohibit further experimentation, much less immunization use.

Clearly, all previous rules ceased to exist. Americans died by the tens of thousands while the CDC simply continued business as usual without even an investigation. Initially, the CDC actually declared that NONE of these deaths, even those within hours of receiving COVID 'vaccine,' were due to the 'vaccine'. Obviously, this constituted severe negligence of responsibility to do what the CDC was created to do, or negligence that was simply criminal at its heart. Once again, we can only conclude COVID-19 is a mere smoke screen or cover story that allows globalists to continue killing people per its depopulation agenda while extorting untold billions or even trillions of dollars from the people and economies of the world and mandating totalitarianism and docility upon all who would accept its agenda as LAW. Many nations succumbed. We would like to believe most Americans have seen and understood what happened, however we fear it may not be the case.

Based on a ton of individual research, reading and studying provable facts written by hundreds of very qualified doctors and scientists, this author sees the lion's share of the information on the Big Tech sites as the real misinformation. Please don't assume that since the information of this book, verified and documented, is false simply on the basis of the disinformation allowed on Big Tech platforms. In light of the known and proven globalist agenda for the New World Order, and what it represents, please do your own homework and ask the Lord for His wisdom in determining real truth. He IS the truth.

> "If any of you lack wisdom, let him ask of God, who gives generously to all without reproach, and it will be given him. But let him ask in faith, with no doubting, for the one who doubts is like a wave of the sea that is driven and tossed by the wind. For that person must not suppose that he will receive anything from the Lord; he is a double-minded man, unstable in all his ways," James 1: 5-8 ESV

> "Jesus said to him, 'I am the way, and the truth, and the life. No one comes to the Father except through Me." Jn 14:6 ESV

Vaccination

Before we proceed to show the extent of 'vaccine' injury and death, we need first to understand that it actually could have been far worse, had the whole program been as successful as they planned. The global narrative was "Get everyone vaccinated and save lives. The narrative said, and to date continues to say, that rumors and conspiracy theories contributed to 'vaccine' hesitancy. Thank God that was true. This author believes, though there was constant lying as to the nature of the 'vaccines,' their history, their emergency production, their toxicity and side effects, and so many more issues, that people weren't as trusting and gullible about the vaccines as the wolves wanted them to be. Supposed 'official' public health spokesmen pounded the narrative out through Big Tech, but the stories didn't all sound exactly alike. Supposed 'facts' about them weren't documented, and their narrative was against a whole lot of highly-suspicious doubters, and rightfully so. The National Institutes of Health received a report from a pre-selected multi-disciplinary team who had reviewed and collected so-called online rumors and conspiracy theories by June 2021 for the time period between 12/21/2019 and 11/30/2020. Quantitative data was extracted for a content analysis of most of Big Tech's entities. The information gleaned was categorized as true, false, misleading, or exaggerated. "We identified 637 COVID-19 related items. 91% were rumors and 9% conspiracy theories from a total of 52 countries. Of the 637 items, only 5% were true, 83% were false, 10% were misleading, and 2% were exaggerated. A 2020 study found that people who were exposed to vaccine-related information on social media were more likely to be misinformed!"[54]

During that same time-frame, Big Tech was doing everything in its power to back the 'vaccine' narrative with what it deemed truth, yet it was only 5%? In addition, all of the entities of global Big Tech were blocking, banning, censoring, and removing truth-tellers from their platforms as fast as they could manage it, but that left only 5% truth? In spite of everything they could do to stop truth from being disseminated, based on actual vaccination rates, more than half of all citizens did NOT believe their idea of truth, or at least were skeptical enough to forego vaccines! Many more who would NOT have taken the 'vaccines' were forced to take them anyway. Despite all claims by official public health, we know the numbers of 'vaccine' adverse events and deaths far surpassed the number of people that died of the disease. We are going to look at many of the things that actually happened first, and then hear from a number of sound medical professionals who were left with the difficult task of trying to rectify 'vaccine' damage. "Officials" claimed 'vaccines' saved the lives of 10 million people OR were those ten million people either dead or 'vaccine'-injured? Clearly there is a massive disconnect of views, but the real facts and numbers speak for themselves. You, dear reader must judge reality for yourselves.

Our Investigative Health Journalist, Jonathan Otto, produced another independent COVID-19 information series entitled "NEW HOPE: How the Elites KNEW the Jabs Would Kill Millions from the Start." In this documentary Jonathan exposed many of the hard facts about the ramifications of the COVID 'vaccines'. To prove the truth of his claims, an article written by Peter and Ginger Breggin entitled, "The Dead Don't Lie: 2 Million Dead from mRNA Jabs," showed just 20,000 of those deaths were actually reported through the VAERS system. "To show the global politics of the 'vaccine', the FDA and the CDC had already pushed out the Johnson & Johnson 'vaccine' after only 9 blood clot deaths because Bill Gates, Klaus Schwab and their collaborators had already decided to invest in and push the Pfizer and Moderna jabs when they announced the 'Decade of Vaccines' in 2010! Currently, more than 60 vaccines are FDA-approved for use in the US for 26 different diseases...since 1990 when VAERS was set up until 2021, a slight but steady rise in the number of vaccine deaths was reported but they never exceeded a few hundred per year. In 2020, before COVID vax came out, 171 deaths were reported for all 60+ vaccines. However, in 2021, when COVID vax was pushed all over the US, the annual number of reported 'vaccine' deaths abruptly skyrocketed from the 171 to

10,544, a 61X increase in one year. COVID mRNA injections were slaughtering people! Worse still, of those 10,544 deaths, 2,958 deaths occurred within the first 3 days of receiving the jabs, a clear confirmation of causality (Almost 30%). It was also a clear signal to the CDC and the FDA that the vaccines were causing an unprecedented onslaught of deaths and MUST be stopped immediately. Instead of admitting to and confronting the mass murder, no one did anything and they continued in denial. The CDC has NEVER yet confirmed ONE SINGLE DEATH due to COVID 'vaccines'. There is NO other logical explanation for this deluge of deaths!"[55]

The New York Times best-selling author, Naomi Wolf, wrote in one of her many excellent books, *The Pfizer Papers*, which refers to the Pfizer clinical trial documents released under court order, about what Pfizer clearly KNEW! "The book shows in high relief that Pfizer's mRNA COVID-19 'vaccine' clinical trial was deeply flawed and that the pharmaceutical company KNEW by November 2020 that its 'vaccine' was neither safe nor effective (a fact that they still claim in every bit of public literature). The reports detail vaccine-induced harms throughout the human body, including the reproductive system; showing women suffer vaccine-related adverse events at a 3:1 ratio. It exposed that vaccine-induced myocarditis is NOT rare, mild, or transient; and, shockingly demonstrated that the mRNA vaccines have created a new category of multi-system, multi-organ disease, which is being called 'COVAX Disease.' Despite the fact that Pfizer committed in its own clinical trial protocol to follow the placebo arm of its trial for a full 24 months, Pfizer vaccinated about 95% of placebo recipients by March 2021, thus eliminating the trial's control group and making it utterly impossible for comparative safety determinations to be made."[56]

An equally important fact the book mentions is how clear it is that the FDA KNEW about all the problems and faults of Pfizer's clinical trials, especially all the more than potential adverse events caused by Pfizer's mRNA COVID vaccine product. This makes it abundantly clear that the FDA completely failed in its mission to protect the public health. It did NOT 'ensure the safety, efficacy, and security of human and veterinary drugs, biological products, and medical devices.' The book gave a thorough picture of how Big Pharma, the US government, and public health entities are completely protected with legal immunity or liability guaranteed to them by the Public Readiness and Emergency Preparedness Act (PREP Act) when creating, prescribing, and administering 'vaccines'. With all this protection, they can do almost anything they want for their bottom lines rather than caring about the health and well-being of all Americans. To date, there are NO Covid 'vaccines' that have been approved by the FDA!! Does anyone still doubt the utter corruption of the federal government, not to mention the control of globalist wolves. The wolves don't even wear sheep's clothing anymore! Their teeth are showing in their salivating mouths!

Another pertinent article written by John Leake with Dr. Peter McCullough was written after 2022 closed. He wrote: "Every day Dr. McCullough and I speak to people who have been injured—or have a family member who has been killed by one of the COVID-19 'vaccines'. Almost every day, the doctor examines one or more patients with 'vaccine' injuries in his clinical practice. He has become a 'go-to' COVID professional for people who are suffering from these syndromes and he views them as distinct individual humans. An associate who is a conservative research analyst focusing on the 148 million Americans between 18-64 who were employed, Ed Dowd's analysis is grim. In addition to the heinous death of a young person, a family and sometimes an entire community is devastated. There were 300,000 excess deaths (over the annual average), 26.6 million injuries, and 1.36 million disabilities in the year 2022. Note that this death count is 5.2 times the number of men killed in ten years of combat in Viet Nam! Dowd added that the most extraordinary thing about these findings is that most Americans have no idea it happened at these levels. Every day young people ARE dying from heart attacks, strokes, and seizures caused by COVID-19 'vaccines'. Worse yet, most of their families and friends are led to believe they just died—suddenly and unexpectedly—of acute conditions that were extremely rare in young people before 2021."[57]

This story represents several hundreds of young, fit, often professional athletes who developed myocarditis after two Pfizer 'vaccine' jabs. "In December, 2021, Oscar Cabrera Adames collapsed on the basketball court during a game and immediately blamed it on vaccine-induced myocarditis. 28-year-old Cabrera Adames died about six months later of an apparent heart attack while undergoing a routine stress test at a health center in the Dominican Republic. He had been previously hospitalized after collapsing. He said, 'I got two doses of Pfizer vaccine because I was coerced to do so as a professional player—it was compulsory or I couldn't work. I knew it—people warned me! I had no health problems, no bad heredity, no asthma, NOTHING. In the middle of a match I almost died. I'm still recovering. I've had eleven different cardiology tests and guess what? They find nothing. I couldn't play for at least five months per my doctors until the heart inflammation went down.' Myocarditis is debilitating and can cause permanent damage to the heart muscle, and cause heart failure. It severely restricts the heart's ability to pump blood, and most cases end in sudden death due to heart failure according to Dr. Peter McCullough. He also said that often these young men (average age of 23 years) are dying suddenly because they are not aware they have myocarditis and these folks should be avoiding exercise. Between March 2021 and March 2022, 769 athletes collapsed on the field during games. The evidence shows the CDC and the FDA knew of myocarditis safety signals as early as February 19, 2020, but HID THAT DATA from the public until after the FDA granted EUA for the vaccine."[58]

Internationally, the same kinds of adverse events were regularly reported as well—it's NOT just the U.S! Most days you can read about another collapsed or dead athlete anywhere in the world. In Germany, Minister of Health Karl Lauterbach, who once claimed COVID-19 vaccines were free of side effects admitted in April of 2023, that he was WRONG…and they can cause 'severe disabilities.' This was after a 17-year-old gymnast who had previously competed in the German Artistic Gymnastics Championships, had been hospitalized for more than one year shortly after receiving the second dose of Pfizer's BioNTech COVID-19 'vaccine'. Lauterbach also admitted that many disabilities were permanent if survived. "The true rate of serious adverse events is about 'one in 100 doses, and for death its one in 1000 doses.' But despite these known figures, Germany did exactly as the US public health/Big Tech has done here, saying, 'however, modern 'vaccines' are safe and adverse effects only occur in sporadic cases.'"[59] So we've seen that governments all cooperate with the globalist propaganda and push 'vaccines' anyway, no matter how much damage they do, and still refuse to recognize they continue to do far more harm than good.

Dr. Elizabeth Lee Vliet, president and CEO of Truth for Health Foundation, reported, "It was already KNOWN that the toxicity of the spike protein and another component of the COVID-19 'vaccine' could cause complications and adverse reactions shortly after the shots were rolled out. Over the first six months after the rollout, I had an entire gamut of patients with all kinds of problems they never had before. The ONLY common denominator was that they all had the 'vaccines'. We've NEVER in the history of the vaccination program worldwide, had an experimental injectable that crosses the blood-brain barrier, gets into the brain itself, and into the nervous system. The COVID gene therapy shots DO that—they also cross the placental barrier…so it's understandable why these experimental gene therapy shots are causing so much damage to developing babies in the womb; also to the brain, and central nervous system in children and adults. Now that doctors understand the mechanism of how the 'vaccines' work, they can use existing medicines to treat adverse effects."[60]

Going back to the docuseries by Jonathan Otto entitled 'NEW HOPE' we now want to bring in some further documentation of what kinds of travesties were seen by first-line caregivers (predominantly nurses) in hospital and clinic settings. Author Ken McCarthy, wrote a book entitled, *What the Nurses Saw: An Investigation into Systematic Medical Murders That Took Place in*

Hospitals During the COVID Panic and the Nurses Who Fought Back to Save Their Patients, (Medical System Corruption). This book does NOT discuss inadvertent human error, like that which every one of us is prone to. One book reviewer, a lawyer, wrote, "This book showcases heart-breaking events in the lives of medical professionals who challenged the top-down directives issued by governmental bureaucrats (CDC, FDA, NIH, WHO) with little or no clinical experience or perspective. The results were catastrophic and likely to continue for decades, all because some pencil-pushers claimed 'settled science' or the 'scientific consensus' of dictated treatment. The narrative is full of haunting, cautionary personal histories that should be read by anyone in the medical business, especially administrators whose job it is to prevent the kind of medical train wreck we experienced during COVID."[61]

What the Nurses Saw—It Was Murder! Calling the failed COVID protocols 'ERRORS' is NOT accurate. These protocols were explicitly ordered by those who took dictatorial control of the medical system early in the pandemic(spring of 2020).Further, when they were shown to be demonstrably failing and harming many thousands of people, experienced healthcare professionals who raised informed concerns were silenced through demotion, firing, and organized campaigns of harassment promoted by the news media and enabled by companies like Google, Facebook, Twitter, and Tik-Tok; in some cases in collaboration with the White House and the Department of Justice's FBI. If this sounds very bad, it's because it is. *What the Nurses Saw* is documentation of what happens in the real world when bureaucrats…in Washington D.C. take literal dictatorial control over the practice of medicine.

"On a pure dollar and cents level, one of every five dollars spent in the U.S. is spent on the products of the medical services industry, as is one of three tax dollars. The U.S., more than any other country in the world, and by a large measure, has been colonized by this industry. As part of this process, the industry and its operatives have corrupted and perverted science, academia, and the news media. Now it's hard at work to weaken and degrade the last pillar that keeps the system even remotely functioning, the integrity of the nursing profession. If we fail to support our good nurses, help them hold the line, and start aggressively turning things around, there is no practical limit to how far this totalitarian medical dictatorship, which we in fact live under, will go in its future abuse and exploitation of human beings."[62] Mr. McCarthy interviewed at least ten nurses and respiratory therapists and documented their names and experiences during the COVID era. Much of the documentation is shocking, egregious, sickening, and even feels extremely threatening to those Americans who have put their unqualified faith in our medical systems.

One obstetrical nurse, interviewed by Jonathan Otto, spoke about her concerns and experiences even BEFORE COVID surfaced. She was very concerned about giving a first Hepatitis B vaccine to brand new infants by law, knowing that these babies' immune systems are fragile. Checking blood sugar levels frequently, and other monitoring procedures felt like they were poking infants constantly. She finally refused to give the vaccine because her hospital was experiencing one baby death in utero per month. Then the COVID 'vax' came out and was given to pregnant mothers. The surge in infant deaths just before or just after birth was averaging one almost every day she worked. While under this pressure, and pushback she was getting, her own mother was hospitalized with COVID, given Remdesiver—and died—she knew drugged to death. In September 2021, an email went out that they'd experienced such an increase in fetal demise, there were 20 in one month. This was reported to the Children's Health Defense (promoting vaccination reform), but she knew that most of the administration had no clue of why this was happening, or were in total denial.[63]

Otto's group of investigators looking at the exponential rise in adverse events with COVID 'vaccines' reported to VAERS, tried to reach out to 'vax' promoters to ask the questions, looking for solutions or potential actions. They refused to meet for any discussion and censored his group instead. They, of course, knew they would get no cooperation from anyone in the mainstream media, but they tried. The US government was hiding actual stats, and there was NO documentation even stating that the 'vaccines' would improve health outcomes. There was no data available correlating vaccination dates with death dates, or if there was, the data was NOT released. Any government agency involved in public health could release the data, but not one of them would. When data were finally released, they proved the 'vaccines' had killed millions.14-71% of the deceased died within 20 days of their vaccinations. A paper was published with irrefutable evidence of the vaccines/heart damage connection, but too often autopsies weren't done, and if they were they were generally NOT thorough enough in taking actual heart tissue to prove the correlation. Interestingly, the 'vaccines' leave a very unique "footprint" that cannot be missed. Despite all of this, the estimates from VAERS data are now 7.7 per 100 actual deaths, not one in 100.

Further, Health and Human Services (HHS) was in league with the US Military Defense programs. There was an exponential number of VAERS cases reported from the military. Verifiable facts don't allow much speculation, but definitely prompted a good deal of buried facts. We know our own Department of Defense (DARPA) was involved in the design of the 'vaccines', as of course was China's military. There is also NO doubt that COVID 'vaccine' IS a biological weapon. Actually Lyme Disease has plenty of evidence of the same, according to the Children's Health Defense. Naturally CHD is not considered a legitimate medical resource by public health agencies, but it definitely encourages good detox programs and also promotes the active classification of viral safety in labs, as #3 and #4 to show how dangerous they are, and that gain-of-function accidents happen far more frequently than have been reported. Even in Nuremburg, Germany, gene therapy technology was not used, even though at least half of the humans in experiments were coerced to be lab rats for their vaccine testing. Their labs did produce some treatments that actually worked, but they lied and hid or destroyed much of what had been done. There have always been lies and deceit surrounding vaccine safety, effectiveness, and side effects.

Further, the so-called 'official' public health agencies like the CDC and the NIH have always been aware of it.

Next, we move to a very well-documented article by Dr. James A. Thorpe and his team regarding reproductive concerns. He has been in obstetric/gynecological practice for over 45 years. When the COVID 'vaccines' rolled out, pregnant moms were coerced into getting them to 'protect their babies.' All the stats became dismal quite quickly. Dr. Thorpe is also a USAF member, professor, writer and has extensively published an estimated 200+ papers—at least 25 of them related to COVID. Based on his practice and study, he took a very unpopular stance on the 'vaccines' for pregnant women and has been viciously attacked by several of the AMA groups of which he was a member. However, "he watched the numbers of complications and high-risk pregnancies increase exponentially, as well as fetal deaths after 20 weeks gestation. This significant study compared numbers with those of influenza vaccines, which were used for 60 years before ever giving them to pregnant women, while the completely experimental EUA-approved, COVID 'vaccines' were given almost as soon as they became available. In addition to the huge increase in fetal deaths, there was a 1,192-fold increase in 120,000 cases of abnormal menstruation, as well as a 57-fold increased risk of miscarriage."[64]

"The study analyzed CDC VAERS data from 1/1/1998 to 6/30/2022. When compared to the influenza vaccines, COVID-19 'vaccines' are associated with a significant increase in adverse events with all proportional reporting ratios of > 2.0 (more than doubled) in ALL of the following: menstrual abnormality, miscarriage, fetal chromosomal abnormalities, fetal malformations, fetal cystic hygroma, fetal cardiac disorders, fetal arrhythmias, fetal cardiac arrest, fetal vascular mal-perfusion, fetal growth abnormalities, fetal abnormal surveillance, fetal placental thrombosis, low amniotic fluid, and fetal death/stillbirth...All COVID-19 'vaccine' adverse effects far exceeded the safety signal on all recognized thresholds. The team concluded that high-risk pregnancies and menstrual abnormalities are significantly more frequent following COVID-19 vaccinations than that of influenza vaccinations. A worldwide moratorium on the use of COVID-19 'vaccines' in pregnancy is advised until randomized prospective trials document safety in pregnancy and long-term follow-up in offspring."[65]

Jonathan Otto interviewed nurse Michele who also did obstetrics. She said, "Big Pharma, the CDC, and all the other 'official' public health agencies lied continuously about a NEED for COVID-19 'vaccines' for pregnant women. In the hospital I worked for, many women came in experiencing all levels of premature labor within a week of taking the 'vaccine'. Premature babies were born, often already stillborn, and many would die not long after birth. Michele was doing her homework, and declared the same was happening every day in other hospitals."[61] Her whistleblowing set her hospital to investigating her for violating HIPPA law in order to fire her, however, in the investigation, they found a 45% increase in fetal demise in that hospital!

One of the most heard and interviewed nurse whistleblowers is Erin Marie Oszewski, RN, BSN. To understand the criminal extent of what hospitals did during the COVID-19 era it is necessary to hear the pain and angst in her testimony as well as the facts of what she witnessed for several months. The interview literally sounds like a horror movie, taking place at Elmhurst Hospital Trauma Center in Queens—New York City. It became known as the Epicenter of the Epicenter of COVID-19. Nurse Erin had retired from the US Army in 2012 after Iraq as a wounded/decorated sergeant and was very experienced in trauma and critical care. Following is a very abbreviated version of what Erin said in this famous interview which shockingly has NOT been scrubbed from the internet as yet: "Knowing NYC's initial COVID-19 hit, I went to Elmhurst as a travel nurse. What I found was a hospital that was literally murdering 90% of its patients, whether accurately diagnosed with COVID-19 or not, by intubating and ventilating them unnecessarily, then overdosing a plethora of dangerous drugs. Very few patients, once on a vent, ever came off. A huge % of the patient population was poor, elderly, and in a minority group. About 50% of patients had negative COVID tests (5+ days for results) documented more than once when they came to the hospital, most with simple shortness of breath, but were marked on charts as 'COVID-confirmed.' Patients were roomed indiscriminately, COVID with Non-COVID patients, then likely to get COVID and treated the same. They had tests that could have results in 45 minutes, but these were too expensive for hospital to use them! Everything done, every decision made came from 'somebody higher up,' and was ALWAYS about money. Trust me, in the army, I saw third-world hospitals and this one was not different. Rooms were filthy, staff was lax with sanitation and personal protective equipment, and hospital-acquired COVID-19 cases were through the roof. It was like the people were all disposable, and any 'mistakes' were a simple 'wash.' Nurses vowed to do everything they could to save patients unless ordered by 'do not resuscitate' (DNR) not to. At Elmhurst, it was nearly impossible to get a written DNR order, so patients would be coded no matter how critical, but when coded, authority figures did little or nothing re: a code. All ventilated patients were so heavily drugged and sedated, it was unlikely to make any difference, but we did call codes without doing codes. I became concerned that I would start to become as calloused to the situation as so many already were, seeming to see nothing wrong with all of it. There were good medical people there, but they were verbally outnumbered. Most cases started out minor, and wound-up dead—they were 'set-up' to die—it was straight up murder, (early in the pandemic and the deadly Remdesivir had not even been introduced yet). There were sensible things that could have been tried if they really wanted to help patients, but it was considered pointless to try them, since 90% would die anyway. Even proven treatments were refused, and ventilators/drugs were the worst possible thing they could do for COVID patients, most of whom were restrained, and had no 'family-allowed' visits."[66]

Erin was so sick of what she had seen and documented per her cell phone for proof, she was seriously considering leaving Elmhurst, because most of the staff knew she spoke truth boldly, and they even made decisions based on her presence or not. One day, she was caring for a younger man who had a tracheotomy for breathing, but he was doing well, she had told his children as much the day before. She was called to the Emergency Room where it was clear she wasn't needed and within a short time she heard a code called in her patient's room—she was stunned. He didn't make it; she couldn't believe he had died so quickly. "Later, she learned that a resident had improperly used an Ambu-bag to resuscitate him when the only thing wrong was a blocked trach. She was absolutely devastated to hear this and knew once again, one of her patients that should NOT have died, did die because of incompetence. The staff had deliberately waited for her to leave before it happened! As of this video broadcast, New York state had made no response to query for compensation for this man's family. Erin wasn't about to stand by and let her patients keep dying on her watch, but she knew telling the truth would not induce people to believe her. She began sharing what she saw and found on social media, and was fired for it. She has now told the whole story in her book entitled, *Undercover Epicenter Nurse*, She is, with many others, demanding justice for those who fell victim to the hospital's greed. Not only must the staff be held accountable for their unethical actions, but also, this kind of corruption MUST be destroyed so that future Americans are not put at risks like this again."[67]

Understand that all of this preceding segment was PRE-Vaccine. Consequently, we have deaths and adverse events by the tens of thousands BEFORE the 'vaccines' even got started. This was all a travesty by itself. But now we have more people dead and damaged from the 'vaccines' than we ever had infected from incurring the COVID19. We may NEVER have an accurate determination of ALL the damage done.

Next we need to look at those professionals in healthcare, public servants, the military, and even people working in a company with over 100 employees because there was so much damage done to people who were coerced to take the 'vaccines' or lose their jobs. Once again, the reality is most of us actually know people who were under those illegal mandates, and either died or continue to suffer the adverse effects they wound up with. This is another travesty beyond belief. The 'vaccine' mandates affected 12 million US employees, about 25% of the total workforce. Up to 61% of employees did NOT want their employer to require the 'vaccines'. If unvaccinated workers were given the choice to take the 'vaccine' or test weekly, almost half said they would do weekly testing. If the only option was the 'vaccine', 72% of adults said they would leave their jobs. What does that say about comfort with 'vaccines'; even if it meant loss of a job? About 59% said they would apply for either a religious or medical exemption. This author personally knows of an RN, who wanted to keep working but was forced to take the jabs to do so. She was very much against the 'vaccines', but decided to go ahead, having rarely been ill. She was very ill after the first shot, didn't want to go ahead with the second, but the response from the hospital system was the same. She took the second and within a few weeks was diagnosed with ALS (Lou Gehrig's Disease) and died of it eleven months later. No one could justifiably deny that the 'vaccine' was the culprit, but refused to admit it as well. Another travesty perpetrated by illegal mandates; they automatically removed Constitutional Informed Consent. The stories that mimic this one are epic and ongoing. There is no way to determine how many more vaccinated people will continue to sicken and die because of the adverse and deadly effects of the 'vaccines' in the future. However, the numbers of young nurses and other workers who were forced to take the jabs are exponentially frequent in all the obituary columns!! This is NOT 'rocket' science, and ANY thinking person can clearly surmise what happened over and over.

"A final consideration besides the loss of a job was the psychological condemnation, and physical abuse on the dissenter for resisting the mandate. Many viewed unvaccinated workers as a potential risk to the workplace. Unbelievably and overwhelmingly, the vast majority of workers accepted and embraced the false science claims about supposed 'vaccine' protection that we know was simply not true. For some, being fired brought some grave consequences. Few were allowed unemployment because they were 'fired for misconduct and not eligible'. Financial hardships came while trying to get a new job."[68] One such instance of abuse by peers is now well-documented. "USAF Senior Airman Lance Castle was at the time an 18year-old, enlisted, active-duty airman who refused the 'Jab'. There is video proof of several other uniformed service members attacking him, jumping on him, holding him down, beating him, and gleefully jailing him, after tearing his shoulder and his MC ligament in the process. Then he was demoted, but charges were later dropped because they found he had done nothing wrong. No one should be subjected to such violence over medical freedom! Subsequently, an entire post about his experience was censored on social media, but Castle was dubbed an 'insider threat', subjected to 60 days pretrial confinement for his 'crime', and that caused him to miss the birth of his first child. After that he was court martialed on an astounding five charges, but was acquitted after being found not-guilty of any of the charges because there was no evidence he had committed any type of crime. Now he struggles with PTSD. Before the original post was scrubbed, many who saw it noted that the way Castle was treated by the Air Force was common throughout the pandemic towards everyone in the military who refused the chemical bioweapon known as COVID 'vaccines.'"[69]

The US Military was hugely affected by the COVID mandates. The military complex has a supposed objective medical data reporting system—the Defense Medical Epidemiology Database (DMED) that saw alarming spikes in several categories right after the rollout of the COVID 'vaccines'. "There were a number of very concerned whistleblowers including: Lieutenant Colonel Theresa Long, MD;

Lieutenant Colonel Pete Chambers, DO; Major Sam Sugoloff, MD; and West Point Grad Dr. Stanton Hom, DC, BS. They were interviewed on Jonathan Otto's, The End of COVID documentary to discuss DMED and the tyranny of the US Department of Defense. This was an active data system, not specific to COVID-19, as proven by the wide variety of ICD medical codes. At first, Dr. Long started seeing very strange things in the data and began running queries and trending them. In 2021, she ran the query for pulmonary embolisms and found them exponentially off the charts. The same was true for dozens of other diagnoses, including super cancers and congenital abnormalities. This team began verifying the overwhelming information with each other and documenting what they found. Issues like malaria were stone-cold normal as always; not changing. The fact that all the exponential increases in certain codes had begun in 2021 with the mandating of COVID 'vaccines', and were consistent across all military branches was eye-opening. They asked a lot of questions of the DOD and received tons of excuses. Then they disclosed the information to Senator Ron Johnson and within hours, Moderna's stock went through the roof at $140 Billion."[70]

"Whistleblower status gives some protection, but Dr. Long was subpoenaed to court in Tampa Bay, FL. She was promptly called by her commander and told she could NOT testify, which was straight-up tampering with a witness. By that time, the panel found a 100% increase in neurological issues. Dr. Long reported to the court that she was ordered NOT to testify which is completely illegal. The DMED is a $100 million system, but it had been 'glitching' often during this time. At first, either DOD was asleep at the switch or they were simply choosing to ignore the real numbers. It did own-up in some small areas, but though it was far beyond enough evidence to stop the vaccinations, they refused to stop them. Then a 2-star General asked about all of this and waited for 47 days for an answer, but within 24 hours, the database went down, and when it came back up, the numbers were all changed! It's called TREASON in the military, where it's tried and if found guilty, EXECUTED! The database then was continually refined and data of the entire fighting force changed by a private company. The original creation of this database was like a sentinel of sorts to be certain the US fighting forces were healthy and fit. But the DMED data and the VAERS data showed the same kinds of problems correlated perfectly. These doctors say the numbers of health concerns in young people continue to show up every day in their individual practices."[71]

Meanwhile, there was a documented 380% increase in helicopter crashes. The "SquawkT100 screeches for every in-flight emergency and it happened frequently, and when investigated were generally pilot-related and NOT equipment issues. Dr. Long was stationed on a border detail for one year and the numbers had been minimal before 'vaccines'. Reportable events for pilots have increased almost five times, and the numbers are consistent across systems. This is dangerous at the least and often deadly, and this was FORCED on our entire fighting forces—absolute insanity. In addition, these treacherous events destroyed morale and created a hostile environment where it's least helpful for 100s of 1000s of men and women. Dr. Sam believes it was possibly bio-weaponry against our own troops; irrational things that doctors NEVER do; were done. It was NEVER about the science, but abuse of power by policy. Many service members and their families have been gaslit and they worry about increased potential of suicides among their friends. There is little available for resources outside the military for them. Dr. Sam has sacrificed so much as a whistleblower that he should have been protected from but mostly wasn't, while the criminals are NEVER held accountable, all the way to the upper echelons of the brass.

Many military observers, some of whom are former military have made a number of statements in the above article that are spot on for the general consensus on US military, including the following:

"Now that you see this, you might understand why people refuse to stay in or even join the force," one commenter wrote after watching the video clip.

Another person who says he served in the Army for 10 years wrote that he will not be letting any of his children serve after him because "this is not the military I used to know."

A retired First Sergeant who served under President Biden and Secretary Austin concurred, adding that the US military "isn't worth serving in."

"The only thing that would get me to serve again is if the nation was militarily invaded," this person added. "But we all know that there's an ongoing illegal alien invasion and that it IS an invasion. Something like that would get me to serve. I would serve the nation, but not the likes of Joe or Austin."

"And it wouldn't be to process them into the country, but to send them back to their own countries and seal the border."

Someone else after watching the video of Castle being persecuted in prison by the US military added to the conversation that everyone who believes the US military would never turn on American citizens should watch the video themselves before coming to such a conclusion. "They are just 'following orders' against one of their own— what do you think they would do to you?"

Still another commented that those seen in the video persecuting Castle are Traitors both to their country and to the Constitution to which they swore an oath. "The revolution will not be fun for many."

"They filtered out the good guys from the military," wrote another. "Now you have politicians saying we should hire illegals and give them weapons and training in return for citizenship. Not too difficult to figure out what they want."[72]

Tens of millions of people continue to suffer debilitating health problems due to having been jabbed for COVID. Find out much more at Chemical Violence.com.

The most disturbing of all the information about all the adverse events and deaths from COVID-19 'vaccines' is that the lethality of the injectable toxins was completely PLANNED! "The full potential of these 'vaccines' was known from animal studies as far back as 2006!! That is precisely because the search for DNA vaccines began as early as 2003 in the midst of the SARS-CoV-1 epidemic. Led by Ralph Baric at UNC-Chapel Hill in North Carolina, researchers were already clear that such a 'vaccine' was absolutely loaded with multiple insurmountable problems. This gain-of-function research was funded by Fauci's NIAID and not only failed to protect, but created immune responses no one wanted. At NO POINT were the researchers able to "FIX" the fatal flaws. Early inoculation of animals caused the same serious illnesses and death caused by the COVID-19 serums. The culprit was always the Spike Protein, made in response to the 'vax' serum. The threat was especially strong for older or impaired animals. It produced severe lung damage including diffuse alveolar damage, hyaline membrane disease, and death. In September of 2020, in the midst of Operation Warp Speed, a major review warned the expedited vaccines could actually exacerbate or worsen COVID-19 disease. The problems were NEVER resolved, and even to date, manufacturers have tweaked the 'vaccines' but issues are not resolved. So, the lethal dangers of these 'vaccines' were documented in 2006 and summarized in a 2020 review article. The Global wolves never even flinched at this news. They pushed the 'vaccines' into production and planned the worldwide distribution of them. Fauci and Gates clearly KNEW the lethal effects were NOT limited to elderly people, or those with co-morbidities and weakened immune systems. They intentionally went right ahead almost certainly BECAUSE they KNEW. They did NOTHING to try to solve the problems and NO MONEY was earmarked for it. Therefore, as previously stated, it was indeed slated to further the globalist goals of eliminating unnecessary people!"[73]

Consequently, globalists were completely satisfied with the pile-up of US and worldwide deaths that far exceeded those of any other vaccine in history. There is simply no other reason why the "official" public health agencies, the WHO, CDC, FDA, NIH and NIAID completely ignored the thousands of deaths and adverse events that were clearly happening all over the globe. Further, any historian will confirm that the idea of "culling" humanity is a concept with a long and honored history among eugenicists, and euthanasia advocates, including many scientists, philanthropist organizations, and political leaders. In the case of COVID-19 and the use of 'vaccines', there clearly has been Nothing Voluntary about them. By all legal standards, it is defined as MASS MURDER! *It* is very little different than that of Adolf Hitler's holocaust, except there was a known end to his travesty. The COVID-19 holocaust is never-ending in its duration, and there has been no attempt at the equivalent of the Nuremberg Trials where international criminals were punished and retribution was at least attempted. With the Globalist agenda, it is also highly unlikely we will ever see anything like that occurring in today's world.

Dangers of the Alien Spike Protein Created in the Body from Vaccination

Besides vaccination deaths and adverse events witnessed by doctors and nurses, we have the additional threat of the permanent presence of the alien spike proteins created in the bodies of all vaxxed people by the 'vaccines'. In December of 2020, two scientific articles were published, showing the spike protein (S protein) alone causes damage and inflammation to the endothelial cells in blood vessels in both the body and brain of animals and humans. Spikes cause both hemorrhages and clotting. To say it succinctly, the same protein that was attached to the SARS-Co-V-2 in the lab in the gain-of-function process to MAKE IT LETHAL, was also incorporated into the 'vaccines'! They KNEW it could ONLY be more harmful for humans. This threat was not only ignored, but embraced in the race to market these toxic 'vaccines'. So the damage from spike proteins comes from incurring COVID-19, and from taking the COVID 'vaccine'. The endothelial damage leads to clotting in the capillaries of the lungs and can be seen clearly on autopsy. Since spike proteins are produced both by the illness and the 'vaccines', it is consistent with reports that many post-vax persons become positive on COVID-19 testing. It also confirms that vaccination either before or after a COVID illness may create or exacerbate a COVID-19 condition. This phenomenon was noted early in the pandemic, but did nothing to induce caution on vaccination.

"More autopsy reports on COVID-19 patients...are helping researchers construct a picture of a virus that damages endothelial cells, causing a clotting disorder that can lead to deep vein thrombosis and pulmonary emboli, a hyper-coagulant state. German researchers looking at 12 autopsies of COVID-19 patients found a substantial number of deaths were related to pulmonary embolism despite the patients having no prior evidence of thrombosis. In the autopsy studies of five centers in the US, Buja and colleagues reported major pulmonary thrombo-emboli with pulmonary infarcts and/or hemorrhage in five of 23 patients and a pattern of cardiac comorbidity similar to what was seen in the German study…All found a preponderance of severe epithelial injury in the COVID-19 lungs, as well as widespread thrombosis with microangiopathy. The damaged endothelial cells showed disruption of inter-cellular junctions, swelling, and loss of contact with the basal membrane."[74] Interestingly, though, the evidence shows significantly more new-vessel growth in the lung than is usually expected from a typical influenza illness by 2.7 times. The growth in the lungs is likely caused by either the endothelial injury and thrombosis or a chronic hypoxic (not enough oxygen) state. It is believed that this phenomenon should spur further research.

By May 31, 2021, Dr. Peter Breggin interviewed German doctor Uwe Alschner, MD who spoke of the disclosure of vital information Pfizer had withheld about its vaccine. It had insisted its vaccine affected the area of an arm that received the vaccination ONLY. However, the internal Pfizer study actually showed their mRNA 'vaccine' forced cells throughout the human body to produce the poisonous artificial spike proteins, exactly as expected! Large concentrations of spike proteins were found in ovaries, after concerns arose that the vaccines caused hormonal disruption in women, posing a potential threat of both current and long-term infertility issues, and a large added threat to children. This conversation got a "first strike" threat of censorship from You Tube over this interview.! Also a review of 'vaccine' information by three doctors stated that pregnant women are NEVER EVER given an untested experimental biological substance. Yet, this 'vaccine', unapproved by the FDA, was pushed rigorously at pregnant women "to protect them," when in reality it held a 100% potential of harm for both mother and child far into their futures.

The COVID vaccines (2024-2025 formulas) to date, are still only approved under the Emergency Use Authorization (EUA) by the US FDA. Therefore, Big Pharma is still by law NOT liable for any untoward adverse events or deaths incurred from receiving them, even though they are still considered "safe and effective" in every bit of written documentation. Clearly, that isn't true, but the propaganda goes on. "The CDC recommends COVID-19 vaccination for everyone ages 6 months and older, including people who are pregnant, breastfeeding, or might become pregnant in the future. Individuals should speak with their health care provider for questions."[74] However, as previously mentioned, changes have been made to policy as of August, 2025. With the globalists still driving this agenda, the propaganda will continue, but anyone who chooses to take another vaccine of ANY KIND, especially COVID-19 or any succeeding genetically manipulated injectables, does so at their own serious risk, as this book is extremely clear about. If any person has had a clear natural case of COVID-19 with its known symptoms, and can get proof of antibodies that produced natural immunity, that person WILL NOT INCUR the disease again! Most COVID-19 tests were also EUA and if a PCR test is done, it will continue to lack reliability. Standard labs now have more accurate tests. Under no circumstance should anyone take another COVID-19 JAB!

There is NO such real determination of either safety or effectiveness. None is even possible, and such statements are deliberate deceit. Documents can only legally say, "may be effective." FDA approval normally requires 8-12 years, and has even taken up to 20 years! These 'vaccines' simply cannot EVER pass legitimate FDA safety standards unless the FDA chooses to do so in corruption. There were/are FORESEEN consequences of "rushing" ahead experimentally, which we have experienced in heinous numbers. All of the adverse events were clearly known BEFORE Operation Warp Speed ever started. The "Breggins' warning to President Trump led him to cancel Fauci's funding to labs. They knew the 'vaccine', when used in ill and elderly animals, not only didn't protect them, but created hyper-harmful responses and death. Early data from New York state reported 50% of deaths were occurring in senior-living facilities. That means the other 50% were dying outside such facilities from vaccines in younger and less incapacitated people. All of the real vaccines at that time were created with DEAD viruses or diluted ones. However, now the 'vaccines' do NOT contain 'inactivated' viruses and because they induce our bodies to make toxic spike proteins, there is NO WAY they should ever be called 'vaccines'. There is exponential risk of a far greater immune response than from traditional vaccines with the additional health risk of spike protein proliferation and this was proven early on. This known toxicity and subsequent damage are a central part of SARS-CoV-2 pathology and may be incurred by the spike proteins ALONE!"[75]

A highly pressing issue in the vaccine industry currently is: "How far will scientists bend the truth to further promote these 'vaccines?" As we saw in an earlier chapter, the answer to that question is a resounding, "Just as far as we must in order to keep the monopoly thriving and making billions more annually than anyone could ever spend!" Bill Gates is the "King of Vaccines" and we know he will stop at nothing. When the World Health Organization (WHO) began making really bad decisions, based on its global relationship with the Chinese Communist Party (the largest globalist concern), the handwriting was on the wall as far as global decisions went. President Trump halted US support to the WHO, so Bill Gates became its largest donor. "WHO proceeded to delete and redefine scientific concepts that promoted Bill Gates, the 'vaccine' industry, and the globalist wolves—China being chief among them. Do you need more proof of this than the ever-changing public health announcements, making us all dizzy:

- Coronaviruses lived on surfaces until they didn't.
- Masks didn't work until they did work, but they still don't work.
- There is asymptomatic transmission, except there isn't.
- Lockdowns are a must to control the virus, except they

don't.

- All these people are sick without symptoms until "oops," they weren't really sick; PCR tests were wildly inaccurate, because they were NEVER intended to be diagnostic tools.
- Everyone was in danger of the virus, except they weren't.
- The virus spreads in schools, except it doesn't.
- It was always one big fishy, inconsistent deception.

After all this, WHO deleted the idea of natural immunity, a long-time, well-established fact—from its entire website. Why? Because Bill Gates and his 'vaccine' industry had NO intention of waiting around for people to get sick and develop their own natural immunity which was exponentially better in every way than the potential acquired immunity of the so-called 'vaccine'. He and his cronies wanted us all to feel so hopeless about the disease globally, we would all come running for his toxic jabs. So the true definition of natural immunity, proven over time and experience was no longer acceptable. According to WHO, the best immunity could only be achieved through immunization. Lies, deception, fraud, disinformation, duplicity, hypocrisy, treachery, flimflam, pretense, and yes, betrayal of 8 billion people took place to sell vaccines. Science had become nothing more than a marketing tool in the hands of Bill Gates and the globalist wolves and just another step closer to the coveted totalitarian rule."[76]

Before we close out this section on the ravages of the vaccines, it might behoove us to look at the special standing of vaccine manufacturers to help us understand how in the world this travesty proliferates. Once again, Dr. Peter Breggin, who has been called 'the conscience of American psychiatry' and has litigated against these companies because of drugs that killed people, knows the extent of their capabilities. He said, "Many professionals told me that vaccine manufacturers are the nastiest of all those in the medical field. This is NOT coincidental! They are making the biggest bucks while among the MOST EGREGIOUS, least regulated, and best protected by federal legislation and a special vaccine court. The manufacturers are so powerful the governmental FDA regulators allow them to test their own vaccines without using placebo-controlled, double-blind clinical trials. They want to RUSH to get vaccines produced however possible under the auspices of the EUA law which promotes an enormous lack of ANY ethical restraints for the drug companies and Big Pharma. These give us a plethora of reasons why we must exercise judicious caution in promoting or using any such products. If you are injured by a 'vaccine', you cannot sue the manufacturer!!! Your only recourse is to sue the US government via a special vaccine 'kangaroo court'![77]

The Pfizer Papers—Summary of Atrocities That Were Known and Hidden, Before the Rollout of Vaccines

One of the most unexpected, though so difficult to attain, revelations of the entire COVID-19 era is that of the Pfizer Papers. Lawsuits against Pfizer (major 'vaccine' manufacturer), by lawyer Aaron Siri to force the FDA's release of internal Pfizer documents were actually WON. These papers "are a stunning revelation of corporate greed and dishonesty, with utter disregard for the law, and Americans' actual health. They are also a stinging indictment of the entire pharmaceutical industry, both globally and especially in the US. Pfizer was relentless in its pursuit of corporate profit, unhampered by ethical, moral, or patriotic considerations. Dr. Naomi Wolf and Amy Kelly were tireless in their pursuit of the truth behind the 'vaccines'. They learned that Pfizer KNEW its 'vaccines' risked causing heart damage in young men, (among a myriad of other treacherous harms). Pfizer did everything it could to keep their documents secret, including stamping 'FDA Confidential' all over them…It is also an indictment of the Trifecta—Big Pharma, mainstream media, and the Washington D.C swamp. It demonstrates how Pfizer's clinical trials for the vaccine were deeply and fatally flawed. By November 2020, before the 'vaccines' rollout, the company KNEW its 'vaccine' was neither safe nor effective. The Pfizer Papers prove the US Food and Drug Administration KNEW about the shortfalls of Pfizer's clinical trials and deliberately looked the other way."[78]

This massive research project of reading and analyzing 450,000 pages of documents written in extremely dense, technical language, was pursued virtually by 3,250 expert volunteers, and is now fully categorized into 34 separate units of adverse events, and has taken from 2022 to the present and continues. This group, under the leadership of Dr. Naomi Wolf and a remarkably gifted project director, Amy Kelly, brought one of the largest and most corrupt institutions in the world, Pfizer, to its knees. It also drove a global pharmaceutical monster to lose billions of dollars in revenue, and hopefully squelched the plans of the most powerful politicians on earth. It even managed to bypass the censorship of the most powerful tech companies on earth. The 'Papers' detail Pfizer's clinical trials, most of which were illegitimate in practice, yet they proved satisfactory for the FDA to award it the coveted EUA approval allowing Pfizer to race right to market with a toxic and experimental, badly tested product. However, the Pfizer Papers also contain documentation of what happened in the 'post-marketing' stage, the three months of December 2020 through February 2021, as the vaccine was thrust upon the mostly unsuspecting public. Reading from what was a well-planned centralized script, all leading spokespeople, and bought-off media proclaimed the vaccine 'safe and effective.' Most people didn't realize it should have taken a minimum of 10-12 years to bring a vaccine to market, and they were effectively being used as guinea pigs. The greatest travesty was that many millions of people submitted to this toxin because they were 'mandated' to do so and threatened with loss of jobs and military positions if they refused. In some states and in other countries they could lose far more rights if they refused, including rights to take transportation, cross borders, go to school or college, receive certain medical procedures, or enter any public buildings. The FDA actually requested of the trial judge that he withhold the release of these documents for 75 Years, but thankfully, the judge refused.[79]

Dr. Wolf spoke about her own warnings to women everywhere

as a career-long writer on women's sexual and reproductive health issues. Menstrual dysregulation was becoming a big problem for women who had taken the jab, and Dr. Wolf saw this as a serious danger signal that such side effects could easily affect fertility. Almost immediately, she was banned from Twitter, Facebook, YouTube, and other platforms and was being attacked globally as an 'anti-vaxxer' and a 'conspiracy theorist.' This effectively halted her work as a best-selling author within the 'legacy media.' No one would talk to her, publish her work, or return her calls. She says she was "unpersoned." Then after two additional, successful law suits in 2023, under AGs for Louisiana and Missouri, she found out the White House, the CDC, and senior leaders of other governmental agencies, including HHS, unlawfully pressured media to remove her health warning, shut her off, and watch for more. This act of suppression is currently pending a Supreme Court Decision on whether this was a First Amendment violation. It was then that Dr. Wolf caught the attention and received significant help and sound advice from Steve Bannon of the War Room. Then Amy Kelly came on board where chaos had reigned and calmly organized the entire project.

There is so much significant information reported from the Pfizer Papers, it would be impossible to write it here, but for a taste to my readers, we will try for a very brief summary of some of the facts. "The first 46 reports published broke huge stories. Within the first three months after the rollout, Pfizer KNEW the vaccines did NOT work to stop COVID. Pfizer's own language was 'vaccine failure' and 'failure of efficacy'. One of the most common 'adverse events' was simply 'COVID'! Pfizer KNEW the vaccine crossed EVERY membrane in the human body—including the blood-brain barrier—and accumulated in the liver, adrenals, spleen, brain, and ovaries for certain, and that there was NO mechanism whereby those vaccine materials leave the body, so that every succeeding injection would pack more and more of those materials into organs.

"Pfizer had to hire 2,400 full-time staffers to help process 'the huge increase of adverse event reports' being submitted to the company's Worldwide Safety database. Pfizer KNEW by April 2021 that the injections damaged the hearts of young people. It KNEW by February 2021 (within 90 days of rollout) that its injection was linked to a myriad of adverse events. Far from its published side effects of fever, chills, and fatigue as the CDC and other authorities claimed, the actual side effects were catastrophically serious. There were 1,233 deaths in the first 3 months of availability. The following adverse events are just a short list of the total: # 1 was muscle pain, #2 was joint pain, #3 was strokes (50% of which happened within the first 48 hours after a jab), and #4 was severe liver damage (also 50% happened within the first 72 hours of a jab). Then came facial paralysis, kidney injury, autoimmune diseases, chilblains, multiple organ dysfunction syndrome (more than one organ system failing at once), activated herpes zoster infections, skin and mucous membrane lesions, multiple respiratory issues including damaged lung structure, failure, acute RDS, SARSCoV-1 (not seen since 2004); industrial-scale blood diseases, blood clots in lungs, legs, brains, hearts, and clotting disease in blood vessels; vasculitis, astronomical rates of neurological disorders including dementias, tremors, Parkinson's, Alzheimer's, seizures and syndromes; and a plethora of cardiac conditions including myocarditis, pericarditis, tachycardia, arrhythmias, etc.; and enormous focus on the disruption of human reproduction which had been planned all along. 72% of adverse events occurred in women with almost 20 % of those involving reproductive disorders. An example of just one such was the destruction of breast milk which actually turned green in many cases. Nine months after the rollout, there was a 13-20% decrease in live births in women who received the jab. For men and boys, it is yet unknown if fertility is greatly decreased or even if masculinity itself will be normal. The worst news of all is that all these figures are NOT universal, but are primarily in North America and Western Europe!"[80] This is clear proof that Globalist Wolves focused heavier destruction and death on the "free world" of the West!

"This information leads us to a clear political context for so much horrific damage perpetrated. The Pfizer pharmaceutical giant KNEW they would be killing babies and significantly harming both women's and men's reproduction. All the information within the documents indicates clearly that damaging human ability to reproduce and causing spontaneous abortions of babies is "Not a bug, it is an intended feature." Pfizer has KNOWN for many years that lipid nanoparticles degrade sexual systems. The Papers also showed the nanoparticles pass through the blood-testes barrier and damage male Sertoli cells, Leydig cells, and germ cells, the factories of masculinity, and also affect the hormones that enable boys' physical changes at adolescence, including deep voices, broad shoulders, and ability to father children. Currently, we have no idea if baby boys born to vaccinated mothers will turn into adults who are recognizably male and fertile. Pfizer counted on the menstrual damages it KNEW was causing thousands of women, ranging from women bleeding every day, having two periods a month, or no periods at all; to hemorrhaging and passing tissue; to menopausal and post-menopausal women bleeding again. Pfizer's scientists calmly observed and noted it all, but no information was given to women about any of it—in other words, there was no informed consent with the vaccine push on pregnant women. Consequently, from the political perspective of this information, the globalist agenda of depopulation has been easily accomplished, particularly in Western nations where the numbers of dissenting citizens to their totalitarian goals are yet too high."[81]

Given all the information in the Pfizer Papers, and there are volumes of reports to cover if the reader has the intestinal fortitude to do so, a number of heinous conclusions can be drawn. This vaccine program is not just caused by abject greed, nor is it a simple oversight. It was and is a carefully contrived and cruelly perpetrated plan using a known bioweapon, and we, especially the people of the still-free Western nations were victimized by a massive attack in a one-sided war. The Bio-N-Tech Pfizer 'vaccine' was manufactured by a German factory whose sole owner is Communist China. It has a signed memorandum of understanding (MOU), a formal, nonbinding agreement between two or more parties that outlines their intentions, roles, and responsibilities, a step in the process of creating a formal contract. It is also filed with the Securities and Exchange Commission (SEC) and is now 100% tech transferred to the Chinese Communist Party (CCP). China has 13 manufacturing sites in Western Europe and two in the United States, ready for all the school children of our nation. Its ALL about killing Westerners either sooner or later. In addition, it's a wholly asymmetric warfare. There was a total of 42,000 adverse events noted. 36,000 of those events were in the United States, leaving a total of 7,000 events in all other nations combined! It is very easy to target set subjects with the 'vaccines' since they are liquid, and the temperature must be very cold to keep nanoparticles from activating before use, and doses can be changed even more easily. A standard Pfizer dose is 30 mcg, but the plan is to use 100mcg for those 'vaccines' intended for children! Now do you understand mandates? We are talking mass murder that could make Hitler's maneuvers look like child's play.[82]

This is a very hard and sickening reality to swallow! But we MUST NOT lose our hope or our vision as Americans. If we even think of giving up, the war has already been won by our many enemies. There is hope in God's truth, in our liberties and freedoms, though they've been sorely challenged, and in our national community. Evil seems to have overtaken the world, especially the free world in lockstep, but our Father God has His own scheduled agenda, and He still has the ultimate control. To close this chapter, here's a fun fact to enjoy: "40 million doses of Pfizer's Bio-N-Tech COVID vaccine expired and had to be completely discarded. In addition, whenever the vaccine is thawed without immediate use, it's discarded."[83] That's a very large chunk of money right into the garbage. We can rejoice in these things!

> "The king's heart is in the hand of the Lord, as the rivers of water: He turneth it whithersoever He will." Proverbs 21:1 KJV

> "Many are the plans in the mind of a man, but it is the purpose of the LORD that will stand." Proverbs 19:21 ESV

"Our God is in the heavens; He does all that He pleases." Psalm115:3 ESV

"The LORD of hosts has sworn: 'As I have planned, so shall it be, and as I have purposed, so shall it stand...'" Isaiah 14:24 ESV

"For Kingship belongs to the LORD, and He rules over the nations," Psalm 22:28 ESV

"The LORD has made everything for its purpose, EVEN the wicked for the day of trouble." Proverbs 16:4 ESV

"For MY thoughts are not your thoughts, neither are your ways MY ways, declares the LORD. For as the heavens are higher than the earth, so are MY ways higher than your ways and MY thoughts than your thoughts. For as the rain and snow come down from heaven and do not return there but water the earth, making it bring forth and sprout, giving seed to the sower and bread to the eater, so shall MY WORD be that goes out from MY mouth; it shall not return empty, but it shall accomplish that which I purpose, and shall succeed in the thing for which I sent it." Isaiah 55:8-11 ESV

"In His hand is the LIFE of every living thing and the breath of ALL mankind." Job 12:10 ESV

"I know that You can do all things, and that no purpose of Yours can be thwarted." Job 42:2 ESV

"I have said these things to you, that in ME you may have peace. In this world you will have tribulation. But take heart; I have overcome the world." John 16:33 ESV

> And said, "O LORD, God of our fathers, are You not God in heaven? You rule over all the kingdoms of the nations. In YOUR hand are power and might, so that none is able to withstand You."
>
> 2 Chronicles 20:6 ESV

> "ALL the inhabitants of the earth are accounted as nothing, and He does according to His will among the host of heaven and among the inhabitants of the earth; and none can stay His hand or say to Him, 'What have You done?'"
>
> Daniel 4:35 ESV

> "Who rules by His might forever, whose eyes keep watch on the nations—let not the rebellious exalt themselves!" Psalm 66:7

Just in case any of you, my dear readers, have any doubts as to the future with all of the current global chaos, please do NOT be fearful or feel hopeless about your future. There is SO much Scriptural assurance for us of our ABBA's provision. Here's the author's favorite takeaway:

> "For God did not give us a spirit of timidity or cowardice or fear, but He has given us a spirit of power and of love and of sound judgment and personal discipline, abilities that result in a calm, well-balanced mind and self-control."
>
> 2 Timothy 1:7 AMP

Chapter 15

Can COVID Vaccine Damage be Treated?

Who Are the Medical/Legal Professionals That Can and Will Help?

In an earlier chapter we mentioned some of the resources available to people who know they need help with the ravages of 'vaccine' adverse events. First and foremost is the recognition that you have been injured by the COVID 'vaccines' or other previous vaccines and have not been diagnosed. Clearly, the most obvious place to go is to your primary care physician. However, you must be aware that if you suspect that your health issues have been caused from taking the COVID 'vaccines,' there are many physicians still promoting them with everything in them, and will not likely be readily willing to admit that your problems are vaccine-related unless you can prove by dates that they occurred after you received the 'vaccines.' Dates of 'vaccines' and dates of onset of new health issues are crucial. If your doctor is one who heavily promotes the 'vaccine' schedules and has a drug for every health issue, you might want to explore other physician options. It was originally estimated that only about 500 medical providers in the United States were willing to look at the vaccine problems from a more realistic perspective. The numbers have increased as more of them have begun to think out of the allopathic medicine box they learned in medical school and seek other potential answers to the problems that are NOT responding to more vaccines and drugs. That is a very healthy development. Other branches of medicine include integrative physicians, functional physicians, naturopathic physicians, chiropractic practitioners, nutritional specialists, and many other alternative specialists who do have some very good information and techniques that offer a wide variety of healthy options.

A next really important step is to have a medical professional help you in reporting your adverse event to the VAERS system. If a medical professional is unable or unwilling to help you submit a report any individual may file one. Surprisingly, the CDC and the FDA do encourage people to do this because it makes the numbers of reports much more valid to verifying the true number of events happening. Since the agencies continue avidly promoting these 'vaccines' in every bit of medical literature, the numbers of adverse events have risen exponentially and will continue to rise irresponsibly. Further assistance may be sought by emailing info @ VAERS.org or phoning 1-800-822-7967. Reports can be submitted online, or you can download a Writable PDF Form and then upload that when completed. Anyone can report and they are NOT limited to how severe the event is or has been. If an adverse effect is listed by the 'vaccine' manufacturer, the 'vaccine' should NOT be given again. In most cases the reporter will receive a confirmation letter and that is all, unless he is contacted for additional information. If the event is classified as serious, a review process ensues. Actions taken are seldom to rare, honestly. However, VAERS data without patient identification is available to the public and specifically to medical providers through a system called CDC's VAERS WONDER because it may be helpful information.

There are also a couple programs that can be of some help entitled the National Vaccine Injury Compensation Program (VICP) and Countermeasures Injury Compensation Program (CICP) available through The Health Resources and Services Administration (HRSA) that may compensate individuals whose injuries may have been caused by certain vaccines. Importantly, these programs operate separately from VAERS. Reporting an adverse event to VAERS does not create a claim for compensation with the VICP or CICP. The person who made the VAERS report must file a claim directly with the VICP or CICP. There are specific reporting requirements for healthcare providers administering COVID-19 and monkeypox 'vaccines'. The VAERS WONDER System can also be accessed on You Tube. When you have a 'vaccine' injury claim, hiring a lawyer to represent you is one of the first steps toward asserting your rights under the VICP. "There are seven factors to consider when choosing a vaccine lawyer:

- Focus on 'Vaccine' Injury Claims
- Experience Negotiating VICP Settlements
- Experience in the Vaccine Court
- Free Resources to Help You Make Informed Decisions
- Nationwide VICP Representation
- Availability and Accessibility
- No-Cost Legal Representation—all lawyers should provide no-cost legal representation for your VICP claim—if they don't you must go elsewhere.[1]

"The National Vaccine Injury Compensation Program (*VICP)* pays hundreds of millions of dollars each year to individuals and families who are suffering due to the effects of vaccine injuries. These injuries result from all types of vaccinations, including the flu shot, TDAP and other CDC-recommended vaccines. In fact, although all CDC-recommended vaccines are generally considered safe, the CDC also warns that "any vaccine can cause side effects." While most of these side effects are minor, unfortunately some vaccine recipients suffer debilitating and life-altering injuries."[2] While this law firm has offered great information, it is only one, yet it is significant to note that just this one firm recovered more than $7.1 million in compensation for its clients in one year, so there is decent potential for legal help with a good lawyer.

More than 270 million Americans have received a COVID-19 vaccine of the 345,426,571 in our total population as of 2024 (about 78%). That is a bit over 75% of Americans that have a strong potential of developing adverse events from COVID-19 'vaccines' over the next several years, based on what we now know of its toxic attributes. There are many people who believe they've suffered serious side effects as a result of their vaccinations and feel "completely ignored, dismissed, and gaslighted." Others feel they have received little support or acknowledgment of their situations. Here is a case in point: "Michelle Zimmerman, 37, said that within minutes of receiving her COVID-19 'vaccine' from Johnson & Johnson, she felt pain racing up her left arm to her left ear and down to her fingertips. Days later, she was extremely sensitive to light and had difficulty remembering simple facts. She has a Ph.D. in neuroscience and until then, was able to ride her bike 20 miles, teach a dance class, and give a lecture on A.I. all in one day. Now, over three years later, she lives with her parents and has been diagnosed with brain damage, unable to work, drive, or stand for long periods of time."[3]

Another case is that of "Shaun Barcavagen, a 54-year-old nurse practitioner in New York City who worked on clinical trials for HIV and COVID-19. He said ever since his first COVID-19 shot, standing up causes his heart to race, a symptom that suggests postural orthostatic tachycardia syndrome—a neurological disorder linked to both COVID-19, and, less often, vaccination. He's also experienced stinging pain in his eyes, mouth and genitals, which has gone away, as well as tinnitus which is still present. He says he's unable to get the government to help him. He is told he's not real, or told he is rare, or even told he's a coincidence!"[3]

A third sufferer is "Renee France, a 49-year-old physical therapist in Seattle, who developed a form of facial paralysis called Bell's palsy as well as a dramatic rash across her face. Bell's palsy is a well-known side effect of some vaccines and has been linked to COVID-19 vaccines in studies. She said doctors were dismissive of any potential connection between her conditions and COVID-19 'vaccines.' The rash, which ended up being a bout of shingles, debilitated France for three weeks, so she reported it to federal databases twice. She thought someone would reach out, but no one ever did."[3]

"Gregory Poland, the editor in chief of the journal '***Vaccine***', said a loud whooshing sound in his ears accompanied every movement since he received his first shot, but his appeals to colleagues at CDC to explore his severe tinnitus haven't led anywhere. He received polite responses, but he gets no sense of any action, and believes that if studies have been done, those studies should be published."[3]

Finally, "Buddy Creech, who led multiple COVID-19 vaccine trials at Vanderbilt University, similarly experience tinnitus and a racing heart for a week after each shot, very similar to what he also experienced during acute COVID in March of 2020. He says it's possible that research might find most reported side effects are unrelated to the 'vaccine'. Regardless, when our patients experience side effects or adverse events that may or may not be related to the vaccine, we owe it to them to investigate it as completely as we can."[3] Former acting FDA Commissioner Janet Woodcock said she believes some recipients of the COVID-19 vaccines had uncommon but "serious" and "life-changing" reactions. She admitted that she feels badly for those people and believes that their suffering should be acknowledged, that they do have real problems, and that they should be taken seriously.[3]

Almost from the very beginning of the COVID-19 pandemic, a group of doctors known as the Frontline Physicians raised many questions of scientific concerns about the whole agenda. They saw a very large concern in the fact that the cherished doctor/patient relationship was already under attack and quality care of sick patients under fire as never before. Powerful forces were undermining the effective practice of medicine by many experienced and highly qualified medical professionals by polarization and heavily biased and even false information. There continues to be censorship on truth from government, media, and Today, it is more difficult, and at times nearly impossible to access true, independent, evidence-based health information to enable patients to make their best-informed decisions about their own health care. Even from the 'programmed' medical establishment. America's Frontline Doctors published a Position Paper on COVID-19 Experimental 'Vaccines' to attempt to warn citizens of their valid concerns. It concluded with a "Call to Action" statement with two simple but all-important life-saving points: "Always use the correct language. These formulations are COVID-19 Experimental 'Vaccines'.

Immediately, now and forever, make it known to ALL that you will refuse to consent to ANY attempt to mandate an experimental vaccine by any employer, school, or business entity."

The Paper also contained a list of safety concerns regarding the COVID-19 Experimental 'Vaccines' including the following:

- They were made using the almost brand-new genetic engineering technology that had barely been tested, and most of the tests prior to this were troublesome and results were NOT marketable.
- There was nothing but failures in making previous coronavirus 'vaccines.'
- There were NO independently published animal studies.
- There were multiple known complications associated with them.
- There were still multiple unknown complications expected.
- Big Pharma companies make a lot of unwise decisions regarding the introduction of new drugs and vaccines and remain completely 'immune' from all liability.
- An Experimental 'Vaccine' is NOT safer than a very low Infection Fatality Rate (IFR). Continued improvement in good treatments bring about an increasingly low IFR which America's Frontline doctors were achieving with medication combos such as Hydroxychloroquine and Ivermectin. However, the CDC and the FDA deliberately banned what had been highly effective because the EUA law would NOT allow the introduction of their new drugs and vaccines unless there was nothing else effective available.

- The data has NOT been independently peer-reviewed and published.
- In addition to the safety concerns, there were at least three very valid questions being asked regarding the effectiveness of the COVID Experimental 'Vaccines':
- Where is the proof that this COVID Experimental 'Vaccine' has actually stopped the transmission of the virus?
- Where is the proof that the mortality and Hospital Admission rates have diminished as a benefit of the so-called 'vaccine?'
- How long does this product last with a high percentage or duration?

In conclusion, for ALL people, contrary to the published narrative even today, the risk of taking mRNA vaccines remains greater than the risk of being without them! The entire contrived 'Vaccine Plot' has turned into a tragic disaster for hundreds of thousands of people, whose proportions of adverse events were and still are developing and the Experimental COVID 'Vaccine' that should NEVER have been initiated, remains available and is still being pushed even onto our infants with the propaganda that it is still 'MOSTLY' safe and effective. Nothing could be further from the truth. An even greater travesty continues because a massive number of mainstream allopathic medical professionals are also still asking, declaring, and avidly pushing the poison onto uninformed patients. They, too, have bought into the whole 'Vaccine' hype because it's easier NOT to do their homework, get informed, and stand against the globalist establishment. From personal experience, this author knows patients, even those with informed decisions made NOT to take the 'vaccines' or worse allow their children to have them, continue to be subjected to the constant propaganda and urging of their providers that they NEED it. Because the information available in offices, from the CDC, online, T.V. Advertisements, etc. is NOT telling the truth, if they succumb to taking the 'vaccines,' they did so without informed consent!

As always, if you take or support the material presented here, and believe it is the truth because it is, you may still be labeled as a conspiracy theorist, and accused of advancing misinformation, just as most of these good doctors have been. It is imperative that you stand your ground and refuse to injure yourself or your family with these highly questionable products.[4]

Where are we today?(from the end of 2022) "According to Dr. Peter McCullough, per the VAERS system we are at 18,000 deaths. Remembering that even the CDC states the VAERS system is notoriously underreported to with totals being estimated at only 10-15% of the adverse events reported. Being ultraconservative with that, the number of deaths in actuality could easily be ten times that number a180,000. VAERS shows 30,000 individuals who are permanently disabled after the vaccine with a conservative estimate of 300,000. There is a vast number of 250,000, estimated 2,500,000 emergency room visits, office visits, and other health care encounters related to the vaccine. Figures from the UK and from Canada show that 50% of the deaths occurred within 48 hours of the shot and 80% of the deaths occurred within a week. We now KNOW that the spike protein produced from these vaccines is produced in the body for an uncontrolled quantity and an uncontrolled duration of time. In fact, the number of antibodies to the spike protein after the vaccine are so high, compared to the actual respiratory infection, we can easily infer that in fact, one gets a much larger dose of the spike protein after vaccination than from an actual illness. Some people simply cannot handle the high spike protein onslaught and die. The vast majority of deaths were in seniors, the very population we supposedly most wanted to protect! An independent researcher, McClacklin, examined and rigorously coded 1,200 of these deaths for causality. He ascertained that 86% of the time there was NO OTHER CAUSE OUTSIDE the VACCINE!"[5] Nearing the end of 2025, an AI summary reported a total death toll from COVID-19 in the US is projected to be around 1.1 million by its end (representing 2020-2025). AI notes it is impossible to count supposed vaccine deaths, because health resources don't admit to vaccine deaths!

There are clear stats on the increased incidence of myocarditis in young men who have taken the 'vaccine.' We already knew there was a normal increased incidence of 80-90% in males in adolescence, though the reason for it is not known, averaging about 4 cases in every million. "Since we know we have approximately 70 million adolescent males in the United States and we multiply that number by 4, we would know about how many boys would get myocarditis normally— 280 potential cases. VAERS reported 13,000 certified cases (but again a possible 130,000 with those unreported) of myocarditis/pericarditis! We also know that about 86% of these kids had to be hospitalized—they are very ill. They have chest pain and EKG changes. Blood testing of enzymes for heart injury is from 10 to 100 times that of a man having a heart attack. These kids have significant heart damage and about 25% are moving into heart failure detected on echocardiograms. Heart failure drugs are required to treat them. They can have NO physical activity because it can trigger sudden cardiac death."[6] The truth is, with the risk in adolescent boys of myocarditis at 80-90% and their risk of dying of COVID-19 at nearly zero %, this is a group that should be automatically omitted from children's scheduled immunization of COVID-19 'vaccine.' Nothing else makes sense. Instead, there is a mere written warning on the vaccine of the potential myocarditis which is both "mild and rare." Since when is the risk of 13,000 healthy young men getting myocarditis considered rare nor mild with 86% hospitalization? How many young adolescent boys do you know that would cheerfully handle NO PHYSICAL ACTIVITY well? There is no wonder so many young men have collapsed and died on athletic fields all over the world, because they don't even know they could be walking corpses looking for a spot to die on! The reality now is that the age of men incurring myocarditis/pericarditis post-'vaccine' is also rising significantly. We do know the spike proteins go to the heart because they are distributed in organs all over the body. Some women are similarly affected. Too often, there is no autopsy, but they would show a clear inflammation load and massive swelling of the heart muscle, as much as double in size. Taking a second 'vaccine' dose would be just like an internal explosion!

In addition to all of the really serious above information, we also have to consider the long-term prognosis of these 13,000 cases reported to VAERS, and since we know reporting is so far behind the actual numbers, there could be conservatively 130,000 cases of myocarditis/pericarditis in the US alone. Since the rate of severity put 86% of cases in the hospital, we know the degree of heart damage has been significant. Can they even hope to recover anything close to normal heart function? According to Dr. McCullough, that is NOT likely. The spike protein in the body is known to last as long as 15 months. However, the recommendation for getting COVID19 boosters is now at every six months. If that happens, the spike protein can NEVER fully leave the body. Progressive accumulation of the spike protein is very worrisome for these progressive organ-injury syndromes. If a person gets by without adverse events after a COVID-19 jab, there is no guarantee the same will be true if he gets another and another. But going back to the long-term prognosis for a young man with myocarditis, even if he NEVER takes another jab, the damage is done. Yes, the heart can be treated with a number of drugs that can allow better function, but the reality is that for many, a return to normal heart function is often elusive. An average of 13% will later develop heart failure or need things like implantable cardio defibrillators or pacemakers, possibly even heart transplants. Obviously, the rate of later cardiac death is much greater as well as a greatly reduced lifespan.

In general, "the treatment for myocarditis would start with 3-6 months of NO physical activity at all. The hyper-inflammation state must be reduced significantly. When the heart pumping mechanism is reduced, doctors use evidence-based beta-blocker drugs and others that can target certain receptors and inhibit others—some of the same drugs that have been used to treat COVID-19 can also be used to treat COVID-19 damage because the spike proteins exist either way. Anti-inflammatory drugs are crucial—like putting out the fire. Some people in danger of losing jobs have asked the question "If I must take the 'vaccine' is there anything that can be potentially taken to mitigate possible damage from the spike proteins?" Dr. McCullough has actually asked his patients in this case, 'If you take the 'vaccine', what do you get? 20 years of employment? Is that employment even a guarantee? Why don't you figure out your social contract BEFORE you take a spin with this 'vaccine?' But in answer to the question on mitigation, there are some things a person could try out of desperation. Again, do whatever you can to reduce inflammation, reduce the tendency toward blood-clotting, and some of the possible organ injury syndromes, if you know of co-morbidities that might be influenced. The reality here is we all make our best decisions based on what we believe to be true and then we will live with that decision or not!!"[7]

Once again, we MUST be very careful where we get our information. For example: Early summer of 2021, the propaganda pushed by people in positions of authority, falsely reported that 99% of the people in the hospital with the Delta variant were NOT vaccinated. This was completely false. At that highest point of the number of people vaccinated, it was guesstimated at 66%. We had the notorious naval cruise where 3700 fully-vaccinated individuals passed the Delta variant to each other! Fully 25% of Americans in the hospital with COVID-19 were fully-vaccinated. Despite the complete falsehood of the claim, officials kept right on lying and people passed the lies. That is supposedly the way you get more people to run right out after all these months and finally get their jabs!

The various medical resources available to those who believe they are 'vaccine' injured are a little trickier to locate, but it's important to know there are professionals who are willing to go above and beyond to help injured people. The Truth for Health Foundation has a wealth of information available online. The website contains a downloadable "Vaccine Injury Treatment Guide: Your Road Map to Recovery." "This booklet does NOT provide individual medical advice or prescribe treatment but is provided as an educational service for patients and their families to know what options are available and widely used for many conditions. Patients should consult the physicians of their choice for individual medical evaluation and recommendations for treatment tailored to individual needs."[8] The following steps are suggested to start the process:

1. Review the experimental COVID shots, how they work, risk issues and safety updates now that we have more data on the outcomes since the COVID shots were released to the public. Go to FACT SHEET 1

2. BEFORE you take any experimental gene therapy COVID shots and boosters, our expert physicians and scientists suggest you read our Patient Guide FACT SHEETS 2-5 to make an informed decision on effective treatment options for vaccine-induced injury.

3. If you have already taken the COVID shot, and do not have any identified adverse effects, we suggest focus on GENERAL PREVENTION STRATEGIES. Go to FACT SHEET 3.

4. If you have taken the COVID shot(s) and boosters and are experiencing puzzling adverse health changes, or have experienced serious side effects, fill out our VACCINE INJURY REPORT on our website. Then consult our VACCINE INJURY TREATMENT options in FACT SHEET 2 and 3 for symptoms, immediate home care steps, and prescription medication options. Then go to FACT SHEET 4 and assess your immediate options to start treatment at home. If your doctor does NOT treat vaccine injuries, check the resources on Truth for Health Foundation for physician resources in APPENDIX.

5. If you are at high risk based on your age, medical conditions, or occupation, we suggest Vaccine-injury testing and medication treatment options. See FACT SHEET 2.

6. The FACT SHEETS listed above are identified below:
    - INTRODUCTION:
    - FACT SHEET 1: Experimental COVID 'Vaccines': Update on Safety
    - FACT SHEET 2: Diagnostic Lab and Imaging Tests for Evaluation of Injury Following COVID Shots
    - FACT SHEET 3: Prevention and Treatment Nutraceutical Options
    - FACT SHEET 4: Prescription Treatment Options for 'Vaccine' Injury
    - FACT SHEET 5: Threats to Pregnancy, Fertility and Endocrine Health
    - APPENDIX: Medical, Legal, and Advocacy Resources

Disclosures: Physicians contributing to this guide for patients are actively treating COVID illness and 'vaccine'-injured patients based on the best available medical evidence, and are focused on early, home-based delivery of medical treatment options unless critical care in a hospital is determined to be urgently needed. Contributors to this guide have no financial ties with any pharmaceutical company or product suggested in the treatment algorithms. All contributors have volunteered their time and expertise as a community service in this pandemic emergency to help inform patients of their options for research-based, peer-reviewed, safe treatments. They have received no remuneration. The opinions expressed in this guide are those of the physician contributors and not those of their institutions listed.

"The experimental COVID shots were rapidly rolled out to the public without the customary 2-7 years of animal and clinical human trials, and with only two months of safety data. We have only recently learned that Pfizer and FDA suppressed trial data from the public, identifying over 1,200 different adverse effects occurred amongst the clinical trial participants. The FDA had requested that this Pfizer data be withheld from the public for the next 75 years...a stunning reversal of all normal procedures for prompt release of clinical trial data for independent review and analysis. Following a Texas federal court ruling, this data was released to the public on March 1, 2022. These adverse effects Pfizer accumulated in the clinical trial are being born out in clinical practice worldwide as physicians are seeing skyrocketing numbers of patients with these problems.

"Safety and effectiveness are now in question worldwide with the rising numbers of vaccine-induced deaths and severe complications. Complications and adverse effects with the experimental COVID shots are primarily occurring because of Inflammation and blood clotting abnormalities, resulting from uncontrolled spike protein production and lipid nanoparticle damage. Immune dysregulation is another critical source of damage from the COVID shots. But there is a hopeful message in all this: Many of the prescription medications we used to treat inflammation and blood clotting in COVID-19 illness syndrome are also effective for treating the adverse effects of the COVID shots. These medications were also approved decades ago in other countries and are in use worldwide, with impressive safety track records in many different ethnic groups and ages. If you use an older, well-established medicine that means you have more information on safety to help guide your decisions.

"We encourage all patients with injuries from the COVID shots to seek comprehensive diagnostic evaluation with laboratory and imaging studies discussed in this guide, in consultation with your personal health professional. We suggest you seek treatment under the supervision of a physician or licensed medical professional who is knowledgeable in the use of the approaches described in this guide. As practicing physicians and health professionals, we have moral, ethical, and fiduciary responsibilities to our patients. It is our duty to do our best to find plausible, medically sound, readily available existing safe medicines, supplements, dietary and other strategies to help patients suffering from severe effects of the COVID shots."[9]

Before we get into some of the Adverse Events in deeper detail, we need to know some "UNPRECEDENTED" information called "Alarming 'FIRSTS' about the COVID Experimental 'Vaccines.'" Many aspects of COVID-19 and subsequent 'vaccine' development are unprecedented for a 'vaccine' deployed for use in the general population. Some of these include the following:

- First to use polyethylene glycol (PEG) in an injection
- First coronavirus vaccine ever attempted in humans
- First to use mRNA vaccine technology against an infectious agent
- First time Moderna has brought any product to market
- First to have public health officials telling those receiving the vaccination to expect an adverse reaction
- First to be implemented publicly with nothing more than preliminary data, no long-term safety data
- First vaccine to make no clear claims about reducing infections, transmissibility, or deaths
- First injection of genetically modified polynucleotides in the general population[10]
- Operation Warp Speed established a few other unprecedented aspects of COVID-19. First, it brought the US Department of Defense into direct collaboration with US health departments with respect to vaccine distribution (Bonsell, 2021). Second, the National Institutes of Health (NIH) collaborated with the biotechnology company Moderna in bringing an unprecedented type of vaccine against infectious disease to market, one utilizing a technology based on messenger RNA (mRNA). The confluence of these unprecedented events has rapidly brought to public awareness the promise and potential of

> mRNA vaccines as a new weapon against infectious diseases into the future. However, at the same time, events without precedent are, by definition, without a history and context against which to fully assess risks, hoped-for benefits, safety, and long-term viability as a positive contribution to public health.

What Are the Main Adverse Event Categories, and Examples?

In the same excellent study, a great deal of effort went into reviewing the occurrence of both autoimmune and inflammatory diseases in patients with COVID-19. They found many instances of a tight homology between viral antigens and self-antigens, as much as 68% of them matched. Autoimmunity is becoming much more widely recognized as a result of COVID-19 disease or vaccine-induction. There are hundreds of reports of previously healthy individuals who developed diseases such as idiopathic thrombocytopenic purpura (ITP), Guillain-Barré syndrome, and hemolytic anemia, systemic lupus erythema (SLE) with cutaneous manifestations. Since COVID-19 antibodies can be found in blood and cerebrospinal fluid (CSF) which may lead to at least some portion of the neurological complications found in many patients. There has also been a high prevalence of autoantibodies against cardiolipin, a kind of lipid in the bloodstream necessary for clotting. This would definitely contribute to the high incidence of blood-clotting pathologies in patients. Cardiolipin is also necessary for proper function of mitochondria (the cells powerhouses). These are just some of the multiple pathological findings of this study, and led these researchers to the conclusion that one of the potential side effects of giving a mass vaccine could be an emergence of autoimmune diseases, especially in individuals who are genetically prone to autoimmunity.

The lipid nanoparticles (LNPs) also known as liposomes encapsulate RNA molecules and with the polyethylene glycol

(PEG) are very stable and almost indestructible. However, this makes them more efficient in increasing the release of cytokines, inducing added inflammatory responses; the probable cause of the many symptoms, such as pain, swelling, fever, and sleepiness that people experience. Muscle cells also enhance immune response and create additional inflammation very rapidly, which explains the rapid pain and inflammation at the injection site, and that quickly advances to fatigue, headache, muscle pain, chills, joint pain, fever, site swelling, redness, nausea, malaise and lymphadenopathy. The PEG used in the lipid nanoparticles amplifies immune responses and may induce anaphylaxis in sensitive people, including cardiac anaphylaxis, especially in succeeding doses. "PEG is a high-risk 'hidden' allergen, usually unsuspected and can cause frequent allergic reactions due to inadvertent re-exposure. Allergy investigation also carries the risk of anaphylaxis and should be undertaken only in specialist drug allergy centers"[11] The more extreme anaphylactic reactions to the COVID-19 'vaccines,' as opposed to previous vaccines, occurred at a rate of 247 per million, more than 21 times greater than the usual.

There is also a very large problem with homologous antibodies of the spike proteins and those of the human system of proteins. There are a wide range of diseases found in association with a prior SARS-CoV-2 infection producing antibodies as well as those of the body's own antibodies from illness or 'vaccine.' Another group of researchers identified 26 heptapeptides (liver) found both in humans and in spike protein. Two of those 26 overlapping heptapeptides were found to be sequential, a strikingly LONG string of identical peptides was found to be in common. They commented, 'this causes the potential for it to drive MANY types of autoimmunity simultaneously. The clinical scenario that emerges is truly upsetting"[12] Antibodies with a high binding affinity to SARS-CoV-2 spike and other proteins also have a high binding affinity with those associated with Celiac Disease, Hashimoto's thyroiditis, Multiple Sclerosis, and several other endogenous (human body) proteins. However, these autoimmune diseases typically take years to manifest symptoms. "In a separate study of the cross-reactivity of antibodies, using human monoclonal antibodies against the SARS-CoV-2 spike protein, the SARS-CoV-2 membrane protein antibody reacted with 18 of 55 tested antigens. These 18 endogenous antigens encompass reactivity to tissue in liver, mitochondria, both the nervous and digestive systems, the pancreas, and elsewhere in the body."[13]

In prior exposures of coronavirus illnesses, especially in children, it is already well-established that the incidence of multi-system inflammatory syndrome (MIS-C) is prevalent, especially where parents with COVID-19 acts as a 'primer' of their immune systems, and even more so if the child is genetically predisposed to such development. Previous infections with other coronaviruses are much more frequent in the pediatric population. Autoimmunity is becoming much more widely recognized as a sequela of consequence of COVID-19. Can you even imagine how critical this can be when the children have also been previously primed from six months of age by the COVID-19 'vaccines.'? There are certainly multiple reports of previously healthy individuals who developed autoimmune diseases after infection with SARS-CoV-2 or after taking the COVID-19 'vaccines.' There are three independent case reports of systemic lupus erythema (SLE) with skin lesions following symptomatic COVID19. In one case a 39-year-old male had SLE onset just two months after outpatient treatment for COVID-19. Another striking case of SLE progressed very rapidly and was fatal.

As discussed previously, autoantibodies are very commonly found in COVID-19 patients' blood and cerebrospinal fluid (CSF). Though the actual virus is not found in the CSF, the autoantibodies created in response to the virus exposure is believed to lead to some portion of the many neurological complications documented in COVID-19 patients. Since we know the exact same virus that causes the COVID-19 has also been used in the 'vaccines' we can see the correlation of the same kinds of symptoms in 'vaccinated' individuals. It is also clear that autoantibodies were present in 52% of hospitalized COVID-19 patients early in the pandemic, which heavily contributed to the high incidence of blood-clotting in these patients. Anticoagulant therapy was used on most hospitalized patients after that discovery during and after the illness; this author being one of those. A high percentage of hospitalized COVID19 patients also had autoantibodies reactive to the plasma membrane of hepatocytes (liver cells) and gastric cells. Knowing all this, it is clear scientifically that one of the potential side effects of giving mass vaccines is an emergence of autoimmune diseases, especially for those who are genetically prone to autoimmunity. Naturally, the same conclusion is true for a range of post or long COVID-19 symptoms, including chronic tachycardia, bradycardia, alopecia (hair loss), attention deficit and brain fog, post-orthostatic tachycardia syndrome (PoTS), various neuropathies, and more.

These diseases could present acutely and over a relatively short time span or could potentially not manifest for months or years following exposure to the spike protein, whether via natural infection or via vaccination. Here is one interesting caveat of possibility if taking COVID-19 'vaccines.' Those folks, and there is believed to be as many as 20% of individuals, are relatively insensitive to SARS-CoV-2 and probably have a very strong innate immune system. "The healthy mucosal barrier's neutrophils and macrophages rapidly clear the viruses, often without the need for ANY antibodies to be produced by the adaptive system. However, the 'vaccine' intentionally completely bypasses the mucosal immune system, both through its injection past the natural mucosal barriers and its artificial configuration as an RNA-containing nanoparticle. Those with a strong innate immune response almost universally experience either asymptomatic infection or only very mild COVID-19 disease presentation. Nevertheless, they could easily face chronic autoimmune disease, as described previously, as a consequence of excessive antibody production in response to the 'vaccine', which was never necessary in the first place!"[14]

With the wide distribution of the COVID-19 'vaccines' came a plethora of VAERS cases of blood-clotting disorders. One of the most dangerous of those is idiopathic thrombocytopenic purpura or ITP. One recorded and prominent case was of "Dr. Gregory Michael, an obstetrician in Miami Beach, who died of a cerebral hemorrhage (stroke) 16 days after receiving his FIRST dose of the Pfizer/BioNTech 'vaccine. Within 3 days of the 'vaccine', he developed ITP, an autoimmune disorder in which the immune cells attack and destroy the platelets. His platelet count dropped precipitously, which caused an inability to stop internal bleeding, leading to the stroke as described in an article in the New York Times...the NYT followed up with a second article discussing several other cases of ITP following the 'vaccine', and several other incidences of precipitous drops of platelets and thrombocytopenia following 'vaccine' also reported in VAERS."[15] Interestingly, it was found that in the biodistribution of the vaccine within the body, the third highest concentration was found in the liver and spleen, coming directly via the lymph system, in the spleen 86.7 ng./ml! Since the spleen is responsible for the storage of most of our blood cells, is it any wonder that the presence of the vaccine in the bloodstream is so rapid. (Remember that the oxygenated red hemoglobin fades out completely within minutes of exposure to the vaccine—completely losing its oxygen-carrying capacity [Fleming]). ITP appears first as petechiae or purpura on the skin and/or bleeding from mucosal membranes. It has a very high risk of fatality through hemorrhaging and stroke and may also come as an immune response.

There are so many other manifestations of illness following COVID-19, we can't begin to cover them all. Just as a brief mention, some of them as reported through VAERS include: the activation of a latent herpes zoster (shingles), rheumatoid arthritis, significant changes to the pulmonary blood vessels including thickening and hypertrophy, and smooth cell changes to the pulmonary artery that causes (pulmonary hypertension, and other lung injuries the author's spouse developed pulmonary fibrosis). Systemic hypertension (high blood pressure), coronary artery disease, stroke, right ventricular heart failure, mitochondrial damage, and other cell damage is common. Neurological issues abound, including loss of blood-brain barrier integrity, and dementia. As previously discussed, there are a plethora of potential problems in both female and male reproductive organs that are well documented. All of the entities discussed in this single section can come just from the spike protein toxicity alone, without any of the previously discussed physical problems. There is also a definitive link to the Prion diseases, such as Mad Cow, as well as significant neurodegenerative diseases such Alzheimer's, Parkinson's, amyotrophic lateral sclerosis (ALS); certain specific proteinaceous infectious particles are linked to these diseases.

A final conversation at this point would be appropriate because of the constant conversation and discussion on it—that is—the potential for permanent incorporation of spike protein genes into human DNA. It has been claimed ad nauseum by Big Pharma, CDC, FDA, etc. that this is impossible. That is because the RNA supposedly cannot become inadvertently incorporated into the human genome. However, "according to most researchers, it is NOT at all clear that it is true. The classic scientific model of DNA -> RNA -> protein is now known to be FALSE. It is now indisputable that there is a large class of viruses called retroviruses that carry genes that reverse transcribe RNA back into complementary DNA (cDNA) in 1975.

Much later it was discovered that this process wasn't even unique to retroviruses. There are known enzymes, particularly transcriptase that convert RNA into DNA and incorporate it into the genome so as to maintain the new gene through future generations. It's essentially a copy / paste process of DNA to a new site in the genome via an RNA enzyme-like tool, while also possibly introducing genetic alterations in the process. A geneticist, Barbara McClintock identified this process some 50 years ago, and won a Nobel prize for it! So, it has now become clear that they can import RNA from an exogenous source into a mammalian host's DNA by recombination. So the implications of this predictable phenomenon are NOT completely clear, but are potentially far-reaching."[16]

There is another phenomenon that is now becoming quite

concerning due to the massive and continued vaccination programs for COVID-19. It is known as Antibody-Dependent Enhancement or ADE. It is an immunological process first described in 1964. The unexpected finding was that, with increasingly high dilutions of the antibody-containing sera being cultured, cell infectivity was enhanced. Lack of a viable explanation for how this could happen is likely responsible for its being largely ignored for almost 20 years. Antibodies are supposed to both directly and indirectly participate in the neutralization of infections. However, "in the case of ADE, low, nonneutralizing levels of either specific or cross-reactive antibodies against a virus are already present at the time of the infection due to prior viral exposure, exposure to a related virus, or to prior vaccination against the virus. Upon reinfection, antibodies in insufficient numbers to neutralize the virus nevertheless still bind to the virus. These insufficient antibodies dock at receptors on cell surfaces, enabling viral entry into the cells and subsequently enhance the virulence or infectivity of the virus."[17] ADE is known to play a role especially in Dengue fever, Zika virus, and Ebola as well as other potential viral infections. These most certainly play a potential role with any vaccinations employed against SARS-CoV-2. Non-neutralizing antibodies form immune complexes with viral antigens that can provoke excessive secretion of pro-inflammatory cytokines, and in the extreme a cytokine storm that causes widespread local tissue damage.

Here is the biggest problem: "At present, there are no known clinical findings, immunological assays or biomarkers that can differentiate any severe viral infection from immune-enhanced disease, whether by measuring antibodies, T cells, or intrinsic host responses. However, preexisting immunoglobulin G antibodies, induced by prior vaccination, are known to contribute to severe pulmonary damage in mammals. There is also evidence that the much more diverse range of prior exposures to coronaviruses experienced by the elderly could certainly predispose them to ADE upon new exposure to SARS-CoV-2. A highly concerning article reported that plasma from 76% of patients who had recovered from severe COVID-19 disease, when added to cultures of SARS-CoV-2 and susceptible cells, exhibited enhanced ability for SARS-CoV-2 viral infection. Therefore it is reasonable to speculate that spike protein-specific antibodies may well contribute to disease severity during SARS-CoV-2 infection."[18] Because all three US vaccine manufacturers are working to continue developing COVID-19 booster shots, this is even more concerning. With tens of millions of young adults and children now having vaccine-induced coronavirus spike protein antibodies, there will always exist the possibility of triggering ADE related either to future SARS-CoV-2 infection or booster injection among the younger population. In all likelihood, time will soon tell. Given evidence only partially reviewed here, there is sufficient reason to suspect that antibodies to the spike protein will contribute to ADE provoked by prior SARS-CoV-2 infection or vaccination, which will manifest as either acute or chronic autoimmune and inflammatory conditions.

Now, in order to understand some of the ways that poisoning from the spike protein can be treated after injury, we need to know its mechanism. The spike protein facilitates entry of the virus into a host cell by binding to ACE2 receptors in the plasma membrane. All by itself, the spike protein causes a signaling response when it binds with the ACE2, going straight to the body's entire vascular/circulatory system with potential widespread consequences, including significant heart and lung damage. So, one of the treatment modalities doctors have used is to find other substances that will do the same thing the spike protein does when it binds with the ACE2, thus preventing the spike from using the ACE2 receptors, whether the spikes are from disease or vaccination. As we speak of some treatment potentials, we will keep this firmly fixed in our minds.

There is so much more evidence of the harm and potential harm inherent in the COVID-19 vaccines and boosters and its mind-blowing. We cannot go further for the purpose of this book, but it suffices to say, there are volumes of books and papers that clearly describe these in far greater detail and all add to the concern that the 'official' health agencies refuse to acknowledge in ANY way. For now, we'll attempt to summarize this segment and move on to treatment for damage incurred.

"Experimental mRNA vaccines have been heralded as having the potential for great benefits, but they also harbor the possibilities of potentially tragic and even catastrophic unforeseen consequences. The mRNA vaccines against SARS-CoV-2 have been implemented with great fanfare, but there are many aspects of their widespread utilization that merit concern...We want to emphasize that these concerns are potentially serious and might NOT be evident for years or even transgenerationally. In order to adequately rule out the adverse possibilities described in these pages, we recommend, at a minimum, that the following research and surveillance practices be adopted:[19]

- A national effort to collect detailed data on adverse events associated with the mRNA vaccines with abundant funding allocation, tracked well beyond the first couple of weeks after vaccination.
- Repeated autoantibody testing of the vaccine-recipient population. The autoantibodies tested could be standardized and should be based upon previously documented antibodies and autoantibodies potentially elicited by the spike protein. These include autoantibodies against phospholipids, collagen, actin, thyroperoxidase (TPO), myelin basic protein, tissue transglutaminase, and perhaps others.
- Immunological profiling related to cytokine balance and related biological effects. Tests should include, at a minimum, IL-6, INF-x, D-dimer, fibrinogen, and C-reactive protein.
- Studies comparing populations who were vaccinated with the mRNA vaccines and those who were not to confirm the

expected decreased infection rate and milder symptoms of the vaccinated group, while at the same time comparing the rates of various autoimmune diseases in the same two populations.

- Studies to assess whether it is possible for an unvaccinated person to acquire vaccine-specific forms of the spike proteins from a vaccinated person in close proximity. (shedding)
- In vitro studies to assess whether the mRNA nanoparticles can be taken up by sperm and converted into cDNA plasmids.
- Animal studies to determine whether vaccination shortly before conception can result in offspring carrying spike-protein-encoding plasmids in their tissues, possibly integrated in their genome.
- In vitro studies aimed to better understand the toxicity of the spike protein to the brain, heart, testes, etc.

Public policy around mass vaccination has generally proceeded on the assumption that the risk/benefit ratio for the novel mRNA vaccines is a "slam dunk." With the massive vaccination campaign well under way in response to the declared international emergency of COVID-19, we rushed into vaccine experiments on a worldwide scale. At the very least, we should have taken advantage of the data that was available from these experiments to learn more about this new and previously untested technology. And, in the future, we urge governments to proceed with far more caution in the face of new biotechnologies.

Finally, as an obvious but tragically ignored suggestion, the government and so-called health authorities should also be encouraging the population to take safe and affordable steps to boost their immune systems naturally. This includes getting out in the sunlight to raise vitamin D levels, and eating mainly organic whole foods rather than chemical-laden processed foods. Also, eating foods that are good sources of vitamin A, vitamin C and vitamin K2 should be encouraged, as deficiencies in these vitamins are linked to bad outcomes from COVID-19. These good health measures would be helpful all the time, whether the appropriate encouragement is available or not![20]

The Voices of the Victims Should Be Loud and Clear.

Unlike today, in 2025, it's a possibility the victims of vaccine injury were simply NOT aware that taking the heavily touted 'vaccines' at the urging of every public health agency, the government, and all the Big Tech entities for the "good of all," must surely be 'safe and effective'. While that seems like an extremely naïve stance, many people desperately wanted to return to "normal." But many victims also did NOT know that if there were 'vaccine' injuries', their government and its agencies were NOT likely to make any recompense for 'vaccine' damage. After all, we live in a fully litigious culture! However, Big Pharma was fully protected from suit for damages by federal law. That was true even if the 'vaccines' were mandated by that same government, that forced you were to take them. One US citizen against the US Department of Justice wouldn't likely experience any compensation any time soon. The following cases are real people with first names only, who were interviewed at length by Jonathan Otto, host of the docuseries: *The End of COVID-19.* He interviewed a number of ladies with stories that, like so many, needed to be heard. In these testimonies, we see the dilemmas these ladies found themselves in with taking or NOT taking the jabs, and the injuries that followed:

Felicity's story—she resides in London, UK. Her boyfriend did not take the 'vaccine', but she didn't want to be an anti-vax voice, didn't want to judge anyone, and believed her choice was important. It was very difficult to find any accurate information about the 'vaccine', both before and after the jab. After taking it, she became 60% disabled and there was no doubt of it being due to the 'vaccine.' She found it extremely difficult, if not impossible, to get any help or receive any compensation. Going back, she took two doses of the Pfizer 'vaccine.' and developed an immediate rash on her arm. She felt very heavy and tired, followed by hugely swollen lymph nodes in that armpit, severe bone pain, and her entire body hurt. She texted her mom and before she could write, went into a seizure and blacked out. The medical advice line was consulted; they told her that a seizure was fine, it was just a side effect! and sent her a medical form to report side effects. From that point she experienced hair loss, horrible dreams and bad sleep. She asked about an exemption from her second shot, but was self-employed and she needed to be able to travel, so she got jab #2. She experienced visual disturbances, and had an average of 10-12 seizures per day. Having severe pain; she could barely stand up with assistance. Doctors assured these symptoms would all "wear off" but they didn't. Then she wasn't walking, scant talking, and tried to call an information line every day for help. She waited four more days before going into the hospital with severe neurological symptoms developing. No one would accept that this was all caused by the jabs. Soon she had forty different symptoms, now including chest pain, constant visual disturbances, skin color changes, paralysis, continued seizures, and had one while she was being interviewed! She stated it changed her entire life. She began speaking and writing about her experiences and was censored for doing so. Finally, her disability was documented as 'vaccine' injury, but it was still censored, she was banned from media, and the medical establishment did essentially nothing but persecute her.

Today, she is still unable to work, and still hadn't received ANY compensation at the time of this interview. She said it literally makes her skin crawl when she hears and sees all the trauma. She and friends she's made with various injuries feel utterly disposable to officials while those responsible are making billions of dollars ignoring what they did to people like her. Felicity's fiancé cares for her no less than 35 hours a week. In the UK, health care is essentially free, but even their rent is far too high-priced. She worries about her long-term health needs. They had to move to her parents for a year because of rent and seizures, and will probably need to do it again. Though she has been considered "disabled," she doesn't meet their qualifications. It was an extremely depressing scenario just hearing her tell her story. One of the hardest things for Felicity to handle is the constant lack of compassion from the medical and governmental entities for her nearly impossible situation and the sense of having to prove her disability. It's like rubbing salt into her wounds. Such a response disturbs her horribly, and the ongoing question is whether anyone will ever step up and actually help her in any way.[20]

- **Sheryl's story—**She knew the media was already hitting hard on anti-vaxxers even before COVID-19. Then her daughter suffered a vaccine injury and she had already stopped vaccinating any of her children. but somehow, it seemed like a different set of circumstances when COVID-19 ensued. Initially, she was still afraid to take the new 'vaccine'. Sheryl went to her doctor to ask questions. There was no good information being offered on it, but the doctor was all about getting the 'vaccine! Still uneasy, she took the first Moderna jab. Within the first 24 hours, her lymph nodes were swollen over most of her body and she was having stroke-like symptoms on her left side. It started what she called, "a fire storm" she is still dealing with two years later. Naturally, she knew immediately it had to be due to the jab. One neurologist actually told her to go ahead and get jab #2, so they could prove it was actually the 'vaccine' that caused the trouble!!! (That one made the entire listening panel gasp in disbelief!) Sheryl vehemently refused, so that neurologist dropped her because she had asked her for a referral to someone else for a second opinion, and told her that if she happened to develop Multiple Sclerosis, she wouldn't treat her! The doctor herself was angry and actually had a bad reaction from her own jab, but refused to believe the 'vaccine' was the cause; she was living in complete denial. A 'friend' told her NOT to even try to share her story, as it wouldn't do any good. Sheryl went ahead and tried to share just one piece of her story on Instagram only, and it was gone the next day! Her husband was censored on You Tube. She decided to keep trying, got increasingly vocal, and was censored often. You can't even share your own story! It hasn't stopped them, however, as she dug in and keeps digging deeper. Sheryl knew about VAERS and asked about it; the doctor said reporting to VAERS was her responsibility. BIG LIE! She didn't try to argue, but started her report. She admitted it was NOT easy to do; it was extremely time-consuming and she had time limitations. She got bumped off the report often and started over four times to get it done. Six months later, she finally received the temporary case number. Then the CDC actually called her and she was on the phone for an hour and a half. They wanted to know if she had any other symptoms, marked her report 'permanently disabled' and was told someone else would contact her. At the time of the interview, no one had ever contacted her again in two full years! She found out from others like her—the CDC actually removed their reports for 'technical' reasons. One reason given was that all the pertinent neurological symptoms were NOT grouped together!

Sheryl admitted she just couldn't live in a victimized state any longer. She gets enraged all over again when it feels like she's "living in the midst of a Steven King novel." She tried to help a group of vax-injured people with another organization called "React-19." It was trying to help them with resources to assist with severe expenses. She said when she thinks of Big Pharma's enormous profits, and NO EFFORTS at ANY kind of compensation, there are "just NO words!" Criminals that aren't punishable! "The sacrifice for the greater good" statement makes her see red! Sheryl was asked what treatments had helped her most. She said it has NOT been a straight-forward, linear path, but loading doses of IV Immunoglobulin have helped. Many natural kinds of things have helped her and others including infrared saunas, various types of detoxes, especially those treating for mold. She believes she is now functioning at nearly 80% on her good days and works to find ways to ignore or set symptoms aside. Her big focus is on her mental/emotional health and says a great support system is so essential. It's important to connect with other vax-injured folks and share hope and ideas on what is working. Sheryl also spoke of just how important her faith in Someone Greater than she has been, so helpful in her healing journey. Her last and possibly most important comment was sharing the fact that our health freedoms are in grave danger and we all must speak out the truth—its power gives courage to keep speaking truth.[20]

- **Brittany's story**—This woman already suffered from an autoimmune disease, but was very worried about getting COVID-19 and how it would jeopardize her health even more if she got it. She researched and couldn't find anything definitive about her situation. She heard all the anti-vaxxers and thought they might be dangerous, but perhaps she judged them. Finally, she took two Moderna 'vaccine' jabs a bit further apart than usual; told she needed the extra protection. After the first shot, her legs felt very heavy and she told her husband she thought something was wrong with her. She was achy and took several baths to ease the discomfort, and then gastro-intestinal symptoms appeared. She had some tests, but they all appeared to be clear. A total of 740 days later (over 2 years), she still struggles with various GI symptoms. Her job was forcing her to get the second jab, while she wanted to stop right there. She 'threw a fit about it,' but wound up taking the second jab anyway. She started calling herself a hypochondriac, but two weeks later, they wound up calling 911 when she couldn't walk! She was numb from her feet upward. The test results this time were really scary. She had pericarditis (heart), brain lesions, meningitis, some evidence of Guillain-Barré syndrome, especially in her face. At the emergency room the GBS stopped and brought a bit of relief. There was extreme pain, and after going to four or five hospitals for help, finally got a Physician's Assistant who would actually listen to her. He did a spinal tap, admitted her to the hospital and gaslit for the next 10 days, because he simply didn't know what to do. She had no seizures, but indescribable pain constantly. Finally a report came back positive for GBS (Guillain-Barré syndrome). The PA said, "You have GBS and you aren't going anywhere!" He said he believed it was 'vax' induced when they finally started to believe her, and she needed to file a VAERS report. She truly thought she was dying and nobody would help her, so she was taking pictures of herself in the hospital for documentation and posting them until she was caught and they called the police on her!! She had 8,000 followers, but when police showed up, they all abandoned her and banned her reports from three Instagram accounts.

Many accused her of doing it for money. It nearly destroyed her family and personal life. It wound up as a court case/legal battle investigating injuries from a so-called motor-vehicle accident, saying she'd made everything up and she was a total fraud. Because it was so skewed against her, she expected to lose the law suit. The censorship went way yonder further than just the online stuff. There were accusations from so many people for everything under the sun, and simply no way to fight it. The mainstream media with their globalist agenda made a habit of destroying victims so they couldn't talk about evidence. The things that happen to people they want to silence are legendary and brutal, and frankly, very hard to believe that anyone would work so hard to make it so. The victims often wind up nearly or fully destroyed, and are void of their once normal lives of personal integrity.

Healing was a long road. Brittany knew there was no quick fix, and there were many setbacks, but she tried everything suggested, knowing it was necessary to do one thing at a time. It required focus, frequent assessment of potential progress for at least two weeks on each trial, and writing everything down. There was an extraordinary amount of detoxing of heavy metals, a huge problem for many post-vax patients. It was hard but worked well. She did Infrared Saunas, some CBD, and the Hyperbaric Oxygen treatments seemed to help her a lot. All detoxing was hard and lengthy but so necessary for healing. Brittany stated that she is a believer in Jesus Christ and her faith in Him was of the maximum importance to her healing. She said she is NOT fully healed but is so much better. She fully agreed with comments made by the other ladies interviewed. She stressed asking questions, again and again and again if necessary, and doing your own homework. You are entitled to the truth and real answers—government agencies are supposed to be working FOR US, not us for them. If you don't want to get educated you are your own problem. A lot of necessary information was withheld from us—now that we are fully aware, we must keep on asking and searching.[20]

- **Pamela's story**—In Pam's case, she was very aware of what was going on, and of the dangers involved in the 'vaccines.' Both she and her husband refused to take the jabs, but were unable to convince their son, Benjamin, even though he had two younger siblings who had suffered vaccine injuries. He didn't want to discuss it or even hear about it, partly because he was heavily involved in show business in New York City, with television (CBS) and Saturday Night Live. Her husband worked at NBC, but there were no mandates for vaccination at the time Benjamin took his 'vaccine.' They had told him he couldn't work without it and he was completely brainwashed. He was also told that if he took the jab there would be no more masking or testing. He was unable to move about freely or travel without it, and the peer pressure was intense. By September of 2020, he had to test daily for both of his jobs. He was convinced he was "helping everyone get back to normal." *On **March 13, 2021***, Benjamin went to a pop-up clinic in downtown NYC and took his first jab, a Johnson & Johnson 'vax', and had not told his parents, but he got a screeching headache, so he told them. From the headache he got severe chills—an anaphylactic reaction. By 3:00 AM, he started seizures. He was rushed to Mt. Sinai Hospital where they said it was "just like his heart had simply exploded." He was pronounced dead at 6:00 AM, less than 12 hours after the jab. His fiancé called them, to tell them he passed. A friend who had gone with Benjamin to get the jab, did NOT get it himself, but he had a copy of his immunization card with the lot # of what had been given.

  At that time, the New York City hospitals were not full, but their Emergency Rooms were FULL of vaccination adverse effects, so reporting all of them to VAERS was NOT a high priority. They wanted an autopsy done and waited for six hours to hear what was happening, full of shock and horror. She talked to everyone she could stop, telling them again and again what had happened, because she knew from her past experience with Benjamin's siblings that they MUST get someone to file a VAERS report. She kept at it until someone finally filed one; she was on a mission to be sure EVERYONE knew what had happened. Both the medical examiner and the pathologist said his heart was 'damaged' and he was 'full of toxicology', but they did report the full truth on his death certificate which was very rare. The "COVID-19 shot caused a body temperature greater than 108 degrees!!" They also filed a VAERS.

Pam went on social media two days later and posted exactly what had happened to Benjamin, because she wanted the truth available to all; that her son had taken one COVID-19 J&J jab and died less than 12 hours later of anaphylaxis and cardiac arrest. He had worked two jobs, was incredibly fit, and was both PCR negative and influenza negative. He had NEVER been sick with anything until the jab!! Pam was censored for reporting her own personal real experience that was labeled as misinformation; incensed and incredibly frustrated she started four different Twitter accounts. They didn't ban his death certificate but remained totally independent of Ben's story, while her husband was vocally 'on the ground real' with everyone he met about their story. With the given lack of any accountability or liability for Pharmacy companies, the grief and frustration were magnified. Pam stated the figures printed in *Forbes* showed Pfizer's 2021 revenues had increased by 95%!!

Pamela was asked how all of this made her feel. She declared that these billions of dollars of profit from the 'vaccine' debacle produced so much anger and it sometimes comes in and out in waves. The systems for compensation, as if there could ever really be compensation for the loss of a child, are worthless. There is no financial help from these companies and rarely from the federal government. Billions of dollars of 'blood' money were made because of the "greed-monster criminals" who will probably NEVER even

> do prison time for negligence, mass malpractice and murder. Some people still say that adverse events are "necessary sacrifices for the greater good" and he "took one for the team," almost as matter-of-factly as if they were speaking of simple every-day events. This attitude and the platitudes would NOT just enrage Pam and her husband, but literally wish that murder was an option. However, she stated that it would also empower her to keep on 'keeping-on.' What an utterly sickening and insensitive thing to say to anyone, let alone a victimized parent.
>
> Worse yet, Pam's husband was fired from his media job for saying that his son died from the COVID-19 'vaccine!' The whole thing is clearly NOT over, even when it's supposed to be "OVER!" Broadway refused even to allow her husband back into his work area to collect Ben's locker contents and tools. Greater than 400 people came to 'Celebration of LIFE service and heard all the details. Pam stated that wherever they are, it still feels like 'the elephant in the room" atmosphere, but at least it's an open 'secret.'[20]

Many other performers have also been 'vaccine'-affected, but most are simply too afraid to talk about it for fear of losing their jobs. In 2024, despite the world basically moving on post-COVID, nothing about these issues is OVER! The government and Big Pharma have all swept damages under a very big rug, but there is NO way it will ever go away, when the issues of greed, control, power, money, and lack of any integrity or morality continue. The 'VACCINES" are still avidly pushed, and the misinformation about them blatantly repeated everywhere. Advertising is as noxious as ever because it's ALL based in deceit. In addition to the COVID-19 'vaccines', there is constant positing of the probability of the next big infection contrived to do exactly what COVID-19 was invented to do, with new drugs and 'vaccines' made exactly the same way, that will be the focus of the next big distraction to maim and kill more people and perpetrate the intended New World Order, brought to you by the Globalist Wolves that have NO intention of stopping any of this until their goal has come fully to fruition.[20]

Detoxification of the Blood/Body from Vaccines or Other Poisons

Once again, we need to return to the wonderful, morally and ethically conscientious physicians and practitioners who have emerged, mostly post-COVID-19 to help heal the victims of vaccine damage. We now look at some of the most tried and effective treatment modalities being used and if possible, why they are working. In the same video "The End of COVID-19" we've mentioned, is another section on this necessary detoxification. Dr. Ana Marie Mihalcea, PhD was one of the presenters on this subject, and the question was asked, "What is happening to Humanity's Blood?" Collectively, the reality is most people do NOT have the mostly untainted blood they were born with, because in our current world environment, there are constantly higher levels of environmental contaminants that should be carefully monitored for our protection, but part of the monitoring process should be both personally and medically cared for as well. "The Environmental Protection Agency (EPA) of the federal government has a "Report On the Environment" (ROE) that shows a total of 80+ Indicators to help answer 23 questions in five theme areas including: Air, Water, Land, Human Exposure & Health, and Ecological Condition. The indicators are simple measures but they help track the state of the environment and human health over time. They are based primarily on measurements of physical or biological conditions within a clearly defined geographic area. Human exposure to environmental contaminants can be measured in the ambient environment (air, water, land), at the point of human contact, or after contaminants have entered the human body through entry portals such as eyes, skin, stomach, intestines, or lungs. There are many different approaches used to measure or estimate the extent of possible human exposure, any of which might be helpful in determining what toxicities a person has encountered."[21]

Dr. Mihalcea said we need to be monitoring human blood regularly for toxicity; whether they are vaccinated or unvaccinated toxicity in some form is a given for everyone. We can only imagine, from what we now know about 'vaccines', just how bad it could look if a person has been vaccinated. Blood was once checked for parasitic issues that are still pertinent, but today, human blood is often far too acidic, and contains features of hydrogels. Heavy metals can be found in abundance both from environmental exposure and of course from 'vaccines.' These can be readily cleared with chelation treatments—blood cleansing with medicine done intravenously, to bind the metals in the blood and remove them through urination. There is a long list of potential metal culprits, including: aluminum, antimony, arsenic, barium, beryllium, bismuth, cadmium, cesium, gadolinium, lead, mercury, nickel, palladium, platinum, tellurium, thallium, thorium, tin, tungsten, and uranium. Each has known reference points of what is allowed, mostly what isn't. The creatinine level of the blood is an indicator of blood toxicity and a high level shows the kidneys are NOT doing an adequate job of clearing it from the body.[22]

Another major problem with the 'vaccines' in particular is that red blood cells are clumping, then clotting; the consistency of the blood begins to take on the appearance of a soup-like sludge, and it's very difficult for hemoglobin to do its proper oxygenation to all body cells. Blood flow can be severely impaired. Aspirin, a traditionally used and easily available blood thinner, is worthless to alleviate the problem. Fibrin is elevated where blood is clotting and blood thinners do NOT help lower the fibrin levels. History of vaccination, along with appropriate blood tests, and pathology of red cells must be done to help ascertain the real cause. Another thing found in blood smears is amyloid and hydrogel formations of a peptide sequence (not from the spike protein). It is a plastic-like, toxic polymer and is completely NOT dissolvable. It can be treated with a specialized form of chelation, EDTA acid chelation which can successfully dissolve this AI-formulated, magnetic hydrogel weapon.[23]

Since we know that the vaccines often cause or contribute to serious neurological issues, with or without symptoms, but especially if symptoms do exist, a functional electroencephalogram (EEG) should be done to determine cause, because an MRI will NOT show damage caused by toxins. An EEG will show low electrical activity in the brain with dementia-like symptoms and the appearance of brain aging by as much as 25 years. A neurologist might diagnose it as early to moderate dementia, due primarily to mitochondrial dysfunction in brain cells. It is autonomic dysfunction, so standard allopathic testing will NOT find the problem. Consequently, one's own primary-care physician could easily miss it and start doling out drugs.[24]

Postural orthostatic tachycardia syndrome (POTS) is another disorder of the autonomic nervous system that can easily occur with toxic damage. It is characterized by abnormally large increases in heart rate upon sitting or standing from a flat position. It can cause a wide variety of symptoms, partially depending on the brain area damaged most. Potential symptoms include: light-headedness, brain fog, visual disturbances, weakness, fatigue, headaches, heart palpitations, exercise intolerance, nausea, diminished concentration, tremors, fainting, coldness, pain, numbness, and tingling of extremities, chest pain, and shortness of breath. Other more severe symptoms include: myalgic encephalomyelitis / chronic fatigue syndrome, migraine headaches, Ehlers-Danlos syndrome (one of 13 connective tissue disorders) asthma, autoimmune diseases, vasovagal syncope (a type of serious dizziness), and mast-cell activation syndrome. POTS symptoms are often treatable with lifestyle changes such as increasing fluids and electrolytes, salt intake, compression stockings, gentle and slow postural changes, avoiding prolonged bed-rest, medication, and physical therapy.[25]

Many people present with what is known as a low lifeforce/ feeling no energy, completely zapped and unable to feel any energy to work with. It is more often seen in folks with "long-COVID" and we now know is often seen in people who received "shedding" from other people or circumstances. Viral shedding is very real and

NOT at all uncommon, as previously touted. Some have been overexposed to the virus by perpetual PCR testing and retesting alone. Other individuals who took the COVID19 'vaccine' experience toxicity from another vax component we know as graphene. Scientists now know with certainty that vaccines produced a graphene-induced embryonic toxicity, that caused stillbirth, fertility problems, and other reproductive issues; very toxic to all reproductive tissues. Graphene is a carbon-based substance consisting of a single layer of atoms arranged in a honeycomb flat nanostructure known for its double bonds. As such it is known for its exceptionally high tensile strength, electrical conductivity and transparency, making it the thinnest two-dimensional material in the world, and on a microscopic scale the strongest material ever measured. That is very important to understand, because it was clearly used in the 'vaccines' for all of those reasons! The global graphene market is booming in the millions because of its intense demand for the research and development of semiconductors, electronics, electric batteries and composites, not to mention production of 'vaccines!'

In the form of graphene oxide, this 'adjuvant', according to all the manufacturers propaganda was used in the COVID-19 'vaccines' "to improve antigen immunogenicity and promote long-lasting immunity...It's properties, such as large surface area, water stability, and high aspect ratio, made it a suitable candidate for delivering biological substances. Due to the limited functionality of some approved human adjuvants for use, the development of new all-purpose adjuvants was urgently required...research on the immunological and biomedical use of graphene oxide (GO) indicates that these nanocarriers possess excellent physicochemical properties, acceptable biocompatibility, and a high capacity for drug loading. However, GO injection can lead to significant oxidative stress and inflammation."[26] This information about a known toxic substance was written and quoted exactly, the National Institutes of Health (NIH) actually admitted it to be a disruptive oxidant that 'could' cause inflammation! Well, of course it does, but we're going to use it anyway, even though it DOESN'T "improve antigen immunogenicity or promote long-lasting immunity" since neither of those things are true of the 'vaccine' either! As we said above, it also kills babies!!The vaccinated person showing graphene poisoning in their blood obviously needs something to neutralize its toxicity first.

So, fulvic acid and humic acid, natural compounds taken from soil, are a natural antidote for graphene, and have been successfully used to treat this problem. These are naturally-occurring substances used as herbal supplements, like mushrooms, that also give immune and brain health benefits. A naturopathic doctor might add other supplements, including antioxidants since the body experienced severe oxidative stress to mitigate the damage of graphene from the 'vaccine.' Many natural substances obtained from various plants and plant derived formulae, known as flavonoids or polyphenols, as well as plant-based foods we may eat often can be used very safely and effectively to restore our bodies to their correct mode of operation, and help neutralize toxins in our bodies. They are used globally and have been used for millennia in many cases. They are either eaten of taken as supplements, teas, elixirs, etc. This author used many of them under the direction of natural medicine practitioners to first detox, and then heal from long-COVID issues very effectively, so this is NOT a pie-in-the-sky approach. Two other groups of natural chemical plant substances known as phenols (polyphenols are many in the same source) and flavonoids (types of phenols). These have been used widely to help neutralize and correct the damage done to our bodies by the toxins of both the disease and the 'vaccines.' "They are also health promoting as well as disease preventing. There are more than 8,000 phenolic compounds naturally occurring from plants—half of these are flavonoids. They are proven effective antioxidants, anticancer, antibacterial, cardioprotective agents, anti-inflammation, immune system promoting, skin protecting from UV radiation, and more. Since a few decades ago (even long before needing it for COVID-19 mitigation), research studies focusing on flavonoids and other phenolic compounds from medicinal plant species have increased considerably, because of their versatile benefits for human health, (not to mention their effectiveness without drug side effects!)"[27]

So many of these compounds have been shown to be naturally potent for treating Long-COVID, Vaccine Injuries, Vaccine Shedding, and Acute COVID prevention and recovery. There are also the compounds known as peptides which are like little protein chains in our bodies. Since the COVID illness and the COVID 'vaccines' (made from the causative SARS-CoV-2) cause such frightful tissue damage, peptides are used to help repair cellular and tissue damage, especially naturally produced peptides. "One of the first examples of peptides discovered was insulin, a peptide containing 51 amino acids, the building blocks of those and the larger proteins. A very large number of synthetic drugs are made to act as peptides today, but natural forms will always be preferred by purists. The problem is the lack of enough naturally-occurring sources for products like insulin; hence the synthetic versions. Nonetheless, they are valuable assets for treating hundreds of issues. Peptides such as Quercetin, Hesperidin, and Luteolin are especially good anti-inflammatory agents and antioxidants, that help reduce the free radicals (particles that harm and even kill cells and cell membranes). It should also be strongly considered that eating nutritionally sound foods can deliver much of the necessary amino acids, peptides, and proteins needed for healing. These noted peptides are also considered anti-aging and can help heal cognitive brain injury. In a way, you can't go wrong, because peptides are necessary electromagnetic donors, meaning they can provide the electrical ionic transfer (charge or spark) needed to help the body move particles throughout our bodies. There are peptides within every system of our bodies specialized to do their work, a very complicated, but exciting field of biochemistry.[28]

Various anti-aging peptides useful in repair processes are mentioned here to validate the importance of these compounds, most of which have long, very complicated names so we use well-recognized acronyms for easier management:

- **Epitalon—*anti-oxidant used to repair DNA*.** Its natural source is the pineal gland, but is synthetically derived from epithalimin. It activates the telomerase enzyme to help elongate the telomeres, thereby causing anti-aging effect. Telomeres are protective structures at the ends of chromosomes made up of repetitive DNA sequences. They prevent chromosomes from fraying or sticking together, which helps maintain the integrity of genetic information during cell division. The longest telomeres are the most protective of age damage. Also called Thymalin.[29] It is also very helpful for degenerative brain and eye disease.
- **GHK Copper (glycyl-histidyl-lysine)—** "the human tripeptide has the potential to positively influence gene expression, essentially 'resetting' the activity of genes in a cell towards a healthier state by regulating various cellular pathways, potentially leading to improved tissue repair and overall health, particularly in the context of aging and disease." It can restore approximately 4,000 genes, about 30% of the human genome, back to health, and also has an anticancer effect. "During human aging there is an increase in the activity of inflammatory, cancer-promoting, and tissue-destructive genes and a decrease in the activity of regenerative and reparative genes. GHK declines also with age, but replacing it does a myriad of reparative functions as well."[30]

Russian scientists have been charged by their leader Vladimir Putin to work diligently on studies promoting the longevity of their people. Khavinson, a leading Moscow professor in particular has spent decades studying anti-aging peptides. There was a specific four-week study done on a group of 90-year-olds using GHK Copper. It claimed to have reversed age by five years, repaired right ventricular heart function, improved heart pumping strength, especially significant in patients with myocarditis, reset the pancreas, and stabilized blood sugars, in a remarkably short period of time. In another study of elderly, GHK regenerated brain tissue 500 to 800%. In patients with symptoms of various dementias it is necessary to start with an EEG, extensive blood pathology, and full nutritional support, to ascertain the degrees of progress made.[31]

- **Vitamin C**—Building the immune system in the elderly is extremely important to help protect them from excessive acute infections and the biggest boon to that building has been shown to be the use of high doses of Vitamin C. Up to 90% of elderly patients demonstrated scurvy-like symptoms due to this lack. Dosing can be up to 10,000 mg as tolerated, remembering that it is a water-soluble vitamin and must be replenished daily. It is also an electron donor.

- **NK—Nattokinase and LK**—Lumbrokinase; These are naturally occurring proteolytic enzymes, meaning they can cleave the bonds in certain proteins. Since we know that many patients, both those who had COVID and those who took COVID 'vaccines' have had severe blood clotting issues due to the spike proteins causing platelet activation and adhesion. They can be treated with anticoagulant therapies and that was a standard part of prophylactic hospital protocol for COVID patients, and for the natural destruction or breakdown of fibrin holding clots together before they could cause more trouble.

  Untreated/unchecked clotting often results in pulmonary embolism, deep vein thrombosis, myocardial infarction, cerebral venous sinus thrombosis, and stroke. These enzymes have been used for centuries in Japan for heart disease. They also have anti-inflammatory properties. Since fibrin is an insoluble protein, it must be broken down to be removed from the system. Additionally, analysis of data by the WHO shows increased clot risk (especially ischemic stroke, CBST) after the mRNA spike protein vaccines which was significantly higher in comparison to the influenza vaccines. The body makes its own Plasmin or Plasminogen primarily in the liver and it circulates in plasma, but the Nattokinase is about four times more potent than plasmin alone and yet still works naturally and more efficiently.[32]

- **GSH or glutathione**—is an antioxidant peptide also made in the body's liver and circulates everywhere, instrumental in protecting against free radicals, peroxides, and heavy metals. "Research has found that GSH can also inhibit human platelet aggregation (clotting). Research has also shown that COVID-19 or associated 'vaccines' decrease GSH synthesis…Decreased GSH leads to a cascade of events, including an inability to mitigate oxidative stress (creating free radicals) and a subsequent increase in platelet activation that contributes to micro-clot formation. Therapies which serve to increase levels of GSH serve a protective role in acute and long COVID as well as vax injured patients."[33] GSH supplementation for these patients has proven beneficial, and the research study backed that usage. GSH is also essential for the immune system's proper functioning and is vital in building and repairing tissues.
- **NAC or N-acetyl cysteine**—Use of high-dose (1000mg DMG); "NAC is an antioxidant glutathione analog and detoxifying agent promoted for medical conditions and pulmonary disorders to alleviate symptoms and can reduce mortality by as much as 50%. Its anti-inflammatory effects work especially well for respiratory support of acute symptoms, and decreasing the excess of mucus production. It is involved with neuroprotection and treatment of neurotoxicity, often in acetaminophen toxicity and in Parkinson's disease. It can alleviate chronic inflammatory pathologies, including any post-viral illnesses, and oxidative stress. Augmentation with GSH is sometimes needed to

boost its effects. The latest research indicates it can protect type-2 diabetics against heart-related pathologies and helps reduce creatinine levels in kidney disease. It has also been proven useful to treat CO poisoning."[34]

- **NO or Nitric Oxide**—Most of us are already deficient in this compound! It is important as a toxic-defense molecule against infectious organisms because it regulates the function, growth, and death of many immune and inflammatory cell types including macrophages, T-lymphocytes, mast cells, neutrophils, and natural killer cells. It increases blood flow to healing areas and reduces blood pressure, thus accelerating wound healing. It is highly effective in opening up blood vessels in the lungs that improves oxygen levels. NO is also a great neurotransmitter of the nervous system and helps send messages all over the body. It should NOT be used without medical supervision because it can be overdosed in other body systems. Much of the food Americans eat frequently depletes NO, but symptoms of depression, fatigue, poor vision, high blood pressure, and memory loss may indicate a lack of NO, particularly post illness. Normally, NO can be easily replenished with a diet full of leafy greens, dark chocolate, walnuts and seeds, beets/beetroot, citrus fruits (vitamin C), watermelon, and pomegranate, but supplementation is easier. NO gas has proven very effective in treating acute COVID-19, but we know that "the mRNA vaccines damage endothelial cells and stiffen arteries, along with a prominent increase in ALL inflammatory markers, especially after a second dose. If there is known endothelial dysfunction and/or clotting abnormalities with low plasma arginine levels, as well as the known graphene, additional NO is indicated. There are also nutritional supplemental support products that when taken will markedly increase the production of NO, especially if the oxygen saturation has been compromised."[35]

- **Various, naturally-occurring supplements** have been utilized for a variety of regenerative reasons as follows:
- **Fisetin or tetrahydroxy flavone**—a **natural flavonoid** found in strawberries, cucumbers, apples, onions, etc. for brain regeneration. It's neuroprotective and cognition-enhancing, enhances object recognition, promotes neuron survival, maintains good mitochondrial function in the presence of oxidative stress. It has exciting potential to reduce age-related decline in brain function, and improve cognitive and behavioral performance."[36]
- **Black Cumin (thymoquinone), Curcumin/Turmeric, Indian**
- **Frankincense, Sweet Wormwood, Boswellia, and Artemesia**—many examples of herbal sources for their anti-inflammatory properties. They are all very effective, however, one may work more efficiently in one person than another and vice versa. As with most natural substances, the user needs to give more time for action than he would to a drug substitute.
- **Methylene Blue**—"an **ultra-violet blue dye** acts as a small molecule inhibitor for protein-to-protein interactions (PPIs), in this case the interaction between the SARS-CoV-2 spike protein and the protein ACE2 receptor which is the first step for viral attachment and system entry. When activated by light, methylene blue inhibits this interaction of the virus's spike protein with the ACE2 receptor. Therefore, it is anti-viral in action, even in the absence of light by blocking this attachment. Better yet, this dye is safe, inexpensive, and readily available. Obviously, with the myriads of spike proteins circulating in the body of a sick or vaxxed person, the more you can prevent this interaction from occurring, the less damage the spike protein can do."[37]

- **EDTA (ethylene diamine tetra acetic acid)**—is the solution used for chelation therapy, generally done intravenously to detoxify the blood of heavy metal poisoning and other toxins. It binds to them enabling the liver and kidneys to dispose of them more readily. This solution, when used with glutathione and vitamin C, is one of the few things found so far that can break down the hydrogel of the COVID-19 vaccines. This type of therapy is especially pertinent for symptoms and illnesses related to neurotoxicity, where gradual removal of the toxic agents can significantly improve the physical prognosis of patients. "There are officially at least 21 heavy metals now considered toxic and most of these are known to induce neurotoxicity. Chronic exposure to lead, for example, induces cognitive dysfunction. Others can modulate the metabolism of energy cell signaling and cell membrane composition, as well as antioxidant and cellular detox systems. There can be damage to both the short and long-term memory. Aluminum has been shown to kill neurons. Nickel has been found in the brain tissue of patients affected with multiple sclerosis and autism. Several have been implicated in inhibition of DNA repair. Air pollution, exposures to radiation and/or electromagnetic fields, pesticides, chemotherapy/drugs, and various pathogens all contribute to the unprecedented environmental toxicity we all are exposed to regularly, and now, the intense exposure to toxic vaccines has multiplied this."[38]

Consider Well-Documented Alternative Health Modalities

Many good medical researchers and scientists have returned to their studies to rethink the values of alternative methods of medical treatment that were known for centuries, even millennia. Folk remedies, tribal lores, and early "medical practitioners actually did learn about things that worked, even when they didn't necessarily know exactly why they worked. When you look at the lists of drug therapies today, you will find that chemists started with tried-and-true plant-based substances and synthetically reproduced them to use for treating some of the same problems; often not nearly as effectively as what God created, and also containing far more side effects or subsequent problems.

One such substance we all know about is Nicotine. Granted, people have smoked it to attain its benefits, and everyone knows smoking is bad for your health. Tobacco contains 7,000 different chemicals, many of which are toxic and cause cancer. However, apart from cigarettes, nicotine has many medicinal properties. The brain functions on neurotransmitters that communicate with its neurons. They help regulate various body functions, as well as memory, learning, focus, and handling stress. Nicotinic acetylcholine receptors stimulate our 'feelgood' neurotransmitters like serotonin and dopamine (like an antidepressant for one).

But guess what? Spike proteins use the same receptors in our body as the nicotine uses. So, those who understood how simple nicotine works, decided to use it in tablet or gum form, and it doesn't take much, to use up the ACE2 receptors and block them from the spike proteins. It has worked like a charm for many postvax patients. Another interesting development that arrived about the same time as COVID-19 vaccines, was a big ad campaign telling all smokers that now was a 'great time to stop smoking!!' Of course they did, because they already knew how well nicotine worked to block their toxic spike proteins! Ivermectin as a COVID treatment also worked like nicotine; one of the many big reasons for banning its use as a treatment. Remember, if they had a treatment that worked, they couldn't bring out another drug to use under the Emergency Use Authorization law![39]

Because the Ivermectin could be used the same way as nicotine, another doctor, Dr. Stella Immanuel began using it for cleansing and rebuilding or repairing the damage done with five consecutive doses. In addition, as a woman of faith, she recommended the fully spiritual side of healing by claiming scripture, especially Psalm 103:12. She said that consenting to the vaccine, which is inherently poison and part of Satan's domain, it was a good idea to take that consent back from him, and repent of it as sin, because God "removes our confessed sin as far as the east is from the west." Once she knew the full list of ingredients in the vaccine, this gave an indication of what things could be used as potential antidotes. If the label ever told you what NOT to do or take after the jab, that was also a good indicator of what might work! [40]

One of the best professionals this author has studied is Dr. Henry Ealy, ND. This man was vaccine-injured years ago himself and has suffered a lifetime of seizures. He had to dig deeply into all that he knew, what he still needed to know, and did it with a great measure of faith in God. First, in terms of healing, Dr. Ealy recommends that each of us "get 'heart-centered and love-focused about the entire COVID debacle and adds it's OK to be angry or upset but be sure the anger is focused on the criminals. The most depraved and evil people that have ever lived are alive and well today. So many individuals were coerced and deceived by these criminals, but we cannot blame or shame the injured; grace must be given and shown. Many found themselves in a lose/lose situation; we can help them by showing kindness and compassion just as much as with our efforts to help them heal physically. Then, be sure that those who are seeking help NEVER take another jab."[41] As Dr. Ealy explained, the average medical student in an allopathic school of medicine receives just 19.6 hours of basic nutritional instruction. It cannot be said in any way that this amount of nutrition education is adequate for the proven importance of good nutrition for good health. Since nutrition is assuredly becoming increasingly key to wellness and healing, good nutritional therapeutic options based on a foundation of solid nutrition are absolutely necessary to practicing adequate medicine. Dr. Ealy has an extensive, high-level education in nutrition of over 20,000 hours. Vaccine-injured people have significantly declined and good nutrition is mandatory.

As a great naturopathic doctor, Dr. Henry knows the necessity of having every fact available about the patient, to make the clearest decisions, and plan the best protocols for that individual. He says it's so important to set the whole case up correctly, knowing what has and has NOT yet been done. It requires vigilant questioning and clarification of those questions. Then the body MUST be nutritionally prepared and detoxed BEFORE the sequential application of therapeutic interventions. There must be solid energy production at the cellular level. This is an extremely time-consuming process requiring constant monitoring and tons of patience. The results or an extremely vaccine-injured person always show well when done this way. There are very few doctors of allopathic medicine that can even come close to this type of healing. Dr. Ealy will NOT be hurried or badgered about the time and attention he gives. This is how medicine should be done, and sadly, it is NOT happening.

One of Dr. Henry's COVID vaccine-injured patients is Liana Rivers, the CEO of the company, Wellness Inspiring Spiritual Health. She didn't feel a personal need to take the jab, but once again, felt compassion toward all the people around her needing protection. Her first jab didn't feel good, but she continued all her normally practiced good-health practices. However, after the second jab, symptoms were horrible. She became short of breath and had difficulty breathing. She had so much allover joint pain as well as systemic pain she could just barely walk. Of course, she knew it was vaccine-induced. She went severely hypothyroid, such that her doctor asked if she'd stopped her medicine. All of her laboratory figures were sky-high and she 'felt like her whole body was shutting down. Her doctor tried a high-vitamin regimen and 3-day water fasts initially, but every attempt she made at re-introduction of foods failed. Dr. Ealy has an immune-priming protocol and it was used as a cycle four separate times, followed by a detox cleanse. Labs showed notably that she had detoxed a lot of heavy metals and toxins, and was gradually starting to keep food down. This protocol focused on reversing the vaccine injuries at the cellular level (from the foundation outward).[42]

There are now so many good doctors using great natural remedies for all different types of vaccine damage so it's difficult to describe even a majority of them. However, one body of evidence for deliberate poisoning via vaccines has been presented by a large number of doctors and scientists, Studies have been done globally, but specifically in France and Italy. The use of purified snake and shellfish venoms has been done long before the SARS-CoV-2 appeared. Snake venom peptides exactly match that of the spike proteins. No fewer than 34 of these peptides have been identified in the COVID vaccines. Naturally, Big Pharma, and all the 'official' health agencies have vehemently denied 'such a horrific accusation', but the proof is there. The kinds of near immediate reactions of people just receiving the vaccine and even some time later, exactly replicate the cessation of heart and lungs seen in a person who has sustained a venomous bite or sting. We've already discussed the reality of the vaccines being made deliberately as bioweapons. Even more to the point, once this was discovered and widely documented, many of the doctors began treating vax-injured patients with the same kinds of antidotes used to treat venomous snake bites. Just as suspected, the antidotes worked in most cases at least to some degree, depending on how much time had elapsed since the jabs. Over 1200 papers have been written on this, and it is NOT easy to procure them, since 'officials' work constantly to destroy all evidence of poisonings as quickly as they can surface.[43]

Almost all of our astute doctors of vaccine damage make some strong, basic statements for prioritizing treatments. All of them agree that most of the damage begins at the cellular levels and so the beginning of all treatments is at the cellular level first. All natural products are definitely the best options. Biochemical medicine begins with the basic biochemical ingredients of good nutrition. After nutritional considerations, in 1988 Dr. Henry Ealy started his naturopathic practice with various other natural therapies, including ozone, hyperbaric oxygen, intravenous nutrient supplementation, various types of fasting techniques which allows the body that God created to go to work doing its divinely-appointed thing and get out of its way to allow nature to heal it. They began studying the five Blue Zones of the world where the best nutritional substances are found. Stress is a huge factor in slowing healing, so physical activity that is enjoyed is optimal. Learning and fun are hugely important in healing. Participation in a community-based church grows the faith of its participants. Basic health measures such as blood pressure and blood sugar levels are monitored closely, inflammation markers in the blood require appropriate natural substances to diminish it. People in Blue Zones also optimize their fiber intake, which may need supplementation. While in the process of detoxification, it's important to monitor known sources of additional toxicity and decrease or eliminate exposures to those. Examples are heavy metals from fires/grilling often, exposure to toxic plastics that shed toxin and particulates everywhere. If many symptoms are neurological, this is especially important. Children should keep their tonsils if at all possible. Colostrum in breast milk is nature's most perfect food, and it can be utilized from banks in adults who must rebuild their immune systems. Knowing that a whopping 90% of the immune system is in our guts, whatever products we put in them should be carefully monitored for potential allergies, like wheat gluten, and questionable products diminished or temporarily eliminated. Think whole, natural foods as much as possible.

Water sources should be monitored for potential contamination and filtered if possible. Good filters eliminate toxins such as chlorine and fluoride. Anything that offers extra hydrogen to the water shares an extra ion, which aids many body processes. Using hydrogen peroxide in ionic baths is beneficial. Infrared saunas with a niacin flush are restorative. Fulvic or Humic acid, as mentioned previously, neutralizes excessive radiation. Regular exercise, even just good movement of the body is underutilized, as is restorative body alignment. Cleanses are the best way to heal the gut. Healing the mitochondria is of course working at the cellular level to restore the energy factories of the cells. There are several specifically formulated protocols for this including Quick Silver, the Colorado cleanse, the Ayurvedic approach of specific herbs like dandelion and milk thistle using homeopathy. When the gut is functioning as it should, hydrogen gas is created, but it is now known that 97% of the public has some level of gut dysfunction; oxidative stress is tied to gut dysfunction because oxygen is decreased. The importance of additional hydrogen to the gut cannot be overstated as proven. There is a tight connection of the brain to the gut—dosing with hydrogen to the gut showed within five minutes on a brain EEG! As we mentioned earlier, we have the 11 days of immune priming with water fasting and proteolytic enzymes. Currently, much is being done using either radio or electromagnetic frequencies because all disease is thought to be caused by a breakdown of signaling. Frequencies are a huge reason for cells to work correctly or not. Much more research needs to be done on this, preferably without any interference from the FDA and Big Pharma. A natural prebiotic called Tributyrin extracted from butter has been shown superior for leaky guts.[44]

If there were half as much money spent on chemical drug/vaccine-making and that money used to further research on all the great natural processes we already know will work, allopathic medicine could be at least put in its proper place! The gigantic problem that's nearly impossible to rectify, is that once all these patients are 'fixed' naturally, there is NO further need of all the drugs/vaccines, and all the money being made on drugs/vaccines dries up. Globalists, drug manufacturers, and all the greedy "official" health agencies and representatives are NEVER going to be willing to see their billions dwindling away! Unfortunately, it means that all the manmade toxicity will continue because few of us have the billions to stop it. This author hopes you the reader can see some of the many natural, holistic approaches to healing. You can begin to read, study, and research the unlimited possibilities that our Father God has provided freely for us to use and enjoy. Clearly, healing does require a holistic approach, but it's important to realize that one size does NOT fit all. Do you remember the Biblical account of the bronze snake wrapped around a pole? The people had sinned against their God and become gravely ill. But He provided a remedy to heal them. They had only to look up at that snake-on-the-pole and live. Jesus Christ Himself used the picture of that snake in His teaching (John 12:32), and the medical profession used the caduceus (snake on s pole) as their symbol of healing. But, today, the caduceus has been replaced by the dollar sign, and the ancient art of healing usurped by the toxic greed of the globalist wolves of the world and their assistants.

Health and Medicine Has Been Sabotaged and Used For Biowarfare.

In the last chapter, we looked at the standard ingredients of the COVID-1 vaccines, but for a better idea of the sum of all ingredients potentially used in all vaccines, there are no fewer than 15, and all 15 of the following are not only identified, but the toxicities and allergies are given:

- **Aluminum**—known to *cause* brain damage at all dosing levels and linked to Alzheimer's disease, dementia, seizures, autoimmune issues, SIDS, and cancer. This TOXIN accumulates in the brain and causes increasing damage with every exposure.
- **Formaldehyde (Formalin)**—known to cause cancer in humans. Probable gastrointestinal, liver, respiratory, immune, nerve, and reproductive system TOXIN. It's been banned from injectables in most European countries.
- **Beta-Propiolactone**—known to cause cancer. Suspected gastrointestinal, liver, nerve and respiratory, skin and sense organ TOXIN.
- **Gentamycin Sulphate & Poly-Myxin B (antibiotics)—Allergic reactions** common for antibiotics can range from mild to anaphylactic, (life-threatening).
- **Genetically Modified Yeast, Bacterial and Viral DNA & Dairy/Egg**

- **Components(GMOs)**—can be incorporated into the recipient's DNA and cause unknown genetic mutations. Eggs and dairy are linked to many allergies.
- **Glutaraldehyde**—Toxic if injected, how would it NOT be toxic if injected? Causes birth defects in animals.
- **Latex Rubber**—can cause life-threatening allergic reactions.
- **Peanut & Soybean Oil**—linked to nut and soy allergies.
- **Human & Animal Cells—Human DNA from aborted babies and animal DNA**. Cells harvested from pig blood, horse blood, rabbit brains, dog kidneys, cow hearts, monkey kidneys, chick embryos, calf serum, sheep blood and more have been verified from labs. It has been linked to childhood leukemia and diabetes.
- *Mercury (Thimerosal)*—One of the most TOXIC substances known to man. Even if a thermometer breaks, the building is cleared and HAZMAT is called for safe disposal. Tiny doses cause damage to the brain, gut, liver, bone marrow, nervous system and/or kidneys. It has been linked to autoimmune disorders and neurological disorders like Autism.
- **Monosodium Glutamate (MSG***)*—a TOXIC chemical that is linked to birth defects, developmental delays and infertility. Banned in Europe.
- **Neomycin Sulphate (antibiotic)**—it interferes with vitamin B6 absorption which can lead to epilepsy (seizures) and brain damage. Allergic reactions can range from mild to anaphylactic (life-threatening).
- **Phenol/Phenoxyethanol ($_2$PE)**—TOXIN used as antifreeze. Toxic to all cells and capable of destroying the immune system.

- **Polysorbate 80 & 20**—Known to cause cancer in animals and linked to numerous autoimmune issues and infertility.
- **Tri (N) Butyl Phosphate**—Suspected TOXIC to the kidneys and nervous system.

The question everyone should be asking themselves with reference to ANY vaccine is: "Is the risk worth the touted benefits that have been outlined for us by the medical community?" Since, the 'official' medical community was so adamant that every infant and child should be fully vaccinated according to the established "schedule" every parent MUST be asking some PERTINENT questions of their children's physicians. You have the RIGHT to Informed Consent, so "asking for the vaccine inserts is NOT a question that should elicit a shaming response from the doctor or any of his/her staff. If it does, find a new doctor posthaste!! Here are three other questions that will clarify the decisions you must make on behalf of your children:

- Why would a parent of a vaccinated child be afraid of an unvaccinated child, if vaccines worked for providing immunity? If their answer is to 'provide herd immunity, well...there are two parts to the immune system. When a vaccine is injected, it artificially stimulates one part of the system while inhibiting the other part; Cell-Mediated immune system and Humoral immune system. Therefore 'vaccines' throw the whole immune system off balance. "Herd immunity cannot be created artificially!"[45]
- If vaccines are safe and effective, why does it declare, ON ALL 'VACCINE' INSERTS, that each 'vaccine' holds the potential to KILL or PERMANENTLY INJURE all vaccine recipients? If they say it doesn't, they haven't read the inserts for themselves!
- Are the companies that make the 'vaccines' held responsible for deaths or injuries? The answer to that question is a clear

and resounding, "NO!" Shouldn't all manufacturers back their products 100%?

Naturally, in most normal allopathic medical practices providing a plethora of vaccines for their patients, these questions will make them very nervous and defensive. They do not have the ability to answer them honestly, and it's very upsetting to them. Just remember, there is a myriad of good honest information available from many antivax sources, and your decisions will have a potentially profound effect on the lives of your children.[46] If you share this information wherever and whenever you can, it will also have a potentially profound effect on the lives of all children—it may even save some lives!

After all that we've discussed about the pandemic, the globalist agenda, Big Pharma, and the extreme toxicities inherent in the vaccines and drugs continually pushed and propagandized to us all, can you, dear reader, begin to understand the enormity of the potential damage that the Governmental/Industrial/Health Complex has done not just to the United States, but globally? It is clear, that all of health and medicine has been sabotaged, reconfigured, and repurposed to be used at ANY given time and place, at the will of the globalist complex for whatever part of the agenda needs it. It is called biowarfare!! It was already enormously successful as such BEFORE the COVID-19 pandemic, and though everything about it did NOT go completely as planned, the lion's share did work, and next time will work even better to aid whatever part of their agenda needs another push. Many of the rules of healthcare and medicine have been revised or destroyed. For example, it has ALWAYS been standard operating procedure to treat an illness as early as possible, knowing that this was the best option for healing and even survival. That was NOT the case with COVID-19 treatment once the 'official' narrative changed. There was a long-understood rule of the FDA that if a vaccine or drug proved dangerous or lethal to many people under the EUA, it would be immediately pulled off the market and investigated. With

COVID-19 and with Remdesivir, the rule and tradition no longer applied. Instead, it was the greatest mass exercise of poisoning ever conducted.

Upwards of 5 billion people globally (of approximately 8 billion), now higher, had at least one suicide shot. The odds of an injury or death were just like playing Russian roulette. The "virus" was not natural, it was manmade in a lab—could be called a Frankenstein virus. The 'vaccine' is NOT a vaccine, but a GMO-like product. After all of this lab-driven manufacture, we wound up with a gamut of unexplained travesty, including super tumors of cancer, some rarely ever seen. Infertility reached an astronomic high. All body systems have been affected, yet the global propaganda rolls on with the well-established lies of "safety and effectiveness." No greater lie has EVER been so well-marketed. We now know that biotechnology has the ability with all of this to use mass poisoning of our air or water sources with conotoxins, animal venoms chemically synthesized, contaminated food sources, and toxic aerosolization. Reality is that for most of these toxins, there are no specific antidotes available. Up until COVID-19 'vaccines', anything suspected of being a bioweapon was outlawed after WW2. Those laws have since been mostly ignored. Consequently, the potential for biological weapons to be used in terrorism is a real possibility. Other manmade pathogens are being developed constantly. All toxins are poisons produced by living organisms. We remember the ricin scares. Unlike pathogens, toxins do NOT produce an infection. Almost all are carcinogens. According to Dr. Ryan Cole, "naturally developing cancers generally take years. All of us have 30 billion T-cells in our bodies that find and break up atypical cells. With spike proteins, those regular processes for finding and breaking up bad cells are knocked out or suppressed. The vaccines start a 'cellular wildfire.'" It has become almost a necessity for our physicians to regularly monitor or surveil our immune systems to see if they've been hit exponentially already and had done so even before COVID. In light of all these things, what else can we citizens be doing to help protect ourselves from so many possible hazards?[47]

We know that our personal levels of body toxicities have been elevated exponentially!

There are a number of modalities that naturopathic doctors and scientists suggest as prevention possibilities. Some of the same things they are using to treat damage, can also help prevent damage. For example, the American public has become very lax in its regular consumption of a balanced healthy diet, filled with whole organic, and sourced foods. We know that a diet like this can be very expensive, especially for larger families. None of our best foods have the quality of the past, our food sources have all been heavily challenged. The subject of supplementation of needed nutrients is controversial, but this would be a great time to learn how to better supply some of our own through gardening, herbal supplementation, foraging, and learning some of the valued skills of our past. There may come a day sooner than later when a lifestyle of such may be necessary to survive. We can all do better with our food choices, and we need to give it some careful consideration. It has become absolutely necessary to take personal responsibility for our own health in every decision we make. We need to understand that the global agenda calls for the deaths of as many global citizens as possible—called depopulation. The ongoing 'vaccine' agenda was placed for that purpose and continues unchecked.

We must decide if we will allow ANY further poison jabs into our bodies, because each one contributes to the overall summary of toxins in our bodies. Reality tells us that even one more jab is foolish and possibly deadly. Americans have far more co-morbidities than the global populations because our lifestyles enable them. Co-morbidities and toxic 'vaccines' are a highly deadly combination. In addition to the 'vaccines', Americans swallow 40% of the world's drugs every day and that is no accident either! They cause liver and kidney failure over time and America has the highest numbers of people on dialysis globally.

"The United States spends more on health care than any other high-income country but still has the lowest life expectancy at birth and the highest rate of people with multiple chronic diseases, as well as the highest obesity rate according to a new report from the Commonwealth Fund, an independent research group. The report...says that compared with peer nations, the US has the highest rates of deaths from avoidable or treatable causes and the highest maternal and infant death rates. Americans are living shorter, less healthy lives because our health system is not working as it should be...to catch up with other high-income countries... the administration and Congress would have to expand access to health care, act aggressively to control costs, and invest in health equity and social services we know would lead to a healthier population. In addition, deaths caused by physical assaults were higher in the US compared with all other peer countries. 100,000 people died in the US in 2020, at least seven times higher than the 2.7% average deaths from physical assault, including gun violence, which occurred at a rate of 7.4 deaths per average in most high-income countries. We are NOT getting the best value for our health care dollar."[48]

"Biological warfare is defined as the intentional use of living organisms such as bacteria, viruses, and fungi with the intent to cause disease, death or environmental damage. Pathogens were classified by the CDC into categories A, B, and C based on ease of transmission, severity of morbidity and mortality, and the likelihood of their use. Category A bio-agents can be easily disseminated or transmitted from person to person, resulting in high mortality rates, and have the potential for major public health impact. This might cause public panic and social disruption, and require special action for public health preparedness. Most of category A agents are considered especially dangerous due to the potential for airborne transmission. Category B bio-agents are regarded as moderately easy to disseminate, may result in moderate morbidity and low mortality, and require diagnostic capacity and enhanced disease surveillance. Category C bio-agents include emerging pathogens that could be engineered for mass dissemination because of availability, ease of production and dissemination, and have the potential for high morbidity and mortality and major health impact.

Toxins are harmful proteins derived from living organisms...owing to their high toxicity, ease of production, and ease of dissemination; there are several toxins regarded as possible bio-terror agents."[49] Given this small bit of information, along with all the evidence presented in this book, and all of the evidence that has surfaced in multitudes of sources since the pandemic, we MUST pay attention! There is simply no doubt that the SARS-CoV-2 virus causing COVID-19 and the associated 'vaccines' made from the same gain-of-function viral pathology/technology, was clearly intended to wreak havoc on humanity then, and forevermore in the future.

Because the nucleic acid (DNA or RNA) of many viruses, including some that are currently not yet known threats, can be manipulated in the laboratory, the potential for genetic engineering remains a serious threat. Biotechnology, which has had a tremendous impact on the development of medicines, vaccines, and technologies needed to counter the threat of naturally-occurring disease, can also be used to modify viruses with unintended consequences or even for the development of novel biological agents. An example involving genetic engineering of viruses is the Mousepox Virus. When researchers investigated virally-vectored, immuno-contraceptive 'vaccines' based on the ectromelia virus, they found mouse pox was causative agent. They recreated a recombination of the virus by genetic engineering to enhance the antibody response. Instead, it altered the host's immune response to the virus resulting in lethal infections in normally genetically resistant lab mice, even those previously immunized against the virus. This led to speculation that similar genetic engineering performed on a different 'pox' virus would create a biological weapon effective against an entire immunized population! Viral agents are extremely prone to genetic variation and mutation, and can be manipulated or created in the laboratory. Unlike bacterial diseases, there are far fewer medical countermeasures to employ when dealing with viral infections.[50]

In the case of the public health 'officials' insisting on COVID-19 vaccination of infants and small children, who are dying in large numbers every day because their immune systems and their nervous systems are never fully developed before the age of three. Worse, just as in the case of abortion, these children have no choice and no voice to thwart this obvious abuse. Mark Crispin Miller, an academic writer from News From the Underground, wrote an article entitled, "In Memory of those who 'died suddenly' in the United States and Worldwide, November 18-25, 2024." He has been doing this tally every week for years, so the public can put faces to the numbers of people that in all likelihood died from getting vaccines. Most of them are infants and very young children, so it's clear their expectant mothers had received the 'vaccines.' Mr. Miller clearly feels the need to summarize the numbers, ages, and any known circumstances listed in a bit of detail so that you, dear reader can begin to grasp the enormity of the 'vaccine' casualties from the United States and Canada in just one week's time! Just one week's worth is so sadly stunning, it absolutely breaks the heart of the reader. This author has seen hundreds of infants who, though she believes they are with Jesus, thinks of those devastated parents and prays for them by name. It's a reality that isn't going away! The articles are printed on his Substack. should you be interested.

In almost every single reported case, the victims "died suddenly" and there was "no cause of death reported." In the US (on this particular week) there were almost 70 deaths in adults from ages 15 to 50 years, the higher majority being less than 35 years. Many were still in their teens and early 20s. Most of these had been 'vaxxed' because of college mandates for admission or military mandates for those entering a military branch. In adults older than 30 and deceased, there were 3 nurses, 5 policemen, 3 firemen, 2 paramedics, 2 educators, and 2 coaches; 9 were killed in 'vaccidents', meaning they had been vaxxed and died of accidents in cars, in water, at work, etc. There were even 3 deer hunters and 2 prison inmates, all within this week of time. Once again, it was known and proven in each case that these adults worked in various jobs that demanded they be vaccinated. Pregnant mothers were instructed to get vaccinated to protect themselves and their babies. In that same week, 62 infants died before they were 6 months old, showing the massive toll this has taken on our mothers and children. Of this number of infants, approximately one third were stillborn or lived just hours. Only one other infant that died lived longer than one year. All 'died suddenly or in their sleep' and 'there was no cause of death reported.' Canada had even more deceased adults, but with similar percentages of those under 50 years. Infant deaths were fewer but percentages of stillbirths and infants under 6 months were similar. In addition, 33 other countries tended to report teen and celebrity deaths mostly, but for all the same reasons. The pandemic lasted three years, and the constant push for mass COVID-19 immunization never diminished. This was due to the clear fact that these 'suicide shots' should never have been allowed to continue, and have never come near to being fully rescinded. The facts of the known adverse events are still almost completely ignored, and the misinformation, is still being perpetrated on the worldwide web.[51]

The reality is that due to all of the various aspects of potential biological weaponry, there is nothing remaining that cannot be created in the biotech laboratory today. The things that were once dreamed up for mass destruction and called science fiction are no longer fictitious. That fact has clearly been proven with the advent of COVID-19. Now that advanced biotechnology and the entire field of genetic manipulation have become everyday concepts, there is no longer any conceivable way that evil perpetration of these abilities, along with the existence of artificial intelligence can be realistically regulated. It has become a Pandora's box, full of the potential to destroy all of mankind with very little effort. Viruses are simply toxic proteins that can be created with AI by the millions. Animal proteins are also toxic to human molecular structure, particularly venomous proteins. Following is the proof of this concept as cited, "The venomous Agent X, or VX, is a deadly nerve agent, an amber, oil-like liquid that can viciously attack the body's nervous system. A single drop on the skin can kill within minutes. In 2017, North Korea is believed to have used VX to assassinate

Kim Jong Un's estranged half-brother in a Malaysian airport. Kim Jong Nam suffered severe paralysis and died in about 20 minutes from this weapon of mass destruction."[52]

"In Geneva, Switzerland, Sean Ekins and his team thought of this VX toxin for a possible experiment needed for a last-minute presentation deadline at the Spiez Laboratory's conference examining how developments in science and technology might affect chemical and biological weapons regimes. As a scientist and CEO of Collaborations Pharmaceuticals, he and colleague Fabio Urbina wanted to flip their AI software, MegaSyn and instead of steering it away from toxicity, try to guide the model toward toxicity. They 'trained' the software with some 2 million molecules from a public database and modeled it for specific, toxic traits. In just 6 hours, the AI generated some 40,000 molecules that met the scientist's toxic criteria, meaning that based on their molecular structure, they ALL looked like toxic chemical agents. The AI designed VX and other known toxic agents and also designed entirely new molecules the scientists had NOT programmed for, creating a sketch for potentially lethal and novel toxic chemical compounds! The team had used only open source, publicly available data, only tweaking the models a tiny bit. Ekins and team were horrified! What they had thought was a silly experiment ended up creating a cookbook for chemically toxic agents—almost anyone could do the same."[53]

Granted, VX is a banned substance and even if it were available, its only reason for existence is to kill. That, however, is not true for many things found in nature, like a virus, or even our own DNA. The experiment did get a lot of attention, particularly among those worried about unregulated biological and chemical warfare. It showed how easily the concept could be applied to almost anything existing around us, and how impossible to tightly control them. It only takes one or a few evil actors with malevolent intentions. As previously discussed, the Biological Weapons Convention (BWC) of 1975 prohibits the production, use, development, stockpiling, of transfer of biological toxins or disease-causing organisms against humans, animals, or plants. This treaty has not always been honored by the 180 signees, and now, in today's hyper-volatile geopolitical scene with this advanced technology, it is clear that this treaty of 50 years is being strained and tested regularly as never before. It is also extremely difficult to determine if any one geopolitical entity is merely involved with their own biological defense mechanisms or are they involved with using the same offensively.

The Citizens' Defense Against All Potential Biowarfare—Awareness

Since there are no official regulations on toxic proteins such as animal venoms, they are and have been used in a wide variety of products for decades. Venom peptides are commercially available online for purchase! The CIA has used them in a variety of ways for a very long time. One way, for example, was revealed to the world in the 1970's and captured the public's imagination—'the heart attack gun.' It was a 'Cold War weapon used for targeted assassinations. "There was almost nothing the CIA wouldn't do to get a leg up on the Soviet Union, from simple operations like intercepting and reading the mail of American citizens to more serious (and equally illegal) acts like dosing 'unwitting, non-voluntary human subjects' with LSD and seeing how well they would hold up to interrogation. We know about these secret efforts because Congress investigated the agency, as well as the FBI, via the National Security Agency (NSA) and IRS, in 1975 it released its findings to the American public. The results of that investigation were, to put it mildly, alarming."[54]

In the early 70s, a Senate Select Committee, led by Idaho Senator Frank Church, studied Governmental Operations with Respect to Intelligence Activities, and became known simply as the Church Committee. A whistleblower revealed the US Army was spying on American citizens at home, and then the discovery was made that the CIA had been spying on Americans suspected of being foreign agents for decades. Incidentally, this was all a mere flash in the pan compared to today's constant surveillance on all of us. The Church

Committee rapidly uncovered the CIA's massive assassination program that had been targeting most anti-American leaders such as the Congo's Patrice Lumumba, Rafael Trujillo of the Dominican Republic, Ngo Dinh Diem of Viet Nam, General René Schneider of Chile, and most famously, Fidel Castro, the dictator of Cuba, who actually survived numerous CIA attempted assassinations! The problem was that attempts to kill world leaders, couldn't look like assassinations!! The CIA MUST find a perfect, undetectable weapon, and found it in shellfish. The extremely potent conotoxin was also a neurotoxin that could be extracted, frozen, and fired from a pistol, killing the target very rapidly with what appeared to be a heart attack. The weapon looked like a Colt M1911 pistol with a scope that fired ,45 caliber toxic frozen pellets silently up to 100 meters away, entering the body through a mere pinprick wound. Interestingly, the Soviet KGB also had a very similar weapon. This all was NOT just shocking because of its ability, but because President Richard Nixon had ordered a ban on biological weapons in 1969 and ordered the CIA to destroy its stockpiles of toxins but the CIA Director Gordon later claimed he never received such an order. Enough of this toxin to kill 5,000 people eventually found its way into a storage room at the CIA headquarters.[55]

Given that such capabilities have been available for over 50 years, and technology is widespread, humanity is in constant danger of potentially poisoning itself. In addition to these capabilities, there are literally tens of thousands of chemical and biological agents being produced every day of our lives. The large-scale production of toxic pollution grows exponentially and regularly and there are no "safety zones" where any of us can live unaffectedly. Though it may not always be instantly noticeable, it doesn't change the fact that our world has been irreparably altered by all the toxic substances that have permeated our air, soil, and groundwater. It has become a global travesty of massive proportions, yet the global community focuses almost ALL of its surveillance efforts on climate change that has never been a real or global threat. As believers in Jesus Christ, climate change is NOT something we need to worry our heads over, but poisoning ourselves is an area for which we should be mindful for many reasons. As citizens of our God-given planet, we do have responsibility to be good stewards of that for which He has entrusted us. Let us take a brief look at the ten major sources of human pollution that we can indeed become more mindful of, not just for the health of our planet, but for the health of every person on it.

In descending order, from least to most important, here are ten of the most important concerns we all must be aware of:

- **The Toxic Byproducts of Computer Waste**—electronic waste is amassing faster than it can be dealt with. Affluent countries create far more than their share of it, then illegally import it to third world countries by means of "donation." But this waste contains lead, cadmium, arsenic, other dangerous substance, and small amounts of precious metals like gold. People, including children, melt the waste down to get to the sellable precious metals, creating viciously toxic fumes and massive air pollution.
- **Massive Amounts of Toxic Waste are Dumped Down our Sinks, ultimately polluting sewage and water supplies**. One enormous culprit is unused prescription drugs dumped down sinks and toilets, but also heavily excreted in human waste. Scientists are becoming more gravely concerned about this ever-increasing toxicity and its effect on public health. Many chemicals are found in drinking water supplies and water treatment facilities; with no way to remove these contaminants—buildup continues.
- **Mercury Poisoning is now a Global Crisis**. There are ever-increasing amounts of mercury, a potent neurotoxin, in even our largest bodies of water. Fish are affected, as we can be if we eat many large fish. The largest source of contamination is coal power plants, which flush mercury into surrounding water sources. The amount of

contamination is NOT diminishing. Discussion of the problem is always about limiting the amount of pollution—not on eliminating it.

- **The Decades Legacy of Lead Paint Continues to Haunt us**. Lead paint was banned in the 70s, but has always remained a problem because it only prevented its use in new construction, but did nothing about the lead poisoning that had already occurred. Previously built homes (before the 70s) still have lead paint, often buried under layers of newer paint. Homes built before the 30s often still have lead pipes. Owners of such homes must disclose knowledge of it to new buyers, but they don't have to fix it—process is very dangerous and expensive. Worse yet, poorer nations still use leaded gasoline. Lead dust and tiny pieces of lead paint are very harmful to children if eaten. Professional disposal is highly recommended.

- **Petroleum 'coke' is Poisoning the Lungs of Chicagoans and others globally.** Residents of Chicago near the Calumet River are exposed to this black byproduct of refining tar sands oil. The dust is greasy and very hard to wash off, traveling on air currents. "Pet coke" is even dirtier to burn than regular fossil fuels, so most is exported to countries like China. This byproduct has not been safely placed in covered storage and is exposed to open air. The oily black dust particles float in the wind of "the windy city." It makes for vicious coughing and trouble for lungs. Regulations are still tardy and easily avoided. The only real relief for those exposed is moving away from it.

- **Asbestos Lawsuits Continue**. It was once utilized heavily as insulation in homes and even large office buildings. Then it was discovered that exposure to its tiny airborne fibers can lead to a form of cancer called mesothelioma that kills rapidly. 1930s findings were largely ignored until the 1960s before being accepted by scientists. By that time a large number of people were heavily exposed. Those who believed their cancers were caused by asbestos sought legal compensation from companies who failed to act on the data. Asbestos suits have been filed now for well over 500,000 people and the cost of resulting litigation at about $1 billion. Some asbestos was placed in a product called vermiculite that was used to pad playgrounds and walkways, also keeping the suits going.

- **Nuclear Waste continues to Pollute our Groundwater and Soil**. Many people believed nuclear power would be the panacea leading us away from 'dirty' energy like coal, while others continue to fear accidental global annihilation. While nuclear power's safety record is actually excellent and incidents very rare, there is still a waste problem. Dangers of radioactive compounds in our drinking water and soil remain serious because of their long-term ramifications. A plutonium facility in Washington was shut down in 1987 for a cleanup process and is still ongoing! 67 of 177 storage tanks are leaking and more will be falling apart soon.
- **Fracking is Ruining our Water Sources**. The term for hydraulic fracturing for extracting natural gas is a form of mining. It uses a combination of water, sand, and chemicals under extremely high pressure to loosen shale rock thousands of feet below the surface, allowing access to the natural gas. The process touted the ability to make energy independence possible for many nations, but it has some serious problems also. There are many cases where fracking polluted nearby water sources. Water can actually be set on fire due to high methane content. Substances like radium and benzene have been found. Some towns near fracking sites have become unlivable. It does also pollute the air around it—one town in Texas found neurotoxins in the air at levels 55 times the recommenced safe amount.

- **The Notorious Ganges River in India is a model of Horror.** Its importance to the people cannot be exaggerated because it is considered "HOLY" by Hindu faith, besides being a vital water source for millions of Indians. The river is so extremely polluted, it's probably too late to be rectified. The millions who rely on it also use it for improper purposes, one being multiple cremation sites on the banks where ashes dump directly into the river. Worse, there is extreme pollution from metallic and other compounds as well as massive electronic waste. Even worse is human and animal waste. Estimates say about 3 billion liters of this waste makes its queasy way into the Ganges every single day, almost all of it untreated. Many farmers are not managing their pesticides while draining water levels. The travesty and utter filth of this river rivals the hopelessness of the bubonic plague in the Middle ages!
- **China's Pollution Problem in its Entirety is Analogous to a Really Bad Sci-Fi Movie.** When Beijing hosted the Olympics, the stories of this problem were legendary. The CCP attempted to cover it up as much as possible for visitors' sake. Beijing is just one major city in China with severe pollution problems, many are far worse. Wearing masks in China is nearly universal and NOT because of COVID! Last year, one city of nearly 7 million people had 129 days of their 365 days when the air quality was so bad it was deemed an emergency. In Xingtai, nearly one-third of their year was spent closed inside due to the incredible air toxicity.[56]

While noting the severity of global poisoning in the above ten ways, we haven't begun to list the remaining tens of thousands of toxic sources in today's world. We tend to think that if we don't live in a huge city of multimillions, we breathe what seems like mostly pure air, our water tastes decent, and we are reasonably careful about the things we live with, we are probably fairly healthy. The reality of that assumption is that it's probably not very accurate. Environmental toxins we don't know about and rarely see or feel, still affect our health. The exposure to endocrine disrupting chemicals (EDCs) in the environment is anywhere and everywhere, or omnipresent. Our endocrine system includes different glands—like the thyroid or pituitary glands—that produce hormones that help regulate body functions. Toxins are artificial chemicals that interfere with the proper functioning of those hormones. "EDCs cause disruption at the cellular level at any point during the hormonal process, from the gland that produces the hormone to the tissue that receives it and many points in between. Studies have linked EDCs to cancer, heart problems and reproductive concerns. We are unknowingly exposed to hundreds of EDCs every day—they are truly everywhere. We know of nearly 800 chemicals that are suspected to be hormone disruptors, so it is definitely safe to say they have become a global health crisis. Our daily touchpoints may include: Air bags, cigarette smoke, cosmetics, foods, detergents, packaging, plastics of all kinds, toys, appliances, fabrics, etc. We know these chemicals are in our bodies because studies detect EDCs in blood, urine, and breast milk—they accumulate over time through consistent exposure to tiny amounts."[57] Research shows EDCs likely play a role in ovarian, prostate, and breast cancers and can disrupt any stage of biological reproduction. There is also evidence that EDCs are linked to diabetes, heart disease, and obesity.

How can we begin to identify and avoid so many environmental toxins? Realistically, we can't, however we can be thoughtful consumers of what we place on or in our bodies and make the effort to decrease or even eliminate known exposure. Many manufacturers are making intentional efforts to avoid known chemical problems. That trend will continue as consumers demand more natural products by buying from responsible producers. "The Environmental Working Group is a trustworthy resource for information and offers consumer guides. When choosing products, look for labels that read: Paraben-free, Phthalate-free, and BPA-free. Drink tap water or filtered water rather than bottled water as tests show bottled water often contains harmful chemicals and bacteria. Avoid pesticides and additives by choosing organic foods when possible. Choose natural cleaning products for your home. These three areas will decrease exposure to chemicals immediately."[58]

Another set of highly damaging chemicals began as PFCs and are now called PFAs (polyfluoroalkyls). One such was the PFOA type used to make the original Teflon, made by DuPont. The company dumped its waste containing the chemical into the Ohio River near Parkersburg, W.Va. for decades, polluting the air and drinking water of tens of thousands of people. As part of a settlement, Dupont funded a study to find out if residents had been harmed by the chemicals. In 2012, its major conclusions were published online and found damning. Evidence from blood samples and health surveys showed a link between PFOA and high cholesterol, ulcerative colitis, thyroid disease, testicular cancer, kidney cancer, and pregnancy-induced hypertension. It reduced antibody counts in vaccinated children. Even today, many Americans, even physicians, are not familiar with PFAs. However, Jamie DeWitt, a professor of pharmacology and toxicology at the Brody School of Medicine at East Carolina University said, "People ARE dying," and citing a report in The Lancet added, "It calculated that about nine million people each year die from chronic diseases caused by environmental pollutants of all kinds. We need prevention, and that means acknowledging that environmental exposures do lead to diseases."

"Over several decades, increasing numbers of Dupont employees and local residents began exhibiting increasing health issues including birth defects as PFAs were detected in the tap water of three additional nearby communities. Eventually, the chemicals were present in virtually everyone in the area, The revelation was basically met with a collective shrug by federal health officials and policymakers. This year, more than 2,800 domestic locations are confirmed to be contaminated with the PFAs—now they are deemed **forever chemicals**, because they don't go away. According to the EPA, tap water typically accounts for only about 20% of a person's overall exposure to these chemicals; we also eat them, inhale them and rub them on our skin. Testing by governmental agencies and watchdog groups have found PFAs in carpets, furniture, nail polish, shampoo, mascara, nonstick cookware, dental floss, raincoats, fast-food wrappers, pizza boxes, microwave popcorn bags, yoga pants, sneakers, sanitary pads, tampons, menstrual cups, bedding, upholstery, children's pajamas, paint, vinyl flooring, and artificial turf. They're in the protective equipment used by firefighters and medical personnel...They are in dust, and the cleaning products used to get rid of the dust. They are in flamingos in the Caribbean and plovers in South Korea. They are in alligators, and Antarctic snow. They've been found in organic eggs, produce, meat, and freshwater fish. They have been found in 45% of tested private wells and public water supplies of our nation's tap water!"[59]

It may seem that this author is a bit over-focused on the degree of toxicity in average, normal-living Americans, but that isn't possible. This author survived a severe bout of COVID-19 illness, only to have it extend into what has been termed "long COVID." It was NOT understood for a number of months until health status became dismal. A consultation with integrative medicine STARTED with a full-body determination of personal toxicity. There was NO history of COVID vaccine, no use of tobacco, alcohol, or recreational drugs in 70+ years, and no known excessive exposures to the multitude of toxicities possible, yet the reports of personal toxicity were extreme in all categories. Thus ensued an 18-month period of full body, supplemental detoxification and nearly perfect nutritional support to attempt a return to a new normal. Time does not allow a complete description of all the body systems' maladies, but suffice it to say, it was a baffling conglomerate of physical malfunction in a medically-trained and health-conscious person who strived for the best health possible before succumbing to COVID-19. It was simply impossible to understand how so much had gone so wrong with the best of health intentions. The answer was massive amounts of cumulative toxicity! As an avid believer in Jesus Christ, the Great

Physician, it was so difficult to accept how badly this earthly house had been betrayed, but through it all, came so much understanding and yes, spiritual growth, that led to writing this book. The Master, through His still small voice, persisted in calling her to write about the things He wanted so many more to learn and understand about these last three years in all our lives.

Many of you dear readers may have a clearer understanding of all potential toxicity than this author had, but if you have experienced a huge lack of physical, mental, emotional, and yes, spiritual health in these last 3+ years during and after COVID-19 and all it brought to humanity, Jesus would have you understand that He wants to restore you to a level of health that hasn't seemed attainable. This author's prayer is that everything you've read here will bring you that desired blueprint for healing. To continue with the investigation on potential toxicity in your life, look closely at your own home and environment. The internet is full of helpful information on how to discover what may be making you sick. Listed here are 35 of the MOST TOXIC household items hiding in our homes along with super-safe alternatives. No home is completely and utterly non-toxic! It's a challenging task but well worth the effort. Be aware that many harmful ingredients may be hidden under unrecognizable or generic terms or disguised by appealing packaging. Also keep in mind that this is an ongoing process of exchanging the toxic for the healthy, and may take some time and budget changes, but that's perfectly fine. Do your inventory, and stay informed about all the products you purchase for your home. Many great alternatives exist. This is not a complete overhaul, but adopt a fun and gradual replacement strategy.

In most of our homes, one of the most potentially toxic groups of items is house-cleaning products. We want our living spaces to be clean, hygienic and fresh-smelling without the health risks of the chemicals they usually contain. Household chlorine bleach is a cheap, reliable, and powerful disinfectant, but it can easily irritate eyes, skin, and respiratory systems. If it is mixed with other chemicals such as ammonia, it can release highly toxic fumes. Other options are ammonia, phthalates, and triclosan but these have been tied to hormone disruption (as above) and antibiotic resistance. The most common household toxin is formaldehyde, a colorless gas with a strong, pungent odor, found in furniture, paints, fabrics and even cosmetics. Its vapors can irritate eyes, nose, and throat and can definitely contribute to respiratory distress. Prolonged exposure has produced more severe health issues and an increased risk of certain cancers. Following is the list of 35 most toxic items in your home:[60]

1. **Non-stick Cookware**—overheating Teflon pans may lead to the release of (PFOA) perfluorooctanoic acid that is a potential carcinogen. Never use them if the coating is scratched or chipped. Consider using coatings like ceramic or stainless steel. Best brands are: Caraway, 360 Cookware, Our Place, GreenPan, and Alva Cookware.

2. **Air Fresheners**—wonderful scents seem so harmless, but many fresheners whether sprays or plugins, release a medley of synthetic chemicals, often volatile organic compounds (VOCs) such as formaldehyde, benzene, toluene, and ethylbenzene. These often trigger headaches, allergies, and asthmatic attacks. Try natural alternatives like essential oil diffusers or homemade room sprays for lovely scent without compromising health. Best Non-Toxic freshener brands: Aera, Enviroscent, Fresh Wave, Grab Green, and Pura.

3. **Scented Candles**—might be one of the most toxic items in your home! Artificial fragrances are similar as for the air fresheners. Prolonged exposure may even pose risks of cancers and birth defects. Switch to natural candles made from soy or beeswax coupled with essential oils. Best Non-Toxic Candles brands: Fontana Candle Co., Be Ambiance Candles, Meaningful Mantras, Mo & Co Home, and Grow.

4. **Electronic Waste (E-Waste)—***is full of* heavy metals like lead and mercury, and poses serious environmental/health risks. When not disposed of properly, these toxins can leach into soil and water, harming ecosystems. Responsibly recycle through

designated programs. The best place to sell or trade electronics is Gizmogo where electronics can be sold or cash.

5. **Furniture**—pressed wood pieces often contain formaldehyde. Flame-retardant chemicals are often found in upholstery and can be released as they begin to break down. Buy solid wood or sustainably sourced furniture like bamboo to create a safer home. Best Non-Toxic Furniture brands: Medley Home, Avocado, Maiden Home, Burrow, and Alabama Sawyer.

6. **Furniture Polish**—many commercial ones contain petroleum-based solvents and chemical fragrances—indoor air pollutants. Natural alternatives are olive oil and lemon juice, citrus or wood oils maintain beauty and health.

7. **Plastic containers and Water Bottles**—culprits of chemical leaching. Plastics with BPA and phthalates contaminate food and drinks. Use glass, or stainless-steel containers or labels on plastics that state chemical free. Best Non-Toxic Food Storage and Reusable Water Bottle brands: Caraway, Xtrema Cookware, W & P Porter, TOMO, and Klean Kanteen.

8. **Oven Cleaners—horribly toxic!!** They often contain corrosive chemicals like sodium hydroxide and butoxyethanol, releasing serious fumes that irritate eyes, nose, and lungs. Choose a mixture of vinegar and baking soda or one of many non-toxic oven cleaners. Best Non-Toxic Oven Cleaner brands: Aspen Clean, Delphis Eco, Clean Environment Cleaner, and Truly Free.

9. **Antibacterial Soaps**—the active ingredient in most is Triclosan, that has been linked to hormone disruption. Opt for non-toxic antibacterial soaps or just regular soap and water. Overuse of antibacterial soaps contributes to antibiotic resistance.

10. **Drain Cleaners**—they can kill you!! They contain harsh chemicals like sulfuric acid or sodium hydroxide. Besides causing skin and eye irritation, they pose heavy environmental risks when flushed into water systems. A safer option is a

mixture of baking soda and vinegar and can be done repeatedly without personal harm and will protect our planet.

11. **Bleach**—it's a standard in whitening and disinfecting, but it does contain potent chemicals like sodium hypochlorite and can easily cause both respiratory issues and skin problems. It actually triggers asthma attacks in this author. Gentler alternatives are hydrogen peroxide and vinegar and both are effective and inexpensive.

12. **Cleaning Products**—most conventional cleaners contain a plethora of chemicals, including ammonia, phthalates, and synthetic fragrances. Longterm exposures cause indoor air pollution and numerous health issues. Create your own safe cleaners with lemon or citrus essential oils, vinegar, and baking soda for a clean and sparkling home. Eco-friendly cleaning product brands include: Branch Basics, Everneat, Common Good, Zero Co, Blueland, and many other home sales companies.

13. **Toilet Bowl Cleaners**—chemical cleaners contain caustic substances like hydrochloric acid that irritate skin, eyes, and respiratory systems while corroding the mechanical parts of your toilet system, requiring more frequent replacements. Again, baking soda and vinegar with essential oils will do the job in good health.

14. **Ammonia**—one of the MOST toxic things found in homes. Exposure to ammonia fumes is almost universally irritating to eyes and mucous membranes. Good cleaning is NOT a good reason to jeopardize our health.

15. **Laundry Detergents**—are not the most toxic of household items, but still cause a wide variety of skin and environmental issues in many people. Most contain synthetic fragrances, phosphates, optical brighteners, etc. which can cause skin problems and contribute to water pollution. Gentler, natural ingredients are easier on people and environments.

16. **Dishwasher Detergents**—often contain phosphates and chlorine-based compounds posing skin and eye irritation, and contributing to water pollution. Natural ingredients like citric acid and borax clean hygienically and safely and do not pollute.

17. **Carpet Cleaner**—commercial carpet cleaners often include perchloroethylene and ammonium hydroxide. These irritate skin and respiratory tracts and leave harmful residues in your living space. Steam cleaning with baking soda and vinegar clean and refresh without polluting air.

18. **Hand Sanitizers**—are we shocked? Many contain high levels of alcohol, fragrance and various additives. Despite convenience, overuse contributes to dry, cracked skin that is vulnerable to infection, as well as development of antibiotic-resistant bacteria. Whenever possible, opt for thorough washing with soap and water.

19. **Perfumes**—fragrances are mixtures of synthetic chemicals, including phthalates and allergens. Many people experience skin problems, respiratory issues, and headaches, even migraines. Consider natural use of essential oils and natural ingredients such as goat milk, beeswax, etc. There are many alternatives among private individual sources.

20. **Sunscreens**—especially if containing Oxybenzone, a chemical linked to hormone disruption and coral reef damage. These are necessary for skin health, but opt for mineral-based sunscreens with zinc oxide or titanium dioxide.

21. **Personal & Beauty Products containing preservatives**—such as parabens and formaldehyde-releasing agents that extend shelf life. These induce skin irritations and hormone disruption. Choose sustainable beauty products labeled as paraben-free. Many companies are becoming more health conscious; for example the products this author uses are all aloe-based, healthy and safe.

22. **Nail Polish**—conventional polishes often contain harmful formaldehyde, toluene, and dibutyl phthalate. Prolonged exposures contribute to respiratory issues and have been linked to reproductive problems. Opt for water-based or "5-free" polishes that exclude these harmful chemicals.

23. **Deodorants/Antiperspirants**—especially those containing aluminum compounds and synthetic fragrances. There are 46 recent studies concluded that aluminum IS a risk factor for the development of Alzheimer's Disease. Use products that are aluminum-free with natural ingredients like baking soda and essential oils. This is a small switch that could make a BIG difference in our health.

24. **Shampoos**—especially containing sulfates, another of the most toxic things in our homes. Sulfates strip hair of natural oils and cause scalp irritation. In addition, some sulfates are contaminated with 1,4-dioxane, a potential carcinogen. Look for sulfate-free shampoos.

25. **Menstruation Products**—MOST traditional tampons and pads contain chlorine, dioxins, and fragrances. Environmentally, they can take up to 800 years to naturally decompose. Choose cups, tampons, and period underwear made from organic cotton or silicone with NO additives.

26. **Paint**—everyone likes freshly painted rooms, but the type of paint we use really matters. Traditional paints are by far one of the most toxic items we could use if they contain volatile organic compounds (VOCs), including chemicals like benzene and formaldehyde. The VOCs are released into the air after painting, causing indoor air pollution. Prolonged exposures cause respiratory issues and headaches, and have been linked to other more severe health issues. Choose either low-VOC or VOC-free paints every time.

27. **Antifreeze**—contains a highly toxic substance, ethylene glycol. Ingesting even miniscule amounts can lead to serious health issues including kidney damage, and even death. It's CRUCIAL to handle it with extreme care, if stored—far from children or pets. Immediate cleanup of spills and proper disposal of used antifreeze is mandatory to prevent environmental contamination and safeguarding all water sources. You can stay clear of risk with a non-toxic formula. (Sidenote: Methamphetamine is illegally made using antifreeze—no wonder the damage to health is so great!!)

28. **Dryer Sheets**—also contain a cocktail of chemicals including synthetic fragrances, benzyl acetate and chloroform, a potential carcinogen. These chemicals can transfer onto clothing, then onto skin. Instead, use wool dryer balls free of chemicals, or create your own small sheets using natural cotton fabric and essential oils.

29. **Mothballs**—though thankfully they are not used as frequently as they once were, they too are among the most toxic items in a home. They contain naphthalene or paradichlorobenzene, both of which release toxic fumes. Prolonged exposure leads to respiratory issues, headaches, and in severe cases, liver and kidney damage. If used, use very sparingly in well-ventilated spaces. Best natural alternatives are cedar sachets that protect clothes and people.

30. **Bedding**—when it contains synthetic materials and dyes. Materials like polyester and those treated with dyes often contain harmful chemicals such as formaldehyde and AZO dyes that make up 60-70% of all fabric colorants. This is a place where alternatives may well be more expensive, however organic and sustainable bedding options made from natural, organic materials and free of harmful dyes create a safer and more comfortable sleep environment; about 33% of your life!

31. **Weed Killers**—a huge source of toxicity from herbicides with active ingredients such as glyphosate. Prolonged exposures have been linked to cancers. Additionally, these chemicals leach into soil and water, seriously impacting ecosystems. Courts of law are teeming with suits from victims of such cancer-causing poison, yet the federal government has refused to act on this travesty in a consistent manner. This affects everyone. There are good, alternative weed control methods like manual weeding, mulching, and eco-friendly herbicides that are safely used in gardens. However, large, competitive agricultural concerns refuse to consider most alternatives in favor of increasing profit margins with glyphosate.

32. **Bug Sprays**—often conventionally containing DEET, toxin which can lead to serious health issues and also has serious environmental implications. On a personal level especially, we choose natural bug spray alternatives containing very effective essential oils like citronella, eucalyptus, or tea tree as well as the natural plant sources of these to effectively repel insects without the chemical risks. Mechanical bug killers are very effective.

33. **Fertilizers**—like 'fast food' for plants, when not abused. They contain high levels of synthetic nitrogen compounds that can lead to nutrient imbalances and harm soil health. When overused, they can accumulate in the soil, affecting microbial activity and possibly harming beneficial organisms. The best natural homemade fertilizers for indoor plants contain nutrients like magnesium, phosphorus, potassium, sulfur, and calcium to maintain the health and structure of plants and soil, that produce the most nutrient rich foods.

34. **Flame Retardants**—commonly are used in products like furniture, mattresses, and electronics. However, they often contain chemicals like polybrominated diphenyl ethers (PBDEs) which have been linked to health issues such as hormone disruption and developmental problems in children. Stay safe

from such dangers by buying only flame-retardant-free products or those with labels assuring the products meet safety standards.

35. **Gas Space Heaters**—can emit carbon monoxide and nitrogen dioxide; both are toxic in high concentrations. Indoor air pollution occurs in poorly ventilated spaces and lead to adverse health effects. Proper ventilation MUST be maintained if using gas heaters. Alternatively, use electric heaters and well-maintained central heating systems to mitigated these risks.

Reducing toxicity in our homes is NOT difficult, and not necessarily expensive, but it does take some thoughtful and conscientious effort based on the clear knowledge of its practical necessity. Failure to do so has already cost many of us some previously good health. There are many excellent ways we can reduce the toxicity in our own home environments and thus improve our own wellbeing, perhaps exponentially. We need to make wise choices in our household product purchases, and always look for the most natural alternatives. We can promote good air circulation by regularly opening windows and doors, relying less on central heating and cooling to do it for us. Good ventilation helps remove indoor air pollutants and bring fresh air in. In cases where family members struggle with respiratory conditions and allergies, good air purifiers with HEPA filters that trap airborne particles, allergens, and pollutants, are particularly beneficial. It might even be a good investment in light of less spending medically. A really big difference was seen in this author's home when we stopped relying on plastic products that too-often contained BPA. We use far more glass, sustainable bamboo, and other better, more durable items, especially for food storage.

Here are a few simple ways to begin your process of identifying potentially toxic items in your home. Like many of us, you have no-doubt heard of any number of known dangerous toxicities, but perhaps have not felt the need to pay too close attention to them, or certainly not taken them seriously enough to make needed changes. However, may we urge you, dear reader to begin to take the information more seriously. It certainly matters far more than most of us ever dreamed, but already felt information overload. Become familiar with the common household toxins that may well have residence in your home. It might be old lead-based paint, or asbestos, such as may be found in the older fixer-uppers that are now so popular. Perhaps you have certain plants you didn't know were harmful to children or pets if ingested. Check the labels of all your cleaning products, detergents, and personal care items for the hazardous chemicals we have informed you about. Many will already have warnings or symbols showing toxicity. Pay attention to any unusual symptoms or health issues being experience by family members, including your pets. A sudden onset of new symptoms might well be new exposure to environmental toxicities. A good habit is to regularly check for product recalls—manufacturers issue recalls for products recently found unsafe or containing hazardous materials. If in any doubt, research and ask questions; consult professionals if necessary. The life you improve, or even save might be your own, or that of a loved one.

There are dozens of other types of environmental toxicities having profound effects on more and more people every day. Once again, awareness is the best way to protect ourselves from the ravages of these toxins, making every effort to minimize their effects on our health and lives. Air pollution is one that has become increasingly serious, particularly in heavily populated cities and states. Pollutants are chemicals, biological or physical agents that contaminate our atmosphere. They are found in vehicle exhaust and industrial emissions, as well as those we found indoors. They often contain particulate matter significantly concerning to public health and contributing to serious health problems. Radon is a naturally occurring radioactive gas invisibly produced from breakdown of uranium, thorium, and radium in soil, rock, and water. Continual construction may free this gas that often seeps into buildings from their exterior surrounds. Carbon monoxide is another silent but deadly gas that can be produced from old or faulty HVAC systems in buildings that should be regularly monitored for its existence. Greater efforts have been made to eliminate second-hand tobacco smoke from public places in recent years, but it remains a major health hazard for all of us, and carries increased risk of lung cancer.

"The Safe Drinking Water Act describes water contaminants as anything other than a water molecule. Some contaminants are considered harmful if consumed at specific levels, while others are considered harmless, however, there are four categories of contaminants that may pose potential health risks when found in drinking water. Those categories are physical, chemical, biological, and radiological. Physical contaminants are sediment from lakes, rivers, and streams and can certainly affect its appearance and taste as well. Chemicals can be natural or man-made, including heavy metals, toxins, nitrogen, bleach, pesticides, and drugs. Biological elements are microbes, and radiological contaminants are also chemical elements in the water that are unstable and emit radiation."[61]

One of the major contaminants in our drinking water is the use of fluoride, which was originally added by governmental authority to prevent dental decay, especially for all who could not afford to supplement it to their families. Even at its outset, the governmental overreach in doing this and affecting everyone, was debated and concerning. Now, after decades of using it, concerns of overall health effects on bones, teeth, and neurological development are frequently raised. Over many years, skeletal fluorosis can result in pain and damage to bones and joints, with increased risk of fractures and impaired mobility. It can also lead to parathyroidism causing depletion of bone calcium. In young children, higher blood levels of fluoride were associated with lower scores on IQ tests due to poorer cognition. In 2014, fluoride, along with ten other industrial chemicals, was documented as a hazardous neurotoxin. It has also been associated with:

- Acne and other skin problems
- Cardiovascular problems, including arteriosclerosis, arterial calcification, hypertension, myocardial (muscle) damage, cardiac insufficiency, and heart failure.

- Reproductive issues, such as lower fertility and early puberty in girls
- Thyroid Dysfunction
- Orthopedic problems affecting joints and bones, arthritis, bone cancer, and temporomandibular joint disorder (TMJ)
- Neurological problems, possibly leading to ADHD
- An 'extreme electron scavenger' with an insatiable appetite for calcium leading to significant calcium deficiencies.

Researchers are calling for the balance of risks and potential benefits to be reconsidered. Fluoride poisoning is possible."[62] Most toothpaste manufacturers also include additional fluoride in their products. This ought NOT to be. If this bothers the consumer, seek out toothpaste that has NO Fluoride added. Most health food and supplement stores will carry it.

When high enough concentrations of toxic chemicals posing a risk to humans or to the ecosystem are found in the soil, it is considered polluted. When agricultural practices and industrial waste (man-made) exceed designated levels in the soil, it is polluted. Agricultural pollutants are pesticides, fertilizers, herbicides, and manure. Industrial pollutants from factories, mills, and refineries producing steel, textiles, drugs, glass, cement, and petroleum can easily leach metals such as lead, arsenic, nickel, copper, and mercury into the soil.

"Contaminants from air, water, and soil are associated with a wide variety of health issues affecting respiratory, cardiovascular, nervous, and reproductive systems, and many contribute to cancers. They are important sources of morbidity and mortality of diseases. Chronic respiratory issues of asthma, allergies, COPD, and general bronchoconstriction cause increased coughing, phlegm, and wheezing even in usually healthy people...there is also increased incidence of cardiovascular issues, especially in people with existing cardiovascular risk. The brain is the MOST affected organ from environmental toxins causing developmental delays, cognitive impairment, autism, ADHD and even seizures. Toxins inhibit mitochondrial activity and cause excessive oxidative stress in all systems. Heavy metal contaminants in particular are associated with infertility and hormonal imbalances. A large number of contaminants are cancer-causing agents through radiation and DNA damage."[63]

Another source of chemical contamination that most of us never spend much time investigating is our food supply, a large percentage of which is processed with various and sundry, and unrecognizable chemicals. They are used for a number of seemingly good reasons, but those reasons are generally NOT healthy. Manufacturers and the FDA simply refer to them as "additives." They are added to lengthen shelf life, provide additional flavor, color, or shine, and even supposedly to augment nutritional value. Our foods should obviously be nourishing and safe to eat, but more than 10,000 chemicals are allowed by the FDA in cereals, snacks, meats, and many other types of food sold in the United States. The ***Environmental Working Group*** (EWG) was established in 1993 to "empower consumers with breakthrough research that enables them to make informed choices and live a healthy life in a healthy environment. It shines the spotlight on outdated legislation, harmful agricultural practices and industry loopholes that pose a risk to our health and the health of our environment."[64]

Chemicals like potassium bromate, propyl paraben, titanium dioxide, and butylated hydroxyanisole are just a few of those 10,000 chemicals that we might even read on the product label, but have no idea what they are or why they were added to our food. "They not only provide no nutritional value, but have been placed there LEGALLY. They have not only been scientifically shown to cause harm to the immune and nervous systems, but trigger changes in the body's hormonal balance, and even increase the risk of cancer. Even more concerning, many of these are found in much of the food marketed especially for children. Candies, sugary breakfast cereals and processed snacks like pizza rolls and mini bagels contain food

colorants and preservatives that have NO nutritional or functional benefits and can harm children's health. The FDA does not review most food additives for safety even when studies show known health risks of tested additives. Under FDA regulations, packaged food manufacturers are even allowed to certify their own ingredients as safe without notifying the government or the public. That means that most additives that could be risky to consume have basically never been meaningfully reviewed by the FDA. The European Union has banned various additives that are used in US food products such as potassium bromate, a carcinogenic chemical added to bread and brominated vegetable oil, a flavor stabilizer used in beverages that can harm the nervous system."[65]

To protect your health and the health of your family, it would be very helpful to check out EWG's 'Guide to Food Additives." Now that you know of all the legalized and hidden dangers in your food, which are not allowed in other Western nations, now is a great time to start giving more attention to food labels, especially those of processed foods. Read ingredients carefully and use your phone's search engine to look some of them up on foods you've purchased regularly. The lengthier the food label is, the more likely the product has far too much junk (maybe toxin) in it. Buy products that don't contain the worst additives and choose fresh, whole foods whenever possible. Join other savvy consumers in urging the FDA to take action on this issue by visiting toxicfreefoodfda.org. for more information. Your family deserves wholesome, nutritional food.

Environmental toxicity and its effects on chronic illness is one of the most important health crises facing us today. While adults are certainly adversely affected, our children are being hurt the most. According to Dr. Leo Trasande, "We are in an epidemic of environmentally mediated disease among American children today. Rates of asthma, childhood cancers, birth defects and developmental disorders have exponentially increased, and it can't be explained by changes in the human genome. So what has changed? All the chemicals we're being exposed to,"[66] (not even to mention the travesty of the excessive immunization schedule.)

Once again, the issue of toxicity in our children was most disturbingly reported by the EWG's release of an investigative report entitled 'Body Burden' in July, 2005. Please note that this report is now two decades old and doesn't even touch today's staggering numbers. "The report revealed that 287 chemicals were detected in the cord blood of newborn babies, 180 of which are known carcinogens, 217 of which are known neurotoxins, and 208 of which have been shown to cause birth defects and abnormal development in animals. This result in newborns is unprecedented in human history and laid the groundwork for a dramatic upswing in chronic illnesses both currently and as these children mature into adulthood. Twenty years ago, the cost of managing chronic illnesses in the US alone was staggering with CDC guesstimating the number at $908 billion per year. Three of every 4 dollars spent were spent on chronic illness (in this older healthcare system)."[67] These figures were considered a crisis greater than terrorism with the stated concern of financial collapse of healthcare systems. It was believed that no amount of healthcare reform could ever resolve this catastrophe. What do you think it looks like today? No wonder the global predators have depopulation as one of their major agenda goals! We know that infants and small children are the most vulnerable to these toxicities, they have increased exponentially in every sector or our society, and now we poison them all deliberately with COVID injections and other vaccines, increasing that vulnerability to high risks of morbidity and mortality EVERY DAY. What does our Father in heaven think about this deliberate criminal treatment of our children, not even mentioning the ones being aborted?

> "Behold, children are a gift from the Lord, they are a reward from Him." Psalm 127:3 NLT. The Holy Scripture also gives a clear statement from Jesus Himself about the necessary protection of His children.

> "Jesus called a little child to him and put the child among them, (His disciples). Then He said, I tell you the truth,

unless you turn from your sins and become like little children, you will never get into the Kingdom of Heaven. Anyone who becomes as humble as this little child is the greatest in the Kingdom of Heaven.

Anyone who welcomes a little child like this one on My behalf is welcoming Me. But if you cause one of these little ones who trusts in Me to fall…it would be better for you to have a large millstone tied around your neck and be drowned in the depths of the sea." Matthew 18: 2-6 NLT.

There is no mistaking how God feels about the abuse and murder of His little children.

Additional Toxicities Becoming Increasingly Problematic.

Finally, there are additional toxicities becoming more and more prevalent in these days, many of which are not as well understood as those previously discussed. We do NOT wish to leave these to a simple cursory mention. One of these we've heard about more frequently is MOLD, that carries with it the real dangers of what we now know are MYCOTOXINS. These are toxic compounds produced by certain molds, usually fungi, that often contaminate food and pose many health risks to humans and animals. These are of concern in agricultural products globally due not only to their impact on food safety, but because of economic losses. The various fungi that produce them create unique characteristics and effects. The main types are known as Aflatoxins, Ochratoxins, Trichothecenes, Fumonisins, and Zearalenone.

Aflatoxins are produced primarily by Aspergillus species and are commonly found in crops such as corn, peanuts, and tree nuts that are heavily influenced by their environment, particularly high humidity and temperature, making tropical climates more susceptible. One type (B1) is carcinogenic, especially to the liver.

Ochratoxins, are produced primarily by Aspergillus and Penicillium species. They are frequently found in cereals, coffee, dried fruits, and wine. The most toxic type (OTA) is known to cause damage to kidneys, both carcinogenic and immuno-suppressive. The unusual stability of these ochratoxins under food processing conditions make them difficult to remove, and require stringent monitoring and control measures. Trichothecenes are produced by various species of Fusarium, a group with over 200 different compounds known. They commonly contaminate grains like wheat, barley, and oats. One of its most well-known (DON) inhibits protein synthesis causing a wide range of effects such as immuno-suppression, stomach disturbances like nausea and vomiting, and even growth retardation. They also thrive in cool, wet climates. Fumonisins are also products of Fusarium species, often infecting maize or corn. They disrupt aspects of cellular metabolism and have been linked to various animal diseases, and the potential of esophageal cancer and neural tube defects in humans.

Fumonisin (B1) is a possible carcinogen. Zearalenone is produced by several Fusarium species, and is known for its effects on human estrogen. It primarily affects cereal crops like maize, wheat, and barley. It actually mimics hormone estrogen causing reproductive issues primarily in livestock.[68]

The detection of mycotoxins is a matter of high technology and precision as it's become increasingly necessary to have accurate and timely identification. Traditional methods take a lot of time and expertise and are not suitable for rapid screening. Recently, enzyme-linked assays are relatively simple and faster as they use antibodies to target specific mycotoxins, and they are more accurate quantitatively on degrees of contamination. Global regulatory agencies have established strict limits on permissible levels of mycotoxins in food and animal feed to minimize exposures and protect public health. The trade and marketability of agricultural products is at stake. Mycotoxin research continuously explores strategies for reducing mycotoxin levels, including the development of resistant crop varieties, but caution is demanded to keep product development from using more chemicals to decrease levels in crops. There must also be continuous efforts to use good agricultural practices that minimize the effects of the environment producing contamination. Research also looks for ways to biologically detoxify crops.

Health of humanity and animals is affected in ways as diverse as the toxins themselves. "When present in food, they can traverse the digestive system, interacting with cells and tissues, potentially leading to an entire spectrum of health issues. Some mycotoxins possess properties toxic to the liver, affecting its overall function, and often leading to liver conditions such as cirrhosis or fibrosis. Since the liver is our primary detoxification organ, it bears the brunt of these toxins, which can result in long-term damage if not managed adequately. Mycotoxins can also compromise the immune system, leaving individuals more susceptible to infections and other diseases. The suppression of the immune system is particularly concerning in populations with already weakened immune defenses, such as children and the elderly. The respiratory system is especially affected when mycotoxin-contaminated dust is inhaled. Exposure is very detrimental to one already having pulmonary issues and can lead to any of the chronic respiratory conditions. This route of exposure underscores the importance of proper handling and storage of agricultural products to minimize airborne contamination. Some mycotoxins have been implicated in cancer development due to their presence in cellular pathways. Their potential to disrupt DNA synthesis and repair mechanisms poses significant risks, especially in geographical areas where exposures are frequent and/or prolonged. Endocrine-disrupting capabilities of some mycotoxins can lead to hormonal imbalances and affect reproductive health and development."[69]

Mold growth can occur either before harvest or after harvest, during storage, on or in the food itself and most often under warm, damp and humid conditions. They are toxic when eaten, absorbed into the skin, or inhaled. Even small amounts are dangerous. Poisoning by mycotoxins is called mycotoxicosis. One easy example of exposure is drinking older coffee that grows mold readily. Mycotoxins grow on nuts, cereals, spices, dried fruit, apples, and coffee beans to name a few. They spread quickly in lower-income countries where many of the crops they thrive on are staple foods and there is far less agricultural regulation. They are very prevalent in coffee, but this can be greatly reduced with the proper storage, transport, and processing of the beans. Roasting the coffee is therefore essential. Symptoms are initially about digestion, especially the digestion of proteins. Symptoms are worsened by frequent alcohol use, malnutrition, and underlying diseases.

Mycotoxins grow most on food surfaces, but can penetrated deeply within the food, but they rarely grow on properly stored, fresh food that is dry and clean. This brings us to good prevention ideas. Perhaps you have heard of the "Dirty Dozen"—a list of mainly fruits and vegetables that require good, intentional washing before consuming them. Apples are one of those. Pay special attention to whole grains, dried fruits, and nuts for signs of mold or decay. Do NOT store or EAT damaged grains. Purchase only fresh dried goods, and store them in air-tight containers. Store foods away from insect, warm, and moist exposures. Date foods and don't store them beyond expiration dates. Eat a wide variety of foods. If you travel to areas of the globe where open markets, and less stringent regulations are used to monitor food, take extra precautions with purchases, and ask good questions of travel guides and reputable citizens. According to the WHO, approximately 25% of the world's agricultural products is contaminated by mycotoxins, and they often occur naturally, which makes their existence easier to miss.[70]

Another health hazard that has been the subject of much controversy and concern for many years is CHEMTRAILS. They are trails of visible particles left behind by aircraft in the sky. They were formerly known as contrails and dismissed as merely condensation, but there are serious questions about their composition and potential health impact on the population. "Reports suggest chemtrails contain a variety of elements and compounds including but not limited to the following: barium, aluminum, radioactive thorium and caesium, copper, titanium, silicon, lithium, cobalt, lead, ethylene dibromide, and various pathogenic agents. Each one of these elements has been linked to various health ailments:

- **Barium**—linked to cardiovascular issues, respiratory problems, and gastrointestinal disturbances.
- **Aluminum**—associated with neurological disorders such as Alzheimer's disease and multiple sclerosis.
- **Radioactive Thorium and Caesium**—exposure to radioactive materials can lead to cancers, genetic mutations, and other serious health conditions.
- **Copper**—overexposure can result in kidney and liver damage, as well as gastro-intestinal symptoms.
- **Titanium**—inhalation of particles may cause respiratory irritation and potential long-term lung damage.
- **Silicon**—prolonged exposure to its dust can lead to respiratory issues such as silicosis.
- **Lithium**—though used in psychiatric meds, excessive exposure can have adverse effects on the nervous system and thyroid function.
- **Cobalt**—linked to respiratory issues, heart problems, and skin irritation.
- **Lead**—known to cause developmental delays in children, as well as neurological and cardiovascular problems in adults.
- **Ethylene Dibromide**—classified as a carcinogen, can lead to cancer and respiratory issues.
- **Pathologic Agents**—presence of bacteria, viruses, and others increases the risks of infectious diseases.[71]

There is an almost continuous presence of chemtrails in our

world that raises concerns about the cumulative effects on general public health. With all of the above increased health risks, how can we NOT be concerned. Reality says they are NOT going away, so this begs the question of how they should be neutralized protectively. There is also not just a human effect, but multiple broader implications for our entire environment, including soil, air, and water contamination, which further increases the health risks of both humans and entire ecosystems. Most people believe these risks simply can't be just ignored as so many other viable concerns have been ignored to our collective detriment. Health officials believe further research and greater public awareness are both essential to examine this serious issue and start mitigating the problem of chemtrail before it becomes a crisis in public health.

The list of toxicities in our world goes on and on, and continues exponentially increasing daily with the sophistication of modern man and all of what he believes to be valuable and even necessary amenities to successful living. We can't even scratch the surface as to the vast complexity of man poisoning man, but we will deal with one more exposure that is massive already and growing daily before we stop. That issue is our almost universal exposure to an invisible web of electromagnetic frequency fields (EMF). Advanced technologies have permeated every area of our lives through smartphones, Wi-Fi routers, laptops, gaming systems, electrical appliances and wireless accessories, keeping us constantly "plugged-in." However, like most good things, we have come to realize there are definite drawbacks to this full-time exposure. *Yes*, we now know it IS hazardous to our health and well-being, especially with no caution or mitigation. In 1996 (nearly 25 years ago), the World Health Organization (WHO) initiated the International EMF Project to "assess health and environmental impacts of EMF, encourage focused research to fill the gaps in knowledge, and to facilitate the development of internationally acceptable standards limiting EMF exposure."

"Electromagnetic fields are areas of energy produced by electrically charged objects, categorized into two main types:

- **Non-Ionizing Radiation**—originates from low-frequency EMFs, such as those from household appliances, Wi-Fi, and cell phones, and are generally considered less harmful.
- **Ionizing Radiation**—originates from high-frequency EMFs, such as X-rays and gamma rays, and have enough energy to remove tightly-bound electrons from atoms, which can cause cellular and DNA damage. Even though non-ionizing EMFs are less powerful, their pervasive presence in our environment has raised increasing concerns about long-term, constant exposure. The term 'exposome' refers to the total environmental exposures a person experiences throughout their lifetime. This includes everything from pollutants in the air to dietary habits, and crucially, EMF exposure. As our reliance on electronic devices grows, so does our cumulative exposure to EMFs."[72]

Dr. Russell Kort, known widely as "Doctor EMF," has done massive research and obtained much insight from his own personal experiences. He admits that chronic exposure to EMFs in today's society is NOT avoidable, our entire environment is filled with EMF sources. This continuous exposure grows in our overall exposure and has subtle, yet potentially significant impacts on our health. Many individuals now attribute a variety of symptoms to EMF exposure, including:

- Headaches—often persistent and otherwise unexplained headaches
- Fatigue—chronic tiredness and lack of energy
- Sleep disturbances—difficulty falling asleep, staying asleep, or lack of good restorative sleep
- Cognitive impairments—memory issues, difficulty concentrating, and brain fog
- Mood changes—increased anxiety, irritability, or depressive symptoms

While all these symptoms can be found in other situations and are somewhat nonspecific in nature, they can and do significantly impact daily life and overall wellbeing. Additionally, long-term exposures have been linked to far more serious health conditions though research continues and can be controversial. Potential risks are:

- **Cancer**—Studies have shown possible links between EMF exposure and certain types of cancer, especially brain tumors.
- **Neurological Disorders**—There are increased risks of neurological diseases, including Alzheimer's and Parkinson's.
- **Cardiovascular Issues**—Potential impacts on heart health include hypertension and arrhythmias.

Definitive causal relationships are difficult, often challenging to establish, *so the precautionary principle says minimizing exposure wherever possible would certainly contribute to better health.*[73]

Given the pervasive, constant exposure to the ever-expanding products we use that we know emit various levels of EMF frequencies, wisdom says that protecting ourselves from all these potential exposures is important. There are suggested strategies to mitigate EMF exposure without much negative effect:

- **Limit Device Usage**—Reduce the amount of time spent on electronic devices, especially an hour or more before sleeping.
- **Optimize Your Living Space**—Arrangement of your home's spaces can help minimize EMF exposure. Use wired internet connections instead of Wi-Fi. As far as possible, electronic devices should be distanced from sleeping areas.
- **Use EMF Shielding Products**—Increasing numbers of products have been designed to shield against EMF radiation; examples are protective cases for smartphones and EMF-blocking fabrics and blankets.

- **Create EMF-Free Zones**—Designate specific areas in your home or office, like the bedroom, or a lounge at work that promotes EMF-free sleep or rest from exposures.
- **Monitor EMF Levels**—Use an **EMF meter** to check the levels of radiation in your home or office and identify "hotspots" that need to be addressed.

The potential dangers of EMFs and their impact on our health are recognized more every day. By our understanding of the problem, being willing to recognize potential symptoms from overexposure, and taking responsibility to minimize the potential exposure and health risk, we can protect ourselves and our families. We can strive for balance and be sure we get plenty of restorative sleep every night. It is possible to find that balance of enjoying the benefits of modern technology while minimizing their possible risks to good health.[74]

Identifying Globalist Hype vs. Real Health/Life Threats

To draw this chapter to its appropriate finish, it is important to show you, the reader, there are myriads of potentially hazardous things in our lives, and we have very little say about them or the addition of the scores more that show up every year. It is impossible to be aware of every one of them, and it's also impossible to know how much of our environmental toxicity is created or manufactured deliberately. The real bottom line in our world is knowing that globalist elite predators remain alive and well. We know beyond the shadow of doubt that one of their major global goals is actual depopulation of our planet to ensure it will be more manageable to govern in the New World Order. There is absolutely no doubt that the vaccine agenda, the unchecked proliferation of the COVID injectables that killed hundreds of people every day, including infants and small children, the corruption of Big Pharma and the FDA in perpetrating the crimes against all of humankind, and the other agendas that help promote them are all being successfully masterminded to that end. Therefore, we must first understand that this worldwide travesty is set to continue and we can't stop it. When we read Scripture thoroughly and study its fulfilled prophecies, we know that those yet to be fulfilled in 'the last days' as we know them, will be fulfilled just as surely. Humankind has run completely amok in its godless perversions and our Father God has already told us He will be the final judge.

A New World Order has not been planned for in a vacuum, and though the Globalists and all their wicked cohorts think they have it all planned to their liking, our God had it planned several millennia ago. Time and space will NOT allow for all of the facts but here are a few that will thwart all the best efforts of those who believe they will be in charge! There will not be a cabal of power-hungry leaders to run this show as they have planned!

> "A king will arise, insolent and skilled in intrigue. His power will be mighty, but not by his own power, and he will destroy to an extraordinary degree and prosper and perform his will; he will destroy mighty men and the holy people. Through his shrewdness he will cause deceit to succeed by his influence; he will magnify himself in his heart, and he will destroy many while they are at ease. He will even oppose the Prince of princes, but he will be broken without human agency." Daniel 8:23-25 NASB

Long before man was created, there was God who first created His angels. One of those, Lucifer, whom we know as Satan or the Devil, decided he would be just like God, his Creator, which of course God would not allow. Satan and a third of the angels were banished from God's heaven, and thrust to Earth, but Satan's greatest ambition has been to rule the world. God is going to allow him that attempt, but it is slated for complete failure. However, to do this, he must first persuade all the nations to cast aside their own nationalism and their differences and come together for the "common good of all." (Have we heard that statement somewhere before?) It's the same spirit behind the World Economic Forum (WEF) and the European Union (EU). We don't know if Satan will utilize any of these groups to achieve his goals, but they've got a mighty start with Satan's constant maneuvering even now, not to mention the mighty men and women of Satan's own forces that have already been operating toward that end for several centuries. One thing is certain—a world empire will form and this Antichrist King will be ruling over it through the power of Satan himself.

> "Then the man of lawlessness will be revealed, but the Lord Jesus will slay him with the breath of His mouth and destroy him by the splendor of His coming. This man will come to do the work of Satan with counterfeit power and signs and miracles. He will use every kind of evil deception to fool those on their way to destruction, because they refuse to love and accept the Truth that would save them. So God will cause them to be greatly deceived, and they will believe these lies." 2 Thessalonians 2:8-11 NLT

All of the major goals that have been established for this New World Order pertain to its rise. Interestingly, another one of those necessities has become the Global Reset and its "cashless society." It's all about total global control, and as we've previously seen, that means the global economy must be controlled. That, too, is predicted in Scripture quite vividly, so it's just another precursor of God's plan. During the plandemic, great strides were made toward this goal. Revelation 6:5-6 speaks of a global financial crisis resulting from hyperinflation resulting from crippling famine. This also has a very familiar ring to it. The implication is that it will take a day's wages just to have a little food to eat; buying and selling will also be life and death. God has never made idle threats. Humankind has NEVER known a global economy as tight-fisted as this one will be, during what is known as the Tribulation. There are a great many other aspects of this time that even the globalist wolves haven't thought of, unless they've read God's Word.

It suffices to say now, that we do want to protect ourselves and our families against the continued specters of the globalists' evil plans. We want to protect our health and well-being, our finances, our homes, our jobs, and be wise stewards of all that our God has entrusted to us. However, if we do all of those things to the very best of our abilities without Jesus Christ in our lives, it will all be for naught. If we miss the greatest provision of all, salvation from our own sin and all of the evil this world owns, through a pure faith in God's Son, Jesus Christ, who died for each of us—-we've lost everything. We only need to trust Him and His shed blood on the cross for each of us, to redeem us from our sin, and accept His gift of eternal life. When He returns for His Church (that global group of people who have accepted Christ's sacrifice on the cross for them and belong to Him) just before this horrible judgment arrives on earth, He will take His believers to Heaven with Him. You and I, as His own, will miss all of the awful things planned only for those who refuse to believe and trust Him. This author made that choice decades ago, but it's never been more urgent to make that choice than it is today! As you may surmise, the time has drawn very short, until all these things come to pass. Don't wait to say "YES" to Jesus.

> "For He says, 'In a favorable time I listened to you, and in a day of salvation I have helped you. Behold, NOW is the favorable time, behold NOW is the day of salvation."
> 2 Corinthians 6:2 ESV

Now that the most important message of this book has been delivered, we want to focus a bit more on how best to live life in today's world, with the best health possible, not just for health and life's sake, but for the sake of the Kingdom of Heaven. It's very difficult to focus on life's needs and the needs of others when we aren't in good health. Globalists would have us believe their agenda is the one of most importance and focus. Nothing could be further from the truth. We have no need to worry about climate change, for example. First, taking care of our planet to the best of our ability pleases our Father who made it, but the kind of protection posited by globalists looks nothing like preservation and maintenance. Our climate has always had temperature and CO2 fluctuations. While man has not always been careful in how he treated his earthly home, any damage is reparable, contrary to globalist beliefs that we must stop doing all the things we've always done to right the wrongs. Our God is still sovereignly in charge of His planet, and even if He should come for us believers today, He has assured us in His Word that this planet will be existing for at least another 1,007 years! He doesn't need us to fix it! All of this hype is nothing but distracting smoke and mirrors to keep our focus off all of the things that really matter, those that are important to our Father.

Understand that the degree of deception perpetrated on us all before, during, and after the plandemic was all about distracting us from what they intended to do and would do so far as we the people allowed. The agenda says no religion, no God, no patriotism to our nation, no democracy, no individual thoughts or ideas, rely on the corporate socialistic government that has never yet been a viable concept. All of these lies didn't come just from their evil hearts—it came from the "father of lies," Satan himself. It now appears that perhaps God has been able to open the eyes of many with the travesties that were visited upon us, and may have given us another chance to right some of the many wrongs we've allowed morally and spiritually. We pray it may be so. However, we must sit up, be alert, pay attention, do our homework, and rely on God himself to show us when deception is near. In short, we need to make every effort to clean up our hearts, our minds, our lives, our families, our homes, and our nation. There is and always has been one very trustworthy, and specific way to do that—it's written in His Word:

> "If My people who are called by My name will humble themselves, and pray and seek My face, and turn from their wicked ways, (repentance) I will hear from heaven, and will forgive their sin and restore their land." 2 Chronicles 7:14 NLT

A final thought that might give us impetus to approach our lives with some degree of urgency is this: The plandemic was a horrendous and unprecedented time in world history that left most of us stunned, confused, and even disabled, not to mention bereaved. Much of the suffering was visited on completely unprepared and unsuspecting people who could do nothing, even had they known what was about to beset us. It was a culture of fear, panic, and death. Many days felt as if life would NEVER be "normal" again. In many ways it still will never be "normal." There are myriads of takeaways in retrospect that have hopefully been instructive. But, as heinous as it was, the day is coming when all that we experienced in the plandemic, and other equally destructive events since then, will all resemble a beautiful walk in the park on a sunshiny day compared to what is yet to come, for those without Jesus. Friend, we beg of you, as did the prophet Isaiah:

> "Seek the Lord while He may be found, call upon Him while He is near." Isaiah 55:6 ESV

Endnotes

CHAPTER 1

1. Wikipedia, "World Economic Forum," Wikipedia—The Free Encyclopedia, last edited January 16, 2025, https://en.wikipedia.org/wiki/World_Economic_Forum

2. Schwab, Klaus (interview), "The Wayback Machine," Financial Times, January 22, 2008, https:/theinternetarchive.enwikipedia.org/wiki/Klaus-schwab

3. Kirsten Salyer, "Live Simulation Exercise to Prepare Public and Private Leaders for Pandemic Response," October 15, 2019, https://www.kirstensawyer@weforum.org

4. Salyer, "Live Simulation"

5. Salyer, "Live Simulation"

6. Salyer, "Live Simulation

7. Peter A. McCollough, MD, MPH, "Pathophysiological Basis and Rationale for Early Outpatient Treatment of SARS-CoV2 (COVID-19) Infection," Video-October 11, 2020, Broadcast- December 7, 2020, Association of American Physicians and Surgeons—Published- August 2020, American Journal of Medicine.

8. David R. Martinez et al., including Ralph Baric, (2021, June 22, initially published online) "Chimeric Spike in mRNA Vaccines Protect Against Sarbecovirus Challenge in Mice," DOI: 10.1126/science. abi4506. https://www.biorxiv.org/content/10.1101/2021.02.11. 434872v 2. Full.

9. Jonathan Iwry, "From 9/11 to COVID-19: A Brief History of FDA Emergency Use Authorization," January 28, 2021. Cross-posted from "COVID-19 and the Law," January 14, 2021, The Petrie-Flom Center Staff/Harvard Law. https://blog.petrieflom.law.harvard.edu/2021/01/28/fda-emergency-use-authorization-history/

10. Jonathan Iwry, "Brief History of FDA/EUA,"

11. Peter R. Breggin, MD and Ginger R. Breggin, COVID-19 and the Global Predators—We Are the Prey! (Lake Edge Press-New York, 11/2021) p. vi, vii

12. Peter R. Breggin, MD, "COVID-19 and the Global Predators." p. vi, vii

13. Peter R. Breggin, MD, "COVID-19 and the Global Predators," p. viii

14. Peter R. Breggin, MD, "COVID-19 and the Global Predators," p. ix

15. Peter R. Breggin, MD, "COVID-19 and the Global Predators," p. x

CHAPTER TWO

1. Klaus Schwab Bio (author unknown), "Klaus Schwab Bio," AAE Speakers, awed January 30, 2024, https://www.allamericanspeakers.com/blog/

2. Klaus Schwab, "The Fourth Industrial Revolution," Encyclopedia Britannica, Original Essay printed 2018.

3. Peter R. Breggin, M.D. and Ginger R. Breggin, "COVID-19 and the Global Predators—We Are Their Prey!" (Lake Edge Press. New York, 2021.)

4. Breggin, MD., "Global Predators"

5. "The Davos Agenda," World Economic Forum. https://www.weforum.org/

6. Breggin, M.D., "Global Predators"

7. Breggin, M.D., "Global Predators"

8. Dawsey, J. and Abutaleb, Y., 2020, October31. "A Whole Lot of Hurt: Fauci Warns of COVID-19 Surge, Offers Blunt Assessment of President Trump's Response," Washington Post, https://www.washingtonpost.com/politics/fauci-covid-winter-forecast/2020/10/31/e3970eb0-1b8b-11eb-bb35-2efdab0a345.story.html.

9. Breggin, M.D., "Global Predators"

10. Xiao, B. and Xiao, L., "The Possible Origins of 2019-nCoV Coronavirus," February 2020. https://www.lifesitenews.com/images/pdfs/the-possible-origins-of-the-2019-ncov-coronavirus.pdf.

11. Breggin, M.D., "Global Predators"

12. Axios Media, "NIH Vaccine—Public Citizen and 'Does Anthony Fauci Own Half of the Patent' For Moderna's COVD Vaccine?" https://www.axios.com/moderna-nih-coronavirus-vaccine-ownership-agreements-22051c42-2dee-4b19-938d-099afd71f6a0.html.

13. The Dispatch Fact Check, "NIH Scientist Who Developed Key COVID Vaccine Technology Says Patent Gives Us Leverage," https://www.commondreams.org/news/2021/04/23/ nih-scientist-who developed-key-vaccine-technology-says-patent-gives-us-leverage

14. Farber, Celia, "AIDS and the AZT Scandal," October 5,2015, SPINS 1989 Feature, "Sins of Omission," https://www.spin.com/featured/aids-and-the-azt-scandal-spin-1989-feature-sins-of-omission/

15. Goodell, Jeff, "Bill Gates: The Rolling Stone Interview," March 13, 2014, reviewed on Wikipedia, updated February 4, 2024, https://en.wikipedia.org

16. Wikipedia. "Bill Gates and Dr. Fauci talk regularly—Here's What They're Discussing Now," CNBC.com. February 11, 2021. Retrieved May 3, 2021, https://en.wikipedia.org

17. Kriss, Sam, "The Truth About Bill Gates", November 1, 2022, First Things, https://www.firstthings.com/article/ 2022/1/11/the-truth-about-bill-gates

18. Gotzsche, Peter, "Deadly Medicines and Organized Crime", Wikipedia, 2013. Review of book Deadly Medicines and Organized Crime—How Big Pharma Has Corrupted Healthcare. https://en.wikipedia.org.

19. Gotzsche, Peter, "Deadly Medicines and Organized Crime," Amazon, 2013. Review of book Deadly Medicines and Organized Crime—How Big Pharma Has Corrupted Healthcare. https://www.amazon.com.

20. Farhat, Yaqub (February 1, 2014). "Reforming Big Pharma," The Lancet. Retrieved December 9, 2018.

21. "Shot/Chasers: "No Wonder the American People Hate Drug Companies," November 10, 2021. https://www.protectourcare.org.

22. Breggin, M.D., "Global Predators"

23. James Comer, Chairman, "COVID Origins Hearing Wrap Up: Facts, Science, Evidence Point to a Wuhan Lab Leak." Dr. Jamie Metzl, PH.D., Mervyn Yan transcript published March 8, 2023. https://oversight.house.gov/release/covid-origins-hearing-wrap-up-facts-science-evidence-point-to-a-wuhan-lab-leak%EF%BF%BC/

24. James Comer, Chairman, "COVID Origins" Nicolas Wade, New York Times.

25. James Comer, Chairman, "COVID Origins" Dr. Robert Redfield, former director of the US CDC.

26. Kania, Elsa B. and Wilson Vorndick, "Weaponizing Biotech: How China's Military Is Preparing for a 'New Domain of Warfare'", August 14, 2019, Defense One, https://www.defenseone.com/ideas/2019/08/china's-military-pursuing-biotech/159167/

27. Kania and Vorndick, "China's Military Weaponizing Biotech."

28. https://www.law.cornell.edu/uscode/text/18/953.

CHAPTER 3

1. Bunker, Theodore, "Climate Czar John Kerry Raked in Millions From Energy Sector," Newsmax, May 3, 2021, https://www.newsmax.com/politics/john-kerry-investments-climate-czar/2021/05/03/id/1019949

2. St. Clair, Jeffrey, "What John Kerry Really Did in Vietnam," CounterPunch, July 26, 2013, https://www.counterpunch.org/2013/07/26/what-john-kerry-really-did-in-vietnam/

3. Breggin, M.D., "Global Predators"

4. Breggin, M.D., "Global Predators"

5. Leubsdorf, Carl P. (September 6, 1987) "Biden Keeps Sights Set on White House," The Dallas Morning News. Archived. Retrieved from the original on June 23, 2021.

6. Dionne, E. J. Jr.—September 18,1987). "Biden Admits Plagiarism in School But Says It Was Not Malevolent." New York Times. Reprinted January 20,2011.

7. Hamilton, Carl. "Daughter of a Man in 1972 Biden Crash Seels Apology from Widowed Senator." Newark Post. January 16, 2017, retrieved March 13, 2017.

8. Levey, Noam M. (August 24, 2008). "In His Home State, Biden is a Regular Joe." Los Angeles Times.

9. Comer, James (Chairman), "The Bidens' Influence Peddling Timeline", Repost of the US House Oversight and Accountability Committee. Dates from 2009 – 2016. (ongoing investigation) Lengthy information is NOT word for word, but is very close due to the legality of this entire document necessary to show the criminality extensively for this chapter.

10. https://x.com/EpochTimes/status/1735491697310843231?s=20

11. Hansler, Jennifer, "Inside Biden's Decision to 'take care of' the Chinese Spy Balloon That Triggered a Diplomatic Crisis," CNN, February 5, 2023, https://www.cnn.com/2023/02/04/politics/china-spy-balloon-tick-tock/index.html

12. Hansler, Jennifer, "Chinese Spy Balloon/Diplomatic Crisis."

13. Shkolnikova,Svetlana, "US Delayed Shooting Down Chinese Spy Balloon Partly to Aid Recovery Efforts, Defense Officials say," Stars and Stripes, February 9, 2023, https://www.stripes.com/theaters/us/2023-02-09/chinese-spy-balloon-military-senate-9090118.html

CHAPTER 4

1. Piccotti, Tyler and Biography.com editors, "LeBron James," Biography, July 26,2024, https://www.biography.com/athletes/lebron-james

2. Yglesias, Matthew (October 7, 2019). "The Raging Controversy Over the NBA, China, and the Hong Kong Protests, Explained," Vox Media.

3. Breggin, Peter, MD. And Breggin Ginger, "COVID-19 and the Global Predators:

We Are the Prey." (Lake Edge Press-NY-2021)

4. Breggin, Peter, M.D., "COVID-19 and Global Predators."

5. Bloomberg News, 2020, November 16, "Black Rock's Fink Calls on Investors to Embrace ESG: NEF Update, yahoo finance. https://finance.yahoo.com/news/blackrock-fink-eskom-ruyter-set-001626898.html

6. Ingraham, Laura, 2020, November 20, Ingraham Angle, Fox News. https://www.foxnews.com/media/laura-ingraham-globalists-bloomberg-forum-world-health-org-bill-gates.

7. Breggin, Peter, M.D., "COVID-19 and Global Predators."

8. Haqqi, Ty, "Top 20 Most Valuable American Companies Today," Yahoo!Finance, updated January, 2025, https://finance.yahoo.com/newss/top-20-most-valuable-american-162016886.html?fr=yhssrp_catchall

CHAPTER 5

1. TIME, 2020, undated online issue, circa late October, The Great Reset. "The Great Reset: How to Build a Better World Post-COVID-19 l TIME

2. Schwab, Klaus, 2020, June 3, "Now is the Time for a 'Great Reset.'" World Economic Forum. https://www.weforum.org/agenda/2020/06/now-is-the-time-for-a-great-reset/.

3. Smith, W., 2020, November 24, "Beware the 'Great Reset'-New World Order." The Epoch Times. https://www.theepochtimes.com/beware-the-great-reset-new-world-order.3584620.html.

4. Smith, W., "Beware the Great Reset-New World Order."

5. https://truthstreammedia.com/2019/10/25/breggin-the-most-important-video-we-have-ever-watched.

6. https://www.theguardian.com/uk-news/2020/06/03/pandemic-is-chance-to-reset-global-economy-says-prince-charles.

7. Breggin, Peter, M.D. "COVID-19 and Global Predators."

8. Clinton, Bill (former President of US.), Intro Speech of Clinton Global Initiative Annual Meeting, September 23, 2024, https://www.clintonfoundation.org/clinton-global-initiative-september-2024-meeting/?ms=lb

9. The quote begins at 1:55 of the video. https://www.bing.com/videos/search?q=Chris+Hedges+and

+George+Soros&docid=607990790830492646&mid=7FE96CBD92B0BA64C

-BA97FE96CBD92B0BA64CBA9&view=detail&FORM=VIRE

10. Zuboff, Shoshana (2019) "The Age of Surveillance Capitalism: The Fight for a Human Future at the New Frontier of Power." Profile Books. ISBN 978-1781256855.

CHAPTER 6

1. Breggin, Peter, M.D., "COVID-19 and Global Predators."

2. Breggin, Peter, M.D., "COVID-19 and Global Predators."

3. Breggin, Peter, M.D., "COVID-19 and Global Predators."

4. Breggin, Peter, M.D., "COVID-19 and Global Predators."

5. Ross, C. 2020, November 23, 'The Wall Street Journal, Washington Post Among Newspapers Paid Millions by Beijing-Controlled News Outlet to Publish Propaganda this Year," The Tennessee Star, https://tennesseestar.com/2020/11/23/the-wall-street-journal-washington-post-among-newspapers-paid-millions-by-beijing-controlled-news-outlet-to-publish-propaganda-this-year/

6. Fitton, T. (2020). "A Republic Under Assault: The Left's Ongoing Attack on American Freedom." New York: Threshold Editions. There are many good examinations of American media economic ties to the Chinese Communist - run nation, including Clark, 2020, May 4, "A Rundown of Major U.S. Corporate Media's Business Ties To China," The Federalist. https://thefederalist.com/2020/05/04/has-china-compromised-every-major-maintstream-media-entity/

CHAPTER 7

1. Kempe, Frederick, CNBC, "Op-ed: A New World Order Is Emerging—and the World is not Ready for it." April 3, 2022, https://www.cnbc.com/2022/04/03/a-new-world-order-is-emerging-and-the-world-is-not-ready-for-it.html.

2. Wikipedia—last edited January 31, 2024. https://en.wikipedia.org /wiki/new-world-order-(conspiracy-theory).

3. Flores, Myles, "The New World Order: The Historical Origins of a Dangerous Modern Conspiracy Theory," Middlebury Institute of International Studies at Monterey, May 30, 2022, https://www.middlebury.edu/institute/academics/centers-initiatives/ctec/ctec-publications/new-world-order-historical-origins-dangerous

4. Shimizu, Yashi (WHO), "Delivering on Commitments: Where Do We Stand Halfway to 2030?" United Nations.org, September, 2023, https://unstats.un.org/sdgs/report//2023/promises-in-peril/

5. Hunter, Greg, "Climate Engineering Must Stop or Humanity is Finished—Dane Wigington," Lioness of Judah Ministry, March 12, 2023, https://www.USAWatchdog.com/GeoEngineeringWatch.org/3/11/2023/

6. Geldard, Rebecca and Ellerbeck, Stefan. "How Much Progress is Being Made on the UN's Sustainable Development Goals," September 11, 2023. Davos Agenda of World Economic Forum. https://www.weforum.org/agenda/2023/09/11/un-sustainable-development-goals-progress-report/

7. Geldard, and Ellerbeck. "Sustainable Development Goals 2023 Report."

8. Guinness World Records. "Best Selling Book of Non-Fiction (of all time)." Wikipedia, original record 15 March, 2015. https://en.wikipedia.org/wiki/list_of-best_selling_books#cite_note_guinnessworldrecords-1.

CHAPTER 8

1. Baric, Ralph S.; Yount, Boyd; Hensley, Lisa; Peel, Sheila; and Chen, Wan; (1997, March), "Episodic Evolution Mediates Interspecies Transfer of a Murine Coronavirus. Journal of Virology, 71(3), 1945-1955 https://jvi.asm.org/content/jvi/71/3/1946.full.pdf

2. Zhang, F, (2004,July 2), "Officials Punished for SARS Virus Leak," China Daily, https://www.chinadaily.com.cn/english/doc/2004-07/02/content 344755.htm

3. https://www.cdc.gov/sars/lab/downloads/nucleoseq.pdf complete genome for Urban SARS corona virus April 17, 2003 submitted to the CDC.

4. Savarino, Andrea; Boelaert, Johan R.; Cassone, Antonio; Majori, Giancarlo; and Cauda, Roberto. (2003, November). "Effects of Chloroquine on Viral Infections: An Old Drug Against Today's Diseases?" Lancet Infectious Diseases 2003; 3: 722-27. https://www.thelancet.com/action/showPdf?pii=S1473-3099%2803%2900806-5.

5. Deming, D. et al. 2006. "Vaccine Efficacy in Senescent Mice Challenged with Recombinant SARS-CoV Bearing Epidemic and Zoonotic Spike Variants." PLoS Med.3:e525.[PMC free article] [PubMed] [Google Scholar]. Vaccine Efficacy in Senescent Mice Challenged with Recombinant SARS-CoV Bearing Epidemic and Zoonotic Spike Variants (plos.org)

6. https://www.gavi.org/investing-gavi/innovative-financing/iffim

7. Immigrant-Founded Moderna Leading The Way In COVID-19 Response (forbes.com).

8. Tseng CT, Sbrana E, Iwata-Yoshikawa N, Newman PC, Garron T, et al. (2012) "Immunization With SARS Coronavirus Vaccines Leads to Pulmonary Immunopathology on Challenge With the SARS Virus." PLOS ONE 7(8):10.1371/annotation/2965cfae-b77d-4014-8b7b-236e01a34592. https://journals.plos.org/plosone/article?id=10.1371/journal.pone.0035421

9. Top 10 Vaccine Manufacturers in the World, (yahoo.com).

10. Press Release, 2010, "Global Health Leaders Launch Decade of Vaccines Collaboration. Bill and Melinda Gates Foundation. https://www.gatesfoundation.org/Media-Center/Press-Releases/2010/12/Global-Health-Leaders-Launch-Decade-of-Vaccines-Collaboration. (The January date is cited in this document.)

11. This "booklet," (Scenarios for the Future of Technology and International Development"), has been expunged from the Rockefeller website but remains available here: https://issuu.com/dueprocesstv/docs/scenario-for-the-future

12. https://www.gatesfoundation.org/Ideas/Media-Center/Press=Releases/2010/12/Global-Health-Leaders-Launch-Decade-of-Vaccines-Collaboration

13. This is goal #3.8 located under "Goal 3. Ensure healthy lives and promote well-being for all at all ages." https://sdgs.un.org/2030agendagrant/https://sustainabledevelopment.un.org/Content/documents/21252030%20Agenda%20for%20Sustainable%20Development%20web,pdf.

14. Bolles, M., et al, (2011), A double-inactivated severe acute respiratory syndrome coronavirus vaccine provides incomplete protection in mice and induces increased eosinophilic proinflammatory pulmonary response upon challenge. J.Virol.85,12201-12215(2011). https://www.ncbi.nlm.nih.gov/pmc/articles/PMC3209347/acknowledgments

15. Lee, Wen Shi et al, September 9, 2020. Nature Microbiology. Re : Operation Warp Speed.

16. https://sph.unc,edu/sphh-news/baric-to-lead-10-million-nih-grant/S

17. https://reporter.nih,gov/search/GCBybhJJPEOJ8Rp15e1Q1A/project-details/98193043-similar-Projects

18. Bill & Melinda Gates Foundation announces $250 million COVID vaccine commitment-ABC News (go.com). "Gates, who had invested in the vaccine technology in 2015, emphasized the importance of messenger RNA (mRNA) vaccines ending this pandemic and potentially ones to come in the future."

19. https://www.business-standard.com/article/current-affairs/scientists-in-china-discussed-weaponising-coronavirus-in-2015-report-121050900916 1.html; https://www.news.com.au/world/coronavirus/leaked-chinese-document-reveals-a-sinister-plan-to-unleash-coronaviruses/news-story/5 3674e8108ad5a655e07e990daa85465;https//www.dailymail.co.uk/news/article-9556415/China-preparing-WW3-biological-weapons-six-years-investigators-say.html;https://www.independent.co.uk/asia/china/china-covid-leak-genetic-weapons-b1844805,html

20. CEPI conceived 2015-Bing

21. The Bill and Melinda Gates Foundation|GAVI, the Vaccine Alliance. https://www.gavi.org/investing-gavi/resource-mobilization-process/gavi-pledging-conference-january-2015. Gavi is the "Global Alliance for Vaccines

22. https:www.scidev.net/global/features/under-fire-critics-challenge-gavi-s-vaccine-spending-practices/

23. https://www.youtube.com/watch?v=6AF6B WYiWI

24. Vineet D.Menachery, Boyd L.Yount, Jr., Kari Debbink1, Sudhakar Agnihothram, Lisa E. Gralinski, Jessica A. Plante, Rachel L. Graham, Trevor Scoby, Xing-Yi Ge, Eric F Donaldson, Scott H. Randell, Antonio Lanzavecchia, Wayne A. Marasco, Zhengli-Li Shi, and Ralph S. Baric. (2015) "A SARS-like Cluster of Circulating Bat Coronaviruses Shows Potential For Human Emergence." Nature Medicine,21(12), 1508-1514, December 2015

25. Breggin, Peter M.D., "COVID-19 and the Global Predators."

26. https://web.archive.org/web20160630124045/https://www.nature.com/nature conferences/viir2016/sponsors.html.

27. History Wuhan Institute of Virology (cas.cnhttps://english.whiov.cas.cn/About Us2016/Directors2016/

28. Homeland Security, 2017, January, "Biological Incident Annex to the Response and Recovery Federal Interagency Operation Plans." Final-January 2017. https://web.archive.org/web/20201104004301/https://www.fema.gov/media-library-data/1511178017324-92a7a7f808b-3f03e5fa2f8495bdfe335/BIA Annex Final 1-23-17 (508Compliant 6-28-17).pdf

29. President Barack Obama. 2019, January 9. The White House. Recommended Policy Guidance for Potential Pandemic Pathogen Care and Oversight | whitehouse.gov (archives.gov). Recommended Policy Guidance for Potential Pandemic Pathogen Care and Oversight (P3CO) | whitehouse.gov (archives.gov)

30. Eleven Days Before Trump Took Office, Obama-Biden White House 'Depopulation' Science Czar Holdren Advised Lifting Gain-of-Function Research Ban; Trump Kept in the Dark—The American Report

31. Secretary Sylvia Mathews Burwell | whitehouse.gov (archives.gov)

32. "Eleven Days Before Trump Took Office, Obama-Biden White House. "The American Report.

33. NOT-OD-17-071: Notice Announcing the Removal of the Funding Pause for Gain-of-Function Research Projects (nih.gov)

34. Breggin, Peter, M.D. "COVID-19 and the Global Predators."

35. https://www.federalregister.gov/documents/2017/01/13/2017-000721/emergency-use-authorization-of-medical-products-and-related-authorities-guidance-for-industry...

36. Monaco, Lisa, 2020, March 3, "Pandemic Disease Is a Threat to National Security," Foreign Affairs Lisa Monaco served as Assistant to the President for Homeland Security and Counter-terrorism from 2013-2017. https://www.foreignaffairs.com/articles/2020-03-03/pandemic-disease-threat-national-secutity

37. CEPI officially launched—CEPI

38. "Bill Gates Warns Tens of Millions Could Be Killed by Bio-terrorism," |Bill Gates| The Guardian.

39. https://www.who.int/medicines/ebolatreatment/ TheCoalitionEpidemicPreparednessInnovations-an-overview.pdf

40. "Rewriting the Genetic Code: A Cancer Cure in the Making |Tal Zaks | TEDxBeacon Street-Bing Video." For commentary, see: https://medicalkidnap.com/2021/03/09/modernas-top-scientist-on-mrna-technology-in-covid-shots-we-are-actually-hacking-the-software-of-life/#:~:-text=Tal%20Zaks%2C%20the%20chief%20medical%officer%20R%20Moderna.we%20

41. Norbert Pardi, Michael J. Hogan, Frederick W. Porter, and Drew Weissman. (2018, April). "mRNA vaccines—a new era in vaccinology." Nature Reviews 17, 261-279, https://www.nature.com/articles/nrd.2017.243.pdf?origin=ppub

42. "TÜBINGEN, Germany / BOSTON—March 15,2020, CureVac AG, a clinical stage biopharmaceutical company pioneering mRNA-based drugs for vaccines and therapeutics, confirmed today that internal efforts are focused on the development of a coronavirus vaccine with the goal to reach, help and to protect people and patients worldwide." https://www.curevac.com/en/2020/03/15/curevac-focuses-on-the-development-of-mrna-based-coronavirus-vaccine-to-protect-people-worldwide/

43. "The Next Epidemic is Coming. Here's How We Can Be Ready." | Bill Gates-gatesnotes.com

44. Crystal Watson, Tara Kirk Sell, Matthew Watson, Caitlin Rivers, Christopher Hurtado, Matthew P. Shearer, Ashley Geleta, and Thomas Inglesby ("Posted October 09, 2018"). "Technologies to Address Global Catastrophic Biological Risks. Johns Hopkins University, Bloomberg School of Public Health, Center for Health Security. Copyright 2018." No sponsors are listed. Technologies to Address Global Catastrophic Biological Risks (centerforhealthsecurity.org) and 181009-gcbr-tech-report.pdf (jhsphcenterforhealthsecurity.s3.amazonaws.com)

45. P. 6 of the JHU report.

46. P.47 of the JHU report.

47. Breggin, Ginger Ross, "COVID-19 and the Global Predators."

48. https://reporter.nih.gov/search/cVFEMwgD-UyuwQkDAvSL8Q/project-details/8674931

49. WEF HGHI Outbreak Readiness Business Impact.pdf (weforum.org)

50. https://health.news/2020-07-08-pandemic-bill-gates-negotiated-contact-tracing-deal-.htm#

51. https://www.congress.gov/bill/116th-congress/house-bill/6666/text. With sponsors: Text-H.R.6666-116th Congress (2019-2020): COVID-19Testing, Reaching, and Contacting Everyone (TRACE) Act | Congress.gov | Library of Congress.

52. https://truepundit.com/exclusive-bill-gates-negotiated-100-billion-contact-tracing-deal-with-democratic-congressman-sponsor-of-bill-six-months-before-coronavirus-pandemic/

53. GPMB annual report 2019.pdf (who.int)

54. https://www,centerforhealthsecurity.org/news/center-news/2020/2020-01-17-Event201-recommendations.html

55. https://www.neweconomyforum.com/2019-new-economy-forum-beijing/

56. Brunson, E.K., Chandler, H., Gronvall, G.K., Ravi, S., Sell, T.K., Shearer, M.P. & Schoch-Spana, M. (2020), "The SPARS Pandemic 2025-2028: A Futuristic Scenario to Facilitate Medical Countermeasure Communication." Journal of International Crisis and Risk Communication Research, 3 (1),71-102. https://doi.org/10.30658/jicrcr.3.1.4; https://stars.library.ucf.edu/jicrcr/vol3/iss1/4/

57. https://www.dailymail.co.uk/news/article-8003713/China-appoints-military- bio-weapon-expert-secretive-virus-lab-Wuhan.html and http://www.asianews.it/news-en/Prof-Tritto-COVID-19-was-created-in-the-Wuhan-laboratory-and-is-now-in-the-hands-of-the-Chinese-military-50719.html

58. https://www.cnas.org/publications/reports/myths-and-realities-of-chinas-military-civil-fusion-strategy

59. https://www.state.gov/wp-content/uploads/2020/05//what-is-MCF—One-Pager.pdf

60. https://www.hindustantimes.com/india-news/journals-retract-two-major-covid-studies/story//EVzDIWf9bUoTgBmVvkRUgVK.html;https://www.theweek.in/ news/sci-tech/2020/02/01/research-paper-by-indian-scientists-on-coronavirus-fuels-bioweapon-theories.html; Prashant Pradhan, Ashutosh Kumar Pandey, Akhilesh Mishra, Parul Gupta, Praveen Kumar Tripathi, Manoj Balakrishnan Menon, James Gomes, Perumal Vivekanandan and Bishwajit Kundu (2020, January 31) Uncanny Similarity of Unique Inserts in the 2019-nCoV Spike Protein to HIV-1 gp120 and Gag.bioRxiv. https://www.biorxiv.org/content/10.1101/2020.01.30.927871v1.full.pdf

61. https://cepi.net/news cepi/cepi-to-fund-three-programs-to-develop-vaccines-against-the-novel-coronavirus-ncov-2019/

62. Headline: "A Coalition Backed by Bill Gates is Funding Biotechs That Are Scrambling to Develop Vaccines for the Deadly Wuhan Coronavirus." https://markets.businessinsider.com/news/stocks/vaccines-for-wuhan-china-coronavirus-moderna-inovio-cepi-2020-1-1028840542?op=1

63. The inside story of how scientists produced an Ebola vaccine (statnews.com) and FDA approves an Ebola vaccine, long in development, for the first time-STAT (statnews.com)

64. https://www.axios.com/moderna-nih-coronavirus-vaccine-ownership-agreements-22051c42-2dee-4b19-938d-099afd71f6a0.html

65. Paules C.I., Marston H.D., Fauci A.S. "Coronavirus Infections – More than Just the Common Cold." JAMA.2020;323(8):707-708. https://pubmed.ncbi.nlm.nih.gov/31971553/

66. National Institutes of Health, Undated. Retrieved May 14, 2021. "Vaccine Development: Behind the Scenes. Years of Research Enable a COVID-19 Vaccine to be Developed In Record Time." https://covid19.nih.gov/news-and-stories/vaccine-development/

67. Breggin, Peter M.D., "COVID-19 and the Global Predators."

68. The CDC Is Still Botching the Coronavirus Testing Process—Reason.com; Early CDC Coronavirus Test Came with Inconsistent Instructions and Cost the U.S. Weeks |WBUR News.

69. https://www.bbc.co.uk/mediacentre/latestnews/2020/coronavirus-trusted-news

70. Trusted News Initiative (TNI) Steps Up Global Fight Against Disinformation with New Focus on US Presidential Election - Media Centre (bbc.co.uk)

71. https://www.who.int/director-general/speeches/detail/who-director-general-s-opening-remarks-at-the-media-briefing-on-covid-19 11-march-2020

72. Ronald Bailey, COVID-19 Mortality Rate 'Ten Times Worse' Than Seasonal Flu, Says Dr. Anthony Fauci. Reason, March 11, 2020. https://reason.com/2020/03/11/covid-19-mortality-rate-ten-times-worse-than-seasonal-flu-says-dr-anthony-fauci/; and Joseph Guzman-Coronavirus 10 times more lethal than seasonal flu, top health official says. The Hill. https://thehill.com/changing-america/well-being/prevention-cures/487086-coronavirus-10-times-more-lethal-than-seasonal-accessed 9.1.2020

73. COVID-19 – Navigating the Uncharted | NEJM

74. https://newlevellers.blogspot.com/2021/03/fauci-shares-stage-with-top-ccp.html. For more about D. Zhong Nanshan: https://www.npr.org/sections/goatsandsoda/2020/04/02/825957192/dr-zhong-is-the-supreme-commander-in-china-s-war-against-coronavirus

75. Fox News' Neil Cavuto Shocked by Trump Hydroxychloroquine Announcement (business-insider.com)

76. Steven Hatfield. How a Single Point Failure Destroyed the National Pandemic Plan-Dr. Steven Hatfill (drstevenhatfill.com) and https://www.kmblegal.com/sites/default/files/NEW%20R.%Bright%20OSC%20C Complaint Redacted.pdf

77. No.202.11: "Continuing Temporary Suspension and Modification of Laws Relating to the Disaster Emergency (ny.gov)

78. Schmad, Robert, "Andrew Cuomo's COVID Policy Killed Thousands—That's What Should Have Ended His Career." Washington Examiner—August 3, 2021. https://www.washingtonexaminer.com/opinion/1167760/andrew-cuomos-covid-policy-killed-thousands-thats-what-should-have-ended-his-career/

79. Fauci, Anthony M. D., "Fact Check: ...Video of Fauci Saying, "There's No Reason to be Walking Around With a Mask." October 8, 2020 https://www.reuters.com/article/idUSKBN26T2T9/

80. Rancourt, D. (2020 April). "Masks Don't Work-A Review of Science Relevant to COVID-19 Social Policy." https://www.algora.com/Algora blog/2020/05/23/masks-dont-work-a-review-of-science-relevant-to-covid-19-social-policy.

81. For the Birx video and transcription: https://www.realclearpolitics.com/video/2020/04/08/dr-birx-unlike-some countries-if someone-dies-with-covid-19-we-are-counting-that-as-a-covid-19-death.html

82. Reuters-April 17, 2020. "True Claim: "Brazilian Chloroquine Study on COVID-19 Patients Was Halted After 11 Deaths. Note: These articles have been flagged multiple times by Facebook to curb misinformation (Big Tech), but it is still on Reuters because it is true!

83. Find the blog and the You Tube presentation by Dr. Breggin that quickly reached 40,000 viewers and exceeded 59,000 on May 24,2020: https://breggin.com/us-chinese-scientists-collaborate on coronavirus/

84. https://investors.modernatx.com/news-releases/news-release-details/moderna-announces-award-us-government-agency-barda-483-million

85. Ren-Di-Jiang, Mei-Qin Liu, Ralph Baric, et al., (2020, July). Pathogenesis of SARS-Co-V-2 in Transgenic Mice Expressing Human Angiotensin-Converting Enzyme 2—Science Direct. https://doi.org/10.1016/j.cell.2020.05.0.

86. https://www.weforum.org/press/2020/07/klaus-schwab-and-thierry-malleret-release-covid-19-the-great-reset-the-first-policy-book-on-the-covid-crisis-globally.

87. https://www.cnn.com/2020/07/22/health/pfizer-covid-19-vaccine-government-contract/index.html

88. U.S. Government Engages Pfizer to Produce Millions of Doses of COVID-19 Vaccine | HHS.gov

89. The paper was originally made available on August 7, 2020 online and then appeared in the printed journal in January 2021; McCullough, P. et al. (2021, January). Pathophysiological Basis and Rationale for Early Outpatient Treatment of SARS-Co-V-2 (COVID-19) Infection. The American Journal of Medicine, Vol 134(1), 16-22.

90. https://www.cdc.gov/nchs/data/health policy/covid19-comorbidity-expanded-12092020-508.pdf

91. Wen Shi Lee, Adam K. Wheatley, Stephen J. Kent, and Brandon J. DeKosky. (2020, October). "Antibody-Dependent Enhancement and SARS-CoV-2 Vaccines and Therapies." Nature Microbiology, 5, 1185-1199, https://www.nature.com/articles/s41564-020-00789-5.pdf

92. Branswell, H. 2020, September 14, "Bill Gates Slams "shocking" U.S. response on COVID-19 Pandemic, STAT." https://www.statnews.com/2020/09/14/bill-gates-slams-mismanaged-u-s-response-to-covid-19-pandemic/

93. Yan, Li-Meng; Kang, Shu; Guan, Jie; Hu, Shanchang. (2020, September 14) "Unusual Features of the SARS-CoV-2 Genome Suggesting Sophisticated Laboratory Modification Rather Than Natural Evolution and Delineation of Its Probable Synthetic Route. Prepublication." https://Breggin.com/coronavirus/The Yan Report.pdf.

94. Yan, Li-Meng, et al., 2020, October 8, "SARS-CoV-2 Is an Unrestricted Bioweapon: A Truth Revealed Through Uncovering a Large-Scale, Organized Scientific Fraud." Republication. https://zenodo.org/record/DOI 10.5281/zenado.4073130.

95. https://breggin.com/wp-content/uploads/1990/01/fluvoxamine.pdf

96. Haskins, Justin, 12/03/2020. The Hill. "John Kerry Reveals Biden's Devotion to Radical 'Great Reset' Movement." https://thehill.com/opinion/energy-environment/528482-john-kerry-reveals-bidens-devotion-to-radical-great-reset-movement/

97. https;//www.wsj.com/articles/china-is-national-security-threat-no.-1-11607019599?mod=article-inline

98. BioNTech in China alliance with Fosun over potential coronavirus vaccine | Reuters

99. The NIH claims joint ownership of Moderna's coronavirus vaccine – Axios

100. Yuyang, et al.,2020. https://www.biorxiv.org/content/biorxiv/early/2020/12/04/2020.12.04.409144.full. pdf

101. Nuovo et al.,2021. https://www.bloomberg.com/news/newsletters/2021-05-01/the-new-economy-saturday-maybe-china-wont-beat-the-U-S-after-all

102. McCullough, P. et al., (2020, December). "Multifaceted, Highly-Targeted, Sequential Multidrug Treatment of Early Ambulatory High-Risk SARS-CoV-2 Infection (COVID-19)." Reviews in Cardiovascular Medicine, 21 (4),517-530. November 2020. DOI: 10.31083/j.rcm.2020.04.264. See the graph at https://breggin.com/coronavirus-research-center/.

103. https://www.mitre.org/news/press-releases/coalition-of-health-technology-industry-leaders-announce-vaccination-credential-initiative

104. https://thecommonsproject.org/commonpass

105. https://www.busiweek.com//pfizer-biontech-and-moderna-to-earn-14.7b-from-covid-19-vaccines-sales-by-2023/

106. Controversy as Israel Stats Report Appears to Suggest 40 Times Higher Deaths in Elderly After First But Before Second Pfizer Dose Than From Covid – NewsRescue.com; As Israel Reopened, 'Whoever Does Not Get Vaccinated Will Be Left Behind' -The New York Times (nytimes.com)

107. South Africa Suspends Use of AstraZeneca's COVID-19 Vaccine After it Fails to Clearly Stop Virus Variant | Science | AAAS (sciencemag.org)

108. The Wuhan Laboratory Origin of SARS-CoV-2 and the Validity of the Yan Reports Are Further Proved by the Failure of Two Uninvited "Peer Reviews" | Zenodo

109. https://www.theepochtimes.com/beijing-seizes-upon-faucis-call-for-solidarity-to-push-covid-19-propaganda 3731620.html; Fauci and the Communists—AIER

110. https://www.worldtribune.com/fauci-makes-nice-with-chinese-communists-at-future-of-health-forum/

111. Congressional Research Service. The PREP Act and COVID-19: Limiting Liability for Medical Countermeasures (congress.gov)

112. https://www.mediaite.com/tv/breaking-former-cdc-director-says-he-believes-coronavirus-escaped-from-wuhan-lab/

113. https://www.msn.com/en-us/news/politics/bidens-climate-duo-puts-us-back-in-global-warming-fight/ar-BB1fJzxM

114. Bill Gates says COVID-19 Vaccine Technology Should Not Be Shared with India, Now There is a Vaccine Shortage – Technology News (indiatoday.in); COVID-19 Vaccine Formulas Shouldn't Be Shared with India: Bill Gates (yahoo.com)

115. https://www.who.int/director-general/speeches/detail/who-director-general-s-opening-remarks-at-the-member-state-information-session-on-who-biohub—-15-april-2021

116. https://www,tge-scuebtust.com/news-opinion/biohub-network-aims-to-advance-sharing-of-pathogens-for-research-68849

117. U.S. Denies India's Request to Lift Ban on Export of COVID-19 Vaccine Raw Materials (jagran-josh.com)

118. https://www.ft.com/content/096dd554-499b-468c-bfa-38b0352941a0?segmentid=a-cee4131-99c2-09d3-a635-873e61754ec6

119. https://www.nbcnews.com/meet-the-press/meet-press-april-25-2021-n1265222

120. https://www.cdc.gov/coronavirus/2019-ncov/vaccines/safety/adverse-events.html. On the second page. These numbers are both hidden and ignored by the CDC which continues to claim there are no proven cases to report, but the best use of CDC's VAERS or the FDA's FAERS is precisely to identify gross patterns like these, whereupon the marketing of the vaccine or drug would, in the past, be stopped, and a massive investigation begun.

121. https://www.cdc.gov/vaccines/covid-19/health-departments/breakthrough-cases.html

122. Coffin, Patrick. "Truth Over Fear Summit" and "Coffin Nation"—a conservative, faith-based media platform; reporting on world events in the church and in the news, exposing media bias and anti-faith agendas. https://www.coffinnation.com

123. Kowarz E, Krutzke L, Reis J, Bracharz S, Kochanek S, Marschalek R. "Vaccine-induced COVID-19 Mimicry Syndrome: Splanchnic Reactions with the SARS-CoV-2 Spike Open Reading Frame Result in Spike Protein Variant that may Cause Thromboembolic Events in Patients Immunized with Vector-based Vaccines. Clinical Infectious Diseases. https://www.researchsquare.com/article/rs-558954/v1

124. https://outlook.live.com/mail/deeplink?popoutv2=1&version=20210426004.07

125. Ofata AF, Cheng C-A, Desjardins M, Senussi Y, Sherman AC, Powell M, et al. "Circulating SARS-CoV-2 Vaccine Antigen Detected in the Plasma of mRNA-1273 Vaccine Recipients." Clinical Infectious Diseases. https://doi.org/10-1093/cid/ciab465. https://www.researchsquare.com/article/rs-558954/v1

126. Seneff S, Nigh G. "Worse Than the Disease? Reviewing Some Possible Unintended Consequences of the mRNA Vaccines Against COVID-19." International Journal of Vaccine Theory, Practice, and Research. 2021;2(1):402-403. Circulating SARS-CoV-2 Vaccine Antigen Detected om the Plasma of mRNA-1273 Vaccine Recipients | Clinical Infectious Diseases | Oxford Academic (oup.com)

127. Hours after clashing with Senator Rand Paul, R-KY, at a Senate hearing Tuesday, Dr. Anthony Fauci called Paul's claim that the National Institutes of Health had funded "gain-of-function" research in Wuhan "preposterous" in an interview with PolitiFact. https://www.politifact.com/article/2021/may/11/united facts-america-fauci-disputes-sen-rand-paul-/

128. Centers for Disease Control and Prevention (CDC), May 12, 2021, Selected Adverse Events Reported after COVID-19 Vaccination | CDC

129. https://www.thedesertreview.com/opinion/letters to editor/ivermectin-for-the-world/article 2aa653ca-b1ae-11eb-903e-a78b2b053ba4.html

130. https://medisolve.org/yellowcard urgentprelimreport.pdf

131. Seneff and Nigh, "Worse Than the Disease?"

132. ACIP Meeting Agenda June 18 2021 (cdc.gov)

133. 'We clearly have an imbalance': CDC holding emergency meeting over COVID vax concern (nypost.com)

134. Voluntary COVID-19 vaccination of children: a social responsibility (bmj. com)

135. 11221-moh-pfizer-collaboration-agreement-redacted.pdf (govextra.gov.il)

136. https://childrenshealthdefense.org/defender/vaers-data-injuries-deaths-vaccinating-5-year-olds/

137. David R. Martinez, Alexandra Schafer, Ralph Baric, et al. (2021, June 22, published online). "Chimeric spike mRNA vaccines protect against Sarbecovirus challenge in mice." DOI: 10.1126 science. abi4506. (Previous Title repeated) Science (sciencemag.org). Acknowledgments and funding awarded to participants in study.

138. Elaine R. Miller, Pedro L. Moro, Maria Cano, and Tom Shimabukuro. (2015, June 26). "Deaths Following Vaccination: What Does the Evidence Show?" Vaccine, 33,3288-3292. The article is from the Immunization Safety Office (ISO), Centers for Disease Control and Prevention (CDC). https://sciencedirect.com/science/article/pii/S0264410X15006556?casa token=dU-jB612SHDQAAAAA:KD0i GcZ74p5wYMAubCcUd-17/ rsvTUleAnB afIofV xNnG6I-e3RRfAPrw8mj4DQ4bKylilVgA

139. https://www.openvaers.com/covid-data.

140. https://www.openvaers.com/covid-data.

141. VAERS may be publicly accessed at https://wwwopenvaers.com/covid-data. Accessed July 9, 2021, by Peter McCullough, MD.

142. https://www.authorea.com/users/414448/articles/522499-sars-cov-2-mass-vaccination-urgent-questions-on-vaccine-safety-that-demand-answers-from-internationa-health-agencies-regulatory-authorities-governments-and-vaccine-developers

143. https://www.ronjohnson.senate.gov/2020/4/open-letter-to-president-trump-urging-action-on-hydroxychloroquine

144. https://aapsonline.org/hcqsuit and https://www.ronjohnson.senate/gov/2020/4/open-letter-to-president-trump-urging-action-on-hydroxychloroquine

145. https://aapsonline.org/preliminary-injunction-sought-to-release-hydroxychloroquine-to-the-public/

CHAPTER 9

1. Berenson, Alex (@AlexBerenson), "Against Hysteria, Satire, Against...," Twitter, April 16, 2020,4:14 AM, available at the Wayback Machine, https://web.archive.org/web/20210324020334/ https://twitter.com/AlexBerenson/status/1250744283012960258.

2. Ehley, Brianna. "CDC: One Quarter of Young Adults Contemplated Suicide During Pandemic." 8/13/2020.Politico. https"//www.politico.com/news/2020/08/13/cdc-mental-health-pandemic-394832

3. Berenson, Alex, "Against Hysteria, Satire, Against...," April 16, 2020.

4. World Health Organization. January 14, 2020. Twitter Post. https:// twitter.com/WHO/status/1217043229427761152

5. W.H. Kellogg, Exec Officer-California Board of Health. "Summary of Conclusions Reached as a Result of the Study of the Control Measures Adapted," 1919. https://boomcalifornia.org/2020/06/18/callifornia-and-the-1918-1920-influenza-pandemic/

6. Kreston, Rebecca, "The Public Health Legacy of the 1976 Swine Flu Outbreak," Discover, September 30, 2013. https://www.discovermagazine.com/health/the-public-health-legacy-of-the-1976-swine-flu-outbreak.

7. Hatchet, Richard J. et al., "Public Health Interventions and Epidemic Intensity During the 1918 Influenza Pandemic," Proceedings of the National Academy of Sciences of the United States of America.104, #18, (May 1, 2007),7582-87. https://www.pnas.org/content/104/18/7583#ref-6.

8. Berenson, Alex, Pandemia: How Coronavirus Hysteria Took Over Our Government, Rights, and Lives. 2021, Regnery Publishing, Washington D.C. (31)

9. Howard, Jacqueline, CNN. "U.S. Surgeon General, Dr Jerome Adams Not Only Wants People to Stop Buying Facemasks to Prevent the Novel Coronavirus, But Warns You Might Actually Increase Your Risk of Infection If Facemasks Are Not Worn Properly." March 2, 2020. https://www.cnn.com/2020/03/02/health/surgeon-general-coronavirus-masks-risk-trnd/index.html

10. Lockhart, Chelsea Bruce, et al., "The Shocking Coronavirus Study That Rocked the UK and US," Financial Times, March 19, 2020. https://www.ft.com/content/16764a22-69ca-11ea-a3c9-1fedcca75.

11. Johns, Stephen, June 10, 2020. "Neil Ferguson Talks Modelling, Lockdown, and Scientific Advice," Imperial College-London. https://imperial.ac.uk/news/198155/neil-ferguson-talks-modelling-lockdown-scientific-advice/

12. Ferguson, Neil and SAGE committee. "Options for Increasing Adherence to Social Distancing Measures," SAGE, March 22, 2020, https://assets.publishing.service.gov.uk/government/uploads/attachment_data/file/882722/25-options-for-increasing-adherence-to-social-distancing-measures-22032020.pdf.

13. Coller, Barry S., "AIDS and Civil Liberties," New York Times, June 26, 1983. https://www.nytimes.com/1983/06/26/nyregion/aids-and-civil-liberties.html.

14. Kossakovski, Fedor, "The Eccentric Scientist Behind the 'Gold Standard' COVID-19 Test," February 19, 2021. National Geographic. https://nationalgeographic.com/science/article/the-eccentric-scientist-behind-the-gold-standard-covid-19-pcr-test

15. Richardson, Safiya; Davidson, Karina, PhD; Libassi, Matthew; et al., "Largest COVID-19 Study of Hospitalized Patients in US Links Comorbidities to Acuity." April 22, 2020. Feinstein Institutes for Medical Research with Hopewell Health. https://feinstein.northwell.edu/news/the-latest/largest-covid-19-study-of-hospitalized-patients-in-us-links-comorbidities-to-acuity.

16. MacMillan, Amanda, "Hospitals Overwhelmed by Flu Patients Are Treating Them in Tents," TIME, January 18, 2018. https://time.com/5107984/hospitals-handling-burden-flu-patients/

17. Berenson, Alex, "Pandemia: How Coronavirus Hysteria Took Over…" 2021.

18. Rodriguez, L.M., Litt, D.M., Stewart, S.H. (2020) "Drinking to Cope with the Pandemic: The Unique Associations of COVID-19-Related Perceived Threat and Psychological Distress to Drinking Behaviors in American Men and Women. Addictive Behaviors,110, 106532. https://doi.org/10.1016/j.addbeh.2020,106532

19. Singman, Brooke, "LA Mayor Garcetti Encourages Residents to Report Violators of Stay-at-Home Order: 'Snitches Get Rewards,'" FOX NEWS, April 3, 2020, https://www.foxnews.com/politics/la-mayor-garcetti-residents-report-violators-stay-at-home-order

20. National Center for Health Statistics. Multiple Causes of Death 2018-2021 on CDC WONDER Database. Accessed February 2, 2023. https://www/cdc.gov/heartdisease/facts.htm

21. Hiltzik, Michael, "Column: COVID-19 May Make Universal Basic Income More Palatable, That's a Good Thing," Los Angeles Times, May 22,2020. https://www.latimes.com/business/story/2020-05-22/covid-19-universal-basic-income-more-palatable/

22. Wolf, Naomi, The Bodies of Others: The New Authoritarians, COVID-19, and the War Against the Human. All Seasons Press, May 31, 2022

23. Feldscher, Karen. "Weighing the Benefits and Costs of COVID-19 Restrictions," October, 2020. Harvard—T.H. Chan School of Public Health. https://www.hsph.harvard.edu/news/features/weighing-the-benefits-and-costs-of-covid-19-restrictions/

24. Feldscher, Karen. "Weighing the Benefits and Costs…" October 2020.

25. Kuhfield, Megan; Soland, Jim; Lewis, Karyn; and Morton, Emily. "The Pandemic (lockdowns) Has Had Devastating Impacts on Learning. What Will it Take to Help Students Catch Up?" Brookings, March 3, 2022. https://www.brookings.edu/articles/the-pandemic-has-had-devastating-impacts-on-learning-what-will-it-take-to-help-students-catch-up/

26. Kane, Tom and Reardon, Sean, News Eds, "New Data Show How the Pandemic Affected Learning Across Whole Communities," Harvard Graduate School of Education, May 11, 2023. https://www.gse.harvard.edu/ideas/news/23/05/new-data-show-how-the-pandemic-affected-learning-across-whole-communities/

27. "COVID-19 Alert No.2: New ICD Code Introduced for COVID-19 Deaths," National Vital Statistics System, Centers for Disease Control, March 24, 2020. https://www.cdc.gov/nchs/data/nvss/coronavirus/alert-2-new-icd-code-introduced-for-covid-19-deaths.pdf.

28. New York Times, June 1, 2021. "Nearly One-Third of U.S. Coronavirus Deaths Are Linked to Nursing Homes." https://www.nytimes.com/interactive/2020/us/coronavirus-nursing-homes.html

Chapter 10

1. Knowles, Eric, MBA. "The REAL Price of the Economic Stimulus," April 7, 2021. The Knowles Group. https://www.theknowlesgroup.org/blog/the-real-price-of-the-economic-stimulus/

2. Knowles, Eric, MBA. "Real Price of Economic Stimulus," April 7, 2021.

3. Vinelli, Andres; Weller, Christian E.; Vijay, Divya. March 2020. "The Economic Impact of Coronavirus in the U.S. and Possible Policy Responses." https://www.americanprogress.org/article/economic-impact-coronavirus-united-states-possible-economic-policy-responses/

4. USC Multidisciplinary Team of Researchers, "USC Study: Mandatory Business Closures Drove the Economic Decline During COVID-19 Pandemic," USC Price School of Public Policy, January 25, 2023, https://priceschool.usc.edu/news/covid-cost-gdp-adam-rose-usc-price/

5. Hlavka,Jakub, PhD; Rose, Adam, PhD. "COVID-19 's Total Cost to the U.S. Economy Will Reach $14 Trillion by End of 2023." May 16, 2023, The Evidence Base. https://www.healthpolicy.usc.edu/article/covid-19s-total-cost-to-the-economy-in-us-will-reach-14-trillion-by-end-of-2023-new-research/

6. Hlavka, Jakub, PhD; Rose, Adam, PhD. "COVID-19 's Total Cost. May 16, 2023.

7. Horowitz, Juliana Menasce; Brown, Anna; and Minkin, Rachel. "A Year Into the Pandemic, Long-Term Financial Impact Weighs Heavily on Many Americans," March 5, 2021, Pew Research Center. https://pewresearch.org/social-trends/2021/03/05/a-year-into-the-pandemic-long-term-financial-impact-weighs-heavily-on-many-americans/

8. Peterson-Withorn, Chase, "How Much Money America's Billionaires Have Made During the COVID-19 Pandemic," April 30, 2021. Forbes. https://www.forbes.com/sites/chasewithorn/2021/04/30/american-billionaires-have-gotten-1.2-trillion-richer-during-the-pandemic/?ish=417ad20af557

9. Bondy, David, "Facebook Shuts Down Group Page Critical of Michigan Stay-at-Home Order," NBC 25 News, May 13, 2020. https://nbc25news.com/news/coronavirus/organizer-of-anti-michigan-quarantine-says/facebook/shut-down-their-group-page.

10. Berenson, Alex. Pandemia: How Coronavirus Hysteria Took Over Our Government, Rights, and Lives. 2021, Regnery Publishing, Washington, D.C.

11. Berenson, Alex. Pandemia: How Coronavirus Hysteria Took Over. 2021.

12. Neilson, Shane, MD. "The Surgical Mask is a Bad Fit for Risk Reduction," NIH-National Library of Medicine and National Center for Biotechnology Information. May 17, 2016. https://www.ncbi.nlm.nih.gov/pmc/articles/PMC4868614/

13. Neilson, Shane, MD. "The Surgical Mask…" 2016.

14. Hayes, Kristin, RN and Lacy, James (fact-checked), "Can Medical Face Masks Prevent Viral Infections?" Very Well Health, February 10, 2021. https://www.verywellhealth.com/can-medical-face-masks-prevent-viral-infections-4798665

15. Centers for Disease Control and Prevention. "Recommendations Regarding the Use of Cloth Face Coverings, Especially in Areas of Significant Community-Based Transmission. https://www.cdc.gov and https://www.verywellhealth.com

16. Howard, Jacqueline, CNN. "WHO Stands by Recommendation to Not Wear Masks if You Are Not Sick or Not Caring For Someone Who Is Sick," World Health Organization, March 31, 2020. https://www.cnn.com/2020/03/30/world/coronavirus-who-masks-recommendation-trnd.index.html

17. Greenberg, Jon, (PolitiFact.com) December 29, 2020, "Did Anthony Fauci Lie About Masks?" Austin American-Statesman. https://www.statesman.com/story/news/politics/2020/12/29/did-anthony-fauci-lie-masks-march-rubio-said/4068162001/

18. Sullum, Jacob, "Anthony Fauci May Not Have 'Lied' About Face Masks, but He Was Not Exactly Honest Either," Reason-Free Minds and Free Markets, June 4, 2021. https://reason.com/2021/06/04/anthony-fauci-may-not-have-lied-about-face-masks-but-he-was-not-exactly-honest-either/

19. Sullum, Jacob, "Anthony Fauci May Not Have Lied, but…," June 4,2021

20. Sullum, Jacob, "Anthony Fauci May Not Have Lied, but…," June 4, 2021

21. Louise, Nickie, "Wearing Mask Outside Offers Little, IF Any, Protection From Coronavirus Infection, New England Journal of Medicine Study Says," July 13, 2020. https://techstartups.com/2020/07/13/ wearing-mask-outside-offers-little-protection- coronavirus-infection-new-england-journal-medicine-study-says/

22. Mansell, Megan, Accommodating Chaos: Correcting Course on a Plague of Misinformation, March 4, 2022/Kindle Edition, https://www.amazon.com

23. Tucker, Jeffrey A., "Why Did They Close the Schools?" June 8, 2020. American Institute for Economic Research (AIER). https://www.aier.org/article/why-did-they-close-the-schools/

24. YPulse, "College Students' Plans for Staying in School Are in Flux," October 7, 2020. https://www.ypulse.com/article/2020/10/07/college-students-plans-for-staying-in-school-are-in-flux/

25. Oster, Matthew E., MD, MPH; Shay, David K., MD, MPH; Su, John R., MD, MPH; et al., "Myocarditis Cases Reported After mRNA-Based COVID-19 Vaccination in the US From December 2020 to August 2021," Journal of the American Medical Association (JAMA), January 25, 2022. https://jamanetwork.com/journals/jama/fullarticle/2788346

26. Haidt, Jonathan, and Lukianoff, Greg. The Coddling of the American Mind: How Good Intentions and Bad Ideas Are Setting Up a Generation for Failure.(New York: Penguin, 2019), p 30.

27. Gibbons, Katic, "Coronavirus Could Age the Brain by 10 Years or Cause IQ to Fall," The Times (London), October 27,2020. https://www.thetimes.co.uk/article/ coronavirus-could-age-the-brain-by-10-years-or-cause-iq-to-fall-v9s273rbs.

28. Morens, David M.; Fauci, Anthony, "Emerging Pandemic Diseases: How We Got COVID-19," CELL 182, September 3, 2020. https://www.cell/pdf/S0092-8674(20) 31012-6.pdf.

29. "Long COVID or Post-COVID Conditions," Centers for Disease Control and Prevention, updated March 14, 2024. https://www.cdc.gov/coronavirus/2019-ncov/long-term-effects/index.html.

30. Robinson, Peter (per interview with Dr. Scott Atlas), "The Doctor Is In: Scott Atlas and the Efficacy of Lockdowns, Social Distancing, and Closings," Uncommon Knowledge with Peter Robinson, June 23, 2020. Hoover Institution. https://www.hoover.org/research/doctor-scott-atlas-and-efficacy-lockdowns-social-distancing-and-closings-1

31. Kulldorff, Martin, MD; Gupta, Sunetra, MD; Bhattacharya, Jay, MD; along with a minimum of at least 50 other professional co-signers, The Great Barrington Declaration, also including 930,000+ global co-signers. https://gbdeclaration.org

32. Sprunt, Barbara, "Don't Be Afraid of It: Trump Dismisses Virus Threat as He Returns to White House," NPR, October 5, 2020. https://www.npr.org/sections/latest-updates-trump-covid-19-results/2020/10/05/920412187/trump-says-he-will-leave-walter-reed-medical-center-monday-night./

33. Berenson, Alex. Pandemia: How Coronavirus Hysteria Took Over Our Government, Rights, and Lives. 2021, Regnery Publishing, Washington, D.C.

34. Abutaleb, Yasmeen; Parker, Ashley; Dawsey, Josh; and Rucker, Philip; "The Inside Story of How Trump's Denial, Mismanagement and Magical Thinking Led to the Pandemic's Dark Winter," The Washington Post, December 19, 2020. https://www.washingtonpost.com/graphics/2020/politics/trump-covid-pandemic-dark-winter/

35. Berenson, Alex. Unreported Truths About COVID-19 and Lockdowns—Part 4: Vaccines. March 23, 2021. Independent, Citizen-funded Journalism. https://alexberenson.substack/com/p/a-poll-should-i-write-a-book-about-the-failure-of-the-mrnas/

36. Andrews, Nick PhD., Tessier, Elise, M.Sc., Stowe, Julia, PhD., et al., "Duration of Protection Against Mild and Severe Disease by COVID-19 Vaccines," New England Journal of Medicine, January 12, 2022, https://www.nejm.org/doi/full/10.1056/NEJMoa2115481

37. Mayo Clinic Staff, "COVID-19 Vaccines: Get the Facts," November 3, 2023. https://www.mayoclinic.org/diseases-conditions/coronavirus/in-depth/coronavirus-vaccine/art-20484859

38. Kalla, Daniel, "The 'Vaccine Hesitant' Are a Threat to Society—But We Must Show Them Compassion," The Globe and Mail, May 7, 2021. https://www.theglobeandmail.com/opinion/article-the-vaccine-hesitant-are-a-threat-to-society-but-we-must-show-them-compassion/

39. Waldrop, Theresa; Andone, Dakin; and Holcombe, Madeline; "Fauci: Vaccinations Will Keep Coronavirus Variants From Emerging," CNN, January 22, 2021. https://www.cnn.com/2021/01/22/health/us-coronavirus-thursday/index.html

40. Srivastava, Mehul, "Israel's COVID Infections Surge as Government Rolls Out Booster Shots," Financial Times, August 10, 2021, https://www.ft.com/content/9e06cb33-38a1-4efe-859e-95008c85a623

41. Gazit, Sivan; Shlezinger, Roei; Perez, Galit ; Lotan, Roni ; et al., "Comparing SARS-CoV-2 Natural Immunity to Vaccine-Induced Immunity: Reinfections Versus Breakthrough Infections," med RX iv, August 25, 2021. https://www.medrxiv.org/content/10.1101/2021.08.24.21262415v1

42. Brueninger, Kevin, "Biden Blames Delta Variant, Unvaccinated People for Weaker-Than- Expected Jobs Report," CNBC, September 3, 2021. https://www. cnbc.com/2021/09/03/biden-blames-delta-variant-unvaccinated-people-for-weaker-than-expected-jobs-report.html

43. Calvan, Bobby Caina, "No Shot, No Proof, No Service: NYC Businesses Begin Checks," AP News, August 17,2021. https://apnews.com/article/lifestyle-business-health-coronavirus-pandemic-0c94e94960b9150668e37599aed3872f

44. Meisel, Hannah, "Unvaccinated COVID Patients Can't Be Denied Insurance Coverage for Hospitalizations as one Dem Lawmaker Wants, But Employers, Including Illinois, Have Other Options," NPR Illinois, December 6, 2021. https://www.nprillinois.org/statehouse/2021-12-06/unvaccinated-covid-patients-can't-be-denied-insurance-coverage-for-hospitalizations-as-one-dem-lawmaker-wants-but-employers-including-ill-have-other-options

45. Lovelace, Jr., Berkeley, "Biden Outlines Plan to Mandate COVID Vaccines For Millions: 'Our Patience Is Wearing Thin,'" CNBC, September 9, 2021. https://www.cnbc.com/2021/09/09/biden-to-detail-new-six-pronged-plan-to-increase-us-covid-vaccination-rates-fight-virus.html

46. Howard, Jacqueline, "Two Departing FDA Leaders Among Scientists Who Say COVID-19 Vaccines Do Not Currently 'Show a Need for Boosting,'" CNN, September 13, 2021. https://www.cnn.com/2021/09/13/health/boosters-not-needed-lancet-review/index.html

47. Baldassaro, Michael; Harbath, Katie; and Scholtens, Michael, "The Big Lie and Big Tech: Misinformation Repeat Offenders and Social Media in the 2020 US Election," The Carter Center, August 2021. https://www.cartercenter.org/resources/pdfs/news/peace_publications/democ racy/the-big-lie-and-big-tech.pdf

Chapter 11

1. Repucci, Sarah and Slipowitz, Amy, "The Global Expansion of Authoritarian Rule," Freedom House/ Freedom in the World-2022. https://freedomhouse.org/report/freedom-world/2022/global-expansion-authoritarian-rule

2. Norman, Donald A., "Being Analog/Making Sense of the World/Humans vsComputers," The Invisible Computer, MIT Press, Cambridge, MA. 1997-98. https://pages.ucsd.edu/-dnorman/DNMss/Being_Analog.html

3. Wolf, Naomi, The Bodies of Others: The New Authoritarians, COVID-19, and the War Against the Human. All Seasons Press, May 31, 2022.

4. Wolf, Naomi, The Bodies of Others… 2022

5. Wolf, Naomi, The Bodies of Others…2022

6. Wolf, Naomi, The Bodies of Others…2022

7. Wolf, Naomi, The Bodies of Others…2022

8. Cuomo, Andrew, "Governor Cuomo Signs the "New York State on PAUSE' Executive Order," Governor's Press Office, Albany, NY, March 20, 2020. https://www.governor.ny.gov/news/governor-cuomo-signs-new-new-york-state-pause-executive-order

9. Schwab, Klaus and Vanham, Peter, "Stakeholder Capitalism: A Global Economy that Works for Progress, People, and Planet," World Economic Forum—Davos Agenda, January 2021. https://www.weforum.org/agenda/2021/01/klaus-schwab-on-what-is-stakeholder-capitalism-history-relevance/

10. Wolf, Naomi, The Bodies of Others…2022

11. Feng, John, "China Culpable in 'Significant' Abuses Against Own People—US Report," Newsweek, March 23, 2023, https://www.newsweek.com/china-human-rights-violations-xinjiang-tibet-state-department-1789880

12. Kazmierczak, Mark and Haneman, Thilo; "China's Biotechnology Development: The Role of US and Other Foreign Engagement," Gryphon Scientific and Rhodium Group, February 14, 2019 prepared for: The National Counterintelligence and Security Center. https://www/dni.gov/files/NCSC/documents/SafeguardingOurFuture/NCSC-China-Genomics-Fact-Sheet-2021revision20210203.pdf

13. Schenker, Jennifer, "China Leaps Ahead in Precision Medicine," The Innovator News, August 27, 2019.

14. Needham, Kirsty, "Special Report: COVID Opens New Doors for China's Gene Giant," Reuters, August 5, 2020.

15. Wolf, Naomi, The Bodies of Others…2022.

16. Wolf, Naomi, The Bodies of Others…2022

17. Clark, Ward, "'We're Going to Get Hit'—China Expert Issues Dire Warning," Red State, December 19, 2024, https://redstate.com/wardclark/2024/12/19/were-going-to-get-hit-china-expert-issues-dire-warning-n2183412

18. Cook, Sarah, "CCP's Media Influence Expands Worldwide: Report Finds Global Rise in Propaganda, Censorship, and Control of Content Delivery Systems," Freedom House. Updated Report: "CCP's Media Influence Expands Worldwide." January 14, 2020. https://freedomhouse.org/article/chinese-communist-partys-media-influence-expands-worldwide.

19. Abrams, Elissa M. MD, MPH; Greenhawt, Matthew MD, MBA, MSc; Shaker, Marcus MD MSc; et al.; "The COVID-19 Pandemic: Adverse Effects on the Social Determinants of Health in Children and Families, Science Direct, October 22. 2021, https://www.sciencedirect.com/science/article/pii/S1081120621011686

20. Carter, D.; Odama, A.; Obi, N.; and Lang, H., "COVID-19 and Its Impacts on Child Abuse and Neglect," Washington University/St. Louis/ CICM, 2021, https://cicm.wustl.edu/items/covid-19-and-child-abuse-and-neglect-brief/

21. Tung, Liz, "'This Was Going to Be a Tidal Wave:' What Makes Pandemic Grief Similar to Violent Death Grief," Why, December 9, 2022. https://whyy.org/segments/pandemic-grief-similar-to-violent-death-grief/

22. Tung, Liz, "This Was Going to Be a Tidal Wave," … December 9, 2022.

23. Vassiliou, Maria (Founder, Philotimo Life), "How to Navigate Grief in the Post-Pandemic Workplace," World Economic Forum, January 31, 2022. https://www.weforum.org/agenda/2022/01/how-to-navigate-grief-in-the-post-pandemic-workplace/

24. Vassiliou, Maria. "How to Navigate Grief in the Pandemic Workplace," January 31, 2022.

25. Lee, Sherman A., and Neimeyer, Robert A., "Pandemic Grief Scale: A Screening Tool for Dysfunctional Grief Due to a COVID-19 Loss," Pub Med/NCBI, December 21, 2020, https://pubmed.ncbi.nim.nih.gov/33349159/

26. Tung, Liz, "This Was Going to be a Tidal Wave,"...December 0, 2022.

27. Weir, Kirsten, "Grief and COVID-19: Mourning our Bygone Lives," American Psychological Association, April 1, 2020 https://www/apa.org/news/apa/2020/grief-covid-19

28. Wolf, Naomi, The Bodies of Others...2022

29. Hippensteel, Chris. "Inside the Push to Open Up Hart Island, NYC's COVID Cemetery," Yahoo News, May 27, 2022. https://www.yahoo.com/news/hart-island-new-york-city-covid-public-cemetery-173916858.html

30. Zhang, Rachel Cohrs. "Andrew Cuomo's COVID-19 Nursing Home Fiasco Shows the Ethical Perils of Pandemic Policymaking," February 26, 2021; https://www.statnews.com/2021/02/26/cuomos-nursing-home-fiasco-ethical-perils-pandemic-policymaking/

31. Select Subcommittee on the Coronavirus Pandemic, "Like Fire Through Dry Grass: Nursing Home Mortality and COVID-19 Policies," Committee on Oversight and Accountability/House of Representatives, May 17, 2023, https://www.congress.gov/118-33/meeting/house/115959/documents/HHRG-118-VC00-Transcript-20230517.pdf

32. Lutz, Brigette, (media contact), "Legality of Mandatory Mask Wearing in the COVID-19 Climate," Marrone Law Firm, LLC, 2024, https://marronelaw.com/white-papers/legality-of-mandatory-mask-wearing-in-the-covid-19-climate/

33. Wolf, Naomi, The Bodies of Others...2022.

34. Wolf, Naomi, The Bodies of Others...2022.

35. Nevradakis, Michael, PhD., and Miller, Brad, "Remdesivir Papers: Drug Used to Treat Service Members Led to Deaths," Children's Health Defense/ The Defender in Depth, October 16, 2024, https://live.children'shealthdefense.org/chd-tv/shows/good-morning-chd/remdesivir-papers-drug-used-to-treat-service-members-led-to-deaths/

36. Oaklander, Mandy; "The Coronavirus Killed the Handshake and the Hug; What Will Replace Them?" Time, May 27, 2020, https://time.com/5842469/coronavirus-handshake-social-touch/

37. Thakur, Ramesh; "Who Killed Granny? Shameless Emotional Manipulation Shaped Too Much of Global COVID Policy, Disastrously," The India Times, February 12, 2021; https://timesofindia.indiatimes.com/blogs/toi-edit-page/who-killed-granny-shameless-emotional-manipulationn-shaped-too-much-of-global-covid-policy-disastrously/

38. Wolf, Naomi, The Bodies of Others…2022.

39. Wolf, Naomi, The Bodies of Others…2022.

40. Gade, Alexander Foss; "Digital Dashboard", AutoPi, 2023, Aalborg, Denmark. https://www.autopi.io/glossary/digitaol-dashboard/

41. Wolf, Naomi, The Bodies of Others…2022.

42. Ealy, Dr. Henry, BSME, ND, BCHN, et al.; "COVID-19: Restoring Public Trust During A Global Health Crisis—An Evidence-Based Position Paper to Ensure Ethical Conduct, including a Formal Grand Jury Petition," (Oregon) Oregon Legislature, February 22, 2021, https://olis.oregonlegislature.gov/liz/2021R1/Downloads/Public Testimony Document/8038

43. Wolf, Naomi, The Bodies of Others…2022.

44. America's Frontline Doctors, "Protecting Your Medical Freedom and Civil Liberties/Honest Healthcare Solutions—From the Ground Up," AFLDS, January 22, 2024, https://americasfrontlinedoctors.org/about-us

45. Boyle, Patrick; "Why Do So Many Americans Distrust Science?" Assoc. of American Medical Colleges, May 4, 2022; https://www.aamc.org/news/why-do-so-many-americans-distrust-science.

46. Wolf, Naomi; The Bodies of Others…2022

47. Wolf, Naomi; The Bodies of Others…2022

48. Miller, Keith, "18 Advantages and Disadvantages of the European Union," Future of Working/ The Leadership and Career Blog, Copyright, 2025, https://futureofworking.com/18-advantages-and-disadvantages-of-the-EU/

49. Wolf, Naomi; The Bodies of Others…2022

50. Nesterak, Max, "Uprooted—The 1950s Plan to Erase Indian Country," American Public Media Reports, November 1, 2019, https://www.apmreports.org/episode/2019/11/01/uprooted—the-1950s-plan-to-erase-indian-country

51. Wolf, Naomi; The Bodies of Others…2022.

52. Dr. Bhattacharya, Jay; Dr. Gupta, Sunetra; and Dr. Kulldorff, Martin; "Why Was the Declaration Written?" The Great Barrington Declaration, October 5,2020. https://gbdelaration.org/why-was-the-declaration-written/

53. The Editorial Board of WSJ, "How Fauci and Collins Shut Down COVID Debate—They Worked with the Media to Trash the Great Barrington Declaration," The Wall Street Journal Opinion, December 21, 2021, https://www.wsj.com/articles/fauci-collins-emails-great-barrington-declaration-covid-pandemic-lockdown-11640129116

54. Official Social Media for Great Barrington Declaration, "Frequently Asked Questions" January 10, 2022, https://gbdeclaration.org/frequently-asked-questions/

55. Wolf, Naomi; The Bodies of Others…2022

56. Romeo, Peter, "Restaurants Push Back on Dining-Room Shutdowns", Restaurant Business, November 17, 2020, https://www.restaurantbusinessonline.com/operations/restaurants-push-back-dining-room-shutdowns

57. Wolf, Naomi; The Bodies of Others…2022

58. Philips, Dr. Patrick, "Dr. Philips Tells His Story of How the Ontario Government Stole His Medical License", Ernest Skinner of Rumble, July 26, 2023, https://rumble.com/v32kl9i-july-26-2023.html

59. Goddek, Dr. Simon, "The Peer Review Process 'Was Rigged' Says Dr. Simon Goddek…Then Twitter Banned Him," Ask Dr. Drew-You Tube. https://www.youtube.com/watch?v=B-YyCbQ4b8E

60. Wolf, Naomi; The Bodies of Others…2022

61. Larson, Dr. Eric, "Understanding PCR in COVID-19 with Kevin McKernan", The Paradocs. (Episode 116, February 18, 2021, https://theparadocs.com/understanding-pcr-in-covid-19-with-kevin-mckernan/

62. Cuomo, Andrew (Governor NY), "Governor Cuomo Announces Wedding Receptions and Catered Events Can Now Resume Statewide," New York State Gov-Albany, NY, March 15, 2021, https://www.governor.ny.gov/news/governor-cuomo-announces-wedding-receptions-and-catered-events-can-now-resume-statewide

63. Bill and Melinda Gates Foundation, "CNN", https://www.gatesfoundation,org/about/committed-grants?q=CNN#committed-grants.

64. Ul Alam, Rezwan, SM; 'In the Era of Social Media, Legacy Media is Indispensable," The Daily Star, April 5, 2024; https://thedailystar.net/opinion/views/news/the-era-social-media-legacy-media-indispensable-3582736

65. Pandolfo, Chris, "Exclusive: The Federal Government Paid Hundreds of Media Companies to Advertise the COVID-19 Vaccines While Those Same Outlets Provided Positive Coverage of the Vaccines," The Blaze.com, March 3, 2022; https://www.theblaze.com/news/review-the-federal-gov-paid-media-companies-to-advertise-for-the-vaccines.

66. Pandolfo, Chris, "Exclusive: The Federal Government Paid Media to Advertise the COVID-19 Vaccines and Provide Positive Coverage," March 3, 2022

67. Grabow, Jeffrey (EY US Venture Capital Leader). "Venture Capital Continues to Exhibit Immunity to the COVID-19 Pandemic," EY-US, February 9,2022. https://www.ey.com/en_us/insights/growth/venture-capital-continues-to-exhibit-immunity-to-the-covid-19-pandemic

68. Bhakdi, Dr. Sucharit "Open Letter from Doctors and Scientists to the European Medicines Agency Regarding COVID-19 Vaccine Safety Concerns," What Do They Know.com, March 17, 2021, https://www.whatdotheyknow.com/en/request/open-letter-from-doctors-and-sci?unfold-1

69. Wolf, Naomi; The Bodies of Others…2022

70. Wolf, Naomi; The Bodies of Others…2022

71. Deoni, Sean CL; Beauchemin, Jennifer; Volpe, Alexandra; D'sa, Viren; and the Resonance Consortium, "The COVID-19 Pandemic and Child Cognitive Development: Initial Findings in a Longitudinal, Observational Study of Child Health," August 11,2021, medRxiv 2021. 08.10.21261846(preprint) https://doi.org/10.1101/2021.08.10.21261846

72. Wolf, Naomi; The Bodies of Others…2022

73. Anweshbiswas, (Product Mgr), "The Meteoric Rise of Zoom!" Medium, October 16, 2023. https://medium.com/@work.anweshbiswas/the-meteoric-rise-of-zoom-f2d7c7140d15

74. Gonzales, Mike and Burke, Lindsey M (PhD), "The Root Cause of the Insanity on College Campuses Is Older Than You Might Think," The Heritage Foundation. November 16, 2023, https://www.heritage.org/progressivism/commentary/the-root-cause-of-the-insanity-on-college-campuses-is-older-than-you-might-think.

75. Hlávka, Jakub, PhD and Rose, Adam, PhD, "COVID-19's Total Cost to the US Economy Will Reach $14 Trillion by End of 2023," The Evidence Base-USCDornsife, May 16, 2023, https://healthpolicy.usc.edu/article/covid-19s-total-cost-to-the-us-economy-will-reach-14-trillion-by-end-of-2023-new-research/

76. Hlávka, Jakub, PhD and Rose, Adam, PhD, "COVID-19's Total Cost…2023

77. Newsroom Staff, "Oregon Senators Call for CDC and FDA Inquiry," NBC—KOBI5, September 22, 2021, https://kobi5.com/news/local-news/oregon-senators-call-for-cdc-and-fda-inquiry-167409/

78. Wolf, Naomi, The Bodies of Others…2022

79. Markowitz, Gayle, "What is a 'Vaccine Passport' and Will You Need One the Next Time You Travel?" World Economic Forum (part of Davos Agenda, May 5, 2022, https://www.weforum.org/agenda/2021/05/what-is-a-vaccine-passport-and-will-you-need-one-the-next-time-you-travel/

80. Flam, F, D. (columnist), "Vaccine Passports Would Get the US Back to Normal Faster," Bloomberg, March 20, 2021, https://www.bloomberg.com/opinion/articles/2021-03-20/covid-vaccine-passports-would-get-the-u-s-back-to-normal-faster

81. Tate, Kristin, "Coming Soon: America's Own Social Credit System," The Hill, August 3, 2021, https://thehill.com/opinion/finance/565860-coming-soon-americas-own-social-credit-system/

82. BBC Staff, "COVID: U.S. Rules Out Federal Vaccine Passports," British Broadcasting CO, April 6,2021, https://www.bbc.com/news/world-u-s-canada-56657194

83. Allocca, Sean; Curcio, Paul; and Tony, David, "Will the US Dollar Become a Digital Currency?" CNN Underscored Money, May 16, 2024, https://www.cnn.com/cnn-underscored/money/will-the-us-dollar-become-a-digital-currency

84. Allocca, Curcio, and Tony, "Will the US Dollar Become…May 16,2024

85. Opeyemi Amure, Tobi, "What Will a U.S. Central Bank Digital Currency Look Like?" Investopedia, June 08, 2024, https://www.investopedia.com/us-cbdc-6740586

86. Zandt, Florian, "Central Bank Digital Currency: The Future of Money?" Statista, June 28, 2023, https://www.statista.com/chart/30296/number-of countries-currency-unions-with-central-bank-digital-currencies-in-advanced-exploration-phases/

87. Benzmiller, Theodore, "China's Progress Towards a Central Bank Digital Currency," Center For Strategic International Studies (CSIS), April 19, 2022, https://www.csis.org/blogs/new-perspective-asia/chinas-progress-towards-central-bank-digital-currency/

Chapter 12

1. Smith, Hazel, "The Legal and Ethical Implications of Using Data HarvestingTools," Time Magazine, December 20, 2024, https://timemagazine.net/the-legal-and-ethical-implications-of-using-data-harvesting-tools/

2. Dickinson, Hunter, "What is a Paywall? Different Types of Paywalls," Whop Blog, October 29, 2023, https://whop.com/blog/what-is-a-paywall/

3. Duggan, Wayne and Adams, Michael, "What Happened to FAANG Stocks? They Became MAMAA Stocks," Forbes Advisor, July 1, 2024, https://www.forbes.com/advisor/investing/faang-stocks-mamaa/

4. Bremmer, Ian, "The Technopolar Moment: How Digital Powers Will Reshape the Global Order," Foreign Affairs, October 19, 2021, https://www.foreignaffairs.com/articles/world/ian-bremmer-big-tech-global-order

5. Bremmer, Ian, "The Technopolar Moment: How Digital Powers Will Reshape…October 19, 2021

6. Lang, Marissa, "There Is No Such Thing as True Privacy in the Digital Age," Government Technology/Cyber Security, 2017, https://www.govtech.com/security/there-is-no-such-thing-as-true-privacy-in-the-digital-age.html

7. Schaake, Marietje, "Big Tech's Coup/How Companies Seized Power from States—and How States Can Claw It Back," Foreign Affairs, September 26, 2024, https://www.foreignaffairs.com/brazil/big-techs-coup

8. Khanal, Shaleen; Zhang, Hongzhou; and Taeihagh, Araz; "Why and How is the Power of Big Tech Increasing in the Policy Process? The Case of Generative AI," Oxford Academic/Policy and Society, March 27, 2024, https://academi.oup.com/policyandsociety/advance-aarticle/doi/10.1093/polsoc/puae012/7636223

9. Anderson, Janna and Rainie, Lee; "3.Themes: The Most Harmful or Menacing Changes in Digital Life that Are Likely by 2035," Pew Research Center, June 21, 2023, https://www.pewresearch.org/internet/2023/06/21/themes-the-most-harmful-or-menacing-changes-in-digital-life-that-are-likely-by-2035/

10. Brenner, Ian, "Big Tech's Big Challenge to the Global Order," Gzero Staff—Ian's Quick Take, October 18, 2021, https://www.gzeromedia.com/quick-take/big-challenge-to-the-global-order

11. Collins, Chuck, "How Billionaire Investors Are Disrupting the US Housing Market," Inequality.Org, October 22, 2024, https://inequality.org/article/how-billionaire-investors-are-disrupting-the-u-s-housing-market/

12. McNeill, Sandra and Card, Kenton with nine graduate students and 14 community partners, "Decommodifying Housing During COVID-19," July, 2020, UCLA Luskin School of Public Affairs, https://www.caclnetwork.org/wp-content/uploads/2020/07/De-Commodifying-Housing-During-COVID-19.pdf

13. González, Silvia R; Loya, José; and Miguel, Miguel; "UCLA Research Reveals Significant Racial and Ethnic Disparities in Los Angeles County's Mortgage Market," UCLA Latino Policy and Politics Institute, June 8, 2023, https://latino.ucla.edu/press/ucla-research-reveals-significant-racial-and-ethnic-disparities-in-los-angeles-countys-mortgage-market/

14. Elmore, Joanna G, MD, MPH, "BIPOC Individuals Bear Greater Post-COVID Health Burdens, New Research Suggests," UCLA Health/Internal Medicine, January 31, 2024, https://www.uclahealth.org/news/release/bipoc-individuals-bear-greater-past-covid-health-burdens-new

15. Reich, Robert, "How the Oligarchy Shrank America's Middle Class (Why American Capitalism is so Rotten, Part 8)," Substack, January 24, 2024, https://robertreich.sustack.com/p/the-declining-power-of-the-middle?utm_source=substack&utm_medium=email&utm_content=share

16. Reich, Robert, "How the Oligarchy Shrank America's Middle Class…" January 24, 2024.

17. Bartlett, Bruce, "Is The Only Purpose of a Corporation to Maximize Profit?" Ritholtz Wealth Management, LLC/ The Big Picture, May 15, 2015, https://ritholtz.com/2015/05/corp-purpose-maximize-profit/

18. Economic Times, Ed., "'Most Billionaire Wealth Is Taken, Not Earned': A New Report Reveals How 60% of World's Wealthiest Are Building Their Fortunes," The Economic Times News, January 19, 2025, https://economictimes.indiatimes.com/news/international/global-trends/most-billionaire-wealth-is-taken-not-earned-a-new-report-reveals-how-60%-of-worlds-wealthiest-are-building-their-fortunes//

19. President Joseph Biden, "Remarks by President Biden on Fighting the COVID-19 Pandemic," The White House, September 9, 2021, https://www/whitehouse.gov/briefing-room/speeches-remarks/2021/09/09/remarks-by-president-biden-on-fighting-the-covid-19-pandemic-3/

20. President Biden, "Remarks on Fighting the Pandemic…September 9, 2021

21. President Biden, "Remarks on Fighting the Pandemic…September 9. 2021

22. National Assembly of France, 1789, "Declaration of the Rights of Man-1789", Yale Law School-Lillian Goldman Law Library, August 26, 1789, https://avalon.law.yale.edu/18th_century/rightsof.asp

23. Glaeser, Edward L.; Ponzetto, Giacomo; and Shleifer, Andrei; "Why Does Democracy Need Education?" National Bureau of Economic Research, March 2006, https://www/nber.org/system/files/working_papers/w12128.pdf

24. Blair, Douglas, "I'm a Former Teacher. Here's How Your Children are Getting Indoctrinated by Leftist Ideology." The Heritage Foundation, August 17, 2020, https://www.heritage.org/education/commentary/im-former-teacher-heres-how-your-children-are-getting-indoctrinated-by-leftist-ideology/

25. Harper, Thomas, "The Marxification of Education: by James Lindsay-Summary and Review," The Marxification of Education-Paulo Freire's Critical Marxism and the Theft of Education", January 21, 2023, https://authortomharper.com/2023/01/21/marxification-of-education-paulo-freire-james-lindsay/

26. Harper, Thomas, "The Marxification of Education…January 21, 2023

27. Cox, Cynthia; Amin, Krutika; Kates, Jennifer; and Michaud, Josh; "Why Do Vaccinated People Represent Most COVID-19 Deaths Right Now?" Peterson-KFF Health System Tracker, November 30,2022, https://www/kff.org/policy-watch/why-do-vaccinated-people-represent-most-covid-19-deaths-right-now/

28. Cox, Amin, Kates, and Michaud, "Why Do Vaccinated People…" 11/30/2022

29. CDC Vaccine Safety, " Historical Vaccine Safety Concerns," CDC, Last reviewed September 4,2020, https://www.cdc.gov/vaccinesafety/concerns/concerns-history.html

30. Bardosh, Kevin; de Figueiredo, Alex; Gur-Ane, Rachel; et al ; "The Unintended Consequences of COVID-19 Vaccine Policy: Why Mandates, Passports and Restrictions May Cause More Harm Than Good," BMJ Global Health, May 26, 2022, https://gh.bgh.com/content/7/5/e008684.info

31. Wolf, Dr. Naomi, The Bodies of Others…, 2022

32. Bor, Alexander; Jorgensen, Frederik; and Petersen, Michael Bang; "Discriminatory Attitudes Against Unvaccinated People During the Pandemic," Nature, December 8, 2022, https://www.nature.com/articles/s41586-022-05607-y

33. U.S. Legal Website, "The Right to (Medical) Treatment," U. S. Legal, 1985, https://healthcare.uslegal.com/patient-rights/the-right-to-treatment/

34. Owermohle, Sarah, "Biden's Top-Down Booster Plan Sparks Anger at the FDA," Politico, August 31, 2021, https://www.politico.com/news/2021/08/31/biden-booster-plan-fda-508149

35. Lybrand, Holmes, "Fack Check: Senator Ron Johnson (again) Misleads on Vaccines and Reported Deaths," CNN, June 28, 2021, https://www.cnn.com/2021/06/28/politics/senator-ron-johnson-vaers-covid-deaths/index.html

36. Bluth, Rachel, " 'My Body, My Choice': How Vaccine Foes Co-opted the Abortion Rallying Cry," National Public Radio Network (NPR), July 4. 2022, https://www.npr.org/sections/health-shots/2022-07/04/1109367458/my-body-my-choice-vaccines

37. Colarossi, Jessica, "Expert Take: Is COVID-19 Still a Pandemic?" The Brink-Boston University, March 4, 2024, https://www.bu.edu/articles/2024/03/04/is-covid-19-still-a-pandemic/

38. Pecotic, Adrian, M.A., and Lancaster, Vanessa (reviewer), "How the Pandemic Has Affected Our Sense of Time," Psychology Today/Synapses, Sanity, Society, May23,2021, https://www.psychologytoday.com/us/blog/synapses-sanity-society/202105/how-the-pandemic-has-affected-our-sense-of-time

39. The Select Committee on the CCP, "What They're Saying about Protecting Americans from the Foreign Adversary-Controlled Applications Act," March 7, 2024, https://selectcommitteeontheccp.house.gov/media/press-releases/what-theyre-saying-about-protecting-american-foreign-adversary-controlled

40. The Select Committee on the CCP, "What They're Saying…March 7, 2024

41. Rosenberg, Scott, "Tech's Globalist Dream is Dying," Axios Business Suite, March 15, 2022, https://www.axios.com/2022/03/15/globalist-dream-dying-russia-china-big-tech

42. Wikipedia, "Endemic (epidemiology)", https://en.wikipedia.org/wiki/Endemic_(epidemilology)#examples

43. Wolf, Dr. Naomi, The Bodies of Others…, 2022

44. Arora, Ashish, "Radicalizing a Nation: How Hitler's Regime Transformed Germany into a Totalitarian State," The World Hour, October 25, 2024, https://theworldhour.com/radicalizing-a-nation-how-hitlers-regime-transformed-germany-into-a-totalitarian-state/

45. Yad Vashem, "Euthanasia Program," Shoah Resource Center, International School for Holocaust Studies, https://www.yadvashem.org/odot_pdf/Microsoft Word-6303.pdf

46. Yad Vashem, "Euthanasia Program…"

47. Robbins, Clair Porter, " How Trudeau Botched the Trucker Protests Response," Foreign Policy Dispatch-the View from the Ground, March 4, 2022, https://foreignpolicy.com/2022/03/04/trudeau-trucker-vaccine-protests-canada-communications/

48. Robbins, Clair Porter, "How Trudeau Botched the Trucker Protests Response," March 4, 2022

49. Farber, Celia, "THE CANADIAN TRUCKERS ACTUALLY WON? 'It Might Just Have Been the Most Successful Individual Protest in Human History,'" The Truth Barrier/Substack, July 26, 2023, https://celiafarber.substack.com/p/the-canadian-truckers-actually-won

50. Boyd, Tim, Cause Unknown: The Epidemic of Sudden Deaths in 2021 and 2022, by Edward Dowd, February 4, 2023, https://www.wesronaprice.org/book-reviews/cause-unknown-by-edward-dowd/#gsc.tab=0

51. Boyd, Tim, Cause Unknown: The Epidemic of Sudden Deaths…2023

52. Boyd, Tim, Cause Unknown: The Epidemic of Sudden Deaths…2023

53. Chung, Frank, "What is SADS? Healthy Young People Dying From Sudden Adult Death Syndrome," News.com.au/Lifestyle, June 8, 2022, https://www.news.com.au/lifestyle/health/health-problems/what-is-sads-healthy-young-people-dying-from-sudden-adult-death-syndrome/news-story/97a476dd99caaf638cd1c15baabbc5d4

54. Instagram Post, "According to International Olympic Committee Data, 'an average of 29 Athletes Under the age of 35 Suffered Sudden Death per year from 1966 to 2004. From March 2021 to March 2022, 769 Athletes Have Died or Suffered Cardiac Arrest,'" Politifact/The Poynter Institute, June, 20, 2022, https://www.politifact.com/factchecks/2022/june/23/instagram-posts/claims-connecting-sudden-death-athletes-covid-19-v/

55. Chong, Dennis, "Political Protest and Civil Disobedience," Science Direct—from Encyclopedia of Applied Ethics, 2012, https://www.sciencedirect.com/topixs/social-sciences/civil-disobedience

56. Wolf, Dr. Naomi, The Bodies of Others…2022

57. Wolf, Dr. Naomi, The Bodies of Others…2022

58. Wolf, Dr. Naomi, The Bodies of Others…2022

59. Wolf, Dr. Naomi, The Bodies of Others…2022

60. Wolf, Dr. Naomi, The Bodies of Others…2022

61. David, Paula and Shoenfeld, Yehuda, of Sheba Medical Center—Tel Aviv University, Israel, "ITP Following Vaccination", 2020, International Journal of Infectious Diseases, https://www.ijidonline.com/article/S1201-9712(20)30629/pdf

62. Balzanelli, Mario, Rastmanesh, Reza, Distratis, Pietro, et al., "The Role of SARS-CoV-2 Spike Protein in Long-term Damage of Tissues and Organs…" PubMed, 2025, https://pubmed.ncbi.nim.nih.gov/38468535

63. Wolf, Dr. Naomi, The Bodies of Others…2022

64. Paik, Dr. Clara, "The Truth Behind COVID-19 Vaccines and Women's Health," UC Davis Health, July 28, 2021, https://health.ucdavis.edu/news/headlines/the-truth-behind-covid-19-vaccines-and-womens-health-/2021/07/28

65. ACOG Practice Advisory et all, "COVID-19 Vaccination Considerations for Obstetric—Gynecologic Care," September 25, 2023, (December, 2020), ACOG Clinical, https://www.acog.org/clinical/clinical-guidance/practice-advisory/articles/2020/12/covid-19-vaccination-considerations-for-obstetric-gynecologic-care

66. Hendler, Carolyn, JD, "FDA Revokes EUA Status for COVID-19 Shots," The Vaccine Reaction—National Vaccine Information Center, September 9, 2025, https://thevaccinereaction,org/2025/9/9/fda-revokes-eua-status-for-covid-19-shots/

Chapter 13

1. Cambridge Advanced Learner's Dictionary & Thesaurus@ Cambridge University Press, "vaccine", (meaning in English), 2024, https://dictionary.cambridge.org/dictionary/english/vaccine

2. The College of Physicians of Philadelphia, "History of Vaccines—Vaccine Timeline—Before Jenner and After COVID-19," 2024, https://historyofvaccines.org/history/vaccine-timeline/overview

3. O'Rourke, Ciara, "George Washington Mandated Smallpox Vaccines (Inoculations) For the Continental Army," POLITIFACT, July 29, 2021, https://www.politifact.com/factchecks/2021/jul/30//viral-image/yes-george-washington-ordered-troops-be-inoculated/

4. Price, Nancy J., "How Louis Pasteur Created the First Rabies Vaccine (1885)," Click Americana Vintage and Retro Memories, December 7, 2019, https://clickamericana.com/topics/health-medicine/how-louis-pasteur-created-the-first-rabies-vaccine-1885

5. College of Physicians of Philadelphia, "History of Vaccines…" 2024

6. Colgrove, James Keith, "The Cutter Incident: How America's First Polio Vaccine Led to the Growing Vaccine Crisis,", Project Muse—Bulletin of the History of Medicine-Johns Hopkins University Press, Volume 81, Number 3, Fall 2007, https://muse.jhu.edu/pub/1/article/220369/pdf

7. Siani, Alessandro, "Vaccine Hesitancy and Refusal: History, Causes, Mitigation Strategies," Springer Nature Link/Integrated Science of Global Epidemics, May 9, 2023, https://link.springer.com/chapter/10.1007/978-3-031-17778-1_23

8. Team Biology Simple, "Natural Active Immunity," Biology Simple, January 10, 2025, https://biologysimple.com/natural-active-immunity/

9. Vaccines Explained Series, "How Do Vaccines Work?" World Health Organization (WHO), December 8,2020, https://www.who.int/news-room/feature-stories/detail/how-do-vaccines-work

10. Food and Drug Administration, "Vaccine Information Fact Sheet for Recipients and Caregivers," FDA, September 11, 2023, https:www.fda.gov/media/144638/download

11. FDA, "Vaccine Information Fact Sheet," 2023

12. CDC Immunization Schedules, "Child and Adolescent Immunization Schedule by Age, (Addendum updated June 27, 2024), National Center for Immunization and Respiratory Diseases, November 16, 2023, https://www.cdc/gov/vaccines/schedules/hcp/imz/child-adolescent.html

13. FDA, "Vaccine Information Fact Sheet," 2023

14. Salmon, Daniel A., and Omer, Saad B., "Individual Freedoms vs Collective Responsibility: Immunization Decision-Making in the Face of Occasionally Competing Values," National Library of Medicine, September 27, 2006, https:// www.ncbi.nim.nih.gov/pmc/articles/PMC1592474/

15. Salmon and Omer, "Individual Freedoms vs Collective Responsibility," 2006

16. Evans, Richard, "A Comprehensive Overview of Kant's Categorical Imperative," Philosophos, August 5, 2023, https://www.philosophos.org/article/a-comprehensive-overview-of-kants-categorical-imperative/

17. National Research Council (US)Committee, Science, Medicine, and Animals, "Safety Testing", National Academies Press, 2004, https://www.ncbi.nim.nih.gov/books/NBK24645/

18. Gallagher, James, "AstraZeneca to Withdraw Covid Vaccine," BBC, May 2024, https://www.bbc.com/news/health-68977026

19. Gentempo, Patrick, DC, et al, "Vaccines Revealed" (DVD Video series), Action Potential Holdings, INC., 2017, https://search.worldcat.org/title/vaccines-revealed/odc/1003298512

20. Golden, Gerald S., MD, "Pertussis Vaccine and Injury to the Brain," The Journal of Pediatrics," June 1990, https://www.jpeds.com/article/50022-3476(05)80640-7/abstract

21. Lund, Danae PhD.LP., "Vaccines and Autism: Separating Facts From Fiction," Sanford Health, November 7, 2021, https://news.sanfordhealth.org/childrens/autism-and-vaccines/

22. Greenfield, Beth, "Parents of Vaccine-Injured Children Speak Out: 'The Guilt is Huge,'" Yahoo!Life, February 17, 2015, https://www.yahoo.com/lifestyle/parents-of-vaccine-injured-children-speak-out-110904439577.html?fr=yhssrp_catchall

23. Wheeler, Marissa, Buttenheim, Alison M., "Parental Vaccine Concerns, Information Source, and Choice of Alternative Immunization Schedules," PubMed Central/Human Vaccines & Immunotherapeutics, July 30, 2013, https://pmc.ncbi.nm.nih.gov/articles/PMC3906282/

24. Smith, Michelle R., "How a Kennedy Built an Anti-Vaccine Juggernaut Amid COVID-19," NBC BOSTON, December 15, 2021, https://www.nbcboston.com/news/local/how-a-kennedy-built-an-anti-vaccine-juggernaut-amid-covid-19/2590911/

25. Wikipedia, "National Childhood Vaccine Injury Act (1986," Wikipedia, The Free Encyclopedia, December 2013, https://en.wikipedia.org/wiki/National-Childhood-Vaccine-Injury-Act

26. Kern, Janet K; Geier, David A; Sykes, Lisa K; Haley, Boyd E; and Geier, Mark R.; "The Relationship Between Mercury and Autism: A Comprehensive Review and Discussion," Science Direct—Journal of Trace Elements in Medicine and Biology, Volume 37, Pages 8-24, September 2016, https://www.sciencedirect.com/science/article/pii/S0946672X16300931

27. Paule, Merle, PhD; Young, John, PhD; et all, "Thimerosal [54-64-8]—Nomination to the National Toxicology Program—Review of the Literature April, 2001, National Institute of Environmental Health/NIH, https://ntp.niehs.nih.gov/sites/default/files/ntp/htdocs/chem_background/exsum-pdf/thimerosal_508.pdf

28. Kern, Janet K; Geier, David A.; Homme, Kristin G.; and Geier, Mark R.; "Examining the Evidence That Ethylmercury Crosses the Blood-Brain Barrier," Science Direct/Environmental Toxicology and Pharmacology, February, 2020, https://www.sciencedirect.com/science/article/abs/pii/S1382668919301875

29. National Center for Immunization and Respiratory Diseases, "Making the Vaccine Decision: Addressing Common Concerns," CDC, Last Reviewed July 19, 2023, https://www.cdc.gov/vaccines/parents/why-vaccinate/vaccine-decision.html

30. Bauer, Julius M.D., "The Tragic Fate of Ignaz Philipp Semmelweis," National Center for Biotechnology Information, Vol 98-No 5-May 1963, https://www.ncbi.nim.nih.gov/pmc/articles/PMC1575625/pdf/califmed00155-0023.pdf

31. Girion, Lisa, "Johnson & Johnson Knew for Decades that Asbestos Lurked In Its Baby Powder," Reuters Investigation, December 14, 2018, https://www.reiters.com/investigates/special-report/johnsonandjohnson-cancer/

32. Gentempo, Patrick, DC, et al, "Vaccines Revealed" (DVD Video series), Action Potential Holdings, INC., 2017, https://search.worldcat.org/title/vaccines-revealed/odc/1003298512

33. Smith, Tara C. and Rubinstein Reiss, Dorit; "Digging the Rabbit Hole, COVID-19 Edition: Anti-Vaccine Themes and the Discourse Around COVID-19," Elsevier-PMC—National Institutes of Health, November 7, 2020, https://www.ncbi.nim.nih.gov/pmc/articles/PMC648494/

34. Gentempo, Patrick, DC, et al, "Vaccines Revealed", 2017

35. McCullough, Peter, MD, "Guide to Early Treatment of COVID-19" Victory Medical Center, January 1, 2020, https://www.victorymed.com/covid-19-precautions/

36. Leake, John and McCullough, Peter A. M.D.,MPH,The Courage to Face COVID-19: Preventing Hospitalization and Death While Battling The Bio-Pharmaceutical Complex, Counterplay Books/Kindle Ed., May 1, 2022.

37. McCullough, Peter A. MD, MPHR, "Fighting for Medical Freedom Through Scientific Data and Analysis, Peter A. McCullough, MD, MPH, (personal website), December 3, 2020, https://www.petermcculloughmd.com

38. McCullough, Peter A. MD, MPHR, "Fighting for Medical Freedom," 2020

39. Renz, Tom, "Jonathan Otto Supports For God, Family, Country," Substacks, December 20, 2024, https://forgodfamilycountry.sustack.com/p/jonathan-otto-supports-for-god-family-country

40. Bruce, Alexandra, "Urgent Warning About Poisonous Jabs," LewRockwell/ Forbidden Knowledge TV, with Stew Peters, July 23, 2021, https://www.lewrockwell.com/2021/07/no_author/dr-peter-mccullough-urgent-warning-about-poisonous-jabs/

41. Kaufman, Andrew, MD, "COVID Reveals Pathology of Scientific Materialism and the Need to ReTHINK Health," Interview with Elisha Celeste on YouTube, 2023, https://www.youtube.com/watch?v=8JPrYNOJOYs

42. Kaufman, Andrew, MD, "COVID-19 Myths—Dr. Andrew Kaufman," Internet Archive, May 18, 2021, updated by newsparadigm, https://archive.org/details/covid-19-myths-dr-andrew-kaufman

43. Goldman, Gary S. MD, and Miller, Neil Z, "Infant Mortality Rates Regressed Against Number of Vaccine Doses Routinely Given; Is There a Biochemical of Synergistic Toxicity?", Sage Journals, May 4, 2011, https://journals.sagepub.com/doi/10.117/0960327111407644

44. Berenson, Alex, "URGENT: Yale Researchers Have Found COVID Spike Protein in the Blood of People Never Infected With COVID—Years After They Got mRNA Jabs,"Unreported Truths/Substack, December 19, 2024, https://alexberenson.substack.com/p/urgent-yale-researchers-have-found

45. Goldman, GS M.D., and King, PG M.D., "Vaccination to Prevent Varicella: Goldman and King's Response to Myers' Interpretation of Varicella Active Surveillance Project Data," Sage Journals/Human Experimenta Toxicology, November 25, 2013, https://journals.sagepub.com/doi/10.1177/0960537113512340

46. Wakefield, Andrew J. MD, foreward by McCarthy, Jenny, Callous Disregard: Autism and Vaccines: The Truth Behind a Tragedy, May 24, 2010, https://www/amazon.com/Callous-Disregard-Autism-Caccines-Tragedy/dp/B0085SCM4G

47. Ragusa, Gina, "What Happens to My Special Needs Child After I Die?" The Street, October 8, 2016, https://www.thestreet.com/personal-finance/what-happens-to-my-special-needs-child-after-i-die-13837716

48. Wakefield, Andrew J. MD, foreward by McCarthy, Jenny, Callous Disregard: Autism and Vaccines: The Truth Behind a Tragedy, May 24, 2010,

49. Renshaw, Jarrett, and Kelly, Stephanie, "RFK Jr. on Abortion, Vaccines, Housing, and Foreign Policy," Reuters, March 20, 2024, https://www.reuters.com/world/us/rfk-jr-abortion-vaccines-housing-foreign-policy-2024-03-20/

50. Gentempo, Patrick, DC et al., "Vaccines Revealed," 2017

51. Gentempo, Patrick, DC et al., "Vaccines Revealed," 2017

52. Park, Jinae with Lipman, Andrew, PhD, "Anatomy of a Public Health Scare: Fear and Accountability in the Creation of Vaccine Courts," Barnard College—Columbia University, April 24, 2020, https://history.barnard.edu/sites/default/files/inline-files/Jinae Park_Final Senior Thesis.pdf

53. Oster, Natalia V.; Williams, Emily C.; Unger, Joseph M.; et all.; "Hepatitis B Birth Dose: First Shot at Timely Early Childhood Vaccination," PubMed Central (PMC), October 1, 2020, https://pmc.ncbi.nlm.nih.gov/articles/PMC6802744/

54. Health Resources and Services Administration, "Frequently Asked Questions," National Vaccine Injury Compensation Program, July 2024, https://www.hrsa.gov/vaccine-compensation/faq

55. Health Resources and Services Admin. "FAQ" NVICP, July, 2024

56. Brogan, Kelly MD, "Own Your Body-Free Your Mind—Experience the Specific Pleasure of Who You Are," ("You're NOT Crazy). 2023. https://www.kellybroganmd.com

57. Brogan, Kelly MD, "A New Approach to Depression" (Integrative), Emerson Ecologics,October18,2017, https://www.emersonecologics.com/blog/post/depression-supplements-psychiatrist

58. Whitaker, Robert, Anatomy of an Epidemic: Psychiatric Drugs and the Astonishing Rise of Mental Illness in America," Ethical Human Psychology and Psychiatry, Vol 7, Number 1, Spring 2005, https://freedom-center.org/pdf/anatomy_of_epidemic_whitaker_psych_drugs.pdf

59. McCullough, Peter MD, "Transcript of Interview with Joe Rogan #1747" You Tube (3 hours censored except for last 1-1/2minute), December 22, 2021, https://www.swellai.com/transcripts/joe-rogan-transcript/-1747-dr-peter-a-mccullough

60. Boyles, Salynn, "VAERS Data Confirm Myocarditis Risk After mRNA Vaccine," Physician's Weekly, January 27, 2022, https://www.physiciansweekly.com/vaers-data-confirm-myocarditis-risk-after-mrna-vaccine/

61. EMLA Councilmember Tupola, "Robert Malone, MD, Pathology; M.S., Virology, Immunology, and Molecular Biology," Honolulu Granicus, October 19, 2021, https://honolulugranicus.com/MetaViewer.php?view_id=3&clip_id=1699&meta_id=207222

62. Malone, Robert W. MD MS, Lies My Gov't Told Me: And the Better Future Coming (Children's Health Defense)—A Guide for the Times—Breaking Down the Lies about COCVID-19 and Shedding Light on Why We Came to Believe Them. Woodcastle Books, December 6, 2022, https://www.amazon.com/Lies_My_Govt_Told_Me/dp/151077324X

63. Malone, Robert W. MD MS, Lies My Govt Told Me…December 6, 2022

64. CDC/COVID-19 staff, "Underlying Conditions and the Higher Risk for Severe COVID-19," CDC/COVID-19, February 6, 2025, https://www.cdc.gov/covid/hcp/clinical-care/underlying-conditions.html

65. Kochhar, Izurieta, Chandler, et al., "Benefit-Risk Assessment of Vaccines," PubMed—NIH Library of Medicine, February 6, 2024, https://pubmed.ncbi.nim.nih.gov/37563049/

66. Kennedy, Robert F. Jr., from the forward to Dr. Joseph Mercola's book, The Truth About COVID-19: Exposing The Great Reset, Lockdowns, Vaccine Passports, and the New Normal, Chelsea Green Publishing, April 29, 2021, https://www.amazon.com/Truth-About-COVID-19-Lockdowns-Passports/dp/1645020886/ref=litb_std_nodl

67. Kennedy, Robert F. Jr., forward to Dr. Joseph Mercola's book, The Truth About COVID-19...April 29, 2021.

68. Thacker, Paul D., "Despite Biden Pardon, Fauci Still Faces Legal Perils. Here They Are," MSN, © 2025, https://www.msn.com/en-us/news/politics/despite-biden-pardon-fauci-stull-faces-legal-perils-here-they-are/ar-AA1xFjOT

69. Mercola, Joseph MD and Cummins, Ronnie, The Truth About COVID-19: Exposing the Great Reset, Lockdowns, Vaccine Passports, and the New Normal, Chelsea Green Publishing, April 2021, https://www.amazon.com/Truth-About-COVID-19-Lockdowns-Passports/dp/1645020886/ref=litb_std_nodl

70. Mercola and Cummins, The Truth About COVID-19...April, 2021

71. Murrow, Edward R., "Edward R. Murrow Quotes,", Goodreads. 2024, https://www.goodreads.com/author/quotes/178884.Edward_R_Murrow

72. Mercola and Cummins, The Truth About COVID-19...April 2021

73. Nilson, Jennifer; Donovan, Joan; and Faris, Rob; "Cloaked Science: the Yan Reports," Taylor & Francis Online—Information, Communication, and Society, Vol 25, April 27, 2022, https://www.tandfonline.com/doi/full/10.1080/13691118X.2022.2027501#extract

74. Federal Department of Foreign Affairs (FDFA), "Biological Weapons", Switzerland's Biological Weapons Conventions, December 1976 (specifically), https://www.eda.admin.ch/eda/en/fdfa/foreign-policy/security-policy/disarmiment-non-proliferation/biologische-waffen.html

Chapter 14

1. Otto, Jonathan, Host; "New Hope—Episode 1-BIOWARFARE: The Prevalence of Biotoxins & How to Protect Your Body from Them," New Hope Docuseries, 2023. Quote of Dr. Brian Ardis, https://newhopeseries.com/episode-1-live/

2. Biology Insights Team, "The Science of Venom: From Stings to Immune Reactions," Biology Insights/Anatomy & Physiology, July 30, 2024, https://biologyinsights.com/the-science-of-venom-from-stings-to-immune-reactions/

3. Otto—Dr. Brian Ardis, "The Prevalence of Biotoxins…" New Hope, 2023

4. Otto—-Dr. Shankara Chetty, "BIOWARFARE", New Hope, 2023

5. Otto, Jonathan, Host; "Patented: Why the Spike Protein Was Designed to Infiltrate in Your DNA," New Hope Docuseries, 2023. Quote from Jonathan Otto Intro, https://newhopeseries.com/episode-bonus1-live/

6. Comer, James (chairman of Committee on Oversight and Accountability), "Hearing Wrap Up: EcoHealth Alliance Should be Criminally Investigated, Formally Debarred," Press Release of Committee Report, May 3, 2024. https://oversight.house.gov/release/hearing-wrap-up-ecohealth-alliance-should-be-criminally-investigated-formally-disbarred/

7. Otto, Jonathan, Host; "Patented: Why the Spike Protein Was Designed…",2023, (Quote from Dr. Peter McCullough)

8. Otto, Jonathan, Host; "Patented: Why the Spike Protein Was Designed…" 2023. (Quote 2 from Dr. Peter McCullogh)

9. Otto, Jonathan, Host; "Patented: Why the Spike Protein Was Designed…" 2023. (Quote from Dr. Brian Ardis)

10. Otto, Jonathan, Host; "Patented: Why the Spike Protein Was Designed…" 2023 (Quote from Dr. Henry Ealy)

11. Otto, Jonathan, Host; "Destruction: The Explosion of mRNA Tech and Its Devastation on Humanity," New Hope Docuseries, 2023. (Quote from Dr. Brian Ardis), https://newhopeseries.com/epidode-2+-live/

12. Otto, Jonathan, Host; "Destruction: The Explosion of mRNA Tech…", 2023 (Quote from Dr. Christina Parks, PhD)

13. Otto, Jonathan, Host; "Destruction: The Explosion of mRNA Tech…", 2023 (Quote from Dr. Seema Nanda, OD)

14. Fuellmich, Reiner Dr; Yeadon, Michael Dr.; Nixon, David Dr.; Mihalcea, Ana Dr.; Yanowitz, Shimon Dr. and Kingston, Karen; "The Nano Structures Found in mRNA Injections," International Crimes Investigative Committee (ICIC)/Rumble, 2024, https://rumble.com/v2dbsdc-dr-mike-yeadon-karen-kingston-dr.mihalcea-dr-nixon—shimon-yanowitz-dr-reine.html

15. Fuellmich, Reiner Dr; Yanowitz, Shimon Dr; et al., "Nano Structures Found in mRNA Injections," ICIC, 2024

16. Fuellmich, Reiner Dr; Yanowitz, Shimon Dr; et al., "Nano Structures Found in mRNA Injections," ICIC, 2024

17. Gary, Major Mike, "About Us,"Truth for Health Foundation, 2024. https://www.truthforhealth.org/2024/08/faith-over-fear-july-30-2024

18. Gary, Major Mike, "About Us,"Truth for Health Foundation, 2024. https://www.truthforhealth.org/2024/08/faith-over-fear-july-30-2024

19. Harari, Yuval Noah, "Humans Are Now Hackable Animals," CNN, November 26, 2019, https://www.cnn.com/videos/world/2029/11/26/yuval-noah-harari-interview-anderson-vpx.cnn

20. Chung, Seokhwan; Chan, Mi Lee; and Zhang, Miqin; "Advances in Nanoparticle-based mRNA Delivery for Liver Cancer and Liver-Associated Infectious Diseases," Royal Society of Chemistry/Nanoscale Horizons, 2023, https://pubs.rsc.org/en/content/articlelanding/2023/nh/d2nh00289b

21. Merritt, Lee Dr; "Dr Lee Merritt's Most Explosive Interview: The International Hyenas," Spreaker/Two Mikes/Freedom First Network, March 15, 2023, https://www.spreaker.com/episode/dr-lee-merritt-s-most-explosive-interview-the-international-hyenas—53215827

22. Maiese, A.; Manetti, A.; La Russa, R.; Di Paulo, M.; et al., "Autopsy Findings in COVID-19-Related Deaths: A Literature Review," Forensic Science, Medicine, and Pathology, October 7, 2020, https://link.springer.com/article/10.1007/s12024-020-00310-8#citeas

23. Addgene, "Optogenetics Guide," 2005-present, https://www.addgene.org/guides/optogenetics/

24. Mothersill, Dr. Carmel and Xiaobing, Dr. Li; "Investigation of Presence and Impact of Radiation-Induced Bystander Effect…" Research Gate, March 2023, https://www.researchgate.net/profile/Carmel-Mothersill

25. Tesla, Nikola, "Nikola Tesla Quote," Pinterest, July 30,2019, https://www.pinterest.com

26. Kerby, Frederick M., "Finds Electricity Can Build Up Brains," Tesla Universe, July 6, 1917, https://teslauniverse.com/nikola-tesla/articles/finds-electricity-can-build-brains

27. Sanchez, Justin (Program Mgr: Brain-Machine Symbiosis), "DARPA's Neurotech Research Resonates with Tesla's Acoustic Mind Control," The Sociable, May 28, 2019, https://sociable.co/technology/darpa-neurotech-research-resonates-tesla-acoustic-mind-control/

28. Karczewska, Ela; "Dr. Pierre Gilbert 1995 Magnetic Vaccines," You Tube, July 10, 2021 (This video has been removed for violating You Tube's Community Guidelines—censored by Big Tech—undoubtedly too true to leave there!) https://www.youtube.com/watch?v=mav2dZqQOcE

29. Sharma, Gaurav (Battelle Sr. Research Scientist), "Battelle Wins DARPA Contract for Injectable Brain Control Technology," Army Technology, May 21, 2019, https://www.army-technology.com/news/darpa-injectaaable-brain-control-technology/?Top-Article-Share-Button-clicked:Share on X&cf-view

30. Liangyu, Ed; "China Unveils Brain-Computer Interface Chip," XINHUANET, September 15, 2024, https://www.xinhuanet.com/english/2019-05-18/c_138069590.htm

31. Giordano, James, PhD; "Weaponizing the Brain: Neuroscience Advancements Spark Debate, " National Defense Magazine/Collins Aerospace, May 11, 2017, https://www.nationaldefensemagazine.org/articles/2017/5/11/weaponizing-the-brain-neuroscience-advancements-spark-debate

32. Willis, Lt, Col. Adam; "Next-Generation Nonsurgical Neurotechnology," Defense Advanced Research Projects Agency (DARPA), February 13, 2021, https://www.darpa.mil/program/next-generation-nonsurgical-neurotechnology

33. Harmsworth, Miles; "How Human Are You? The Internet of Bodies is Here, But Are We Ready?" Taylor Wessing, January 30, 2023, https://www.taylorwessing.com/en/interface/2023/Iot—next-gen/how-human-are-you-the-internet-of-bodies-is-here-but-are-we-ready

34. Wikipedia, " Biography of Julian Huxley," Wikipedia Foundation,Inc, last edited August 27, 2024, https://en.wikipedia.org/wiki/Julian_Huxley

35. McKie, Robin (Science Editor), "No Death and an Enhanced Life: Is the Future Transhuman?" The Guardian/Observer, May 6, 2018, https://www.theguardian.com/technology/2018/may/06/no-death-and-an-enhanced-life-is-the-future-transhuman

36. Gorey, Colm, "Scientists Propose Putting Nanobots in our Bodies to Create 'Global Superbrain,'" Silicon Republic, April 12, 2019, https://www.siliconrepublic.com/machines/brain-cloud-interface-nanobots-global-superbrain

37. Reedy, Christianna, "Kurzweil: By 2030, Nanobots Will Flow Throughout Our Bodies—This Fleet of Tiny Robots Would Keep You Healthy and Connected to the Cloud," Futurism, April 24, 2017, https://futurism.com/kurzweil-by-2030-nanobots-will-flow-throughout-our-bodies

38. Vassanelli, Stefano, "Brain-Chip Interfaces: The Present and The Future," ELSEVIER/Science Direct, December 20, 2011, https://www.sciencedirect.com/science/article/pii/S1877050911006855

39. Versaggi, Charles PhD, "Injectable Body Sensors Take Personal Chemistry to a Cell Phone Closer to Reality," Profusa Inc, March 19, 2018, https://profusa.com/injectable-body-sensors-take-personal-chemistry-to-a-cell-phone-closer-to-reality/

40. Craig, Lev; Laskowski, Nicole; and Tucci, Linda; "What is AI (Artificial Intelligence)?" Tech Target, May 1, 2024, https://www.techtarget.com/searchenterpriseai/definition/AI-Artificial-Intelligence

41. Multiple authors/text, Principles of Biology,/ LibreTexts. January, 2024, file:///C:/Users/grame/Downloads/Full.pdf

42. Mansouri, Maysam and Fussenegger, Martin, "Electrogenetics: Bridging Synthetic Biology and Electronics to Remotely Control the Behavior of Mammalian Designer Cells," Science Direct, June, 2022, https://www.sciencedirect.com/science/article//pii/S1367593122000369

43. Costandi, Mo, "Genetically Engineered 'Magneto' Protein Remotely Controls Brain and Behavior," The Guardian/Neurophilosophy Science, March 24, 2016, https://www.theguardian.com/science/neurophilosophy/2016/march/24/magneto-remotely-controls-brain-and-behavior

44. Rosenkranz, Sina C.; Shhaposhnykov, Artem; et al., "TRPV4-Mediated Regulation of the Blood Brain Barrier Is Abolished During Inflammation," PubMed Central, August 27, 2020, https://pmc.ncbi.nim.nih.gov/articles/PMC7481434/

45. Zhang, Feng PhD; "CRISPR: Gene Editing Tools Launch Biotech Revolution," McGovern Institute for Brain Research/MIT, July, 2021, https://betterworld.mit.edu/crispr-gene-editing-tools-launch-biotech-revoltion/

46. Kohn, Donald B.; Porteus, Matthew H.; and Scharenbeg, Andrew M.; "Ethical and Regulatory Aspects of Genome Editing," Ash Publications, May 26, 2016, https://ashpublications.org/blood/article/127/21/2553/35191//ethical-and-regulatory-aspects-of-genome-editing

47. Patent # KR20210028065A, "Physiological Saline Containing Graphene Dispersion and Corona Virus Vaccine Using the Same," Espacenet (Patent Search), November 3, 2021(pub), https://worldwide.espacenet.com/patent/search/family/075143358/publication/KR 20210028065A?q=pn%3D

48. Elmore, Susan et al., "Apoptosis: A Review of Programmed Cell Death," Sage Journals/Toxocologic Pathology, Vol 35-Issue 4, First Pub, June 2007, https://journals.sagepub.com?doi/10.1080/01926230701320337

49. Stevenson, Ian Max, "Idaho Capitol, Says His Speeches 'Cost Me My Career,'" Idaho Statesman, March 22, 2024, https://www.idahostatesman.com/news/local/community/boise/article286983160. html

50. Dean, Laura, et al., "Red Blood Cell," Wikipedia, September 4, 2024 (last edit), https:// en.wikipedia.org/wiki/red-blood-cell

51. Bussel, Dr. James; Connors, Dr. Jean; Cines, Dr. Douglas; et al., "Vaccine-Induced Immune Thrombotic Thrombocytopenia," American Society of Hematology/COVID-19 Resources, May 9, 2022, httpps://www.hematology.org/covid-19/vaccine-induced-immune-thrombotic-thrombocytopenia

52. Fleming, Dr. Richard, PhD, JD; "Faith, Health, and Hope Global COVID Summit," AAPS/NTD Live, November 13, 2021, https://www.ntd.com/live/faith-health-and-hope-global-covid-summit-kansas-city_700963.html

53. Centers for Disease Control and Prevention (CDC), "COVID-19 Vaccine: Addressing Concerns," UCLA Health Pub, September 10, 2024, https://wwwuclahealth.org/treatment-options/covid-19-info/covid-19-vaccine-addressing-concerns

54. Islam, Dr. Saiful; Kamal, Abu-Hena Mostofa; Kabir, Alamgir; Southern, Dorothy, et al., "COVID-19 Vaccine Rumors and Conspiracy Theories: The Need for Cognitive Inoculation Against Misinformation to Improve Vaccine Adherence," NIH/PMC Published Central, May 12, 2021, https:www.nvbi.nim.nih.gov/pmc/articles/PMC8115834/

55. Breggin, Dr. Peter and Breggin, Ginger; "The Dead Don't Lie: Two Million Dead From mRNA Jabs!" Breggins' Alerts: Exposing Global Preditors, April 12, 2024, https://www.substack.com/bregginsalerts.exposingglobalpreditors

56. The War Room/Daily Clout/ Pfizer Docs Analysts; Wolf, Dr. Naomi (Ed); and Kelly, Amy (Ed); The Pfizer Papers: Pfizer's Crimes Against Humanity, War Room Books/Amazon, October 15, 2024, https://www.amazon.com/Pfizer-Papers-Pfizers-Crimes-Against-Humanity/dp/1648210376/ref=pd

57. Leake, John and McCullough, Dr. Peter; "Analysis: COVID Vaccines Caused 300,000 Excess Deaths in 2022 Alone," Health Viewpoints/EPOCH Health, April 1, 2023, https://www.epochtimes.com/health/analysis-covid-vaccines-caused-300,000-excess-deaths-in-2022

58. Baletti, Brenda; "28 -Year-Old Pro Basketball Player Dies of Heart Attack," The Defender-Children's Health Defense/ Health Viewpoints for Epoch Times, April 7, 2023, https://www.theepochtimes.com/health/28-year-old-pro-basketball-layer-dies-of-heart-attack/

59. Duchamps, Lorenz and Kietlinska, Ella; "COVID-19 Vaccines Can Cause 'Permanent Disabilities' : German Health Minister," NTD News/The Epoch Times, April 13,2023, https://www.theepochtimes.com/article/covid-19-vaccines-can-cause-permanent-disabilities-German-health-minister/

60. Duchamps and Kietlinska; "COVID-19 Vaccines Can Cause 'Permanent Disabilities'...per Dr. Elizabeth Lee Vliet quote, April 23, 2023.

61. Reviewer CF, "Scorching Reproval of the Medical Industry During the COVID Epidemic," Amazon Review, reviewed in the US on April 9,2924, https://www.amazon.com/what-nurses-saw-investigation-corruption

62. McCarthy, Ken, What the Nurses Saw: An Investigation into Systemic Medical Murders That Took Place in Hospitals During the Covid Panic and the Nurses Who Fought Back to Save Their Patients. (Medical System Corruption Brasscheck Press—December 6, 2023, https://www.amazon.com/what-nurses-saw-investigation-corruption/ dp/BOCPQVTDR/ ref=pd_rhf_dp_s_pd_sbs_ rvi_d_scci_1_1/145-6421443-1124729?pd

63. McCarthy, Ken, What the Nurses Saw:...December 6, 2023

64. Thorp, Dr. James A; Rogers, Dr. Claire; McCullough, Dr. Peter; et al., "COVID-19 Vaccines: The Impact on Pregnancy Outcomes and Menstrual Function," Creative Commons CC BY license/PrePrints, September 28, 2022, file:///C:/Users/grame/Downloads/preprints202209.0430.v1.pdf

65. Otto, Jonathan, Host; "New Hope—Episode 1-BIOWARFARE: The Prevalence of Biotoxins & How to Protect Your Body from Them," New Hope Docuseries, 2023. https://newhopeseries.com/episode-1-live/

66. Olszewski, RN Erin Marie; "The Epicenter Nurse—A Conversation with Erin Marie Olszewski," Interviewed by John Kirby/The Press and Public Project-Ep 9, You Tube/Journeyman Pictures, May 14, 2020, https://www.youtube.com/watch? V=UIDsKdeFOmQ

67. Olszewski, RN Erin Marie, BSN; Undercover Epicenter Nurse: How Fraud, Negligence, and Greed Led to Unnecessary Deaths at Elmhurst Hospital, Tantor & Blackstone Publishing—March 1, 2021, https://www.amazon.com/Undercover-Nurse-Negligec-Unnecessary/dp/B08ZBJFGVM

68. Hsu, Andrea; "Thousands of Workers Are Opting to Get Fired, Rather than Take the Vaccine," National Public Radio (NPR), October 24, 2021, https://www.npr.org/2021/10/24/1047947268/covid-vaccine-workers-quitting-getting-fired-mandates

69. Huff, Ethan; "USAF Senior Airman Lance Castle ABUSED in Prison, Court-Martialed for Refusing COVID 'Vaccine'," Natural News, April 16, 2024, https://www.naturalnews.com/2024-04-16/usaf-lance-castle-abused-prison-court-martial.html

70. Long, Dr. Theresa, MD; Chambers, Dr. Pete, DO; Sugoloff, Major Sam, MD; and Horn, Dr. Stanton, DC, BS; "The End of COVID Docuseries," Jonathan Otto, Host, 2023, https://theebdofcovidseries.com/episode7-part2live/

71. Long, Chambers, Sugoloff, and Horn; "The End of COVID Docuseries…2023.

72. Huff, Ethan; "USAF Senior Airman Lance Castle Abused in Prison…"; 2024.

73. Peter R. Breggin, M.D. and Ginger R. Breggin, "COVID-19 and the Global Predators—We Are Their Prey!" (Lake Edge Press. New York, 2021.)

74. McKeown, L.A.; "COVID-19 Autopsies Put Endothelial Damage, Angiogenesis in the Spotlight," TCTMD, May 26, 2020, https://www.tctmd.com/news/covid-19-autopsies-put-endothelial-damage-angiogenesis-spotlight

75. US Food & Drug Administration, "COVID-19 Vaccines for 2024-2025," September 03, 2024, https://www.fda.gov/emergency-preparedness-and-response/coronavirus-disease-2019-covid-19-vaccines-2024-2025

76. Peter R. Breggin, M.D. and Ginger R. Breggin, "COVID-19 and the Global Predators…2021.

77. Peter R. Breggin, M.D. and Ginger R. Breggin, "COVID-19 and the Global Predators…2021.

78. Breggin, Dr. Peter and Ginger; "Cover-up of COVID 'Vaccine' Deaths and Injuries," Breggin.Com, June 19, 2023, https://breggin.com/article-detail/post_detail/Cover-Up-of-COVID-Vaccine-Deaths-and-Injuries

79. Bannon, Stephen K., Foreward for The Pfizer Papers: Pfizer's Crimes Against Humanity; Authors: Wolf, Dr. Naomi and Kelly, Amy; Skyhorse Publishing, Inc. and War Room Books, LLC, 2024, https://www.google.com/books/edition/The_Pfizer_Papers/OjzkEAAAQBAJ?hl

80. Wolf, Dr. Naomi--Introduction to The Pfizer Papers: Pfizer's Crimes Against Humanity; Skyhorse Publishing, Inc. and War Room Books, LLC, 2024

81. Wolf, Dr. Naomi—Introduction to The Pfizer Papers…2024.

82. Wolf, Dr. Naomi; "What's in the Pfizer Documents?" Guest Speaker @ CCA IV: Big Pharma conference @ Hillsdale College, March 6, 2023, https://freedomlibrary.hillsdale.edu/programs/CCA-IV-big-pharma/what-s-in-the-pfizer-documents?

83. Wolf, Dr. Naomi; "What's in the Pfizer Documents?"2023.

Chapter 15

1. Law Office of Leah V. Durant & Assoc., "How Do You Choose a Lawyer to File a Vaccine Injury Claim?", Vaccine Law, 2024, https://vaccinelaw.com/how-do-you-choose-a-lawyer-to-file-a-vaccine-injury-claim/

2. Leah V. Durant & Assoc Law Office, "How to Choose a Lawyer to File a Vax Injury Claim"—2024

3. Daily Briefing of Advisory Board, "Thousands Believe They Suffered Serious Side Effects from COVID-19 Vaccines," COVID-19 Vaccine Communications Readiness Assessment, May 6, 2024, https://www.advisory.com/daily-briefing/2024/05/06/covid-vaccine-side-effects

4. America's Frontline Doctors, "America's Frontline Doctors White Paper on Experimental Vaccines for COVID-19," Course Hero/Palo Alto College, April 19, 2021, https://www.coursehero.com/file/89304771/Vaccine-PPpdf/

5. McCullough, Dr Peter, interviewed by Joe Rogan, "Transcript of Interview #1747," Candid and Detailed Discussion on all things COVID-19. Spotify, August 21, 2024, https://www.swellai.com/transcripts/joe-rogan-transcript/-1747-dr-peter-mccullough

6. McCullough, Dr. Peter, "Joe Rogan interview transcript #1747," 2024.

7. McCullough, Dr. Peter, "Joe Rogan interview transcript #1747," 2024.

8. Vliet, Dr. Elizabeth Lee, M.Ed.; Landers, Nicole, RN, BSN, CCN, LNC; and Constantine Chambers, Lt. Col. Peter (US Army Ret.) DO; "Your 'Road Map' for Using This Guide," Truth for Health Foundation, April 29,2022, https://www.truthforhealth.org/wp-content/uploads/2022/05/2022-VaccineInjuryTreatmentGuide_4-29-22-FINAL.pdf

9. Vliet, Landers, and Constantine Chambers; Introduction to "Your 'Road Map' for Using This Guide," Truth for Health Foundation…2022

10. Seneff, Stephanie and Nigh, Greg; "Worse Than the Disease? Reviewing Some Possible Unintended Consequences of the mRNA Vaccines Against COVID-19," International Journal of Vaccine Theory, Practice, and Research (IJVTPR), May 10, 2021 https://dpbh.nv.gov/uploadedFiles/dpbhnvgov/content/Boards/BOH/Meetings/202 1/SSeneff-1.PDF

11. Sellaturay, P., Nasser, S., and Ewan, P., "Polyethylene Glycol (PEG)-Induced Systemic Allergic Reactions (Anaphylaxis)," The Journal of Allergy and Clinical Immunology: In Practice-9(2):670-675, 2020, https://doi.org/10.1016/j.jaip.2020.09.029.

12. Ehrenfeld, M., Tincani, A., Andreoli, L., et al., "COVID-19 and Autoimmunity," Autoimmunity Reviews 19(8):102597, 2020, https://www.ncbi.nlm.nih.gov/pnc/articles/PMC7289100/

13. Vojdani, A., Vojdani, E., and Khaarrazian, D., "Reaction of Human Monoclonal Antibodies to SARS-CoV-2 Proteins with Tissue Antigens: Implications for Autoimmune Dieseases," Frontiers in Immunology 11:3679, 2021, https://doi.org/10.3389/fimmu.2020.617089

14. Carsetti, R., Zaffina, S., Piano Mortari, E., et al., "Different Innate and Adaptive Immune Responses to SARS-CoV-2 Infection of Asymptomatic, Mild, and Severe Cases," Frontiers in Immunology 11,3365. 2020, https://www.frontiersin.org/articles/10.3389/fimmu.2020.610300/full

15. Grady, D., and Mazzei, P., "Doctor's Death After COVID Vaccine is Being Investigated," New York Times, January 12, 2021, https://nytimes.com/2021/01/12/health/covid-vaccine-death.html.

16. McClintock, Barbara, "Components of Action of the Regulators Spm and Ac," Carnegie Institute of Washington, Yearbook 64:527-536. 1965, https://repository.cshl.edu/id/eprint/34634/.

17. Wan, Y., Shang, J., Sun, S., et al., "Molecular Mechanism for Antibody-Dependent Enhancement of Coronavirus Entry," Journal of Virology, 94(5), 2020, https://doi.org/10.1128/JVI.02015-19.

18. Wu, F., Yan, R., Liu, M and Z., et al., "Antibody-Dependent Enhancement (ADE) of SARS-CoV-2 Infection in Recovered COVID-19 Patients: Studies Based on Cellular and Structural Biology Analysis," MedRxiv Preprint, 2020, https://doi.org/10.1101/2020.10.08.20209114.

19. Seneff and Nye, "Worse Than the Disease? Reviewing Some Possible Unintended Consequences of the mRNA Vaccines Against COVID-19," IJVTPR, 2021.

20. Seneff and Nye, "Worse Than the Disease?" IJVTPR, 2021.

21. Otto, Jonathan, Host; "The Voices of the Victims," End of COVID" docuseries, 2024, Voices of Felicity Jackson, Sheryl Ruttgers, Pamela Goodman, and Brittany Gavin, https://endofcovidseries.com/episode-part1-live/2024

22. U.S. Environmental Protection Agency, "Exposure to Environmental Contaminants: What Are the Trends in Human Exposure to Environmental Contaminants?" EPA, September 10, 2024, https://www.epa.gov/report-environment/exposure-environmental-contaminants

23. Yazdani, Armand N.; DeMarco, Nathaniel; Patel, Parth; et al.; " Adverse Hematological Effects of COVID-19 Vaccination and Pathomechanisms of Low Acquired Immunity in Patients with Hematological Malignancies," PubMed Central, March 15, 2023, https://pmc.ncbi.nim.nih.gov/articles/PMC10058097/

24. Chatterjee, Aparajita and Chakravarty, Ambar, "Neurological Complications Following COCVID-19 Vaccination, PubMed Central, November 29, 2022, https://pmc.ncbi.nim.nih.gov/articles/PMC9707152/

25. Blitshteyn, Svetlana and Fedorowski, Artur, "The Risks of POTS after COVID-19 Vaccination and SARS-CoV-2 Infection: More Studies Are Needed," Nature Cardiac Research, December 12,2022, https://www.nature.com/articles/s44161-022-00180-z

26. Vakili, Bahareh; Karami-Darehnaranji, Mahboubeh; Mirzaei, Esmaeil; Hosseini, Farnaz; and Nezafat, Navid; "Graphene Oxide as Novel Vaccine Adjuvant," PubMed, October 23, 2023, https://pubmed.ncbi.nim.nih.gov/37866317/

27. Tungmunnithum, Duangjai; Thongboonyou, Areeya; Pholboon, Apinan; and Yangsabai, Aujana; "Flavonoids and Other Phenolic Compounds from Medicinal Plants for Pharmaceutical and Medical Aspects: An Overview," PubMed Central—National Library of Medicine (NIH), August 25, 2018, https://pmc.ncbi.nlm.nih.gov/articles/PMC6165118/

28. Tungmunnithum, et al., "Flavonoids and Other Phenolic Compounds..." 2018.

29. Klavinson, V Kh; Bondarev, IE; Butyugov, AA; "Epithalon Peptide Induces Telomerase Activity and Telomere Elongation in Human Somatic Cells," PubMed/National Library of Medicine, June 2003, https://pubmed.ncbi.nlm.nih.gov/12937682

30. Pickart, Loren; Vasquez-Soltaro, Jessica; and Margolina, Anna; "GHK and DNA: Resetting the Human Genome to Health," Biochemistry Research International/PubMed Central, September 11, 2014, https://pmc.ncbi.nim.nih.gov/articles/PMC4180391/

31. Klavinson, Vladimir; Bondarev, IE; and Butyugov, AA; "Anti-Aging Bioregulator Peptides: How They Work and Peptide Stacks," The Synthesis of Wellness, August 20, 2023, https://www.synthesisowellness.com/post/anti-aging-bioregulator-peptides-how-they-work-peptide-stacks

32. Tanikawa, Takashi; Kiba, Yuka; Yu, James; et al., "Degradative Effect of Nattokinase on Spike Protein of SARS-CoV-2," PubMed Central/Molecules, August 24, 2022, https://pmc.ncbi.nim.nih.gov/articles/PMC9458005

33. Venketaraman,Vishwanath; Norris, Brandon; Chorbajian, Abraham; Dawi,John; et al., "Evaluation of Glutathione in Spike Protein of SARS-CoV-2 Induced Immuno-thrombosis and Cytokine Dysregulation," MDPI/Antioxidants, February 22, 2024, https://www.mdpi.com/2076/3921/13/3/271

34. Goodarzi, Azadeh; Atefi, Najmolsadat; Behrangi, Elham; et al., "NAC and Coronavirus Disease-2019: May it Work as a Beneficial Preventive and Adjutant Therapy? A Comprehensive Review Study," PubMed Central/Journal of Research in Medical Sciences, November 26, 2020, https://pmc.ndbi.nim.nih.gov/articles/PMC8019127/

35. Meyer, Dr. Jim, PharmD; "Recovering from Post COVID and Post Vaccine Syndromes," People Rx—Austin's Wellness Headquarters, March 1, 2023, https://peoplesrx.com/post-covid-and-post-vaccine-syndromes/

36. Gao, Xueqin; Huard, Johnny; Huard, Charles; Dey Hazra, Maria E.; et al., "Effects of Fisetin Treatment on Cellular Senescence of Various Tissues and Organs of Old Sheep," PubMed Central/Antioxidants, August 21, 2023, https://pmc.ncbi.nim.nih.gov/articles/PMC10451965/

37. Buchwald, Peter; Bojadzic, Damir; and Alcazar, Oscar; "Methylene Blue Inhibits the SARS-CoV-2 Spike—ACE2 Protein-Protein Interaction—A Mechanism That Can Contribute to its Antiviral Activity Against COVID-19 (and vaccines)," Frontiers (In Pharmacology, January 12, 2021, https://www.frontiersin.org/journals/pharmacology/articles/10.3389/fphar.2020. 600372/full

38. Fulgenzi, Alessandro; and Ferraro, Maria Elena; "EDTA Chelation Therapy for the Treatment of Neurotoxicity," MDPI/Molecular Sciences, February 26, 2019, https://www.mdpi.com/1422-0067/20/5/1019

39. Ardis, Dr. Brian; "The Other 'N' Word," The Dr. Ardis Show/Podcast, April 10, 2024, https://podtail.com/podcast/the-dr-ardis-show-podcast/the-dr-ardis-show-4-10-2024-the-other-n-word/

40. Kirsch, Steve with Dr. Stella Immanuel, M.D., "Spirituality and Medicine with Dr. Stella Immanuel M.D., VSRF Live, September 12, 2024, https://www.vacsafety.org/episode-143-spirituality-and-medicine-with-dr-stella-immanuel-m-d/

41. Ealy, Dr. Henry, ND, PhD; "How We Can Heal the Hurt: Autophagocytosis and DNA Repair," Energetic Health Institute/Founder, January 11, 2022, https://www.bitchute.com/video/Rc7BeeeU1yjs/

42. Otto, Jonathan, Host; "Destruction: The Explosion of mRNA Tech and Its Devastation on Humanity," New Hope Docuseries, 2023. (Dr. Henry Ealy) https://newhopeseries.com/epidode-2+-live/

43. Otto, Jonathan, Host: "Unbreakable Truth: Hidden COVID Facts They've Tried to Bury," Bonus Episode #1 of Unbreakable Docuseries, featuring Dr. Richard Bartlett, MD and Dr. Brian Ardis, 2023

44. Otto, Jonathan, Host, "How We Can Heal the Hurt: Contributors: Ardis, Bartlett, Buttar, Mikovits, Ealy, Marz, Tapper, Greenfield, Barattiero, Merritt, Braun, and Marble. 2023.

45. Blaylock, Dr. Russell, MD; "The Deadly Impossibility of Herd Immunity Through Vaccination" Vaccination Council, February 18, 2018, https:www.vaccinationcouncil.org/2012/0218/the-deadly-impossibility-of-herd-immunity- through-vaccination-by-dr-russell-blaylock/

46. Meschuk, Jodie, "What the 'Hokey Pokey' Is Really About: Vaccine Information," Ebook/The Warrior Center, 2024, https://tribe.thewarriorcenter.com/

47. Blaylock, Dr. Russell L. MD, "Ignored Dangers of the COVID-19 Injections," PubMed Central. National Library of Medicine, November 3, 2023, quote: Dr. Ryan Cole, pathologist, https://pmc.ncbi.nim.nih.gov/articles/PMC10695344/

48. Howard, Jacqueline, CNN, "US Spends Most on Health Care But Has Worst Health Outcomes Among High-Income Countries, New Report Finds," CNN Health, January 31,2023, https://www.cnn.com/2023/01/31/health/us-health-care-spending-global-perspective/index.html

49. Berger,Tamar; Eisenkraft, Arik; Bar-Haim, Erez; et al., "Toxins as Biological Weapons for Terror—Characteristics, Challenges and Medical Countermeasures: A Mini-Review," Biomed Central/Disaster and Military Medicine, April 29, 2016, https://disastermilitarymedicine.biomedcentral.com/articles/10.1186/s40696-016-0017-4

50. Morse, SA and Meyer, RF; "Viruses and Bioterrorism," PubMed Central/NIH National Library of Medicine, October 31, 2016, https://pmc.ncbi.nih.gov/articles/PMC7157459/

51. Miller, Mark Crispin, "In Memory of Those Who 'Died Suddenly' in the United States and Worldwide, November 18-25, 2024," News From the Underground (NFU)/Substack, November27, 2024, https://www.markcrispinmiller@substack.com

52. Kirby, Jen, "Can a 50-Year-Old Treaty Still Keep the World Safe From the Changing Threat of Bioweapons? (How Geopolitics and Technological Advances Are Making This a Riskier World for Bioweapons,)" VOX Media, April 28, 2023, https://www.vox.com/future-perfect/23700801/bioweapons-biological-weapons-convention-united-nations-covid-coronavirus-russia-biology.

53. Kirby, Jen, "Can a 50-Year-Old Treaty Still Keep the World Safe…" April, 2023.

54. Stilwell, Blake, "The CIA's 'Heart Attack Gun': A Cold War Weapon for Targeted Assassinations, American Military History, November 14, 2024, https://www.military.com/history/cias-heart-attack-gun-cold-war-weapon-targeted-assassinations.html

55. Stillwell, Blake, "The CIA's 'Heart Attack Gun,'"...November 14, 2024

56. Myers, Gregory, "Ten Cases of Massive Environmental Poisoning," LISTVERSE/ Science—Our World, June 5, 2014, https://listverse.com/2014/06/05/10-cases-of-massive-environmental-poisoning/

57. Avadhanula, Dr. Shirisha, MD (Endocrinologist), "How Environmental Toxins Can Impact Your Health," Cleveland Clinic/Health Essentials, August 14, 2020, https://health.clevelandclinic.org/how-environmental-toxins-can-impact-your-health

58. Avadhanula, Dr. Shirisha, MD, "How Environmental Toxins Can Impact Your Health," August 14, 2020.

59. Tingley, Kim, "'Forever Chemicals' Are Everywhere. What Are They Doing to Us? PFAS lurk in so much of what we eat, drink, and use. Scientists are only beginning to understand how they're impacting our health—and what to do about them...The New York Times Magazine, August 16, 2023, https://www.nytimes.com/2023/08/16/magazine/pfas-toxic-chemicals.html

60. Antoniadou, Konstantina, "35 Most Toxic Household Items Hiding in Your Home," Sustainably Kind Living, UD December 31, 2024, https://sustainablykindliving.com/most-toxic-items-hiding-in-your-home/

61. Khakham, Dr. Chil MBA, NMD, "Understanding Environmental Toxins and Their Impact on Health," Rupa Health Magazine, September 17, 2024, https://www.rupahealth.com/post/understanding-environmental-toxins-and-their-impact-on-health

62. Brazier, Yvette/Medically reviewed by Cross, Karen, FNP, MSN, "Why Do We Have Fluoride in Our Water?" Medical News Today, February 21, 2018, https://www.medicalnewstoday.com/articles/154164

63. Khakham, Dr. Chil, "Understanding Environmental Toxins…" September 17, 2024

64. Environmental Working Group, "Food Additives: More Than You May Have Bargained For," (Consumer Guides), September 18, 2024, https://www.ewg.org/areas-focus/toxic-chemicals/food/chemicals

65. Environmental Working Group, "Food Additives…", September 18, 2024.

66. Schauss, Mark, "Toxicity and Chronic Illness," Weston A. Price Foundation for Wise Traditions in Food, Farming, and the Healing Arts, June 30, 2015, https://www.westonaprice.org/health-topics/environmental-toxins/toxicity-and chronic-illness/#gsc.tab=0

67. Environmental Working Group, "Body Burden: The Pollution in Newborns," Know Your Environment-Protect Your Health, July 14, 2005, https://www.ewg.org/research/body-burden-pollution-newborns.

68. Biology Insights Team, "Understanding Mycotoxins: Types, Detection, and Health Effects," Biology Insights, January 9, 2025, https://biologyinsights.com/understanding-mycotoxins-types-detection-and-health-effects/

69. Biology Insights Team, "Understanding Mycotoxins…, January 9, 2025.

70. Omotayo, Oluwadara Pelumi, et al., "Prevalence of Mycotoxins and Their Consequences on Human Health," PubMed Central—Toxicological Research, January 18, 2018, https://pmc.ncbi.nlm.nih.gov/articles/PMC6354945/

71. Hemmler, Kenneth, "The Health Risk of Chemtrails—Examining the Evidence," Greater Good—Health & Healing, May 5, 2024, https://greatergoodhealth.substack.com/p/the-health-risk-of-chemtrails.

72. Leigh, Tricia, "The Hidden Dangers of EMFs: Understanding Exposure and Its Impact on Health," Mojo Health, June 4, 2024, https://www.mojohealth.org/post/hidden-dangers-of-emfs-understanding-exposure-and-its-impact-on-health.

73. Leigh, Tricia, "The Hidden Dangers of EMFs…" June 4, 2024.

74. Leigh, Tricia, "The Hidden Dangers of EMFs…" June 4, 2024

www.ingramcontent.com/pod-product-compliance
Lightning Source LLC
Chambersburg PA
CBHW062308240926
51846CB00013B/617